Interventional and Neuromodulatory Techniques for Pain Management

VOLUME **4**

Spinal Injections and Peripheral Nerve Blocks

VOLUME

4 Spinal Injections and Peripheral Nerve Blocks

Volume Editors

Marc A. Huntoon MD

*Professor of Anesthesiology, Department of Anesthesiology,
College of Medicine, Mayo Clinic, Rochester, Minnesota*

Honorio T. Benzon MD

*Professor of Anesthesiology and Senior Associate Chair for Academic Affairs,
Feinberg School of Medicine, Northwestern University
Chief, Division of Pain Medicine, Northwestern Memorial Hospital, Chicago, Illinois*

Samer Narouze MD, MSc, DABPM, FIPP

*Clinical Professor of Anesthesiology and Pain Medicine, OUCOM
Clinical Professor of Neurological Surgery, OSU
Associate Professor of Surgery, NEOUCOM
Chairman, Center for Pain Medicine, Summa Western Reserve Hospital, Cuyahoga Falls, Ohio*

Video Editor

Samer Narouze, MD, MSc, DABPM, FIPP

Series Editor

Timothy R. Deer, MD, DABPM, FIPP

*President and CEO, The Center for Pain Relief
Clinical Professor of Anesthesiology, West Virginia University School of Medicine
Charleston, West Virginia*

ELSEVIER
SAUNDERS

1600 John F. Kennedy Blvd.
Ste 1800
Philadelphia, PA 19103-2899

SPINAL INJECTIONS AND PERIPHERAL NERVE BLOCKS   ISBN: 978-1-4377-2219-2
(Volume 4: A Volume in the Interventional and Neuromodulatory Techniques
for Pain Management Series by Timothy Deer)

Library of Congress Cataloging-in-Publication Data

Interventional and neuromodulatory techniques for pain management.
    p. ; cm.
  Includes bibliographical references and indexes.
  ISBN 978-1-4377-3791-2 (series package : alk. paper)—ISBN 978-1-4377-2216-1 (hardcover, v. 1 : alk. paper)—ISBN 978-1-4377-2217-8 (hardcover, v. 2 : alk. paper)—ISBN 978-1-4377-2218-5 (hardcover, v. 3 : alk. paper)—ISBN 978-1-4377-2219-2 (hardcover, v. 4 : alk. paper)—ISBN 978-1-4377-2220-8 (hardcover, v. 5 : alk. paper)
  1. Pain—Treatment. 2. Nerve block. 3. Spinal anesthesia. 4. Neural stimulation. 5. Analgesia. I. Deer, Timothy R.
  [DNLM: 1. Pain—drug therapy. 2. Pain—surgery. WL 704]
  RB127.I587 2012
  616′.0472—dc23
                                                                    2011018904

Acquisitions Editor: Pamela Hetherington
Developmental Editor: Lora Sickora
Publishing Services Manager: Jeff Patterson
Project Manager: Megan Isenberg
Design Direction: Lou Forgione

Printed in China

Last digit is the print number: 9 8 7 6 5 4 3 2 1

For Missy for all your love and support.

For Morgan, Taylor, Reed, and Bailie for your inspiration.

To those who have taught me a great deal: John Rowlingson, Richard North, Giancarlo Barolat, Sam Hassenbusch, Elliot Krames, K. Dean Willis, Peter Staats, Nagy Mekhail, Robert Levy, David Caraway, Kris Kumar, Joshua Prager, and Jim Rathmell.

To my team: Christopher Kim, Richard Bowman, Matthew Ranson, Doug Stewart, Wilfredo Tolentino, Jeff Peterson, and Michelle Miller.

Timothy R. Deer

I would like to acknowledge my wife Elizabeth, who has been a tremendous blessing to me personally, an ardent supporter of my career, and "editor-in chief" for all of my writing projects.

Marc A. Huntoon

To my family—Juliet, Hazel, Hubert, Paul, and Annalisa.

Honorio T. Benzon

To my family, Mira, John, Michael, and Emma, the true love and joy of my life.

Samer Narouze

Contributors

Honorio T. Benzon, MD
Professor of Anesthesiology and Senior Associate Chair for
Academic Affairs, Feinberg School of Medicine, Northwestern
University; Chief, Division of Pain Medicine, Northwestern
Memorial Hospital, Chicago, Illinois
Chapter 16, Pulsed Radiofrequency
*Chapter 22, Musculoskeletal Injections: Iliopsoas, Quadratus
Lumborum, Piriformis, and Trigger Point Injections*

Abram H. Burgher, MD
The Pain Center of Arizona, Peoria, Arizona
*Chapter 11, Therapeutic Epidural Injections: Interlaminar and
Transforaminal*

Allen W. Burton, MD
Houston Pain Associates, Houston, Texas
Chapter 19, Vertebral Augmentation

Kiran Chekka, MD
*Chapter 22, Musculoskeletal Injections: Iliopsoas, Quadratus
Lumborum, Piriformis, and Trigger Point Injections*

Jianguo Cheng, MD, PhD, FIPP
Professor of Anesthesiology, Cleveland Clinic Lerner College of
Medicine, Case Western Reserve University; Director of Cleveland
Clinic Pain Medicine Fellowship Program, Departments of Pain
Management and Neurosciences, Cleveland, Ohio
*Chapter 12, Facet (Zygapophyseal) Intraarticular Joint Injections:
Cervical, Lumbar, and Thoracic*

Christopher M. Duncan, MD
Instructor of Anesthesiology, Department of Anesthesiology,
Mayo Clinic, Rochester, Minnesota
Chapter 6, Upper Extremity Peripheral Nerve Blockade

Jerald Garcia, MD
Fellow, Pain Medicine, Department of Anesthesiology, University
Hospitals Case Medical Center, Case Western Reserve University,
Cleveland, Ohio
Chapter 4, Differential Diagnostic Nerve Blocks

Stanley Golovac, MD
Co-Director, Space Coast Pain Institute, Merritt Island, Florida
*Chapter 3, Fluoroscopy, Ultrasonography, Computed Tomography,
and Radiation Safety*
Chapter 17, Discogenic Pain and Discography for Spinal Injections

Sean Graham, MD
Chapter 8, Cervical and Lumbar Sympathetic Blocks

Manfred Greher, MD
Medical Director and Head of the Department of Anesthesiology,
Perioperative Intensive Care and Pain Therapy, Sacred Heart of
Jesus Hospital, Vienna, Austria
Chapter 20, Ultrasound-Guided Lumbar Spine Injections

Basem Hamid, MD
Chapter 19, Vertebral Augmentation

Craig Hartrick, MD, FIPP
Departments of Anesthesiology, Biomedical Sciences, and Health
Sciences, Oakland University
William Beaumont School of Medicine, Rochester, Michigan
Chapter 14, Radiofrequency Rhizotomy for Facet Syndrome

Salim M. Hayek, MD, PhD
Associate Professor, Department of Anesthesiology, Case Western
Reserve University; Chief, Division of Pain Medicine, University
Hospitals, Case Medical Center, Cleveland, Ohio
Chapter 4, Differential Diagnostic Nerve Blocks

Marc A. Huntoon, MD
Professor of Anesthesiology, Department of Anesthesiology,
College of Medicine, Mayo Clinic, Rochester, Minnesota
*Chapter 2, Therapeutic Agents for Spine Injection: Local
Anesthetics, Steroids, and Contrast Media*
*Chapter 11, Therapeutic Epidural Injections: Interlaminar and
Transforaminal*

Mark-Friedrich B. Hurdle, MD
Assistant Professor of Physical Medicine and Rehabilitation,
College of Medicine, Mayo Clinic, Rochester, Minnesota
*Chapter 23, Ultrasound-Guided and Fluoroscopically Guided Joint
Injections*

Robert W. Hurley, MD, PhD
Associate Professor; Chief of Pain Medicine; Director of UF Pain
and Spine Center; Departments of Anesthesiology, Neurology,
Psychiatry, and Orthopedics and Rehabilitation Medicine,
University of Florida, Gainesville, Florida
Chapter 9, Nerve Destruction for the Alleviation of Visceral Pain

Sheryl L. Johnson, MD
Assistant Professor, Department of Psychiatry and
Anesthesiology, University of Virginia, Charlottesville, Virginia
Chapter 1, History of Spine Injections

Leonardo Kapural, MD, PhD
Professor of Anesthesiology, Wake Forest University, School of
Medicine; Director, Pain Medicine Center, Wake Forest Baptist
Health, Winston-Salem, North Carolina
*Chapter 18, Minimally Invasive Intradiscal Procedures for the
Treatment of Discogenic Lower Back and Leg Pain*

Arno Lataster, MSc
Clinical Anatomist and Vice Head, Department of Anatomy and
Embryology, Maastricht University, Maastricht, The Netherlands
Chapter 14, Radiofrequency Rhizotomy for Facet Syndrome

Padraig Mahon, FCARCSI, MSc, MD
Regional Anesthesia Fellow, Sunnybrook Health Sciences Centre, Toronto, Ontario, Canada
Chapter 7, Lower Limb Blocks

Khalid Malik, MD
Assistant Professor, Department of Anesthesiology, Northwestern University Feinberg School of Medicine; Staff Anesthesiologist, Northwestern Memorial Hospital, Chicago, Illinois
Chapter 16, Pulsed Radiofrequency

Colin J.L. McCartney, MBChB, FRCA, FRCPC
Associate Professor, Sunnybrook Health Sciences Centre, University of Toronto, Toronto, Ontario, Canada
Chapter 7, Lower Limb Blocks

Anne Marie McKenzie-Brown, MD
Chapter 22, Musculoskeletal Injections: Iliopsoas, Quadratus Lumborum, Piriformis, and Trigger Point Injections

Nagy Mekhail, MD, PhD, FIPP
Department of Pain Management, Cleveland Clinic, Cleveland, Ohio
Chapter 14, Radiofrequency Rhizotomy for Facet Syndrome

Kacey A. Montgomery, MD
Resident, Department of Anesthesiology, University of Florida, Gainesville, Florida
Chapter 9, Nerve Destruction for the Alleviation of Visceral Pain

Samer Narouze, MD, MSc, DABPM, FIPP
Clinical Professor of Anesthesiology and Pain Medicine, OUCOM; Clinical Professor of Neurological Surgery, OSU; Associate Professor of Surgery, NEOUCOM; Chairman, Center for Pain Medicine, Summa Western Reserve Hospital, Cuyahoga Falls, Ohio
Chapter 5, Head and Neck Blocks
Chapter 8, Cervical and Lumbar Sympathetic Blocks
Chapter 21, Ultrasound-Guided Cervical Spine Injections

Vinita Parikh, MD
Chapter 13, Medial Branch Blocks: Cervical, Thoracic, and Lumbar

Philip Peng, MBBS, FRCPC
Director of Anesthesia Chronic Pain Program, University Health Network, Wasser Pain Management Center, Mount Sinai Hospital, University of Toronto, Toronto, Canada
Chapter 10, Peripheral Applications of Ultrasonography for Chronic Pain

Tristan C. Pico, MD
Fellow, Pain Medicine, Department of Pain Medicine, UT MD Anderson Cancer Center, Houston, Texas
Chapter 19, Vertebral Augmentation

Matthew J. Pingree, MD
Division of Pain Medicine, Departments of Anesthesiology and Physical Medicine and Rehabilitation; Assistant Professor of Physical Medicine and Rehabilitation, College of Medicine, Mayo Clinic, Rochester, Minnesota
Chapter 2, Therapeutic Agents for Spine Injection: Local Anesthetics, Steroids, and Contrast Media

Jason E. Pope, MD
Pain Medicine Fellow, Department of Pain Management, Cleveland Clinic, Cleveland, Ohio
Chapter 12, Facet (Zygapophyseal) Intraarticular Joint Injections: Cervical, Lumbar, and Thoracic

Dawood Sayed, MD
Associate Professor, The University of Kansas, Department of Anesthesiology and Pain Medicine, Kansas City, Kansas
Chapter 13, Medial Branch Blocks: Cervical, Thoracic, and Lumbar

Hugh M. Smith, MD, PhD
Assistant Professor of Anesthesiology, Department of Anesthesiology, Mayo Clinic, Rochester, Minnesota
Chapter 6, Upper Extremity Peripheral Nerve Blockade

Dawn A. Sparks, DO
Assistant Professor of Anesthesiology, Dartmouth Medical School, Dartmouth-Hitchcock Medical Center, Lebanon, New Hampshire
Chapter 18, Minimally Invasive Intradiscal Procedures for the Treatment of Discogenic Lower Back and Leg Pain

Maarten van Eerd, MD, FIPP
Staff Anesthesiologist, Department of Anesthesiology and Pain Management, Amphia Ziekenhuis, Breda, The Netherlands; PhD Fellow, Department of Anesthesiology and Pain Management, University Medical Centre Maastricht, Maastricht, The Netherlands
Chapter 14, Radiofrequency Rhizotomy for Facet Syndrome

Maarten van Kleef, MD, PhD, FIPP
Professor and Chairman, Department of Anesthesiology and Pain Management, University Medical Centre Maastricht, Maastricht, The Netherlands
Chapter 14, Radiofrequency Rhizotomy for Facet Syndrome

Jan Van Zundert, MD, PhD, FIPP
Chairman, Multidisciplinary Pain Centre, Ziekenhuis Oost-Limburg, Genk, Belgium; Scientific Consultant, Department of Anesthesiology and Pain Medicine, University Medical Centre Maastricht, Maastricht, The Netherlands
Chapter 14, Radiofrequency Rhizotomy for Facet Syndrome

Pascal Vanelderen, MD, FIPP
Staff Anesthesiologist, Department of Anesthesiology, Intensive Care Medicine, Multidisciplinary Pain Centre, Ziekenhuis Oost-Limburg, Genk, Belgium; PhD Fellow, Department of Pain Management and Palliative Care Medicine, Radboud University Nijmegen Medical Centre, Nijmegen, The Netherlands
Chapter 14, Radiofrequency Rhizotomy for Facet Syndrome

I. Elias Veizi, MD, PhD
Clinical Fellow, Department of Anesthesiology, Division of Pain Medicine, Case Western Reserve University, University Hospitals Case Medical Center, Cleveland, Ohio
Chapter 4, Differential Diagnostic Nerve Blocks

Kevin E. Vorenkamp, MD
Assistant Professor, Department of Anesthesiology and Pain Medicine; Medical Director, Pain Management Center; Director, Pain Medicine Fellowship, University of Virginia, Charlottesville, Virginia
Chapter 1, History of Spine Injections

Seth A. Waldman, MD
Director, Division of Musculoskeletal and Interventional Pain Management, The Hospital for Special Surgery; Clinical Assistant Professor, Anesthesiology, Cornell University Medical College, New York, New York
Chapter 13, Medial Branch Blocks: Cervical, Thoracic, and Lumbar

Bryan S. Williams, MD, MPH
Assistant Professor of Anesthesiology, Division of Pain Medicine, Rush Medical College, Rush University Medical Center, Chicago, Illinois
Chapter 15, Sacroiliac Joint Injections and Lateral Branch Blocks, Including Water-Cooled Neurotomy

Steve J. Wisniewski, MD
Assistant Professor of Physical Medicine and Rehabilitation, Mayo Clinic, Rochester, Minnesota
Chapter 23, Ultrasound-Guided and Fluoroscopically Guided Joint Injections

Preface

Volume 4 of *Interventional and Neuromodulatory Techniques for Pain Management* is focusing on therapeutic, diagnostic regional anesthesia procedures put together by Tim Deer, who deserves credit for attracting significant and knowledgeable professionals to further the best interest of our patients and physicians. Looking through this book, it is obvious that we have to learn new things and must keep up with new developments. It is also obvious that studies without the expertise and experience do not necessarily lead us to avoiding problems. Very few if any studies show us major disasters; yet, we must learn how to avoid major disasters. The field is growing and is attracting more and more physicians without appropriate training to get involved and do procedures on their patients, which is a reality of our time. Additionally, there are others who feel that interventional pain procedures and neuromodulation are not exclusively in the realm of trained interventional pain physicians but are available to anybody who can acquire the skills, which again is unacceptable. The better trained the physician, the better the outcome. Volume 4, with its systematic approach to covering the field, is worthy of spending time, sitting down and getting familiar with each topic, and adding the new pieces of information to the knowledge base of the individual physician. Interventional pain procedures are forever expanding and basic principles need to be utilized to avoid problems that come from placing medications, putting needles that do not just inject but also cut and end up in structures and areas that were never intended, and this is where the evaluation of the skill of the physician is highly recommended and encouraged. Three-dimensional skills that these procedures often demand need clarification and guidance, oftentimes with fluoroscopy, CAT scan, or now the expanding ultrasonic guidance for the more superficial procedures. Volume 4 has 23 chapters, even though there are possibly 75 to 100 procedures that are utilized to take care of patients. The individual patient needs to have overriding importance in the selection of the treatment modality that the experienced physician may recommend. This volume also includes procedural videos, which can be viewed on the companion website at www.expertconsult.com.

This book will serve the reader in the intent to improve patient care and expand the knowledge that we use in taking care of our patients. It is becoming more and more common for patients to research individual physicians' credentials and qualifications on the Internet, and it is advisable for the interventional physician to show evidence of having been evaluated in the field of interventional pain medicine. Therefore, taking an examination such as ABIPP (American Board of Interventional Pain Practice) of the American Society of Interventional Pain Physicians or FIPP (Fellow of Interventional Pain Practice) of the World Institute of Pain is gaining wider and wider recognition of the physician preparing and passing the examination where the three-dimensional skills have been evaluated and found to be adequate by the examining peers.

The interventional pain practice is growing because it works, reduces the use of narcotics, gets patients back to functional recovery, and reduces the incidence of costly surgical interventions. The highly trained interventional pain physician is carrying out these procedures because the patients need them and the physicians can do them.

By Gabor Bela Racz, MD, FIPP, ABIPP
Co-Director International Pain Center
Grover Murray Professor
Professor and Chair Emeritus, Anesthesiology
Texas Tech University Health Sciences Center

Acknowledgments

I would like to acknowledge Jeff Peterson for his hard work on making this project a reality, and Michelle Miller for her diligence to detail on this and all projects that cross her desk.

I would like to acknowledge Lora Sickora, Pamela Hetherington, and Megan Isenberg for determination, attention to detail, and desire for excellence in bringing this project to fruition.

Finally, I would like to acknowledge Samer Narouze for his diligent work filming and reviewing the procedural videos associated with all of the volumes in the series.

Timothy R. Deer

Contents

SECTION I   General Considerations

1 History of Spine Injections   3
   Sheryl L. Johnson and Kevin E. Vorenkamp

2 Therapeutic Agents for Spine Injection: Local
   Anesthetics, Steroids, and Contrast Media   16
   Matthew J. Pingree and Marc A. Huntoon

3 Fluoroscopy, Ultrasonography, Computed
   Tomography, and Radiation Safety   28
   Stanley Golovac

SECTION II   Peripheral Nerve Blocks

4 Differential Diagnostic Nerve Blocks   37
   Jerald Garcia, I. Elias Veizi, and Salim M. Hayek

5 Head and Neck Blocks   46
   Samer Narouze

6 Upper Extremity Peripheral Nerve Blockade   58
   Hugh M. Smith and Christopher M. Duncan

7 Lower Limb Blocks   63
   Padraig Mahon and Colin J.L. McCartney

8 Cervical and Lumbar Sympathetic Blocks   76
   Samer Narouze and Sean Graham

9 Nerve Destruction for the Alleviation of
   Visceral Pain   88
   Kacey A. Montgomery and Robert W. Hurley

10 Peripheral Applications of Ultrasonography
    for Chronic Pain   101
    Philip Peng

SECTION III   Injections for Back Pain

11 Therapeutic Epidural Injections: Interlaminar
    and Transforaminal   121
    Marc A. Huntoon and Abram H. Burgher

12 Facet (Zygapophyseal) Intraarticular Joint
    Injections: Cervical, Lumbar, and Thoracic   129
    Jason E. Pope and Jianguo Cheng

13 Medial Branch Blocks: Cervical, Thoracic,
    and Lumbar   136
    Seth A. Waldman, Vinita Parikh, and Dawood Sayed

14 Radiofrequency Rhizotomy for Facet
    Syndrome   148
    *Jan Van Zundert, Pascal Vanelderen,
    Maarten van Eerd, Arno Lataster, Craig Hartrick,
    Nagy Mekhail, and Maarten van Kleef*

15 Sacroiliac Joint Injections and Lateral
    Branch Blocks, Including Water-Cooled
    Neurotomy   164
    Bryan S. Williams

16 Pulsed Radiofrequency   174
    Khalid Malik and Honorio T. Benzon

17 Discogenic Pain and Discography for
    Spinal Injections   178
    Stanley Golovac

18 Minimally Invasive Intradiscal Procedures
    for the Treatment of Discogenic Lower
    Back and Leg Pain   184
    Leonardo Kapural and Dawn A. Sparks

19 Vertebral Augmentation   193
    Tristan C. Pico, Basem Hamid, and Allen W. Burton

20 Ultrasound-Guided Lumbar Spine Injections   200
    Manfred Greher

21 Ultrasound-Guided Cervical Spine Injections   210
    Samer Narouze

22 Musculoskeletal Injections: Iliopsoas,
    Quadratus Lumborum, Piriformis, and
    Trigger Point Injections   216
    *Anne Marie McKenzie-Brown, Kiran Chekka,
    and Honorio T. Benzon*

23 Ultrasound-Guided and Fluoroscopically
    Guided Joint Injections   224
    Steve J. Wisniewski and Mark-Friedrich B. Hurdle

Index   233

I General Considerations

Chapter 1 History of Spine Injections

Chapter 2 Therapeutic Agents for Spine Injection: Local Anesthetics, Steroids, and Contrast Media

Chapter 3 Fluoroscopy, Ultrasonography, Computed Tomography, and Radiation Safety

1 History of Spine Injections

Sheryl L. Johnson and Kevin E. Vorenkamp

CHAPTER OVERVIEW

Chapter Synopsis: Similar to many medical procedures used today, spinal injection for the control of pain originally arose from a misunderstanding. James Leonard Corning first injected cocaine into the spinal cord in 1885 with the aim of producing regional anesthesia. He targeted interspinal blood vessels, which of course do not exist. But his efforts likely produced epidural anesthesia in a human subject and spinal anesthesia in a dog, paving the way for future experiments. Spinal injection procedures have come a long way in the time since then; this chapter chronicles their evolution. By the turn of the twentieth century, more than 1000 reports of spinal anesthesia had been published. Not surprisingly, intrathecal injections of cocaine were often lethal, but epidural injections were more successful. In the 1930s, injection of steroids gained favor for a number of indications. Throughout the early and mid-twentieth century, spinal injection treatments proliferated, but placebo controls and follow-up data were limited. Treatment of a common side effect—postdural puncture headache—also evolved with these early investigations, ultimately culminating in the epidural blood patch. Early understanding of variations in neuronal fiber diameter laid the foundation for differential spinal block, which has proved more informative than functional. The more recent development of diagnostic tools for back pain are also described, including medial branch block for zygapophysial joint pain, injection of the sacroiliac joint for low back pain, and disc stimulation. These studies led to a better understanding of the myriad sources of back pain.

Important Points:
- In 1884, cocaine was first used as topical anesthetic.
- From 1885-1901, epidural, intrathecal, and caudal procedures were described.
- In 1899, Bier described "cocainization of the spinal cord."
- In 1925, treating sciatica with caudal epidural was first described.
- From 1938-1960, techniques of SI joint injection, discography, epidural blood patch, and differential spinal blockade were described.
- In 1964, chemonucleolysis with chymopapain was described.
- From 1971-1975, Rees and Shealy reported "facet rhizolysis."
- In 1980, Bogduk described medial branch neurotomy.
- In 1984, C2 vertebroplasty was performed.
- From 1998-2011, IDET, nucleoplasty, and various techniques of SI joint denervation were described.

Neuraxial Injections

In review of the history of spinal injections for pain management, it is clear that the procedures have been developed and expanded from their original use in anesthesia (**Fig. 1-1**). After the publication of evidence in 1884 that cocaine could be used to render the cornea insensate for ophthalmologic procedures,[1] interest in the ability to anesthetize only the region to be operated upon grew. In 1885, the neurologist James Leonard Corning first described spinal anesthesia,[2] which was interestingly a result of a misunderstanding of the anatomy and physiology of the spine and its contents. His intention was to inject cocaine into the interspinal blood vessels, so that it could be delivered to the spine via the communicating vessels in the spinal cord. No such vessels exist, although the correct anatomy had been described in *Gray's Anatomy* by 1870.[3]

Corning used a hypodermic needle with the goal of injecting cocaine into the interspinous vessels. He wrote: "I hoped to produce artificially a temporary condition of things analogous in its physiological consequences to the effect observed in transverse myelitis or after total section of the cord."[2]

In his report, he describes injecting 120 mg of cocaine into a male human subject and 13 mg of cocaine into a dog. By description of onset and effects, it appears that the injections probably resulted in epidural anesthesia in the man and spinal anesthesia in the dog. The doses used far exceeded the potential toxic doses, but

fortunately, there were no significant complications. Corning had been searching for treatment for neurological diseases but noted that the procedure certainly could have surgical implications.[4]

Documentation of intentional dural puncture was introduced by Dr. Essex Wynter in 1891. Using a Southey's tube and trocar, he placed the tube between the lumbar vertebrae after making an incision in the skin for the purpose of draining the fluid in tuberculous meningitis. He noted temporary relief and no complications with the procedure, although none of the patients survived the tuberculous meningitis.[5]

Six months later, Heinrich Irenaeus Quincke wrote "Die Lumbalpunction des Hydrocephalus."[6] He based his approach on the knowledge of the lumbar anatomy of the continuous subarachnoid space and the end of the spinal cord at approximately L2, which allows for the introduction of a needle below that point, avoiding spinal cord injury. The procedure was introduced for the treatment of hydrocephalus. Quincke improved the technique by the use of needles that were 0.5 to 1.2 mm in diameter, including a stylet in the larger needles. The initial description is a paramedian approach, starting 5 to 10 mm from midline.

The application of the procedure for spinal anesthesia rather than a therapeutic option was developed by a surgeon, Dr. August Bier. He published his findings in 1899 with the title "Versuche uber Cocainisirung des Ruckenmarkes" ("Research on Cocainization of the Spinal Cord").[7] His goal was to use minimal amounts of

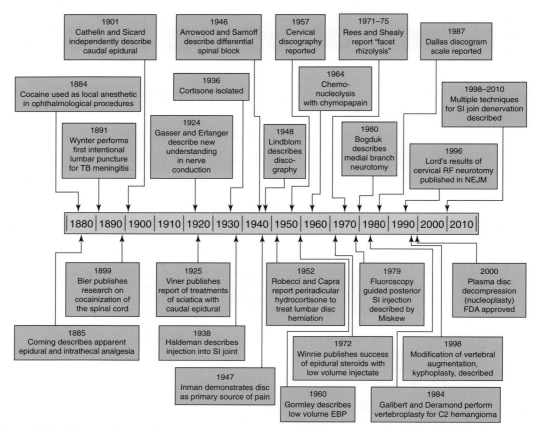

Fig. 1-1   Timeline outlining history of spine injections (1884-2010). EBP, epidural blood patch; FDA, Food and Drug Administration; *NEJM, New England Journal of Medicine*; RF, radiofrequency; SI, sacroiliac; TB, tuberculosis.

medication to anesthetize a large region. News and promise of the technique spread quickly, and by October of 1899 Drs. Dudley Tait and Guido Caglieri had tried the approach in San Francisco, becoming the first to do so in the United States.[8] By January 1901, a report in *The Lancet* stated that there were already almost 1000 published reports of spinal anesthesia.[9]

In 1901, Fernand Cathelin demonstrated the ability to gain access to the epidural space via the caudal approach. He noted that fluids rose in a fashion that was proportional to the volume and speed of the injection.[10] Both Cathelin and Dr. John Sicard presented a paper on epidural injections the same year (1901), but the two physicians were working independently.

De Pasquier and Leri attempted intrathecal injections of 5 mg of cocaine at the lumbar level but noted in their results "toxic cocaine accidents . . . to the bulbar and cerebral centers." Using a rubber band "gently tightened around the neck," they tried to prevent the flow of cocaine to the brain but were unsuccessful. They claimed a better level of success with sacral epidural injections.[11]

W. Stoeckel[12] published his experience in obstetrical care with the caudal epidural method in 1909 after modifying the method by using the less toxic procaine rather than cocaine. He was interested in the possible spread of medication in the epidural space from a caudal injection and used colored fluid in cadavers to document the extensive spread, including through the sacral foramina.

In 1925, Dr. Norman Viner[13] published his experience in treating intractable sciatica with caudal epidural injections. He described his technique of injecting first 20 cc of 1% Novocain followed by 50 to 100 cc of sterile Ringer's solution, normal saline, or liquid petrolatum. These injections were typically repeated three to four

times at weekly intervals. He notes that "liquid petrolatum is frowned on by some on account of the remote possibility of fatty embolism" but goes on to note the overall low risk. He concludes his paper by suggesting the procedure be tried with many other conditions because he believed it could be very successful in the treatment of sciatica.

Cortisone (called Compound E) was discovered in 1936.[14,15] Hench et al[16,17] reported in a 1950 publication that it could treat rheumatoid arthritis, rheumatic fever, and other conditions as well. A longer acting steroid, Compound F (hydrocortisone) was noted by Hollander[18] to reduce the synovial membrane inflammation histologically but even then the author was cautious to state that the action of the steroid was palliative, not curative. The use of steroids to treat many conditions became common during this period.

Claiming that patients' sciatic pain was a result of inflammation, Robecchi and Capra[19] reported using "periradicular" hydrocortisone to treat lumbar disc herniation in 1952. Lievre et al[20] described caudal epidural injections as being effective when five of 20 patients improved. No data were reported more than 3 weeks after the injections, and no control subjects were used, so placebo and the natural history of the problem were not addressed. The popularity of caudal epidural injections appears to have increased after this report.

"Pressure caudal anesthesia" was advocated by Brown,[21] who used 50 to 70 cc of mixtures of lidocaine, normal saline, and steroid. He noted improved success (100% vs. 32 of 38) when a steroid was added to the normal saline and local anesthetic. Again, however, the lack of control subjects and structured follow-up is notable.

The first clinical description of the technique for a paramidline lumbar approach is credited to Pagés in 1921.[22] The procedure then modified to include the loss of resistance technique, introduced by Dogliotti in 1933.[23] Gutierrez suggested the hanging drop technique by using the negative pressure of the epidural space in the same year.[24] Dogliotti was also the first to describe an epidural injection into the cervical region.[23]

During the middle of the twentieth century, investigators experimented with treatments using both intrathecal and epidural injections. In the 1950s, there was interest in treating patients with multiple sclerosis with intrathecal steroids, but no control subjects or follow-up were included in these trials.[25-27] In later reports,[28,29] excitement about the procedure waned as persistent improvement was seen in only a limited portion of the patients.

In the early 1960s, Gardner et al[30] tried high-volume epidural injections (20 cc of 1% procaine and 125 mg hydrocortisone) in 239 patients with sciatica. About half of the subjects had failed to obtain relief with surgery. After 57% of the patients failed to get pain relief with the epidural injections, the investigators started using an intrathecal approach with 80 mg of methylprednisolone acetate and 40 mg of procaine. Sixty percent of the 75 subjects noted relief of the sciatic pain for more that 4 months. By 1963, Sehgal and Gardner[31] and Sehgal et al[32] had treated more than 1000 patients with intrathecal steroids for diverse conditions, but no improvement data or control group was reported.

The transition back to epidural injections began in response to data published by Winnie et al in 1972.[33] At the time, there continued to be controversy as to the aspect of the procedure that produced pain relief. The theories proposed were therapeutic benefit from the injections resulted from lysis of adhesions by large volumes of injectate, interruption of the sympathetic reflex mechanisms by the local anesthetic, or the antiinflammatory effect of the steroid. By demonstrating success of epidurals with low-volume injectate, Winnie et al[33] proposed that the effect seemed to be from the steroid itself. They further suggested that the success of an injection seemed to be related to the proximity of the injection to the pathology causing the patients' complaint.

The more recent modifications of epidural injections have occurred as a result of the concern regarding accurate delivery of the medication to the site of pathology. Multiple studies[34,35] show that the loss of resistance technique in a lumbar epidural steroid injection results in inaccurate needle placement up to 30% to 40% of the time. The use of fluoroscopy has been encouraged by some to improve accuracy in epidural injections for chronic pain in recent years.[36,37] Fredman and Nun[38] reported a lower incidence of inaccurate placement into the epidural space during "blind" epidural injections (8.3% failure rate) than previous reports but noted that the intended level of the injection was missed in 53% of the cases. Interestingly, in the cases in which the needle placement was correct, the contrast reached the level of the pathology in only 26% of the patients, largely because of altered anatomy. This study was done on patients with failed back surgery syndrome and highlights the potential difficulty of injections in this population.

The other major modification of the procedure is the transforaminal approach to the epidural space. This technique mandates the use of fluoroscopy. This technique was developed with the recognition that in caudal and translaminar approaches, the medication is delivered into the dorsal aspect of the spinal canal. The dorsal median epidural septum can stop the spread of the medication to the contralateral side.[39] The translaminar technique delivers the medication to the ventral aspect of the nerve root sleeve and to the dorsal aspect of the disc herniation.[40,41] Although the transforaminal technique is commonly used, one complication that has

been particularly concerning is inadvertent arterial injection of particulate steroid, which has resulted in devastating consequences. To decrease the risk, nonparticulate steroid and digital subtraction imaging can be used. Some practitioners have abandoned the procedure altogether because of this risk, particularly in the cervical region.

The epidural steroid injection is the most common spinal procedure performed in pain management today, but the effectiveness is unclear. Although many studies suggest pain relief in the short term, long-term effectiveness has been disappointing. The ability of epidural injections to decrease the rate of subsequent spinal surgery has also been questionable.

Epidural Blood Patch

It is interesting to note that the development of a dural puncture headache was described very early in the development of spinal procedures. Quincke,[6] while noting some improvement of patients with hydrocephalus after lumbar puncture, also reported that some patients complained of a pattern of pain for several days that would seem consistent with a postdural puncture headache (PDPH). Multiple punctures with a large-bore needle had been used. The observation of edema in the surrounding tissues seems to be evidence of continued cerebrospinal fluid (CSF) leaks.

It was not, however, until 1898 that August Bier[42] clearly made the association between dural punctures and subsequent headaches that appeared to have unique characteristics. He reported that three of his first six patients in whom he performed the procedure complained of a headache shortly after the procedure. As an experiment, Dr. Bier and his clinical assistant went on to perform spinal anesthesia on themselves and then developed classical symptoms of PDPH. They documented their personal experience in what makes both interesting and somewhat comical reading today.

> After performing these experiments on our own bodies we proceeded without feeling any symptoms to dine and drink wine and smoke cigars. I went to bed at 11 p.m., slept the whole night, awoke the next morning hale and hearty and went for an hour's walk. Towards the end of the walk I developed a slight headache, which gradually got worse as I went about my daily business. By 3 p.m. I was looking pale and my pulse was fairly weak though regular and about 70 beats per minute. In addition, I had a feeling of very strong pressure on my skull and became rather dizzy when I stood up rapidly from my chair. All these symptoms vanished at once when I lay down flat, but returned when I stood up. Towards the evening I was forced to take to bed and remained there for nine days, because all the manifestations recurred as soon as I got up. ... The symptoms finally resolved nine days after the lumbar puncture.[42]

By January 1901, in the almost 1000 published reports of spinal anesthesia, physicians continued to note concern about the common occurrence of PDPH. Investigation into the etiology and treatment of PDPH quickly followed the early reports.

Treatment of PDPH historically can be viewed as using one of several different approaches. One approach focused on replacing the lost CSF volume to restore the intracranial pressure. Infusions of normal saline into the intrathecal space were attempted, which tended to provide temporary relief but also produced a second dural puncture. The intracranial hypotension would return with the painful symptoms shortly after the infusion was stopped with redistribution of the fluid and pressure.[43-47] Such efforts were abandoned in the 1950s. Attempts to increase CSF production by using hypotonic intravenous saline infusions and intramuscular pituitary extract resulted in perhaps some relief for a portion of patients but again did not produce consistent or dramatic results.[48,49]

In attempt to produce a "splint" type of effect, the second of the approaches, epidural infusions were used.[50] This technique avoided the second dural hole in theory but failed to produce long-term pain relief because again the pain would return with redistribution of the fluid shortly after the infusion was stopped.[51]

The third approach is the one that we are still working with today. The principle is to plug to hole in the dura that is allowing for escape of the CSF. Dr. James Gormley was a general surgeon in the truest sense in a time (1950s and 1960s) when surgeons were also directly involved in the anesthetic care of the patient. Spinal anesthesia was attractive because the surgeon could perform the block and allow the patient to maintain his or her own airway while performing surgery and supervising the nurse for management of vital signs. One of his observations was that bloody taps seemed to result in a lower incidence of PDPH. Also important was the idea that blood in the central neuraxis did not appear to result in disaster as previously believed.[4] He published a report of seven cases in which 2 to 3 mL of autologous blood was injected into the epidural space for the treatment of PDPH in 1960.[52] He was actually one of these subjects who presented with a PDPH after a myelogram. Although later studies have refuted the notion that bloody taps decrease the incidence of PDPH, it was a fortunate mistaken idea.

In 1960, Dr. Anthony DiGiovanni, having just read Gormley's letter in *Anesthesiology*, was asked to help in the care of a woman on the obstetric ward who had a severe headache after a spinal anesthetic. Because the anesthesiologist who did the initial procedure had attempted the injection at multiple levels and could not remember the level of the successful block, Dr. DiGiovanni decided to use a volume of 10 mL of autologous blood, thinking that the higher volume could possibly cover several levels. This resulted in the resolution of the patient's headache, and Dr. DiGiovanni continued to treat patients presenting with PDPH with this volume as a result of this initial success.[4] In subsequent years, he trained many other anesthesiologists in this technique and published his experience with the procedure in 1970.[53]

This procedure, quite understandably, was met with resistance by many in the field, particularly because of concerns about safety. Animal studies as well as prospective data accumulated with time and suggested that the technique was not only effective but also very safe.[54] This led to the general acceptance of the blood patch in the treatment of PDPH.

Progress has certainly been made in reducing the occurrence of PDPH with the use of smaller gauge needles and "pencil point" tips (versus the prior use of "cutting" needles). Some physicians have tried to prevent PDPH with prophylactic blood patches at the time of the dural puncture. The evidence does not, however, support this practice.

Given the long history and the well-accepted practice of performing blood patches for PDPH, it is interesting to note the relative lack of evidence from randomized, controlled clinical trials. Van Kooten et al[55] published such a study in 2007 that strongly supports the current practice and is interesting to review.

Differential Spinal Blockade

Clinically, the etiology of a patient's pain is sometimes difficult to define. This has remained true despite recent advances in medicine. In the 1920s, Gasser and Erlanger[56,57] published some groundbreaking work in the area of neural conduction. Although incorrect about the site of conduction (mistaking it to be within the axoplasm), they established the idea that fiber size was related to conduction velocity and fiber function. They were able to define three classes (A, B, and C) of nerve fibers and subdivided class A fibers into 4 groups (α, β, γ, and δ). Working with cocaine, they were able to demonstrate that the fibers types appeared to have different sensitivities to local anesthetic.

This understanding was the basis for the differential spinal block developed by Sarnoff and Arrowood.[58,59] Noting prior animal experimentation suggesting that a low concentration of procaine could selectively abolish the carotid sinus reflex without affecting respiration or motor function, they proceeded to test this principle in patients with varying diagnoses (residual limb pain, herpes zoster, sciatic nerve pain, and inguinal hernia repair pain). The 1948 publication is focused on patients with stump pain or phantom limb pain, with the goal of the study to decipher if the pain was of a local origin or whether it was related to a projection from the sensory cortex. If it were found to be of local origin, the investigators wanted to know if interruption of the sympathetic nervous system would result in pain relief. An initial bolus of 0.2% procaine was injected into the subarachnoid space. This was followed by an infusion of the same concentration, and observations were made regarding pain relief and neurological examination results. The results of the procedure were intended to aid in surgical planning. **Table 1-1** shows their results, demonstrating their ability to block some nerve fibers and spare others.

If the smaller fibers were successfully blocked without relief of pain, full spinal anesthesia was induced to test if the pain had a local origin. This technique was further modified to the conventional technique as described by Winnie and Candido.[60] This technique involved four sequential injections (normal saline, 0.25% procaine, 0.5% procaine, and 5% procaine). If the patient responded to the normal saline, the pain was classified as "psychogenic." Response to 0.25% procaine was interpreted to mean that the pain was sympathetically mediated because the concentration is usually sufficient to block B fibers but not A-δ and C fibers. No response to the first two injections but pain relief with 0.5% procaine was interpreted as consistent with a somatic pain diagnosis as such a concentration is usually able to block B, A-δ and C fibers without blocking A-α, A-β, and A-γ fibers. The solution of 5% procaine blocked all fiber types, and failure to respond to that solution was interpreted as having a "central mechanism," the possibilities of which include a central lesion, psychogenic pain, encephalization, and malingering.

Because this type of investigation is clearly time consuming and made with the assumption of a "typical" minimum blocking concentration response for each patient when clinically there is variation, a modification was proposed.[61-64] The newer technique requires only two injections, the first with normal saline and the second with 2 cc of 5% procaine. The pain response and neurological

Table 1-1: Fibers That Are and Those That Are Not Blocked by the Introduction of 0.2% Procaine Hydrochloride in Large Amount into the Subarachnoid Space

Differential Spinal Block	
Fibers Blocked	**Fibers Spared**
Vasomotor	Touch
Sudomotor	Position sense
Visceromotor	Vibration sense
Pinprick sensation	Pain, types other than pinprick
Stretch afferents	Somatic motor

examination are then followed with the return of function of the different nerve fibers. This decreases the time for the procedure and does not rely on an average minimal concentration response of the nerve fibers. After a patient recovers sensation, only the sympathetic fibers remain blocked. Pain relief that remains after recovery of sensation suggests a sympathetically mediated pain.

Raj[65] presented a similar differential block strategy using the epidural space in 1977. The technique is limited, however, because of the even slower onset of the blockade and even less clear distinctions of the appropriate dose and concentration of local anesthetic for any particular patient compared with the intrathecal approach. In theory, however, the technique has the advantage of avoiding dural puncture.

The theory behind the differential spinal block was challenged by other investigators, including Fink.[66] He found that the size of the fiber did not truly explain the differential blockade and proposed the "bathed length principle." To block conduction of a nerve, at least three consecutive nodes must have adequate local anesthetic exposure. He reasoned that thicker axons have larger intermodal distances, and this decreases the likelihood of blocking the larger axons compared with the smaller fibers. He was also able to explain the differential block of the sympathetic nerves was a result of decremental block. Fink[66] explained some of the phenomenon noted during a spinal epidural differential block and contributed to a better understanding of the clinical observations noted during a differential spinal block.

The true utility of these blocks have been questioned in recent years, and the use of the technique has certainly declined. There is a significant range of conduction speed and fiber size within a fiber type. A lack of correlation of size and necessary anesthetic concentration for blockade within a group creates an overlap of the fiber types that seems to "negate any possibility of obtaining steady state differential interruption" by local anesthetics.[67,68] The vulnerability of the fiber type to diffusion of the local anesthetic also seems to play a significant role in explaining the timing of the neural blockade.[69] The clinical result of the overlap is that a partial block of the A fibers has already occurred by the time C fiber activity is blocked.[70]

The complex nature of pain often makes interpretation of even well-designed techniques difficult. The differential spinal blocks are a good reminder of not only the complexity of the nervous system but also the important role of performer bias, reliable and valid measurement, placebo response, and patient expectations. Although some authors[60] continue to promote the use of this procedure to establishing more accurate diagnosis, others[70,71] suggest significant caution in their use and applications.

Injections and Procedures Targeting the Zygapophysial (Facet) Joints

Lumbar medial branch blocks (MBBs) were first described in the late 1970s and were supported by anatomical studies showing that these branches of the lumbar dorsal rami were a valid and accessible target.[72-75] The sole purpose of the lumbar MBB is to determine if the patient's pain is relieved by anesthetizing the nerves targeted. Because the lumbar zygapophysial joints (Z-joints) account for 15% to 40% of low back pain[76] and because the lumbar medial branches send an intraarticular branch that supplies these joints, by convention a positive response to the MBB suggests the pain is arising from the Z-joints (facet joints). Although there was a flurry of literature describing intraarticular facet joint corticosteroid injections in the 1980s, the literature suggests that these did not provide lasting relief in the majority of studies. Studies by Dreyfuss et al[77] and Kaplan et al[78] showed that lumbar MBBs were

target specific and a valid test of zygapophysial joint pain. Lumbar medial branch neurotomy has emerged as the treatment of choice for patients with pain arising from the lumbar zygapophysial joints.

Radiofrequency (RF) neurotomy has been used successfully for the treatment of trigeminal neuralgia since the pioneering work by White and Sweet in 1969.[79] Early studies by Rees[80,81] and Shealy[80-85] reporting neurotomy or rhizolysis of the "facets" sparked interest in the Z-joint as a source of pain and target for treatment. Subsequent analysis of their technique, however, lead to conclusions that they were unsuccessful in severing the nerves to the lumbar zygapophysial joints.[72,73,86] After this, a modified technique targeting the correct nerve locations was reported in 1980,[87] and subsequent studies showed good benefit. Analysis of the lesion created with RF neurotomy[88] led to a modification in technique that placed the needle and therefore lesion parallel to the target nerve.[89] A study using controlled diagnostic blocks as a diagnostic step and lesions created parallel to the target nerve demonstrated significant benefit for patients with chronic lumbar zygapophysial joint pain.[90] Pulsed RF (PRF) treatment has also been proposed as an alternative to conventional RF, although overall, there is less supportive evidence.

In the cervical spine, the premise for cervical MBBs as a diagnostic test for cervical zygapophysial joint pain also appears justified. The technique of selective blockade of the cervical dorsal rami was first suggested in 1980.[91] Anatomical studies again led to further refinement and description of blockade of the cervical medial branches[92] rather than their parent nerve. Diagnostic utility of cervical MBBs was established with studies for head pain and neck pain beginning in 1985. Pain referral maps were created that enabled practitioners to better predict the segmental level of painful joints.[93,94] In the early 1990s, a series of papers argued the importance of comparative diagnostic blockade and the shortcomings of single diagnostic blocks. Epidemiological studies that followed reported a high prevalence of pain arising from the cervical zygapophysial joints, especially in patients with head or neck pain from whiplash injuries. Injecting cervical zygapophysial joints with corticosteroids did not provide any additional benefit over anesthetizing the joint.

The first descriptions of cervical medial branch neurotomy appeared in the 1970s in papers focused predominantly on low back pain, and the first studies focusing exclusively on neck pain appeared in the early 1980s. Over the following decade, several more studies appeared, but similar to the lumbar treatments, the selection criteria and techniques varied, resulting in only fair overall results. The publications between 1995 and 2003 on cervical medial branch RF neurotomy demonstrated significant and prolonged benefit, most notably with the publications by Lord et al[88] and Govind et al[95] on patients with neck and head pain, respectively.

Pain arising from the thoracic zygapophysial joints account for 34% to 48% of chronic thoracic pain.[96-99] Thoracic MBBs have also been described as analogs to the diagnostic blocks in the cervical and lumbar regions, but few studies have described their application in clinical practice. In one study of 46 patients with chronic thoracic pain, 48% had relief with the diagnostic blocks.[98] A subsequent study by the same authors showed that 71% had relief that persisted for several months or even years with or without the inclusion of corticosteroids.[99] There is great variability in the location of the medial branch nerves, especially in the midthoracic region (T5-T8). Two papers have reported thoracic referred pain patterns.[100,101] Thoracic intraarticular zygapophysial joint blocks were first reported for relief of chronic thoracic pain in 1987.[102] One prospective study showed significant pain relief persisting for 12 months after thoracic RF medial branch neurotomy.[103]

Sacroiliac Joint Injections and Procedures

Appreciation that the sacroiliac joint could be a source of low back pain fluctuated throughout the twentieth century. There were no validated tests to confirm the diagnosis of pain arising from the sacroiliac joint. The first description of injection of medication into the sacroiliac joint for diagnosis and treatment was described by Haldeman and Soto-Hall in 1938.[104] Later studies[105] suggested that the likelihood of medication entering the sacroiliac joint with a blind injection was approximately 22%. The first description of using fluoroscopic guidance to secure entry in the sacroiliac joint was described in 1979.[106] Three years later in the same journal, Hendrix et al[107] described the use of contrast medium to confirm intraarticular spread of injectate. Both of these descriptions involved using a posterior approach to the joint, which has since been replaced with the recommended inferior approach to the joint. This inferior approach was first described in 1992[108] with numerous modifications and descriptions until the simplified approach that is currently used in clinical practice was described in 2000.[109] With the ability to confirm needle entry into the sacroiliac joint with use of fluoroscopy and contrast, it was now possible to more accurately diagnose sacroiliac joint pain. Sacroiliac joint pain has now become a recognized source of pain in the low back with an estimated incidence of 13% to 19%[110,111] based on response to controlled diagnostic blocks. Pain referral patterns after injections were created to better elicit which patients were likely to possess sacroiliac joint pain based on history and physical examination findings, including use of provocative maneuvers. Numerous studies have demonstrated that no single clinical feature is predictive to response of diagnostic blockade.[112-114]

The sacroiliac joint has a diffuse and variable innervation that cannot be reliably blocked using selective nerve blocks. The exact pattern of innervation is disputed but likely involves a possible anterior component from the ventral rami of L5-S2 and via branches from the sacral plexus and a posterior component from the lateral branches of the S1-S4 dorsal rami and possibly involving the L5 and even L4 dorsal rami. Numerous studies have targeted the sacral lateral branches as diagnostic tests and for RF ablation of these same nerves. Others have targeted extraarticular structures, including the deep interosseus ligament and the posterior sacroiliac ligaments.[115-117] In fact, targeting these structures has shown promise for both RF ablation procedures and for corticosteroid injections.

After the sacroiliac joint has been confirmed as the source of the patient's pain, then the most common treatment involves injection of corticosteroid in the same fashion as the diagnostic block. Injections of corticosteroids into the sacroiliac joint have been shown to be efficacious in the treatment of sacroiliitis caused by various spondyloarthropathies.[118-121] Other studies demonstrate efficacy with extraarticular corticosteroid injections[104,122-124] or a combination of both intra- and extraarticular techniques.[116] One study reported moderate relief of sacroiliac joint pain after injection of phenol (6%) into the sacroiliac joint.[125]

Numerous techniques have been described for RF denervation of the sacroiliac joint and contributing structures. Ferrante et al[126] described performing bipolar strip lesions along the inferior pole of the sacroiliac joint. This provided significant benefit to only a small percentage of patients. Because of the variable innervation to the joint, the treatments also offer some variability but generally target the lateral branches of S1-S3 and may include the lateral branch of S4 and the dorsal rami of L5 and even L4.[114,127-129] The most recent innovations that show promising results include cooled RF treatment[130-132] and use of a single multilesion RF probe.[133] Both of these techniques involve creating larger sized lesions than has been reported with conventional RF approaches directed at the sacroiliac joint and contributing structures.

Disc Stimulation (Provocation Discography)

Lumbar disc stimulation was developed in the late 1940s as a technique for diagnosing herniation of lumbar intervertebral discs, and the first published description appeared in 1948.[134] This corresponded with the published belief in 1947 that the disc could be a primary source of pain,[135] a notion that was supported by subsequent intraoperative studies.[136-138] Nevertheless, the disc as a primary source of pain ran contrary to conventional wisdom until the 1980s.

Despite a key paper by Massie & Stevens[139] in 1967 reinforcing that the pain reproduction is the essential element in distinguishing symptomatic discs from similarly degenerated ones, there remained skepticism and controversy surrounding the procedure. Again, many of the critics who offered negative reviews failed to recognize that it was the stimulation portion that was critical to identifying the symptomatic disc.[140] This led to an executive statement from a major spine society, the North American Spine Society,[141] in 1988, again emphasizing that the pain response to disc stimulation is the key component to the procedure. Studies demonstrated that discography did improve surgical results when interpreted and performed correctly.[142-145] At the same time, there was an explosion of studies between 1980 and 1992 showing that the disc can be innervated and a source of pain.

After the reports of computed tomography discography in 1986 to 1987,[146,147] the Dallas discogram scale was reported[148] and subsequently modified.[149] Studies correlated pain reproduction with the extent of annular disruption,[150] and the term *internal disc disruption* emerged.[151] Use of manometry led to a classification system based on observational studies.[145,152] Risks associated and reported with the procedure include infection (discitis) and reaction to medication. A recent prospective study demonstrated accelerated progression of degenerative changes in the lumbar disc 7 to 10 years after "discography" compared with those who did not undergo the procedure.[153]

The history of disc stimulation in the cervical spine parallels that of the lumbar region. The technique for cervical discography was first published in 1957[154] and was followed by more published reports over subsequent years. Intraoperative disc stimulation (mechanical and electrical) verified the notion that the cervical disc itself could be a source of pain and may by mediated by sinuvertebral nerves,[155] a notion that was confirmed by anatomical studies.[156-159] Many of the same critics of lumbar discography argued that the morphological changes seen on discography did not correlate with the reproduction of pain.[160,161] They again missed the notion that the primary objective of discography is to detect reproduction of concordant pain. A 1996 study demonstrated that stimulation of cervical discs in asymptomatic volunteers is either painless or minimally painful.[162] A prior study[163] had shown a "false-positive" response to cervical disc stimulation in patients who had positive relief with diagnostic blockade of the cervical zygapophysial joints. Grubb and Kelly[164] showed that many patients had positive responses at multiple levels and argued that disc stimulation should be performed at all levels from C2-C3 to C6-C7 when technically feasible. Others[152] had modified this approach to exclude C2-C3 if head pain was not a major component based on pain referral distribution maps based on prior studies.[162,164] Observational studies suggest that cervical discography does help surgeons select (and avoid) segmental levels that should (not) be fused and may lead to avoidance of surgery altogether if multilevel disease is present.[164]

Risks and complications associated with cervical disc stimulation are similar to the lumbar spine with the noted difference that high pressures may accentuate disc bulging or prolapse, especially in patients with spinal stenosis or impingement on the spinal cord.[165,166] Additionally, the larynx may obstruct access to the disc at C2-C3, and the apex of the lung may intervene at C7-T1. Before utilization of antibiotic prophylaxis, the incidence of discitis reported was 0.64% per patient,[165] possibly related to the proximity of the pharynx and esophagus. A recent review[167] reported an overall incidence of discitis of 0.44%, but there were no cases of discitis noted in the only two studies (2140 patients) that consistently gave intradiscal antibiotics.

Thoracic disc pathology is far less common than in the lumbar or cervical regions. Accordingly, there is less reporting on thoracic provocation discography. The first published series of 100 patients was published in 1994,[168] and this was followed by a prospective study in 1999.[169] The principles are the same as for the lumbar and cervical regions, but thoracic provocation discography is a technically challenging procedure with the added risk of pleural puncture that should only be performed by expert physicians.

Anesthetic discography was described by Roth in 1976[170] but has gained little attention until recently. A subsequent study reported that the authors only achieved an anesthetic response to anesthetizing the disc in seven of 34 patients with painful cervical discs.[163] Functional anesthetic discography (FAD) is an emerging new technique for establishing pain reproduction and evaluating potential relief after injection of local anesthetic into the disc. The clinical utility and safety of this test are yet to be determined; however, preliminary presentations suggest that it may further stratify patients with positive pain provocation with conventional disc stimulation into those who do or do not gain relief from FAD.[171,172]

Intradiscal Treatments

Numerous intradiscal treatments have been reported for patients with discogenic pain or disc herniation or protrusion. These include chemonucleolysis with chymopapain[173,174] and intradiscal injection of corticosteroid,[175,176] ozone,[177] hypertonic dextrose,[178] etanercept,[179] and methylene blue.[180] Additionally, mechanical and electrical means have been used, including high-voltage intradiscal PRF,[181] intradiscal RF,[182] intradiscal electrothermal annuloplasty (IDET),[183-194] RF annuloplasty,[191,195] intradiscal biacuplasty,[196-199] percutaneous lumbar discectomy,[200] and plasma disc decompression (nucleoplasty).[201-211]

IDET is a treatment in which a flexible electrode is introduced into a lumbar intervertebral disc and delivers heat to the annulus fibrosus in an attempt to relieve pain stemming from the disc. The mechanism of action remains unclear but may work to strengthen the collagen and seal radial tears or by denervating nerve endings near painful fissures, thereby sealing the fissures against fresh exudates entering from the nucleus pulposus. Saal and Saal[183,184] first presented the IDET treatment in 1999, and several observational studies were reported over the first few years of introduction. The procedure has demonstrated good benefit in a number of observational studies[185-191] and in one of two placebo-controlled trials.[192,193] A meta-analysis demonstrated compelling evidence for the efficacy and safety of the procedure.[194] Outcomes from IDET have been reported to be similar to those from surgical fusion but with fewer complications.[190] Other thermal treatments have also been performed with similar goals of denervating symptomatic nerve endings. One such treatment termed *RF posterior annuloplasty* has

been performed but with far less benefit compared with IDET, including a head-to-head study of the two treatments. In that study, both treatments provided benefit, but the pain and disability scores were both significantly better in the IDET group.[191,195] A new treatment termed *intradiscal biacuplasty* has been performed for patients with internal disc disruption.[196] This treatment consists of placing bilateral RF probes in the posterolateral annulus and delivering bipolar cooled RF energy to create a precise and reproducible lesion. By placing the probes directly into the annulus, this treatment avoids having to navigate a thermoelastic coil around the annulus, which can prove difficult. A few early studies have been quite promising in demonstrating benefits in pain scores in patients with discogenic pain who underwent intradiscal biacuplasty.[196-199]

The second area of focus for intradiscal procedures is for contained disc protrusions or herniations causing radicular or axial pain complaints (or both). Chemonucleolysis with chymopapain was initially described in 1964 as a management option for contained disc herniations without sequestration or extrusion.[173] Chymopapain is a proteolytic enzyme that was derived from papaya and is thought to catalyze hydrolysis of proteins in the nucleus pulposus. A number of studies have demonstrated benefit compared with placebo but possibly inferior results when compared with surgical discectomy. A meta-analysis of 22 eligible clinical trials found that chemonucleolysis with chymopapain was superior to placebo and was as effective as collagenase in the treatment of lumbar disc prolapse. The summary data comparing chemonucleolysis with surgery were heterogenous, showing both options to be equivalent in their effectiveness.[174] After a number of patients were reported to have developed anaphylaxis and died after chymopapain injection, the substance was banned for a short time in the mid-1970s by the Food and Drug Administration, and reinjection continues to be prohibited in the United States for fear of sensitization and anaphylaxis. Collagenase has also been associated with allergic reactions.

Newer techniques have focused on percutaneous manual decompression by mechanical (automated percutaneous lumbar discectomy [APLD], DeKompressor) or electrical (plasma disc decompression) means. Use of APLD was first published in the early 1990s and showed mixed results. Later, a mechanical high-RPM device (DeKompressor probe) was introduced. It was designed to extract the nuclear material through an introducer cannula using an auger-like device that rotates at high speeds. A number of studies demonstrated improvement in pain and function,[200] but overall, the evidence was limited. Percutaneous disc decompression (PDD) with nucleoplasty (coblation technology) is performed with RF energy to dissolve nuclear material through molecular dissociation with resultant intradiscal pressure reduction.[201] The proposed advantage of the coblation technology is production of a controlled and highly localized ablation with minimal thermal damage to surrounding tissues. Additionally, there is avoidance of injection of chemicals that may predispose the patient to allergic reaction or anaphylaxis as is seen with chemonucleolysis. Although a number of prospective studies have demonstrated benefit,[202-208] overall the evidence is limited. This treatment has also been proposed as an alternative to IDET for patients with discogenic pain, although the results appear less dramatic than for radicular pain.[209] Cervical PDD has also been reported with good benefit,[210] including a recent randomized trial.[211]

Vertebral Augmentation

In the early twentieth century, chemist Otto Röhm developed and marketed a substance with unique structural properties and good biocompatibility called polymethyl methacrylate (PMMA)[212,213] registered under the brand name Plexiglas. In 1936, commercially viable production of acrylic safety glass began. The acrylic glass was used for submarine periscopes, windshields, and gun turrets for airplanes in World War II.[214] The biocompatibility of the substance was noted when splinters from the side windows of the Supermarine Spitfire fighters (made of PMMA) caused almost no rejection reaction in the eyes of soldiers compared with the glass splinters of aircraft such as the Hawker Hurricane.[215] Sir John Charnley started using PMMA as bone cement for fixation of the femur and acetabulum in total hip arthroplasty in the 1960s. The same substance has been used for decades in dentistry as part of dentures and in filling materials. PMMA is used as a grout material to fill in the gaps between the prosthesis and bone. The substance has been found to be stable for long-term implantation.[212,213]

PMMA has been used extensively in the spine as well. Historically, it has been used to stabilize motion segments with posterior applications,[216] fill defects in open corpectomy procedures for spinal tumors,[217,218] and improve hardware stability in osteoporotic bone.[219]

The first percutaneous use of PMMA, however, was not until 1984, when Deramond et al[220] used this material as part of a treatment for a patient with an aggressive C2 hemangioma. Treatment of aggressive hemangiomas was the first major indication for the procedure, now known as vertebroplasty. PMMA was then injected in a similar percutaneous manner with fluoroscopic guidance into vertebral compression fractures (VCFs) secondary to osteoporosis.[221] After the initial experience was documented in Europe, the procedure was introduced and expanded by the neuroradiology interventionalists at the University of Virginia starting in 1994.[222] Jensen et al[222] published the results of the treatment of 47 painful vertebral fractures related to osteoporotic fractures a few years later in an English language journal, concluding that vertebroplasty could provide pain relief and early mobilization in appropriately selected patients. The paradigm of "benign neglect" of VCFs to active intervention started to shift.[223]

Most of the North American data are related to the use of vertebral augmentation for the treatment of osteoporotic fractures, although the European literature demonstrates extensive experience in the setting of metastases and myeloma as well. The procedure offers a minimally invasive option of pain control because patients with VCFs are typically poor candidates for surgical correction. Poor bone quality limits effective healing, and the patients' comorbidities often make surgical options unattractive. Patients for whom surgery may be indicated include those with significant spinal instability or neurological consequences of the VCF.

The mechanism in which pain relief occurs with the introduction of PMMA into fractured vertebral bodies has been debated for years. The polymerization of the cement is exothermic, and temperatures can reach 122° C.[224,225] Some investigators have suggested that thermal necrosis and chemotoxicity of the intraosseous pain receptors as well as restored mechanical stability could be responsible for the pain relief. Animal data, however, suggests that PMMA causes relatively little necrotic exothermic effect.[226]

The complication rate of vertebroplasty is low, with most of the concerns focused on leakage of the PMMA into nearby structures. The majority of cases of cement extravasations are asymptomatic and occur in areas of cortical destruction, fracture lines, or into the epidural and paravertebral venous complexes.[227,228] Murphey and Deramond[229] divided the risk by indication for the procedure and found a complication rate of 1.3% for osteoporosis, 2.5% for hemangiomas, and 10% for neoplastic disease. Another issue of concern has been an increased risk for fracture in an adjacent vertebral body,[230] but some data from cadaveric studies have suggested that it is the result of the natural progression of the disease rather than a result of vertebral augmentation.[231]

The procedure modifications over the past couple of decades have included larger bore needles and additional barium in the PMMA mixture. The larger bore needles allow for a more viscous cement mixture, and additional barium allows for a well-monitored injection under live fluoroscopy of the PMMA, both theoretically limiting the risk of extravertebral and vascular migration of the PMMA.

Another technique modification to decrease the extravasations risk was a modified use of an angioplasty balloon, a technique first performed by Mark Reiley, an orthopedic surgeon, in 1998.[232] In this procedure, called kyphoplasty, the inflatable balloon is used to create a cavity in the fractured vertebral body. The cavity is then filled with PMMA. This allows for a lower pressure injection and the use of a more viscous cement mixture than is possible with vertebroplasty. The additional benefit of kyphoplasty over vertebroplasty is the possibility of partial restoration of the height of the vertebral body. This normalization of the vertebral column could potentially decrease the complications of vertebral fractures such as pulmonary dysfunction.

The consensus statement from 2009[233] concluded that vertebroplasty resulted in significant pain reduction and improved function and quality of life in the setting of osteoporotic fractures and vertebral fractures related to metastatic cancer. Although fewer studies have investigated the efficacy of kyphoplasty compared with vertebroplasty, the position of the committee was that the efficacy appeared equivalent. There was no evidence of additional benefit of either procedure in regard to pain relief, vertebral height restoration, or complication rate.

References

1. Koller C: On the use of cocaine for producing anaesthesia on the eye. *Lancet* 2:990, 1884.
2. Corning JL: Spinal anaesthesia and local medication of the cord with cocaine. *NY Med J* 1885;42:483.
3. Gray H: *Anatomy: descriptive and surgical*, ed 5, Philadelphia, 1870, Henry C. Lea, pp 572-574.
4. Harrington BE: Postdural puncture headache and the development of the epidural blood patch. *Reg Anesth Pain Med* 29:136-163, 2004.
5. Wynter WE: Four cases of tubercular meningitis in which paracentesis of the theca vertebralis was performed for the relief of fluid pressure. *Lancet* 1:981-982, 1891.
6. Quincke H: Die lumbalpunction des hydrocephalus. *Berliner Klinische Wochenschrift* 28:929-933, 1891.
7. Bier A: Versuche uber Cocainisrung des Ruckenmarkes. *Dtsch Z Chir* 5151:361, 1899.
8. Tait D, Caglieri G: Experimental and clinical notes on the subarachnoid space, *Trans Med Soc State Cal* 30:266-271, 1900.
9. Anonymous: Surgical anaesthesia by the injection of cocaine into the lumbar sub-arachnoid space. *Lancet* 12:137-138, 1901.
10. Cathelin MF: Mode d'action de la cocaine injectee dans l'espace epidural par le procede du canal sacre. *CR Soc Biol (Paris)* 53:478-479, 1901.
11. De Pasquier M, Leri M: Injections intra et extra-durales de cocaine a dose minime dans le traitement de la sciatique. Valeur comparee des deux methods: resultats immediats et Tardifs. *Bull Gen Ther* 142:192-223, 1901.
12. Stoeckel W: Ueber sakrale Anasthesie. *Zentralbl. Gynaekol* 33:1, 1909.
13. Viner N: Intractable sciatica: the sacral epidural injection: an effective method of giving relief. *Can Med Assoc J* 15:630-634, 1925.
14. Mason HL, Myers CS, Kendall EC: The chemistry of crystalline substances isolated from the suprarenal gland. *J Biol Chem* 114:613-631, 1936.

15. Mason HL, Myers CS, Kendall EC: Chemical studies of the suprarenal cortex II. The definition of a substance which possesses the qualitative action of cortin; its conversion into a diketone closely related to androstenedione. *J Biol Chem* 116:267-276, 1936.

16. Hench PS, Kendall EC, Slocumb CH, et al: Effects of cortisone acetate and pituitary ACTH on rheumatic fever and certain other conditions. *Arch Intern Med* 85:545-566, 1950.

17. Hench PS, Kendall EC, Slocumb CH, et al: The effect of a hormone of the adrenal cortex (17-hydroxy-11-dehydrocorticosterone: compound E) and of pituitary adrenocorticotropic hormone on rheumatoid arthritis; preliminary report. *Proc Staff Meet Mayo Clin* 24:181-197, 1949.

18. Hollander JL: The local effects of compound F (hydrocortisone) injected into joints. *Bull Rheum Dis* 2:3-4, 1951.

19. Robecchi A, Capra R: [Hydrocortisone (compound F); first clinical experiment in the field of rheumatology]. *Minerva Med* 2:1259-1263, 1952.

20. Lievre JA, Block-Michel H, Pean G, et al: L'hydrocortisone en injection locale, *Revue du Rhumatisme et des Maladies Osteo-articulares* 20:310-311, 1953.

21. Brown JH: Pressure caudal anesthesia and back manipulation. *Northwest Med* 59:905-909, 1960.

22. Pagés E: Anestesia metamerica. *Rev Sanid Mil Madr* 11:351, 1921.

23. Dogliotti AM: Segmental peridural anesthesia. *Am J Surg* 20:107, 1933.

24. Gutierrez A: Valor de la aspiracion liquada en al espacio peridural en la anesthesia peridural. *Rev Circ* 12:225, 1933.

25. Kamen GF, Erdman GL: Subdural administration of hydrocortisone in multiple sclerosis: effect of ACTH. *J Am Geriatr Soc* 1:794-804, 1953.

26. Boines GJ: Remissions in multiple sclerosis following intrathecal methylprednisolone acetate. *Del Med J* 33:231-235, 1961.

27. Boines GJ: Predictable remissions in multiple sclerosis. *Del Med J* 35:200-203, 1963.

28. Goldstein NP, McKenzie BF, McGuckin WF, et al: Experimental intrathecal administration of methylprednisolone acetate in multiple sclerosis. *Trans Am Neurol Assoc* 95:243-244, 1970.

29. Nelson DA, Vates TS, Thomas RB: Complications from intrathecal steroid therapy in patients with multiple sclerosis. *Acta Neurol Scand* 49:176-188, 1973.

30. Gardner WJ, Goebert HW, Sehgal AD: Intraspinal corticosteroids in the treatment of sciatica. *Trans Am Neurol Assoc* 86:214-215, 1961.

31. Sehgal AD, Gardner WJ: Place of intrathecal methylprednisolone acetate in neurological disorders. *Trans Am Neurol Assoc* 88:275-276, 1963.

32. Sehgal AD, Tweed DC, Gardner WJ, et al: Laboratory studies after intrathecal corticosteroids. *Arch Neurol* 9:64-68, 1963.

33. Winnie AP, Hartman JT, Meyers HL, et al: Pain Clinic II: intradural and extradural corticosteroids for sciatica. *Anesth Analg* 51:990-999, 1972.

34. White AH, Derby R, Wynne G: Epidural injections for the diagnosis and treatment of low back pain. *Spine* 5:78-86, 1980.

35. Weinstein SM, Herring SA, Derby R: Contemporary concepts in spine care: epidural steroid injections. *Spine* 20:1842-1846, 1995.

36. el-Khoury G, Ehara S, Weinstein JN, et al: Epidural steroid injection: a procedure ideally performed with fluoroscopic control. *Radiology* 168:554-557, 1988.

37. Stojanovic MP, Vu T, Caneris O, et al: The role of fluoroscopy in cervical epidural steroid injections: an analysis of contrast dispersal patterns. *Spine* 27:509-514, 2002.

38. Fredman B, Nun MB, et al: Epidural steroids for treating "failed back surgery syndrome": is fluoroscopy really necessary? *Anesth Analg* 88:367-372, 1999.

39. O'Neil C, Derby R, Knederes L: Precision injection techniques for the diagnosis and treatment of lumbar disc disease. *Semin Spine Surg* 11:104-118, 1999.

40. Derby R, Bogduk N, Kine G: Precision percutaneous blocking procedures for localizing spinal pain: part 2. The lumbar neuroaxial compartment. *Pain Diag* 3:175-188, 1993.

41. Derby R, Kine G, Saal JA, et al: Responses to steroid and duration of radicular pain as predictors of surgical outcome. *Spine* 17(suppl):176-183, 1992.

42. Bier A: Versuche ueber cocainisirung des rueckenmarkes, *Deutsche Zeitschrift fuer Chirurgie* 51:361-368, 1899.

43. Jacobaeous HC, Frumerie K: About the leakage of the cerebrospinal fluid after lumbar puncture. *Acta Med Scandinav* 58:102-108, 1923.

44. Pickering GW: Experimental observations on headache. *Br Med J* 1:907-912, 1939.

45. Ahearn RE: Management of severe postlumbar puncture headache. *NY State J Med* 48:1495-1498, 1948.

46. Ekstrom T: Treatment of headache after spinal anesthesia with intraspinal injection of physiological saline solution. *Acta Chir Scand* 101:450-456, 1951.

47. Glesne OG: Lumbar puncture headaches. *Anesthesiology* 11:702-708, 1950.

48. Solomon HC: Raising cerebrospinal fluid pressure. *JAMA* 82:1512-1515, 1924.

49. Weed LH, Cushing H: Studies on cerebrospinal fluid. VIII. The effect of pituitary extract upon its secretion (choroidorrhoea). *Am J Physiol* 36:77-103, 1915.

50. Heldt TJ, Moloney JC: Negative pressure in epidural space. Preliminary studies. *Am J Med Sci* 175:371-376, 1928.

51. Heldt TJ: Lumbar puncture headache. *Med J Rec* 129:13613-13619, 1929.

52. Gormley JB: Treatment of postspinal headache. *Anesthesiology* 21:565-566, 1960.

53. DiGiovanni AJ, Dunbar BS: Epidural injections of autologous blood for postlumbar-puncture headache. *Anesth Analg* 49:268-271, 1970.

54. DiGiovanni AJ, Galbert MW, Wahle WM: Epidural injection of autologous blood for postlumbar-puncture headache. II. Additional clinical experiences and laboratory investigation. *Anesth Analg* 51:226-232, 1972.

55. Van Kooten F, Oedit R, Bakker SLM, Dippel DWJ: Epidural blood patch in post dural puncture headache: a randomized, observer-blind, controlled clinical trial. *J Neurol Neurosurg Psychiatry* 79:553-558, 2008.

56. Gasser HS, Erlanger J: The compound nature of the action current of nerve as disclosed by the cathode ray oscilloscope. *Am J Physiol* 70:624, 1924.

57. Gasser HS, Erlanger J: The role played by the size of the constituent fibers of a verve trunk in determining the form of its action potential wave. *Am J Physiol* 80:522, 1927.

58. Sarnoff SJ, Arrowood JG: Differential spinal block. I. *Surgery* 20:150-159, 1946.

59. Sarnoff SJ, Arrowood JG: Differential spinal block. V. Use in the investigation of pain following amputation. *Anesthesiology* 9:614-622, 1948.

60. Winnie AJ, Candido KD: Differential neural blockade for the diagnosis of pain. In Waldman SD, editor: *Pain management*, Philadelphia, 2007, Saunders, pp 155-166.

61. Akkineni SR, Ramamurthy S: *Simplified differential spinal block.* Presented at the Annual Meeting of the American Society of Anesthesiologists, New Orleans, October 15-19, 1977.

62. Winnie AP: Differential diagnosis of pain mechanisms. *ASA Refresher Courses in Anesthesiology* 6:171, 1978.

63. Ramamurthy S, Winnie AP: Diagnostic maneuvers in painful syndromes. *Int Anesth Clin* 21:47, 1983.

64. Ramamurthy S, Winnie AP: Regional anesthetic techniques for pain relief. *Semin Anesth* 4:237, 1985.

65. Raj PP: *Sympathetic pain mechanism and management.* Presented at the Second Annual Meeting of the American Society of Regional Anesthesia, Hollywood, FL, March 10-11, 1977.

66. Fink BR: Mechanisms of differential axial blockade in epidural and subarachnoid anesthesia. *Anesthesiology* 70:851-858, 1989.

67. Fink BR, Cairnes AM: Lack of size related differential sensitivity to equilibrium conduction block among mammalian myelinated axons exposed to lidocaine. *Anesth Analg* 66:948-953, 1987.

68. Raymond SA: Subblocking concentrations of local anesthetic: effects on impulse generation and conduction in single myelinated sciatic nerve axons in frog. *Anesth Analg* 75: 906-921, 1992.

69. Torebjork HE, Hallin RG: Perceptual changes accompanying controlled preferential blocking of A and C fibre responses in intact human skin nerves. *Exp Brain Res* 16:321-332, 1973.

70. Hogan QH, Abram SE: Neural blockade for diagnosis and prognosis: a review. *Anesthesiology* 86:216-241, 1997.

71. Raja SN: Nerve blocks in the evaluation of chronic pain: a plea for caution in their use and interpretation. *Anesthesiology* 86:4-6, 1997.

72. Bogduk N, Long DM: The anatomy of the so-called 'articular nerves' and their relationship to facet denervation in the treatment of low back pain. *J Neurosurg* 51:172-177, 1979.

73. Bogduk N, Long DM: Percutaneous lumbar medial branch neurotomy. A modification of facet denervation. *Spine* 5:193-200, 1980.

74. Bogduk N, Wilson AS, Tynan W: The human dorsal rami. *J Anat* 134:383-397, 1982.

75. Bogduk N: The innervation of the lumbar spine. *Spine* 8:286-293, 1983.

76. Schwarzer AC, Wang S, Bogduk N, et al: Prevalence and clinical features of lumbar zygapophysial joint pain: a study in an Australian population with chronic low back pain. *Ann Rheum Dis* 54:100-106, 1995.

77. Dreyfuss P, Schwarzer AC, Lau P, et al: Specificity of lumbar medial branch and L5 dorsal ramus blocks: a computed tomographic study. *Spine* 22:895-902, 1997.

78. Kaplan M, Dreyfuss P, Halbrook B, et al: The ability of lumbar medial branch blocks to anesthetize the zygapophysial joint. *Spine* 23:1847-1852, 1998.

79. White JC, Sweet WH: *Pain and the neurosurgeon*, Springfield, IL, 1969, CC Thomas, pp 193-197.

80. Rees WES: Multiple bilateral subcutaneous rhizolysis of segmental nerves in the treatment of intervertebral disc syndrome. *Ann Gen Pract* 16:126-127, 1971.

81. Rees WES: Multiple bilateral percutaneous rhizolysis. *Med J Aust* 1:536-537, 1975.

82. Shealy CN: Facets in back and sciatic pain. *Minn Med* 57:199-203, 1974.

83. Shealy CN: The role of the spinal facets in back and sciatic pain. *Headache* 14:101-104, 1974.

84. Shealy CN: Percutaneous radiofrequency denervation of spinal facets. *J Neurosurg* 43:448-451, 1975.

85. Shealey CN: Facet denervation in the management of back sciatic pain. *Clin Orthop* 115:157-164, 1976.

86. Bogduk N, Colman RRS, Winer CER: An anatomical assessment of the "percutaneous rhizolysis" procedure. *Med J Aust* 1:397-399, 1977.

87. King JS, Lagger R: Sciatica viewed as a referred pain syndrome. *Surg Neurol* 5:46-50, 1976.

88. Lord SM, Barnsley L, Wallis B, et al: Percutaneous radiofrequency neurotomy for chronic cervical zygapophyseal joint pain. *N Eng J Med* 335:1721-1726, 1996.

89. Bogduk N, Macintosh J, Marsland A: Technical limitations to the efficacy of radiofrequency neurotomy for spinal pain. *Neurosurgery* 20:529-535, 1987.

90. Dreyfuss P, Halbrook B, Pauza K, et al: Efficacy and validity of radiofrequency neurotomy for chronic lumbar zygapophysial joint pain. *Spine* 25:1270-1277, 2000.

91. Sluijter ME, Koetsveld-Baart CC: Interruption of pain pathways in the treatment of the cervical syndrome. *Anesthesia* 35:302-307, 1980.

92. Bogduk N: The clinical anatomy of the cervical dorsal rami. *Spine* 7:319-330, 1982.

93. Dwyer A, April C, Bogduk N: Cervical zygapophyseal joint pain patterns I: a study in normal volunteers. *Spine* 15:453-457, 1990.

94. April C, Dwyer A, Bogduk N: Cervical joint pain patterns II: a clinical evaluation. *Spine* 15:458-461, 1990.

95. Govind J, King W, Bailey B, et al: Radiofrequency neurotomy for the treatment of third occipital headache. *J Neurol Neurosurg Psychiatry* 74:88-93, 2003.

96. Manchikanti L, Boswell MV, Singh V, et al: Prevalence of facet joint pain in chronic spinal pain of cervical, thoracic, and lumbar regions. *BMC Musculoskelet Disord* 5:15, 2004.

97. Manchukonda R, Manchikanti KN, Cash KA, et al: Facet joint pain in chronic spinal pain: an evaluation of prevalence and false positive rate of diagnostic blocks. *J Spinal Disord Tech* 20(7):539-545, 2007.

98. Manchikanti L, Singh V, Pampati V, et al: Evaluation of the prevalence of facet joint pain in chronic thoracic pain. *Pain Physician* 5:354-359, 2002.

99. Manchikanti L, Manchikanti KN, Manchukonda R, et al: Evaluation of therapeutic thoracic medial branch block effectiveness in chronic thoracic pain: a prospective outcome study with minimum 1-year follow up. *Pain Physician* 9(2):97-105, 2006.

100. Dreyfuss P, Tibiletti C, Dryer SJ: Thoracic zygapophyseal joint pain patterns. A study in normal volunteers. *Spine* 19:807-811, 1994.

101. Fukui S, Ohseto K, Shiotani M: Patterns of pain induced by distending the thoracic zygapophyseal joints. *Reg Anesth* 22:332-336, 1997.

102. Wilson PR: Thoracic facet syndrome—a clinical entity? *Pain Suppl* 4(suppl):S87, 1987.

103. Stolker RJ, Vervest ACM, Groen GJ: Percutaneous facet denervation in chronic thoracic spinal pain. *Acta Neurochir* 122:82-90, 1993.

104. Haldeman KO, Soto-Hall R: The diagnosis and treatment of sacroiliac condition by the injection of procaine. *J Bone Joint Surg* 20:675-685, 1938.

105. Rosenberg J, Quint T, de Rosayro A: Computerized tomographic localization of clinically-guided sacroiliac joint injections. *Clin J Pain* 16:18-21, 2000.

106. Miskew DB, Block RA, Witt PF: Aspiration of infected sacro-iliac joints. *J Bone Joint Surg Am* 61(suppl A):1071-1072, 1979.

107. Hendrix RW, Lin PP, Kane BJ: Simplified aspiration or injection technique for the sacroiliac joint. *J Bone Joint Surg Am* 64(suppl A):1249-1252, 1982.

108. April CN: The role of anatomically specific injections into the sacroiliac joint. In Vleeming A, Mooney V, Snijders C, Dorman T, editors: *First Interdisciplinary World Congress on Low Back Pain and its Relation to the Sacroiliac Joint*, San Diego, November 5-6, 1992, Rotterdam, ECO, 1992, pp 373-380.

109. Dussault RG, Kaplan PA, Anderson MW: Fluoroscopy-guided sacroiliac joint injections. *Radiology* 214:273-277, 2000.

110. Schwarzer AC, April CN, Bogduk N: The sacroiliac joint in chronic low back pain. *Spine* 20:31-37, 1995.

111. Maigne JY, Aivaliklis A, Pfefer F: Results of sacroiliac joint double block and value of sacroiliac pain provocation tests in 54 patients with low back pain. *Spine* 21:1889-1892, 1996.

112. Fortin JD, Dwyer AD, West S, et al: Sacroiliac joint pain: pain referral maps upon applying a new injection/arthrogram technique. Part I: asymptomatic volunteers. *Spine* 19:1475-1482, 1994.

113. Fortin JD, April CN, Ponthieux B, et al: Sacroiliac joint: pain referral maps upon applying a new injection/arthrography technique. Part II: clinical evaluation. *Spine* 19:1483-1489, 1994.

114. Dreyfuss P, Michaelson M, Pauza K, et al: The value of history and physical examination in diagnosing sacroiliac joint pain. *Spine* 21:2594-2602, 1996.

115. Yin W, Willard F, Carreiro J, et al: Sensory stimulation-guided sacroiliac joint radiofrequency neurotomy: technique based on neuroanatomy of the dorsal sacral plexus. *Spine* 28(20):2419-2425, 2003.

116. Borowsky CD, Fagen G: Sources of sacroiliac region pain: insights gained from a study comparing standard intra-articular injection with a technique combining intra- and peri-articular injection. *Arch Phys Med Rehabil* 89:2048-2056, 2008.

117. Dreyfuss P, Henning T, Malladi N, et al: The ability of multi-site, multi-depth sacral lateral branch blocks to anesthetize the sacroiliac joint complex. *Pain Med* 10(4):679-688, 2009.

118. Maugers Y, Mathis C, Vilon P, et al: Corticosteroid injection of the sacroiliac joint in patients with seronegative spondyloarthropathy. *Arthritis Rheum* 35:564-568, 1992.

119. Maugers Y, Mathis C, Berthelot J: Assessment of the efficacy of sacroiliac corticosteroid injections in spondyloarthropathies: a double-blind study. *Br J Rheum* 35:767-770, 1996.

120. Braun J, Bollow M, Seyrekbasan F, et al: Computed tomography guided corticosteroid injection of the sacroiliac joint in patients with spondyloarthropathy with sacroiliitis: clinical outcome and follow up by dynamic magnetic resonance imaging. *J Rheumatol* 23:659-664, 1996.

121. Bollow M, Braun J, Taupitz M, et al: CT-guided intra-articular corticosteroid injection into the sacroiliac joints in patients with spondyloarthropathy: indication and follow up with contrast enhanced MRI. *J Comput Assist Tomo* 20:512-521, 1996.

122. Luukkainen R, Nissila M, Asikiainen E, et al: Periarticular corticosteroid treatment of the sacroiliac joint in patients with seronegative spondyloarthropathy. *Clin Exp Rheum* 17:88-90, 1999.

123. Norman GF: Sacroiliac disease and its relationship to lower abdominal pain. *Am J Surg* 116:54-56, 1968.

124. Schuchmann JA, Cannon CL: Sacroiliac strain syndrome: diagnosis and treatment. *Tex Med* 82:33-36, 1986.

125. Ward S, Jenson M, Royal M, et al: Fluoroscopy-guided sacroiliac joint injections with phenol ablation for persistent sacroiliitis: a case series. *Pain Pract* 2(4):332-335, 2002.

126. Ferrante FM, King LF, Roche EA, et al: Radiofrequency sacroiliac joint denervation for sacroiliac syndrome. *Reg Anesth Pain Med* 26(2):137-142, 2001.

127. Bujis E, Kamphuis E: Radiofrequency treatment of sacroiliac joint-related pain aimed at the first three sacral dorsal rami: a minimal approach. *Pain Clin* 16(2):139-146, 2004.

128. Cohen SP, Abdi S: Lateral branch blocks as a treatment for sacroiliac joint pain: a pilot study. *Reg Anesth Pain Med* 28(2):113-119, 2003.

129. Burnham RS, Yasui Y: An alternate method of radiofrequency neurotomy of the sacroiliac joint: a pilot study on the effect on pain, function and satisfaction. *Reg Anesth Pain Med* 32(1):12-19, 2007.

130. Kapural L, Nageeb F, Kapural M, et al: Cooled radiofrequency (RF) system for the treatment of chronic pain from sacroiliitis: the first case-series. *Pain Pract* 8(5):348-354, 2008.

131. Cohen SP, Hurley RW, Buckenmaier CC, III, et al: Randomized placebo-controlled study evaluating lateral branch radiofrequency denervation for sacroiliac joint pain. *Anesthesiology* 109(2):279-288, 2008.

132. Kapural L, Stojanovic M, Bensitel T, et al: Cooled radiofrequency (RF) of L5 dorsal ramus for RF denervation of the sacroiliac joint: technical report. *Pain Med* 11:53-57, 2010.

133. Starr B, Dahle N, Vorenkamp KE: *Radiofrequency lesioning of the SI joint with the Simplicity III probe: a case series. Proceedings of the American Society of Regional Anesthesia and Pain Medicine*, San Antonio, TX, 2009, Annual Fall Pain Meeting.

134. Lindblom K: Diagnostic disc puncture of intervertebral discs in sciatica. *Acta Orthop Scandinav* 17:231-239, 1948.

135. Inman VT, Saunders JB: Anatomicophysiological aspects of injuries to the intervertebral disc. *J Bone Joint Surg Am* 29:461-475, 1947.

136. Falconer MA, McGeorge M, Begg AC: Observations on the cause and mechanism of symptom-production in sciatica and low-back pain. *J Neurol Neurosurg Psychiatry* 11:13-26, 1948.

137. Wiberg G: Back pain in relation to the nerve supply of intervertebral discs. *Octa Orthop Scandinav* 19:211-221, 1949.

138. Hirsch C, Ingelmark BE, Miller M: The anatomical basis for low back pain. *Acta Orthop Scandinav* 33:1-17, 1963.

139. Massie WK, Stevens DB: A critical evaluation of discography. *J Bone Joint Surg Am* 49(suppl A):1243-1244, 1967.

140. Holt EP: The question of lumbar discography. *J Bone Joint Surg Am* 50(suppl A):720-725, 1968.

141. Executive Committee of the North American Spine Society: Position statement on discography. *Spine* 13:1343, 1988.

142. Colhoun E, McCall IW, Williams L, et al: Provocation discography as a guide to planning operations on the spine. *J Bone Joint Surg Am* 70(suppl B):267-271, 1988.

143. Grubb SA, Lipscomb HJ, Guilford WB: The relative value of lumbar roentgenograms, metrizamide myelography, and discography in the assessment of patients with chronic low-back-syndrome. *Spine* 12:282-286, 1987.

144. McFadden JW: The stress lumbar discogram. *Spine* 13:931-933, 1988.

145. Derby R, Howard MW, Grant JM, et al: The ability of pressure-controlled discography to predict surgical and non-surgical outcomes. *Spine* 24:364-372, 1999.

146. McCutcheon ME: CT scanning of lumbar discography: a useful diagnostic adjunct. *Spine* 11:257-259, 1986.

147. Videman T, Malmivaara A, Mooney V: The value of the axial view in assessing discograms: an experimental study with cadavers. *Spine* 12:299-304, 1987.

148. Sachs BL, Vanharta H, Spivey MA, et al: Dallas discogram description: a new classification of CT/discography in low-back disorders. *Spine* 12:287-294, 1987.

149. April C, Bogduk N: High intensity zone: a diagnostic sign of painful lumbar disc on magnetic resonance imaging. *Br J Radiol* 65:361-369, 1992.

150. Vanharanta H, Sachs BL, Spivey MA, et al: The relationship of pain provocation to lumbar disc deterioration as seen by CT/discography. *Spine* 12:295-298, 1987.

151. Crock HV: Internal disc disruption: a challenge to disc prolapse fifty years on. *Spine* 11:650-653, 1986.

152. Bogduk N, editor: *Practice guidelines for spinal diagnostic and treatment procedures*, San Francisco, 2004, International Spinal Intervention Society, pp 20-46.

153. Carragee E, Don A, Hurwitz E, et al: Does discography cause accelerated progression of degeneration changed in the lumbar disc: a ten-year matched cohort study. *Spine* 43(21):2338-2345, 2009.

154. Smith GW, Nichols P: The technic of cervical discography. *Radiology* 68:718-720, 1957.

155. Cloward RB: The clinical significance of the sinu-vertebral nerve of the cervical spine in relation to the cervical disk syndrome. *J Neurol Neurosurg Psychiatry* 23:321-326, 1960.

156. Bogduk N, Windsor M, Inglis A: The innervation of the cervical intervertebral discs. *Spine* 13:2-8, 1989.

157. Groen GJ, Baljert B, Drukker J: Nerves and nerve plexuses of the human vertebral column. *Am J Anat* 188:282-296, 1990.

158. Mendel T, Wink CS, Zimny ML: Neural elements in human cervical intervertebral discs. *Spine* 17:132-135, 1992.

159. Stuck RM: Cervical discography. *Am J Roentgenol Radium Ther Nucl Med* 86:975-982, 1961.

160. Sneider SE, Winslow OP, Pryor JH: Cervical diskography: is it relevant? *JAMA* 185:163-165, 1963.

161. Holt EP: The fallacy of cervical discography. *JAMA* 188:799-801, 1964.

162. Schellhas KP, Smith MD, Gundry CR, et al: Cervical discogenic pain. Prospective correlation of magnetic resonance imaging and discography in asymptomatic subjects and pain sufferers. *Spine* 21:300-312, 1996.

163. Bogduk N, Aprill C: On the nature of neck pain, discography and cervical zygapophysial joint blocks. *Pain* 54:213-217, 1993.

164. Grubb SA, Kelly CK: Cervical discography: clinical implications from 12 years of experience. *Spine* 25:1382-1389, 2000.

165. Connor PM, Darden BV: Cervical discography complications and clinical efficacy. *Spine* 18:2034-2038, 1993.

166. Laun A, Lorenz R, Agnoli AL: Complications of cervical discography. *J Neurosurg Sci* 25:17-20, 1981.

167. Kapoor SG, Huff J, Cohen SP: Systematic review of the incidence of discitis after cervical discography. *Spine J* 10(8):739-745, 2010.

168. Schellhas KP, Pollei SR, Dorwart RH: Thoracic discography: a safe and reliable technique. *Spine* 19:2103-2109, 1994.

169. Wood KB, Schellhas KP, Garvey TA, et al: Thoracic discography in healthy individuals. A controlled prospective study of magnetic resonance imaging and discography in asymptomatic and symptomatic individuals. *Spine* 24:1548-1555, 1999.

170. Roth DA: Cervical analgesic discography. A new test for the definitive diagnosis of the painful-disk syndrome. *JAMA* 235:1713-1714, 1976.

171. Anitescu M, Patel A, Simon A: Benefit of functional anesthetic discography, a double-blinded, prospective surgery outcome study. *Proceedings of the American Society of Anesthesiology 2009 Annual Meeting*, New Orleans, 2009.

172. Luchs J, Cho M, Demoura A: Preliminary experience with (functional anesthetic discography) FAD. Proceedings of the NASS 22nd Annual Meeting, Orlando, FL. *Spine J* 7(suppl):635, 2007.

173. Smith L: Enzyme dissolution of nucleus pulposus in humans. *JAMA* 187:137-140, 1964.

174. Couto JMC, de Castilho EA, Menezes PR: Chemonucleolysis in lumbar disc herniation: a meta-analysis. *Clinics (São Paulo)* 62(2):175-180, 2007.

175. Feffer HL: Treatment of low-back and sciatic pain by the injection of hydrocortisone into degenerated intervertebral discs. *J Bone Joint Surg Am* 38(suppl A):585-590, 1956.

176. Khot A, Bowditch M, Powell J, et al: The use of intradiscal steroid therapy for lumbar spinal discogenic pain: a randomized controlled trial. *Spine* 29:833-836, 2004.

177. Buric J, Molino Lova R: Ozone chemonucleolysis in non-contained lumbar disc herniations: a pilot study with 12 months follow-up. *Acta Neurochir Suppl* 92:93-97, 2005.

178. Miller MR, Mathews RS, Reeves KD: Treatment of painful advanced internal lumbar disc derangement with intradiscal injection of hypertonic dextrose. *Pain Physician* 9:115-121, 2006.

179. Cohen SP, Wenzell D, Hurley RW, et al: A double-blind, placebo-controlled, dose-response pilot study evaluating intradiscal etanercept in patients with chronic discogenic low back pain or lumbosacral radiculopathy. *Anesthesiology* 107:99-105, 2007.

180. Peng B, Zhang Y, Hou S, et al: Intradiscal methylene blue injection for the treatment of chronic discogenic low back pain. *Eur Spine J* 16:33-38, 2007.

181. Teixeira A, Sluijter ME: Intradiscal high-voltage, long-duration pulsed radiofrequency for discogenic pain: a preliminary report. *Pain Med* 7(5):424-428, 2006.

182. Van Kleef M, Barendse GAM, Wilmink JT: Percutaneous intradiscal radiofrequency thermocoagulation in chronic non-specific low back pain. *Pain Clin* 9:259-268, 1996.

183. Saal JS, Saal JA: Intradiscal electrothermal annuloplasty (IDET) for chronic disc disease: outcome assessment with minimum one year follow-up. *Proceedings of the 14th Annual Meeting of the North American Spine Society*, 1999, pp 75-76.

184. Saal JA, Saal JS: Intradiscal electrothermal annuloplasty (IDET) for chronic multi-level discogenic pain: prospective one year follow-up outcome study. *Proceedings of the 14th Annual Meeting of the North American Spine Society*, 1999, pp 78-79.

185. Saal JA, Saal JS: Intradiscal electrothermal treatment for chronic discogenic low back pain. A prospective outcome study with minimum 1-year follow-up. *Spine* 25:2622-2627, 2000.

186. Derby R, Eek B, Chen Y, et al: Intradiscal electrothermal annuloplasty(IDET): a novel approach for treating chronic discogenic back pain. *Neuromodulation* 3:82-88, 2000.

187. Singh V: Intradiscal electrothermal therapy: a preliminary report. *Pain Physician* 3:367-373, 2000.

188. Kapural L, Mekhail N, Korunda Z, et al: Intradiscal thermal annuloplasty for the treatment of lumbar discogenic pain in patients with multilevel degenerative disc disease. *Anesth Analg* 99:472-476, 2004.

189. Assietti R, Morosi M, Block JE: Intradiscal electrothermal therapy for symptomatic internal disc disruption: 24-month results and predictors of clinical success. *J Neurosurg Spine* 12(3):320-326, 2010.

190. Andersson GB, Mekhail NA, Block JE: Treatment of intractable discogenic low back pain. A systematic review of spinal fusion and intradiscal electrothermal therapy (IDET). *Pain Physician* 9:237-248, 2006.

191. Kapural L, Hayek S, Malak O, et al: Intradiscal thermal annuloplasty versus intradiscal radiofrequency ablation for the treatment of discogenic pain: a prospective matched control trial. *Pain Med* 6:425-431, 2005.

192. Pauza KJ, Howell S, Dreyfuss P, et al: A randomized, placebo-controlled trial of intradiscal electrothermal therapy for the treatment of discogenic low back pain. *Spine J* 4:27-35, 2004.

193. Freeman BJ, Fraser RD, Cain CM, et al: A randomized, double-blind, controlled trial: intradiscal electrothermal therapy versus placebo for the treatment of chronic discogenic low back pain. *Spine* 30:2369-2377, 2005.

194. Appleby D, Anderson G, Totta M: Meta-analysis of the efficacy and safety of intradiscal electrothermal therapy (IDET). *Pain Med* 7:308-316, 2006.

195. Kvarstein G, Måwe L, Indahl A, et al: A randomized double-blind controlled trial of intra-annular radiofrequency thermal disc therapy—a 12-month follow-up. *Pain* 145:279-286, 2009.

196. Kapural L, Ng A, Dalton J, et al: Intervertebral disc biacuplasty for the treatment of lumbar discogenic pain: results of a six-month follow-up. *Pain Med* 9(1):60-67, 2008.

197. Kapural L: Letter to the editor: intervertebral disk cooled bipolar radiofrequency (intradiskal biacuplasty) for the treatment of lumbar diskogenic pain: 12 month follow up of the pilot study. *Pain Med* 9:407-408, 2008.

198. Kapural L, Cata JP, Narouze S: Successful treatment of lumbar discogenic pain using intradiscal biacuplasty in previously discectomized disc. *Pain Pract* 9(2):130-134, 2009.

199. Kapural L, Sakic K, Boutwell K: Intradiscal biaculoplasty (IDB) for the treatment of thoracic discogenic pain. *Clin J Pain* 26(4):354-357, 2010.

200. Alò KM, Wright RE, Sutcliff J, et al: Percutaneous lumbar discectomy: clinical response in an initial cohort of fifty consecutive patients with chronic radicular pain. *Pain Pract* 4(1):19-29, 2004.

201. Chen YC, Lee SH, Chen D: Intradiscal pressure study of percutaneous disc decompression with nucleoplasty in human cadavers. *Spine* 28:661-665, 2003.

202. Sharps LS, Isaac Z: Percutaneous disc decompression using nucleoplasty. *Pain Physician* 5:121-126, 2002.

203. Singh V, Piryani C, Liao K, et al: Percutaneous disc decompression using coblation (nucleoplasty) in the treatment of chronic discogenic pain. *Pain Physician* 5:250-259, 2002.

204. Gerszten PC, Welch WC, King JT, Jr: Quality of life assessment in patients undergoing nucleoplasty-based percutaneous discectomy. *J Neurosurg Spine* 4:36-42, 2006.

205. Masala S, Massari F, Fabiano S, et al: Nucleoplasty in the treatment of lumbar diskogenic back pain: one year follow-up. *Cardiovasc Intervent Radiol* 30:426-432, 2007.

206. Mirzai H, Tekin I, Yaman O, et al: The results of nucleoplasty in patients with lumbar herniated disc: a prospective clinical study of 52 consecutive patients. *Spine J* 7:88-92, 2007.

207. Yakovlev A, Tamimi MA, Liang H, et al: Outcomes of percutaneous disc decompression utilizing nucleoplasty for the treatment of chronic discogenic pain. *Pain Physician* 10:319-328, 2007.

208. Gertszten P, Smuck M, Rathmell JP, et al: Plasma disc decompression compared with fluoroscopy-guided transforaminal epidural steroid injections for symptomatic contained lumbar disc herniation: a prospective, randomized, controlled trial. *J Neurosurg Spine* 12(4):357-371, 2010.

209. Gerges FJ, Lipsitz SR, Nedeljkovic SS: A systematic review on the effectiveness of the Nucleoplasty procedure for discogenic pain. *Pain Physician* 13(2):117-132, 2010.

210. Nardi PV: Percutaneous cervical nucleoplasty using coblation technology. Clinical results in fifty consecutive cases. *Acta Neurochir Suppl* 92:73-78, 2005.

211. Cesaroni A, Nardi PV: Plasma disc decompression for contained cervical disc herniation: a randomized, controlled trial. *Eur Spine J* 19(3):477-486, 2010.

212. Mathis JM, Maroney M, Fenton DC, et al: Evaluation of bone cements for use in percutaneous vertebroplasty (abstract). In Proceeding of the 13th Annual Meeting of the North American Spine Society, San Francisco, CA, October 28-31, 1998, Rosemont, IL, North American Spine Society, 1998, pp 210-211.

213. DiMaio FR: The science of bone cement: a historical review. *Orthopedics* 25(12):1399-1407, 2002.

214. Acrylic plastic: how products are made, accessed from http://www.enotes.com/how-products-encyclopedia/acrylic-plastic.080515enotes.com.

215. Basak SK: Birth centenary of Sir Harold Ridley (10th July1906-25th May 2001). *Indian J Ophthalmol* 54:219-220, 2006.

216. Panjabi MM, Goel VK, Clark CR, et al: Biomechanical study of cervical spine stabilization with methylmethacrylate. *Spine* 10:198-203, 1985.

217. King GJ, Kostuik JP, McBroom RJ, Richardson W: Surgical management of metastatic renal carcinoma of the spine. *Spine* 16:265-271, 1991.

218. McAfee PC, Zdeblick TA: Tumors of the thoracic and lumbar spine: surgical treatment via the anterior approach. *J Spinal Disorders* 2:145-154, 1989.

219. Kostuik JP, Errico TJ, Gleason TF: Techniques of internal fixation for degenerative conditions of the lumbar spine. *Clin Orthop* 203:203-231, 1986.

220. Deramond H, Depriester C, Galibert P, Le Gars D: Percutaneous vertebroplasty with polymethylmethacrylate: technique, indications, and results. *Radiol Clin North Am* 36:533-546, 1998.

221. Bascoulergue Y, Duquesnel J, Leclercq R, et al: Percutaneous injection of methy methacrylate in the vertebral body for the treatment of various diseases: percutaneous vertebroplasty [abstract]. *Radiology* 169P:372, 1988.

222. Jensen ME, Evans AJ, Mathis JM, et al: Percutaneous polymethylmethacrylate vertebroplasty in the treatment of vertebral body compression fractures: technical aspects. *Am J Neuroradiol* 18:1877-1904, 1997.

223. Lewiecki M: Augmentation procedures for osteoporotic vertebral fractures—an ongoing experiment or emerging standard of care. *Southern Med J* 99:449-450, 2006.

224. San Millan Ruiz D, Burkhardt K, Jean B, et al: Pathology findings with acrylic implants. *Bone* 25(2 suppl):85S-90S, 1999.

225. Jefferiss CD, Lee AFC, Ling RSM: Thermal aspects of self-curing polymethylmethacrylate. *J Bone Joint Surg* 57B(4):511-518, 1975.

226. Togawa D, Kovacic J, Bauer TW, et al: Radiographic and histologic findings of vertebral augmentation using polymethylmethacrylate in the primate spine: percutaneous vertebroplasty versus kyphoplasty [abstract]. *Spine* 31:E4-E10, 2006.

227. Cotton A, Dewatre F, Cortet B, et al: Percutaneous vertebroplasty for osteolytic metastasis and myeloma: effects of the percentage of lesion filling and the leakage of methyl methacrylate at clinical follow-up. *Radiology* 200:525-530, 1996.

228. Jenson ME, Dion JE: Percutaneous vertebroplasty in osteoporotic compression fractures. *Neuroimaging Clin North Am* 10:547-568, 2000.

229. Murphy KJ, Deramond H. Percutaneous vertebroplasty in benign and malignant disease. *Neuroimaging Clin N Am* 10:535-545, 2000.

230. Grados F, Depriester C, Cayrolle G, et al: Long-term observations of vertebral osteoporosis fractures treated by percutaneous vertebroplasty. *Rheumatology (Oxford)* 39:1410-1414, 2000.

231. Ananthakrishnan D, Berven S, Deviren V, et al: The effect on anterior column loading due to different vertebral augmentation techniques. *Clin Biomech* 20:25-31, 2005.

232. Garfin SR, Yan HA, Reiley MA: New technologies in spine: kyphoplasty and vertebroplasty for the treatment of painful osteoporotic compression fractures. *Spine* 26:1511-1515, 2001.

233. Jensen ME, McGraw JK, Cardella JF, et al: Position statement on percutaneous vertebral augmentation: a consensus statement developed by the American Society of Interventional and Therapeutic Neuroradiology, Society of Interventional Radiology, American Association of Neurological Surgeons/Congress of Neurological Surgeons, and American Society of Spine Radiology. *J Neuro Intervent Surg* 1:181-185, 2009.

CHAPTER

2 Therapeutic Agents for Spine Injection: Local Anesthetics, Steroids, and Contrast Media

Matthew J. Pingree and Marc A. Huntoon

CHAPTER OVERVIEW

Chapter Synopsis: Spinal and epidural injections may be performed for therapeutic, diagnostic, and imaging purposes. This chapter explores the evolution of these techniques and the injectable agents in particular. Historically, the local anesthetic procaine was the most commonly injected drug followed by a wave of corticosteroid injection that began in the 1960s in Europe. Fluoroscopic guidance with injected dyes followed. Among local anesthetics, amide-type drugs have become the preferred class, which includes lidocaine and bupivacaine. Metabolism of the ester-type anesthetics (including procaine) produces para-aminobenzoic acid as a byproduct and presents greater risk of adverse allergic reaction. Local anesthetic systemic toxicity presents a separate serious complication risk. Glucocorticoids are useful in the control of pain because of their inhibitory action on inflammatory agents. Complication risks include Cushing's syndrome—a suppression of the hypothalamic–pituitary–adrenal axis—and infarct from particulate steroids. Other more specific blockers of cytokines and other inflammatory mediators have also been investigated for epidural injection. Contrast media injected to aid in fluoroscopic imaging typically contain iodine. Adverse events are for the most part mild and easily treated. Anxiety can play a significant role in adverse reactions from injection of any substance.

Important Points:
- Local anesthetics are rarely associated with immediate hypersensitivity (allergic) reactions, and the amide-type local anesthetics are particularly safe.
- Local anesthetic systemic toxicity is an emergency that requires additional help and may be ameliorated with lipid emulsion therapy.
- Corticosteroid agents for spinal injection have significant dose-related complications with repetitive use. Users should be aware that multiple practitioners may be using these agents, with no consistent dosing guidelines.
- Particulate steroids have been associated with catastrophic spinal cord and brainstem infarcts, presumably from embolization into critical arteries, and caution suggests that nonparticulate agents may be more appropriate in specific procedures (e.g., cervical transforaminal epidurals).
- Patients with iodine or shellfish allergies are not at greater risk for adverse reactions to contrast agents.
- In cases of previous reaction to iodinated contrast, gadolinium is an acceptable alternative with extremely low incidence of adverse reactions.
- Patients with previous anaphylactoid reactions, those with asthma, and certain food allergies may benefit from pretreatment with histamine receptor 1 and 2 antagonists and systemic steroids.

Clinical Pearls:
- In patients who have had prior anaphylaxis due to contrast dyes, one might consider not injecting contrast agent if it is not critical to the outcome.
- Because local anesthetic injection does not contribute to the long-term therapeutic outcome in most spinal injections, and may cause toxicity or fall risk, its use should be limited.
- Doses of corticosteroid are not standardized, and thus dose selection should always be the lowest possible to achieve a therapeutic effect.

Clinical Pitfalls:
- Practitioners need not ask about shellfish allergies, as the information has little clinical significance when choosing contrast agents.
- Particulate corticosteroids should be avoided for most anterior and lateral cervical injections.

Introduction

Therapeutic spinal injections date back to the early part of the twentieth century before World War II. Over the past several decades, corticosteroids have emerged as the preferred class of spinally administered drugs for presumed inflammatory causes of pain. Common usage has been based largely on case series demonstrating efficacy and select double-blind placebo controlled trials (see Chapter 1). Surface landmark–based technique has also changed over time, with most authors currently endorsing very specific fluoroscopically controlled and contrast-proven injections. Despite these proscriptions, there have been no large-scale head-to-head trials that demonstrate outcome-based superiority of the more technologically advanced techniques. This chapter focuses on the agents that are commonly being used to perform therapeutic epidural and spinal injections, as well as the appropriate and safe use of contrast media (e.g., iohexol or gadodiamide agents) and some of the experimental agents being considered for future use.

History

One of the first reports of spinal injections for pain control was trans-sacral (caudal) injections of the local anesthetic procaine.[1] The first use of epidural corticosteroids came out of the European literature.[2] One of the first large series was published in 1961, in which Goebert and colleagues[3] administered 121 injections to 113 patients spanning a 5-year period. The majority of these injections were caudal epidural injections with only three cervical epidural injections. Large-volume injections of a mixture of 1% procaine with 125 mg of hydrocortisone acetate in 30-mL volumes were administered over a consecutive 3-day period.[3] Subsequently, in the modern era after the 1970s, interlaminar epidural injections became standard. Winnie and colleagues[4] published recommendations that are still popular today, including corticosteroid dose limitations, 2-week dosing intervals, and three epidural procedures in series. Later, many physicians adopted a transforaminal fluoroscopically guided approach.

Local Anesthetics

Local anesthetics block voltage-gated sodium channels and interrupt propagation of axonal impulses, but their action is not only limited to those biological actions. There are two classes of local anesthetics based on structure–activity relationships: amino esters and amino amides. Because of the popularity and much more common use of amide-type local anesthetics for spinal diagnostic and therapeutic procedures, the focus of this review is mainly on the amide-type local anesthetics lidocaine and bupivacaine.[5,6]

Important properties of local anesthetics that pertain to clinical use include potency, speed of onset, and duration of action. The potency of a local anesthetic is related to its lipid solubility, which is usually defined by the octanol-buffer coefficient. The molecule must diffuse into the nerve membrane and bind at a partially hydrophobic site on the sodium channel.[7] The more hydrophobic or lipophilic the local anesthetic, the more quickly it will permeate neuronal membranes, which increases its sodium channel binding affinity. Bupivacaine, for example, is many times more lipophilic than lidocaine (**Table 2-1**).

The speed of onset of most local anesthetics directly relates to the dissociation constant, or pKa, of the compound as well as the pH of the local tissues. The pKa is the pH at which half of the compound is ionized or protonated; the other half is in the un-ionized or neutral form that more readily crosses the nerve membrane. This makes the local anesthetic with the pKa that is closest to physiological pKa of faster onset. The pH of the local anesthetic preparation also affects the onset time, and some commercially available preparations containing a vasoconstrictor (e.g., epinephrine) have an adjusted pH that is acidic because of the addition of hydrochloric salts, enhancing the stability of the vasoconstrictor (**Table 2-2**).[8,9] In vivo, other factors such as dose or concentration can also affect the onset of action.[7] If faster onset is desired, then the addition of a small amount of sodium bicarbonate (1:20 $NaHCO_3$-to-anesthetic volume) can help adjust the pH closer to physiological conditions. Caution should be taken not to adjust the pH greater than 7 because of the possibility that drug precipitation will increase.

Defining the duration of action is somewhat more difficult because it depends on multiple variables such as the location of injection, the lipophilicity of the local anesthetic, the dose, and the presence or absence of a vasoconstrictor. Longer acting local anesthetics are more lipophilic and are more slowly "washed out" from the lipophilic membrane.[10] In humans, the peripheral vascular effects of the local anesthetics themselves also affect duration. Many agents have a biphasic effect on vascular smooth muscle with a vasoconstrictive response at low concentrations and vasodilatation at higher concentrations. These effects are complex and vary according to the concentration, time, and location of injection.[7] In

Table 2-1: Effects of pKa and Hydrophobicity on Local Anesthetic Action

Drug	Relative Conduction Blocking Potency	pKa*	Hydrophobicity*
Bupivacaine	8	8.1	3420
Lidocaine	2	7.8	366

*pKa and hydrophobicity at 36° C hydrophobicity equals the octanol-buffer partition coefficient of the base. Values are ratios of concentrations. From Strichartz GR, Sanchez V, Arthur GR, et al: Fundamental properties of local anesthetics. II. Measured octanol: buffer partition coefficients and pKa values of clinically used drugs, *Anesth Analg* 71:158-170, 1990.

Table 2-2: Pharmacology of Selected Amide Local Anesthetics

Agent	Available Concentrations (%)	Onset	Duration (hr)	pKa (25° C)	pH of Plain Sol.	Max Single Dose without Epinephrine
Bupivacaine	0.25, 0.5, 0.75	Slow	2-4	8.1	4.5-6.0	175
Lidocaine	0.5, 1, 1.5, 2, 5	Fast	1-2	7.8	6.5	300

From Covino BG, Wildsmith JAW: Clinical pharmacology of local anesthetic agents. In Cousins MJ, Bridenbaugh PO, editors: *Neural blockade in clinical anesthesia and management of pain*, ed 3, Philadelphia, 1998, Lippincott-Raven, pp 97-128.

general, the more vascular the location, the more rapidly the agent is absorbed, metabolized, and excreted.

Metabolism of local anesthetics, not surprisingly, is dependent on its amide or ester structure. Ester type agents undergo rapid metabolism via plasma pseudocholinesterase, of which para-aminobenzoic acid (PABA) is a by-product. The ester type local anesthetics include procaine and benzocaine, which are two of the more commonly used agents. Conversely, amide-type agents such as lidocaine and bupivacaine are metabolized through the hepatic cytochrome P450 enzyme system as well as via conjugation. The byproduct of the ester-type metabolism, PABA, is thought to be an allergen involved in many local anesthetic allergic reactions. Moreover, given the dependence on the liver for the metabolism of amide-type local anesthetics, caution should be exercised when using these agents in patients with liver dysfunction.

Adverse Reactions

Reactions involving the use of local anesthetics can result from a number of different sources, including toxicity from the medication itself, a reaction to a preservative or added vasoconstrictor, or even an allergic reaction. Outside of the discussion of PABA as a potential allergen, immediate hypersensitivity reactions to amide local anesthetics and their pathomechanism remain largely unidentified. Clinically, the allergic response corresponds with anaphylaxis (manifesting as tachycardia; hypotension; and feelings of weakness, heat, or vertigo) even though immunologically mediated reactions have rarely been observed. Other ingredients in the local anesthetic commercial preparations such as certain preservatives or even anxiety need to be considered as potential sources of the adverse reaction as well.[11]

Toxicity, especially systemic toxicity, is usually the result of inadvertent intravascular injection, overdosage, or increased uptake from the area of injection. Systemic toxicity is a significant source of morbidity and mortality in the practice of anesthesia and especially the subspecialty regional anesthesia. Recently, the American Society of Regional Anesthesia and Pain Medicine published a practice advisory dealing with local anesthetic systemic toxicity (LAST). LAST was first recognized in the 1880s with the introduction of cocaine into clinical practice. Today, there is a focus on the development of less cardiotoxic local anesthetics based on structural changes or chirality (e.g., ropivacaine or levobupivacaine) as well as new and improved treatment for the cardiovascular effects of LAST with lipid emulsion therapy.

Epidemiological studies report a range of incidence of LAST that varies from 0 to 79 per 10,000.[12-14] In general, the cardiac toxicity results from the binding and inhibition of sodium channels, however, and correlates with local anesthetic potency especially in regards to inhibition of cardiac conduction. In addition, there is a vast array of other inotropic and metabolic signaling systems as well as mitochondrial metabolism implicated as potential targets for local anesthetics that would help explain the local anesthetic agents variable role in LAST.[15]

One way to reduce the incidence of LAST is to prevent it. Unfortunately, there is no single intervention that has proven to prevent this potentially life-threatening response. Obviously, using the least amount of local anesthetic required, incremental injection, frequent aspiration looking for the return of blood, using an intravascular marker such as epinephrine, and the use of ultrasound guidance are all recommended to try to prevent LAST.[15]

Classically, LAST presents in a predictable sequence with subjective central nervous system (CNS) symptoms of auditory changes, circumoral numbness, and metallic taste. Signs can then progress to seizures, coma, respiratory arrest, and ultimately cardiac

toxicity that include cardiac excitation followed by cardiac depression at greatly increased blood concentrations. Unfortunately, in reality, the presentation can be extremely variable and is atypical in about 40% of cases with LAST. Even with an atypical presentation, the first symptoms presented in less than 5 minutes after injection 75% of the time. Seizure was the most common presenting symptom, and fewer than 20% of these seizures presented without any of the classic prodromal symptoms.[15]

Treatment of LAST, given the possible serious morbidity, should be quick and aggressive. Priorities include obtaining an airway, circulatory support, and diminishing the systemic effects as much as possible. Seizures should be rapidly treated with benzodiazepines if possible. Initiating the clinical algorithm as part of advanced cardiac life support (ACLS) is also important, although LAST presents a very different clinical scenario than that usually addressed by ACLS. The cause of circulatory arrest in LAST means that vasopressin and epinephrine may have less of a role or not be recommended. In fact, animal studies indicate that lipid emulsion treatment had better outcomes than both epinephrine and vasopressin.[15,16] (Please refer to the Practice Advisory sheets included in **Table 2-3**.)

Corticosteroids

Cortisone as a purified glucocorticoid preparation was first introduced in 1949; later, in 1952, its application was described for epidural use.[17-19] Since then, the use of steroids has been applied in the field of interventional pain management with varying degrees of success and complications.

Table 2-3: Practice Advisory on Treatment of Local Anesthetic Systemic Toxicity for Patients Experiencing Signs or Symptoms of Local Anesthetic Systemic Toxicity
• Get help
• Initial focus
• **Airway management:** ventilate with 100% oxygen
• **Seizure suppression:** benzodiazepines are preferred
• **Basic and advanced cardiac life support (BLS/ACLS)** may require prolonged effect
• Infuse 20% lipid emulsion (values in parenthesis are for a 70-kg patient)
• **Bolus 1.5 mL/kg** (lean body mass) IV over 1 min (~100 mL)
• **Continuous infusion at 1.25 mL/kg/min** (≈18 mL/min; adjust by roller clamp)
• Repeat bolus once or twice for persistent cardiovascular collapse
• Double the infusion rate to 0.5 mL/kg/min if blood pressure remains low
• **Continue infusion** for at least 10 min after attaining circulatory stability
• Recommended upper limit: ≈10 mL/kg lipid emulsion over the first 30 min
• **Avoid** vasopressin, calcium channel blockers, β-blockers, and local anesthetics
• **Alert** the nearest facility with cardiopulmonary bypass capability
• **Avoid propofol** in patients with signs of cardiovascular instability
• **Post the LAST event** at www.lipidrescue.org and report use of lipid to www.lipidregistry.org

Neal JM, Bernards CM, Butterworth JF IV, et al: ASRA practice advisory on local anesthetic systemic toxicity. *Reg Anesth Pain Med* 35:152-161, 2010.

IV, intravenous; LAST, local anesthetic systemic toxicity.

Glucocorticoids, of which the injectable corticosteroids are a part, are produced in the zona fasciculate of the adrenal cortex and function under negative feedback from the hypothalamus and pituitary gland as part of the hypothalamus–pituitary–adrenal axis.[20] Glucocorticoids are used in interventional pain procedures because of their effects on inflammation. Glucocorticoids have significant inhibitory effects on cytokines and chemokines that are generated at sites of inflammation, as well as suppressive effects on leukocyte concentration, distribution, and function. Glucocorticoids have potential effects on most cells of the body through interactions with glucocorticoid receptors. Normally, intracellular glucocorticoid receptors are in a stabilized form coupled with two elements of heat-shock protein 90 (HSP90) and other proteins. Binding of glucocorticoid to its receptor allows the glucocorticoid to enter the cell where dissociation of the proteins occurs, and the glucocorticoid–receptor complex binds to the glucocorticoid response element of a target gene. Resultant transcription activity via RNA polymerase is thus altered, eventually leading to alterations in messenger RNA (mRNA) and new protein production, which leads to the hormonal response.[21]

Table 2-4 lists the antiinflammatory potency of some of the more commonly used neuraxial steroids.

Complications

Multiple complications of corticosteroids are possible and largely relate to unwanted side effects (e.g., iatrogenic Cushing's syndrome). Tuel and colleagues[22] described a case of iatrogenic Cushing's syndrome occurring in a 24-year-old man after a single dose of 60 mg of methylprednisolone. Laboratory evidence of suppression of the hypothalamic–pituitary axis, 20-lb weight gain, and cushingoid features (moon facies, stria) persisted for 12 months. In another report, two doses of 80 mg of methylprednisolone resulted in Cushing's syndrome with peripheral edema, moon facies, a "buffalo hump," and purpura in a 63-year-old woman.[23] These cases illustrate that doses that are well within the normal guidelines for epidural steroid injections may still result in adverse consequences.

Perhaps the most dreaded recent complications have been attributed to particulate steroids. A large survey of members of the American Pain Society[24] identified 78 cases of either spinal cord or brainstem infarcts that were known of by those members that responded to the survey. Of these, 14 were fatal cases, and all involved particulate steroids. Tiso et al[25] and Benzon, et al[26] both studied the microscopic appearances of commonly used steroids. Although discrepancies exist between the two studies, they are useful to any discussion of the potential pathophysiology of injury. One notable difference is that dexamethasone was found to be nonparticulate in the study by Benzon et al[26] (**Fig. 2-1**). A subsequent animal study demonstrated that dexamethasone acted like a nonparticulate in that direct, intentional injection of the vertebral artery in a porcine model resulted in ischemic brain injury only in the animals receiving particulate steroids.[27]

Although particulate size and aggregation have received much attention, other arguments exist regarding the etiology of steroid toxicity to the nervous system. One source of potential toxicity is the multiple chemical entities used in the formulation of epidural

Table 2-4: Antiinflammatory Potency of Commonly Used Neuraxial Steroids			
Drug	**Equivalent Dose (mg)**	**Epidural Dose (mg)**	**Antiinflammatory Potency**
Hydrocortisone	20	NA	1
Depo-methylprednisolone (Depo-Medrol)	4	40-80	5
Triamcinolone acetonide (Kenalog)	4	40-80	5
Betamethasone (Celestone Soluspan)	0.6	6-12	33
Dexamethasone (Decadron)	0.75 mg	8-16	27

From Manichikanti L: Pharmacology of neuraxial steroids. In Manchikanti L, Singh V, editors: *Interventional techniques in chronic spinal pain.* ASIPP Publishing: Paducah, KY, pp 167-184, 2007.
NA, not applicable.

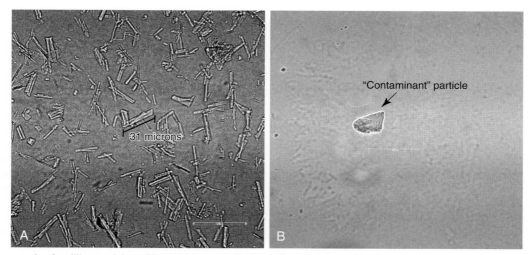

Fig. 2-1   A, Micrograph of rodlike particles of betamethasone. **B,** A small contaminant in otherwise clear dexamethasone solution. (From Sen S, Mantilla C, Mayo Clinic Department of Anesthesiology.)

Table 2-5: Chemical Entities Used in the Formulation of Epidural Steroids

| | Depo-Medrol | | Kenalog | Celestone | Decadron | Nonparticulate Celestone |
	Methylprednisolone		Triamcinolone Acetonide	Betamethasone, Preservative Free	Dexamethasone Sodium Phosphate	Betamethasone Sodium Phosphate
Amount of steroid (mg/mL)	40	80	40	6	4	6
Polyethylene glycol 3350	29.1	28.2	—	—	—	—
Polysorbate 80	1.94	1.88	0.4	—	—	—
Monobasic sodium phosphate	6.8	6.59	—	3.4	—	3.0
Benzyl alcohol	9.16	8.8	9	—	—	—
Dibasic sodium phosphate	—	—	—	7.1	—	6.0
Edentate disodium	—	—	—	0.1	—	—
Benzalkonium chloride	—	—	—	0.2	—	—
Sodium sulfite	—	—	—	—	1 mg	—

From Manichikanti L: Pharmacology of neuraxial steroids. In Manchikanti L, Singh V, editors: *Interventional techniques in chronic spinal pain*. ASIPP Publishing: Paducah, KY, pp 167-184, 2007.

steroids, including benzyl alcohol, polyethylene glycol, and so on (**Table 2-5**). The ingredient with the most controversy is benzyl alcohol, which is used in Depo-Medrol, Aristocort, and Kenalog.[20] Benzyl alcohol has been implicated in one case of flaccid paralysis of 16 months' duration.[28] Multiple other studies in different models on different steroids have been performed with variable results. Bogduk and Cherry,[29] however, concluded that none of the literature provides direct evidence of the steroid itself or their preservatives causing neurotoxicity in the lumbar region.

Other side effects from the use of neuraxial steroids may be delayed for months or even years.[30] The list of possible side effects not discussed above includes adrenal suppression, osteoporosis, avascular necrosis of the bone, fluid retention, adverse gastrointestinal effects, muscular effects, subcapsular cataracts, vision loss, dural puncture, and others. In-depth review of each of these is beyond the scope of this chapter, but essentially, all of these side effects can best be mitigated by minimizing the dose of steroids, using alternative therapies when able, and carefully monitoring the total dosage. Unfortunately, there is no consensus among pain practitioners regarding type, dosage, frequency, or total number of injections; however, a limitation of 3 mg/kg of body weight or 210 mg/year in the average patient with a total lifetime exposure of 420 mg of steroid has been advocated without any supporting scientific data.[20]

For many years, it was assumed that glia were simply structural supports for the varied neuronal cells in the CNS. In the past decade, it has become increasingly evident that glia are intricately involved in the development of persistent pain states and that glial expression of cytokines and other neurotransmitter substances play key roles. Sciatic constriction injury models in animals have provided significant clues as to the time course of glial activation. There are two main types of glial cells: microglia and macroglia (oligodendrocytes and astrocytes). Resting microglia become activated in the presence of injury and are drawn to the local source of adenosine triphosphate (**Fig. 2-2**). After being activated, microglia can produce various cytokines, neurotransmitters, and neurotrophins. Astrocytes become activated about 4 to 7 days after injury and are suspected to be involved in development of persistent pain (**Fig. 2-3**).[31] Cytokines include tumor necrosis

factor α, interleukin-1β (IL-1β), interleukin-6 (IL-6), and many others. Several cytokine antagonists exist, which include corticosteroids, disease-modifying anti-rheumatic drugs (DMARDs), and clonidine.

Initial studies of systemic infliximab and etanercept seemed to be promising, but randomized trials did not demonstrate a difference in the treatment of sciatica.[32-34]

Based on the failed randomized trial of infliximab, Cohen and colleagues[35] suggested that precise local delivery to the area of nerve involvement might be necessary. In the first trial of perineural etanercept in humans, etanercept was injected via the transforaminal epidural route to three groups each of six patients with increasing doses of 2, 4, and 6 mg, respectively, and compared with a sham saline injection group in a 3:1 ratio. Because previous safety testing was incomplete, concurrent histological studies were performed in beagle dogs to evaluate for any functional deficits. Cohen and colleagues[35] found etanercept to be effective compared with saline for several months in their study, and there were no histological trends or magnetic resonance imaging changes in human subjects that warranted study termination.

Etanercept has immune modulation properties that carry some risks. These risks include anaphylaxis, immune deficiency, sepsis, tuberculosis (reactivation or novel infection), and rarely lymphoma. A black box warning was submitted in May 2008 by the U.S. Food and Drug Administration to warn of these occurrences.[36] Etanercept is an interesting therapy that seems to have some promise, but it should undergo further study before clinical use, due to potentially infectious outcomes. Another anticytokine drug with established safety profiles could emerge, however.

Clonidine is another drug that may have some promise for the treatment of sciatica.[37] Clonidine has recently been studied in a randomized, controlled, double-blind study comparing it with the active control triamcinolone. Both drugs were equally effective in decreasing pain over the 6-week period of study, but functional improvement was more apparent with triamcinolone. It is possible that clonidine's short duration of action might require longer exposure of drug at the dorsal root ganglion. Clonidine is an antagonist of IL-1β and other cytokines but for only a few days (**Fig. 2-4**).

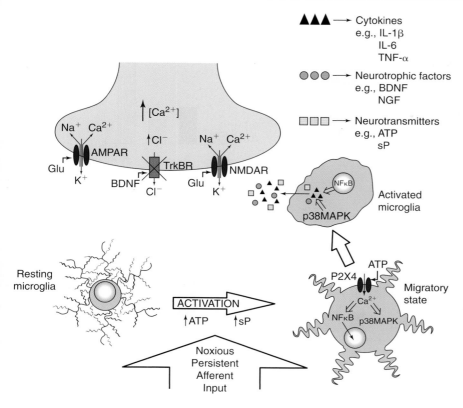

Fig. 2-2 Glial activation occurs in the presence of noxious afferent stimulation. Activated microglia migrate to sources of adenosine triphosphate, activate purinergic receptors (P2X4), and induce calcium influx, which causes translocation of nuclear factor κB into the nucleus and activates p38 MAP kinase. These activated microglia move to the dorsal root ganglion and other areas and induce production of cytokines, neurotransmitters, and neurotrophins. (Modified from Vallejo R, Tilley DM, Vogel L, Benyamin R: The role of glia and the immune system in the development and maintenance of neuropathic pain, *Pain Pract* 10:167-184, 2010.)

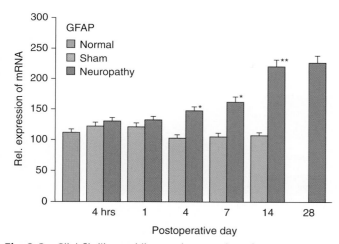

Fig. 2-3 Glial fibrillary acidic protein, a marker of astrocyte activation and the time course of messenger RNA expression, is depicted in a rat model. Astrocyte activation becomes significant after 4 to 7 days and remains elevated for 28 days. This suggests that early microglial activation-initiated pain sensitization is replaced by astrocyte maintenance of chronic pain sensitization. (Modified from Tanga FY, Raghavendra V, DeLeo JA: Quantitative real-time RT-PCR assessment of spinal microglial and astrocytic activation markers in a rat model of neuropathic pain. *Neurochem Int* 45:397-407, 2004.)

Contrast Agents

The radiopaque nature of contrast media is one method to assist in confirming correct needle position. This in turn can improve the safety of the procedure. There continues to be an emerging number of case reports describing catastrophic injuries from presumed injection of medication in the intravascular, subdural, or even intrathecal (IT) space.[24] By using a radiopaque contrast media before injection of local anesthetic or steroid, the risk of any procedure should be reduced.[38] Because needle misplacement is a common complication associated with percutaneous spinal injections, utilization of a safe contrast medium is essential.[39]

Iodine is an element commonly used in contrast medium, and iodine-based contrast agents have proven to be satisfactory for visualization, yet provide no therapeutic effect. The iodine atom in contrast media provides its radiopaque aspect because iodine atoms provide more attenuation than the tissue surrounding them. The level of attenuation is known as the *attenuation coefficient* for that tissue.[10] First-generation contrast agents loosely bound the iodine molecules, resulting in a highly osmolar compound that increased its toxicity. For this reason, they are referred to as *high-osmolality contrast media* (HOCM). Second-generation agents, referred to as *nonionic* or *low-osmolality contrast media* (LOCM), tightly bind the iodine atoms to a benzene ring but still provide the needed ratio of iodine to non-iodine particles that leads to an appropriate attenuation profile while maintaining an almost physiological osmolality.

Pharmacology

The different types of iodine-based contrast media can be placed into four different varieties, which are ionic monomers, nonionic monomers, ionic dimers, and nonionic dimers. All types are readily redistributed upon injection and rapidly excreted through the kidneys (90% within 12 hours of administration). These agents come in a range of concentrations that correlate with their radiopacity. The more concentrated the solution, the more iodine and the more radiopaque.[38] Osmolality plays an important role in the safety of contrast media. Osmolality is the number of particles of solute in a solution and is highest in ionic contrast agents by way of a tri-iodinated benzoate anion. The hyperosmolality of some "ionic" agents directly relates to toxicity in the form of hemodynamic effects and patient discomfort.[10] The nonionic agents

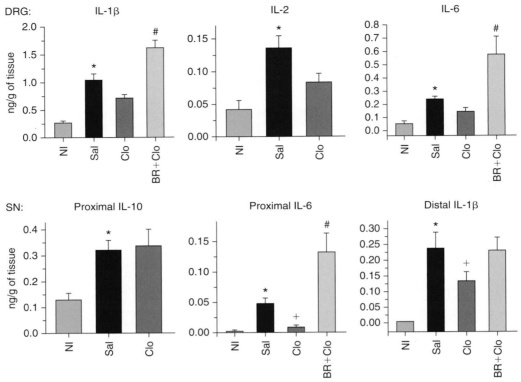

Fig. 2-4 Effects of clonidine for the treatment of sciatica.
Upper panel: Cytokine release is increased in sciatic nerve—injured animals at the nerve level (SN) or dorsal root ganglion (DRG) compared to normal animals (NI). Saline treatment is compared to clonidine or BRL 44408, a specific antagonist of alpha-2A receptor.
Lower panel: Clonidine has no effect on IL-10, a "good" cytokine that has antiinflammatory effects, while it decreases expression of both IL-1β and IL-6. (Modified from Romero-Sandoval A, Eisenach JC: Perineural clonidine reduces mechanical hypersensitivity and cytokine production in established nerve injury, *Anesthesiology* 104:351-355, 2006.)

contain iodine atoms tightly attached to a benzene ring, making the osmolality closer to physiological conditions, while at the same time preserving a high attenuation coefficient because of the amount of iodine atoms. The majority of pain clinicians now almost exclusively use the non-ionic monomers.

The most frequently used non-ionic monomers include iohexol (Omnipaque) and iopamidol (Isovue-M). Each agent is commercially available in varying concentrations and osmolality (**Fig. 2-5**). Each is rapidly absorbed into the bloodstream from paraspinal, epidural, and IT locations (**Fig. 2-6**). There is minimal deiodination, biotransformation, or metabolism.[40,41]

Adverse Events: Incidence

The actual incidence of adverse effects related to the use of iodinated contrast medium is difficult to quantify because of coadministration with other medications that may be responsible for an adverse reaction. The majority of the data regarding adverse events are related to intravascular injection of contrast medium, which usually involves larger doses of contrast medium compared with the amount injected for spinal procedures. There is even disagreement regarding how to classify adverse reactions. One method classifies reactions by their severity (**Table 2-6**). The incidence of adverse reactions was reported to be as high as 15% with the use of HOCM. The use of LOCM has a significantly lower incidence of adverse reactions, especially those of a non–life-threatening nature. In reports reviewing many contrast injections at multiple institutions in large numbers of patients, the incidence varied from 0.2% to 0.7%.[42,43] Serious reactions occurred in one to two per

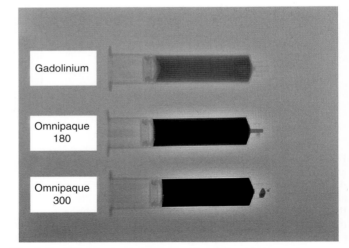

Fig. 2-5 Different types of contrast in a 10-cc syringe demonstrating the relative opacities.

10,000 IV injections of LOCM. Fatalities associated with IV contrast media in the time when HOCM was being used were quoted as one per 40,000 IV injections. However, a Japanese study reported no fatality in more than 170,000 intravenous (IV) injections with the use of both LOCM and HOCM.[44] As a result, the conservative estimate of incidence of one per 170,000 has been quoted, with the

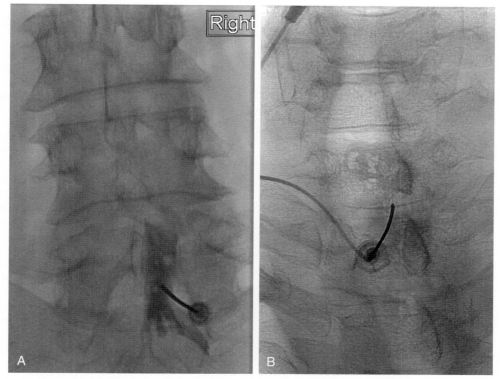

Fig. 2-6   Lumbar epidural (**A**) using iodinated contrast and cervical epidural (**B**) using gadolinium-based contrast.

true incidence likely even less frequent, especially because of the use of LOCM and more effective treatment of reactions.

Adverse Events

Importantly, the majority of adverse events are mild, not life-threatening, and easily treated with observation, reassurance, and support. Severe adverse events may have a mild presentation, but nearly all life-threatening reactions occur with the first 20 minutes of contrast injection.[45]

These reactions can be further divided into three categories: allergic, chemotoxic, and osmolar. Although the exact pathogenesis of many of the reactions is not well known, certain causes can be identified. Hypotension and tachycardia are posited by some to be related to hypertonicity. Pulseless electrical activity and associated cardiac arrest are thought to be related to a sudden decrease in serum-ionized calcium. All of these events have decreased in incidence and severity with the use of LOCM. Vasovagal reactions characterized by hypotension and bradycardia related to increased vagal tone from the CNS are also relatively common. Vasovagal reactions are related to anxiety and can occur pre-procedurally or during the procedure and usually present with feeling of apprehension and diaphoresis. Most vasovagal episodes are mild and self-limited and should be treated and observed until completely resolved.

The incidence of adverse events has been reduced with time but not eliminated. The presentation of a severe allergic response can appear identical to an anaphylactic reaction, but because no antigen–antibody complex has been identified, these reactions are characterized as "anaphylactoid," although treatment is identical to that of an immune-mediated anaphylactic reaction. Potentially, there are multiple possibilities and even combinations of possibilities, including the involvement of a variety of vasoactive mediators as well as a process effecting histamine release. Suffice it to say that

an in-depth review of the mechanisms is beyond the scope of this text. Specific chemical formation of the contrast media being used can provide more explanation.

Unfortunately, predicting a contrast reaction with any great accuracy is not possible, although there are definitely patients who are at greater risk than others. An obvious risk factor for adverse reaction is a prior allergy-like reaction to contrast media, which increases the chance of subsequent reaction by five fold.[44] In fact, any specific allergy may predispose the patient to an allergic-type reaction when exposed to contrast. Although difficult to explain, the proceduralist's focus should be aimed at patients with a prior major anaphylactic response to other allergens. Allergies to shellfish or dairy products, which in the past have been purported to be a predictor of contrast media allergy, have proven to be unreliable.[46,47] There is no evidence that the practice of questioning patients about this type of allergy provides any useful clinical information.[48,49]

A history of asthma may be indicative of an increased likelihood of reaction to contrast medium.[44,50] Significant cardiac disease, including symptomatic angina and congestive heart failure as well as severe aortic stenosis and primary pulmonary hypertension or even well-compensated cardiomyopathy, may have an increased risk of adverse reaction. Care should be given to limiting the volume and osmolality of the contrast given to these patients.

Anxiety is another risk factor that can contribute to adverse reactions. Hopper et al[51] studied the effect that informed consent had on anxiety level for patients undergoing injection of IV contrast media and found no significant difference in adverse reactions between the groups; the majority of patients in each group had an equally elevated level of anxiety when graded using a validated index of anxiety. Care should be taken to provide supportive measures to calm the patient as much as possible. In some cases, this may require mild IV sedation. However, in the name of patient

Table 2-6: Classification of Severity and Manifestations of Adverse Reactions to Contrast Media*

Mild

Signs and symptoms appear self-limited without evidence of progression (e.g., limited urticaria with mild pruritus, transient nausea, one episode of emesis) and include:

- Nausea
- Altered taste
- Itching
- Rash
- Hives
- Warmth
- Nasal stuffiness
- Headache
- Flushing
- Swelling: eyes, face
- Dizziness
- Shaking

Treatment: Requires observation to confirm resolution or lack of progression but usually no treatment. Patient reassurance is usually helpful.

Moderate

Signs and symptoms are more pronounced. Moderate degree of clinically evident focal or systemic signs or symptoms, including:

- Tachycardia or bradycardia
- Bronchospasm
- Wheezing
- Hypertension
- Laryngeal edema
- Generalized or diffuse erythema
- Mild hypotension
- Dyspnea

Treatment: Clinical findings in moderate reactions frequently require prompt treatment. These situations require close, careful observation for possible progression to a life-threatening event.

Severe

Signs and symptoms are often life-threatening, including:

- Laryngeal edema (severe or rapidly progressing)
- Convulsions
- Profound hypotension
- Unresponsiveness
- Clinically manifest arrhythmias
- Cardiopulmonary arrest

Treatment: Requires *prompt* recognition and aggressive treatment; manifestations and treatment frequently require hospitalization.

*These classifications (mild, moderate, severe) do not attempt to distinguish between allergic-like and non–allergic-like reactions. Rather, they encompass the spectrum of adverse events that can be seen after the intravascular injection of contrast media.
From American College of Radiology: *Manual on contrast media*, ed 7, American College of Radiology: Reston, VA, 2010. Online only. http://www.acr.org/SecondaryMainMenuCategories/quality_safety/contrast_manual/FullManual.aspx.

safety, the patient should not be sedated to the point that he or she cannot provide feedback during the procedure.

Contrast-induced nephrotoxicity (CIN) is another concern when using iodine-based contrast (**Table 2-7**). In a patient with normal renal function, the risk of developing CIN is extremely low. In Byrd and Sherman's[52] review of significant risk factors for developing CIN, they highlighted preexisting renal insufficiency (serum creatinine level ≥1.5 mg/dL), diabetes mellitus, dehydration, cardiovascular disease with diuretic use, age older than 70 years, multiple myeloma, hypertension, and hyperuricemia. More recent studies have indicated that the patients at highest risk for CIN are those with a combination of diabetes mellitus and preexisting renal insufficiency.[52-54] Other less common conditions that may put patients at risk for renal involvement include paraproteinemias, particularly multiple myeloma, which likely predispose patients to renal failure because of protein precipitation and aggregation; however, these data are based on HOCM-related data. Also, the use

of β-blocking agents in some retrospective studies may lower the threshold, increase the severity, and reduce the response to treatment of contrast reactions with epinephrine.[52] Additional even less commonly encountered clinical situations such as the use of papaverine or other intraarterial injections or patients with pheochromocytoma, hyperthyroidism, or carcinoma of the thyroid with possible iodine-131 treatment planned may require extra consideration of the risk-to-benefit ratio before an elective pain procedure is performed.

Delayed reactions to contrast media have also been described in the literature and have been reported with both iodinated and gadolinium-based contrast types. Concerns about gadolinium-based contrast adverse reactions are addressed elsewhere. Various types of signs and symptoms have been reported as delayed reactions, including nausea, vomiting, drowsiness, headaches, and pruritus, which are almost always self-limited and require no treatment other than reassurance. The delayed cutaneous reactions are the most important because they may recur (reported anecdotally ≤25%) and may have serious sequelae. The incidence of delayed adverse cutaneous reactions ranges from 0.5% to 9%, are more common in patients being treated with IL-2 therapy, and may present 3 hours to 7 days after contrast exposure. The cutaneous reactions are usually macular and self-limited; however, in rare instances, they have progressed to resemble Stevens-Johnson syndrome, toxic epidermal necrolysis, or even cutaneous vasculitis, with one fatality being reported.[45]

Premedication

"At-risk" patients who require contrast media may require premedication in an effort to avoid an adverse reaction. The exact mechanism by which the anaphylactoid reaction occurs is not completely understood; similarly, the role IV steroids play in reducing the risk of the reaction likewise is not completely understood. Evidence suggests that allergic contrast reactions are related to mediators released by basophils and that histamine and basophil counts are reduced by IV steroids as soon as 1 hour after administration with increasing effect at 4 and 8 hours (16 patients). Therefore, premedication is considered to be most effective at least 4 to 6 hours before injection.[55-57] Premedication does not prevent all reactions, and given the possible risks, premedication should be reserved for those who have had moderately severe to severe contrast reactions in the past. No randomized controlled studies have demonstrated that premedication protects against severe life-threatening reactions, but it does reduce those that are less severe.[57-59] Oral prednisone or methylprednisolone premedication regimens used with diphenhydramine, with or without a histamine-2 receptor blocker, have been described with approximately equal success.[60,61] Alternatively, the use of a different contrast agent may also be protective (HOCM to LOCM), although changing from one LOCM to another has little, if any, benefit.[62] Again, pretreatment does not prevent all breakthrough reactions, which most likely will present similarly to the original reaction,[63] and the proceduralist should be prepared to treat that reaction.

Gadolinium

Gadolinium-based contrast media (GBCM) has been in use since the 1980s. Osmolality, viscosity, and stability mark the differences among the different agents without any difference in their reported effectiveness. Currently, it is common for pain proceduralists to use GBCM in patients with previous allergic responses to iodinated contrast material.[64] Shetty et al[65] recently published a review of

Table 2-7: Iodine-Based Intrathecal Contrast

Product	Chemical Structure	Anion	Cation	% Salt Concentration	% Iodine Concentration	Iodine+ (mg/mL)	Viscosity+ 25° C (cps)	Viscosity+ 37° C (cps)	Osmolality (mOsm/kg H$_2$O)
Omnipaque 240 (GE Healthcare)	Iohexol	Nonionic	None	24	24	240	5.8*	3.4	520
Omnipaque300 (GE Healthcare)	Iohexol	Nonionic	None	30	30	300	11.8*	6.3	672
Isovue-M 200 (Bracco)	Iopamidol	Nonionic	Nonionic	None	20	200	3.3*	2.0	413
Isovue-M 300	Iopamidol	Nonionic	Nonionic	None	30	300	8.8*	4.7	616

Magnetic Resonance Contrast Media

Product	Chemical Structure	Anion	Cation	Viscosity+ 25° C (cps)	Viscosity+ 37° C (cps)	Osmolality (mOsm/kg H$_2$O)
Magnevist (Bayer Healthcare)	Ionic linear	Gadopentetate	Dimelglumine	4.9*	2.9	1960
Omniscan (GE Healthcare)	Gd-DTPA-BMA linear	Nonionic		2.0	1.4	789

Gd-DTPA-BMA, Gadolinium,[5,8-bis[(carboxy-kO)methyl}-11-[2-(methylamino)-2-(oxo-kO)ethyl]-3-(oxo-kO)-2,5,8,11-tetraazatridecan-13-oato93-)-kN5,kN8,kN11,kO13].

*Measured at 20°C.

From American College of Radiology: *Manual on contrast media*, ed 7, American College of Radiology: Reston, VA, 2010. Online only. http://www.acr.org/SecondaryMainMenuCategories/quality_safety/contrast_manual/FullManual.aspx.

2067 epidural steroid injections over a 25-month period in which 38 of those used GBCM to confirm needle placement. They found that, based on a radiologist's review of the saved spot image, contrast spread as compared to iodinated contrast images resulted in significantly greater confidence of needle placement. In addition, they also found that GBCM was a useful confirmatory test to help localize the needle tip in patients in whom GBCM was used.[65] This difference in visualization between iodinated contrast medium and GBCM would not be unexpected given the relatively low concentration of gadolinium in the available commercial preparations compared with the iodinated compounds. It is also important to note that similar to the use of intraarterial and power-injected gadolinium, the use of epidural gadolinium represents off-label use at this time.[65] The authors of that study found and would suggest (which would be confirmed by our experience at our institution) that the use of digital subtraction would improve the visualization of gadolinium in the epidural space.

Adverse Reactions

GBCM is extremely well tolerated and safe. The literature reports that the overall incidence of acute adverse events at approved IV dosing ranges from 0.07% to 2.4%. Similar to other contrast media reactions, the vast majority of reactions are mild. The symptoms include coldness or warmth at the injection site, nausea, headache, paresthesias, dizziness, or pruritus. An allergic-like reaction does occur but is rare with an incidence of 0.004% to 0.7%; this presents with rash, hives, and urticaria and less commonly, bronchospasm. Life-threatening anaphylactoid reactions also occur but are extremely rare (0.001% to 0.01%) but include fatal reactions.

The frequency of acute reactions of GBCM is eight times higher in those with a known previous reaction to GBCM. Second reactions tend to be more severe. Patients with asthma and other allergies, including those to certain foods, are also at greater risk, reported to be as high as 3.7%.[45] In relation to patients with an allergy to iodinated contrast media, there is no known cross-reactivity, although a previous allergic-type reaction would place

them in previously mentioned category of 3.7%. Similar recommendations for premedication and trying an alternative agent also apply to the patient with a previous allergic reaction to GBCM. Gadolinium has no known nephrotoxicity at the approved IV magnetic resonance dosing. It is also noted that initially there was some concern with GBCM's promoting a sickle cell disease–related vaso-occlusive event[66]; however, at the approved dosage, there is no evidence to withhold GBCM from patients with sickle cell disease.

Nephrogenic systemic fibrosis (NSF) is a fibrosing disease of the skin and subcutaneous tissues and was first described in 2000 and noted to occur primarily in patients with end-stage chronic kidney disease, especially those on dialysis. In 2006, a number of reports emerged that noted a strong association with GBCM to patients with advanced renal disease and the development of NSF.[67,68] Much about NSF and its development is unknown such as the causation, exact risk of developing NSF after GBCM, and why some at-risk patients develop NSF and others do not. It does appear that not all agents have the same risk of developing NSF. A recent report by the American College of Radiology Committee on Drugs and Contrast Media placed GBCM into three categories with gadodiamide (Omniscan) and gadopentetate dimeglumine (Magnevist) in the group associated with the greatest number of NSF cases, which likely reflects a number of different factors, including market share as well as agent toxicity.[45,69-73] Risk factors include high cumulative dose or even a single dose of GBCM, although up to 50% of NSF occurred after one dose and usually occurred in days to 6 months after exposure. Patients with chronic kidney disease with a glomerular filtration rate (GFR) of less than 30 L/min/1.73 m^2 and patients with acute kidney injury have a reported 1% to 7% risk[45,67-69,73-76] of developing NSF.[77] Recommendations include GFR screening within 6 weeks of the procedure and consideration of alternative procedures whenever possible in "at-risk" patients.

All of what has been reported above relates to the use of GBCM delivered in up to nine times the volume used in most spinal procedures, which likely reduces the practical risk of GBCM-related adverse events. In regard to diagnostic and therapeutic spine procedures performed by pain specialists, there are few reports that specifically report on the use of gadolinium and its safety. In a study by Safriel et al[39] that reviewed 527 procedures in which GBCM was used and included a wide variety of procedures from cervical discograms to lumbar facet injections, they reported one documented IT injection without sequelae and two patients who required admission to the intensive care unit. These two patients who underwent cervical procedures (multilevel discogram and cervical epidural unspecified type) experienced headache, nausea, and seizures and required intensive care admission. In both cases, all symptoms completely resolved, and both were documented to have IT gadolinium observed on postprocedure imaging.[39] In another report of four allergic reactions to gadolinium in patients with reported allergy to iodinated contrast, one underwent a lumbar facet injection, and the other three underwent lumbar transforaminal injections. Each of the four presented with a rash, and the fourth also experienced fever. Three of the four had also been exposed to gadolinium previously without difficulty. All four did not require hospitalization.[64] The study mentioned earlier by Shetty et al[65] reported no adverse reactions in the 38 patients who received GBCM. Overall, for patients with an known iodine contrast allergy and normal renal function, the use of GBCM appears to have a relatively low incidence of adverse events GBCM, but based on the small numbers, further study is warranted.

References

1. Evans W: Intrasacral epidural injections in the treatment of sciatica. *Lancet* 1225-1229, 1930.
2. Robecchi A, Capra R: [Hydrocortisone (compound F); first clinical experiments in the field of rheumatology]. *Minerva Med* 43:1259-1263, 1952.
3. Goebert HW, Jr, Jallo SJ, Gardner WJ, Wasmuth CE: Painful radiculopathy treated with epidural injections of procaine and hydrocortisone acetate: results in 113 patients. *Anesth Analg* 40:130-134, 1961.
4. Winnie AP, Hartman JT, Meyers HL, Jr, et al: Pain clinic. II. Intradural and extradural corticosteroids for sciatica. *Anesth Analg* 51:990-1003, 1972.
5. Abbott Laboratories: *Product information: bupivacaine hydrochloride injection*, North Chicago, 1999, Abbott Laboratories.
6. Abbott Laboratories: *Product information: lidocaine hydrochloride injection*, North Chicago, IL, Abbott Laboratories.
7. Miller RD: *Miller's anesthesia*, ed 7, Philadelphia, 2010, Churchill Livingstone, pp 3084-3089.
8. DiFazio CA, Carron H, Grosslight KR, et al: Comparison of pH-adjusted lidocaine solutions for epidural anesthesia. *Anesth Analg* 65:760-764, 1986.
9. Ririe DG, Walker FO, James RL, Butterworth J: Effect of alkalinization of lidocaine on median nerve block. *Br J Anaesth* 84:163-168, 2000.
10. Benzon HT: *Essentials of pain medicine and regional anesthesia*, ed 2, Philadelphia, 2005, Elsevier-Churchill Livingstone.
11. Ring J, Franz R, Brockow K: Anaphylactic reactions to local anesthetics. *Chem Immunol Allergy* 95:190-200, 2010.
12. Auroy Y, Benhamou D, Bargues L, et al: Major complications of regional anesthesia in France: the SOS Regional Anesthesia Hotline Service. *Anesthesiology* 97:1274-1280, 2002.
13. Brown DL, Ransom DM, Hall JA, et al: Regional anesthesia and local anesthetic-induced systemic toxicity: seizure frequency and accompanying cardiovascular changes. *Anesth Analg* 81:321-328, 1995.
14. Ireland PE, Ferguson JK, Stark EJ: The clinical and experimental comparison of cocaine and pontocaine as topical anesthetics in otolaryngological practice. *Laryngoscope* 61:767-777, 1951.
15. Neal JM, Bernards CM, Butterworth JF IV, et al: ASRA practice advisory on local anesthetic systemic toxicity. *Reg Anesth Pain Med* 35:152-161, 2010.
16. Weinberg GL, Di Gregorio G, Ripper R, et al: Resuscitation with lipid versus epinephrine in a rat model of bupivacaine overdose. *Anesthesiology* 108:907-913, 2008.
17. Coursin DB, Wood KE: Corticosteroid supplementation for adrenal insufficiency. *JAMA* 287:236-240, 2002.
18. Hench PS, Slocumb CH, Polley HF, Kendal EC: Effect of cortisone and pituitary adrenocorticotropic hormone (ACTH) on rheumatic diseases. *JAMA* 144:1327-1335, 1950.
19. Williams RH, Wilson JD: *Williams textbook of endocrinology*, ed 9, Philadelphia, 1998, Saunders.
20. Manichikanti L: Interventional techniques in chronic spinal pain. In Manchikanti L, Singh V, editors: *Interventional Techniques in Chronic Spinal Pain*, Paducah, KY, 2007, ASIPP Publishing, pp 167-184.
21. Katzung BG: *Basic & clinical pharmacology*, ed 9, New York, 2004, Lange Medical Books/McGraw Hill.
22. Tuel SM, Meythaler JM, Cross LL: Cushing's syndrome from epidural methylprednisolone. *Pain* 40:81-84, 1990.
23. Stambough JL, Booth RE, Jr, Rothman RH: Transient hypercorticism after epidural steroid injection. A case report. *J Bone Joint Surg Am* 66:1115-1116, 1984.
24. Scanlon GC, Moeller-Bertram T, Romanowsky SM, Wallace MS: Cervical transforaminal epidural steroid injections: more dangerous than we think? *Spine (Phila Pa 1976)* 32:1249-1256, 2007.
25. Tiso RL, Cutler T, Catania JA, Whalen K: Adverse central nervous system sequelae after selective transforaminal block: the role of corticosteroids. *Spine J* 4:468-474, 2004.
26. Benzon HT, Chew TL, McCarthy RJ, et al: Comparison of the particle sizes of different steroids and the effect of dilution: a review of the relative neurotoxicities of the steroids. *Anesthesiology* 106:331-338, 2007.
27. Okubadejo GO, Talcott MR, Schmidt RE, et al: Perils of intravascular methylprednisolone injection into the vertebral artery. An animal study. *J Bone Joint Surg Am* 90:1932-1938, 2008.
28. Craig DB, Habib GG: Flaccid paraparesis following obstetrical epidural anesthesia: possible role of benzyl alcohol. *Anesth Analg* 56:219-221, 1977.
29. Bogduk C, Cherry D: *Report of the Working Party on Epidural Use of Steroids in the Management for Back Pain*, Caberra, Australia, 1994, National Health and Medical Research Council, pp 1-76.
30. Neal JM, Rathmell JP: *Complications in regional anesthesia and pain medicine*, ed 1, Philadelphia, 2007, Saunders/Elsevier.
31. Vallejo R, Tilley DM, Vogel L, Benyamin R: The role of glia and the immune system in the development and maintenance of neuropathic pain. *Pain Pract* 10:167-184, 2010.
32. Genevay S, Stingelin S, Gabay C: Efficacy of etanercept in the treatment of acute, severe sciatica: a pilot study. *Ann Rheum Dis* 63:1120-1123, 2004.
33. Korhonen T, Karppinen J, Malmivaara A, et al: Efficacy of infliximab for disc herniation-induced sciatica: one-year follow-up. *Spine (Phila Pa 1976)* 29:2115-2119, 2004.
34. Korhonen T, Karppinen J, Paimela L, et al: The treatment of disc herniation-induced sciatica with infliximab: results of a randomized, controlled, 3-month follow-up study. *Spine (Phila Pa 1976)* 30:2724-2728, 2005.
35. Cohen SP, Bogduk N, Dragovich A, et al: Randomized, double-blind, placebo-controlled, dose-response, and preclinical safety study of transforaminal epidural etanercept for the treatment of sciatica. *Anesthesiology* 110:1116-1126, 2009.
36. Bongartz T, Sutton AJ, Sweeting MJ, et al: Anti-TNF antibody therapy in rheumatoid arthritis and the risk of serious infections and malignancies: systematic review and meta-analysis of rare harmful effects in randomized controlled trials. *JAMA* 295:2275-2285, 2006.
37. Romero-Sandoval A, Eisenach JC: Perineural clonidine reduces mechanical hypersensitivity and cytokine production in established nerve injury. *Anesthesiology* 104:351-355, 2006.
38. Benzon HT, Raj PP: *Raj's practical management of pain*, ed 4, Philadelphia, 2008, Mosby-Elsevier.

39. Safriel Y, Ang R, Ali M: Gadolinium use in spine pain management procedures for patients with contrast allergies: results in 527 procedures. *Cardiovasc Intervent Radiol* 31:325-331, 2008.

40. Nycomed: *Product information: Omnipaque, Iohexol*, Princeton, NJ, 1996, Nycomed.

41. Bracco Diagnostics: *Product information: Isovue iopamidol*, Princeton, NJ, 1999, Bracco Diagnostics.

42. Cochran ST, Bomyea K, Sayre JW: Trends in adverse events after IV administration of contrast media. *AJR Am J Roentgenol* 176:1385-1388, 2001.

43. Wang CL, Cohan RH, Ellis JH, et al: Frequency, outcome, and appropriateness of treatment of nonionic iodinated contrast media reactions. *AJR Am J Roentgenol* 191:409-415, 2008.

44. Katayama H, Yamaguchi K, Kozuka T, et al: Adverse reactions to ionic and nonionic contrast media. A report from the Japanese Committee on the Safety of Contrast Media. *Radiology* 175:621-628, 1990.

45. American College of Radiology: *Manual on contrast media*, ed 7, Reston, VA, 2010, American College of Radiology. Online only. http://www.acr.org/SecondaryMainMenuCategories/quality_safety/contrast_manual/FullManual.aspx.

46. Coakley FV, Panicek DM, Iodine allergy: an oyster without a pearl? *AJR Am J Roentgenol* 169:951-952, 1997.

47. Lieberman PL, Seigle RL: Reactions to radiocontrast material. Anaphylactoid events in radiology. *Clin Rev Allergy Immunol* 17:469-496, 1999.

48. Beaty AD, Lieberman PL, Slavin RG: Seafood allergy and radiocontrast media: are physicians propagating a myth? *Am J Med* 121:158:e151-e154, 2008.

49. Boehm I: Seafood allergy and radiocontrast media: are physicians propagating a myth? *Am J Med* 121:e19, 2008.

50. Shehadi WH: Adverse reactions to intravascularly administered contrast media. A comprehensive study based on a prospective survey. *Am J Roentgenol Radium Ther Nucl Med* 124:145-152, 1975.

51. Hopper KD, Houts PS, TenHave TR, et al: The effect of informed consent on the level of anxiety in patients given i.v. contrast material. *AJR Am J Roentgenol* 162:531-535, 1994.

52. Byrd L, Sherman RL: Radiocontrast-induced acute renal failure: a clinical and pathophysiologic review. *Medicine (Baltimore)* 58:270-279, 1979.

53. Parfrey PS, Griffiths SM, Barrett BJ, et al: Contrast material-induced renal failure in patients with diabetes mellitus, renal insufficiency, or both. A prospective controlled study. *N Engl J Med* 320:143-149, 1989.

54. Schwab SJ, Hlatky MA, Pieper KS, et al: Contrast nephrotoxicity: a randomized controlled trial of a nonionic and an ionic radiographic contrast agent. *N Engl J Med* 320:149-153, 1989.

55. Lasser EC: Pretreatment with corticosteroids to prevent reactions to i.v. contrast material: overview and implications. *AJR Am J Roentgenol* 150:257-259, 1988.

56. Lasser EC, Berry CC, Mishkin MM, et al: Pretreatment with corticosteroids to prevent adverse reactions to nonionic contrast media. *AJR Am J Roentgenol* 162:523-526, 1994.

57. Morcos SK: Review article: acute serious and fatal reactions to contrast media: our current understanding. *Br J Radiol* 78:686-693, 2005.

58. Brockow K, Christiansen C, Kanny G, et al: Management of hypersensitivity reactions to iodinated contrast media. *Allergy* 60:150-158, 2005.

59. Tramer MR, von Elm E, Loubeyre P, Hauser C: Pharmacological prevention of serious anaphylactic reactions due to iodinated contrast media: systematic review. *BMJ* 333:675, 2006.

60. Dunsky EH, Zweiman B, Fischler E, Levy DA: Early effects of corticosteroids on basophils, leukocyte histamine, and tissue histamine. *J Allergy Clin Immunol* 63:426-432, 1979.

61. Greenberger PA, Patterson R, Tapio CM: Prophylaxis against repeated radiocontrast media reactions in 857 cases. Adverse experience with cimetidine and safety of beta-adrenergic antagonists. *Arch Intern Med* 145:2197-2200, 1985.

62. Davenport MS, Cohan RH, Caoili EM, Ellis JH: Repeat contrast medium reactions in premedicated patients: frequency and severity. *Radiology* 253:372-379, 2009.

63. Freed KS, Leder RA, Alexander C, et al: Breakthrough adverse reactions to low-osmolar contrast media after steroid premedication. *AJR Am J Roentgenol* 176:1389-1392, 2001.

64. O'Donnell CJ, Cano WG: Allergic reactions to gadodiamide following interventional spinal procedures: a report of 4 cases. *Arch Phys Med Rehabil* 88:1465-1467, 2007.

65. Shetty SK, Nelson EN, Lawrimore TM, Palmer WE: Use of gadolinium chelate to confirm epidural needle placement in patients with an iodinated contrast reaction. *Skeletal Radiol* 36:301-307, 2007.

66. Brody AS, Sorette MP, Gooding CA, et al: AUR memorial Award. Induced alignment of flowing sickle erythrocytes in a magnetic field. A preliminary report. *Invest Radiol* 20:560-566, 1985.

67. Grobner T: Gadolinium—a specific trigger for the development of nephrogenic fibrosing dermopathy and nephrogenic systemic fibrosis? *Nephrol Dial Transplant* 21:1104-1108, 2006.

68. Marckmann P, Skov L, Rossen K, et al: Nephrogenic systemic fibrosis: suspected causative role of gadodiamide used for contrast-enhanced magnetic resonance imaging. *J Am Soc Nephrol* 17:2359-2362, 2006.

69. Collidge TA, Thomson PC, Mark PB, et al: Gadolinium-enhanced MR imaging and nephrogenic systemic fibrosis: retrospective study of a renal replacement therapy cohort. *Radiology* 245:168-175, 2007.

70. Harrington, RA, Chair, FDA Advisory Committee: Gadolinium-based contrast agents & nephrogenic systemic fibrosis. FDA Briefing Document. Joint Meeting of the Cardiovascular and Renal Drugs and Drug Safety and Risk Management Advisory Committee, 2009. Online at http://www.fda.gov/downloads/AdvisoryCommittees/CommitteesMeetingMaterials/Drugs/DrugSafetyandRiskManagementAdvisoryCommittee/UCM190850.pdf.

71. Peak AS, Sheller A: Risk factors for developing gadolinium-induced nephrogenic systemic fibrosis. *Ann Pharmacother* 41:1481-1485, 2007.

72. Thomsen HS, Marckmann P, Logager VB: Nephrogenic systemic fibrosis (NSF): a late adverse reaction to some of the gadolinium based contrast agents. *Cancer Imaging* 7:130-137, 2007.

73. Wertman R, Altun E, Martin DR, et al: Risk of nephrogenic systemic fibrosis: evaluation of gadolinium chelate contrast agents at four American universities. *Radiology* 248:799-806, 2008.

74. Broome DR, Girguis MS, Baron PW, et al: Gadodiamide-associated nephrogenic systemic fibrosis: why radiologists should be concerned. *AJR Am J Roentgenol* 188:586-592, 2007.

75. Sadowski EA, Bennett LK, Chan MR, et al: Nephrogenic systemic fibrosis: risk factors and incidence estimation. *Radiology* 243:148-157, 2007.

76. Shabana WM, Cohan RH, Ellis JH, et al: Nephrogenic systemic fibrosis: a report of 29 cases. *AJR Am J Roentgenol* 190:736-741, 2008.

77. Wahba IM, Simpson EL, White K: Gadolinium is not the only trigger for nephrogenic systemic fibrosis: insights from two cases and review of the recent literature. *Am J Transplant* 7:2425-2432, 2007.

CHAPTER

3 Fluoroscopy, Ultrasonography, Computed Tomography, and Radiation Safety

Stanley Golovac

CHAPTER OVERVIEW

Chapter Synopsis: A detailed, accurate picture of the body's internal environment is key for a clinician guiding a needle to a targeted location within the spine, extremities, or viscera. This chapter considers imaging technologies that aid in this guidance for the diagnosis, confirmation, and/or treatment of pain. Ultrasound (US) technology sends very high-pitched sound waves into the body, which are reflected differently depending on the tissue's makeup, thereby providing a picture of the internal environment and good resolution images of soft tissue structural relationships. US is limited, however, by lack of clarity of many deeper spinal targets because of bone shadowing. Computed tomography scans can provide high-resolution images of the internal environment, including the spine and deeper targets, but carries additional risk from radiation exposure, particularly in children. In addition, most CT techniques are delayed, thus real-time guidance of the needle is not always possible. Fluoroscopy, which utilizes x-rays and is usually portable, is perhaps the most versatile tool. Fluoroscopy does not provide resolution for soft tissues, but instead relies on bone images and the use of real-time contrast dye administration for procedural guidance in interventional pain. Although available in some centers, the use of magnetic resonance imaging (MRI) guidance is not discussed due to the complexity and cost of this modality. The relative merits of US, CT, and fluoroscopic image guidance are emphasized in this chapter, along with known safety concerns.

Important Points:
- At the present time, multiple forms of radiological imaging devices are used to evaluate and confirm the diagnosis of clinical conditions.
- Safety is still a very real concern, and awareness of risk that is taken with each procedure is important.

Clinical Pearls:
- Interventional pain procedures are now required to be performed with the use of radiological guidance in most situations. Without imaging, patients may be placed at greater risk unnecessarily.
- Minimizing radiation exposure is still most important. MRI or US allows the performance of evaluations without radiation exposure, and may be considered in specific situations.

Clinical Pitfalls:
- Careless use of and overexposure to radiation can compromise the health and well-being of both the operator and the patient being examined. Careful attention to lead apron quality, sizing, and regular safety inspections of all equipment are important.
- The use of pulsed or reduced dose techniques of fluoroscopy are important safety measures to consider, particularly in higher dose procedures such as spinal cord stimulation electrode placement.
- The effects of US gel are not well known, and efforts to limit the introduction of gel internally are important.

Introduction

In the last three decades, image guidance for interventional pain management procedures has become standard, replacing the less accurate and less reproducible use of surface landmark–based techniques. There are many reasons for this evolution in procedural therapy, including the advent of new procedures (e.g., transforaminal epidural injections largely replacing interlaminar epidural injections); increases in both the number of procedures performed and an associated rise in the number of complications; and the need for image storage to ensure the appropriateness of the diagnostic and therapeutic procedures that were performed. First used in 1895, fluoroscopy has become the most popular technique for image-guided procedures, particularly for those procedures in the cervical, thoracic, and lumbar spine. It is one of many different forms of imaging, including ultrasonography, computed tomography (CT), and magnetic resonance imaging (MRI), all of which can be used to help guide needle placement to diagnose, confirm, and treat areas believed to be the pain generators.

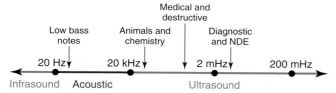

Fig. 3-1 Ultrasound kilohertz. NDE, Nondestructive evaluation.

Box 3-1 Ultrasound Gel

- Ingestion: nonsignificant
- Eye contact: flush with water for 15 minutes
- Overexposure: reddening or blistering of the eyes
- Carcinogenicity: none
- OSHA regulated: no
- Boiling point: >212° F
- Specific gravity: 1.1^2

Ultrasound

Ultrasound is cyclic sound pressure with a frequency greater than the upper limit of human hearing. Although this limit varies from person to person, it is approximately 20 kHz (20,000 Hz) in healthy, young adults, and thus 20 kHz serves as a useful lower limit in describing ultrasound (**Fig. 3-1**).

The production of ultrasound is used in many different fields, typically to penetrate a medium and measure the reflection signature or supply focused energy. The reflection signature can reveal details about the inner structure of the medium, a property also used by animals such as bats for hunting. The most well-known application of ultrasound is its use in sonography to produce pictures of fetuses in the human womb. There are a vast number of other applications as well.

In diagnostic ultrasonography, also known as sonography, the physician or technician places a *transducer*, or ultrasound probe, in or on the patient's body. Pulsed ultrasound waves emitted by the transducer pass into the body and reflect off the boundaries between different types of body tissue. The transducer receives these reflections, or echoes. A computer then assembles the information from the reflected ultrasound waves into a picture on a video monitor. The frequency, density, focus, and aperture of the ultrasound beam can vary. Higher frequencies produce more clarity but cannot penetrate as deeply into the body. Lower frequencies penetrate more deeply but produce lower resolution, or clarity. For uses in the spine or deeper tissues such as the hip joint, a curvilinear (low frequency) probe is generally used. Bone structures such as the posterior elements and lamina reflect sound waves back, causing darker "hypoacoustic" areas, effectively shadowing many soft tissue targets such as spinal nerves in the foramina that may be deeper than these bones, thus the bones obscure the reflected echoes from the nerves. In many cases, the use of color Doppler will add additional clarity by rendering blood flow in either red or blue color to delineate vascular structures from other anatomical tissues in the visual field.

Disadvantages of Ultrasound

Unfortunately, the use of ultrasonography does not confirm contrast spread to enhance structures that need to be identified. This is important in techniques such as transforaminal epidural injections where the desire is to ensure that medications and particulate steroids not be injected intravascularly. Ultrasonography allows visualization of tissue density and depth but not unlike fluoroscopy one cannot see radiographic contrast enhancement. Deep spinal injections utilizing ultrasound are particularly difficult and require a large learning curve to become proficient, compared to the relatively simple use of fluoroscopy techniques.

Safety Concerns

Most infants now born in the United States are exposed to ultrasonography before birth, and in Germany, Norway, Iceland, and Austria, all pregnant women are screened with ultrasonography. To date, researchers have not identified any adverse biological effects clearly caused by ultrasonography, even though 3 million babies born each year have had ultrasound scans in utero. This is an enviable safety record. However, the National Council on Radiation Protection and Measurements advocates continued study of ultrasound safety, improvements in the safety features of ultrasound systems, and more safety education for ultrasound system operators.[1] Because of the sheer number of people exposed to ultrasonography, any possibility of a harmful effect must be investigated thoroughly.

Ultrasound gel is intended only for external use. If a needle becomes contaminated with gel, every effort should be made to remove the needle and replace it with a sterile new one. Even though the gel initially is sterile, the substance itself may irritate structures either in the epidural space or even intrathecally. Either way, one should err toward needle replacement. Remember, ultrasound gel contains propylene glycol, glycerine, phenoxyethanol, and FD&C Blue #1. For properties and side effects of ultrasound gel, see **Box 3-1**.

Computed Tomography

CT was discovered independently by a British engineer named Sir Godfrey Hounsfield and Dr. Alan Cormack. Cormack was the first to analyze the possibility of such an examination of a biological system, in 1963 and 1964, and to develop the equations needed for computer-assisted x-ray reconstruction of pictures of the human brain and body. It has become a mainstay for diagnosing medical diseases. For their work, Hounsfield and Cormack were jointly awarded the Nobel Prize in 1979.

CT scanners first began to be installed in hospitals around 1974. Currently, 6000 scanners are in use in the United States. Advances in computer technology have vastly improved patient comfort because CT scanners are now much faster. These improvements have also led to higher resolution images, which improve the diagnostic capabilities of the test. For example, the CT scan can show doctors small nodules or tumors, which they cannot see on radiography.

The CT scanner is an expensive yet sophisticated way to guide needle placement (**Fig. 3-2**). It is somewhat expensive for the routine use of image-guided procedures, especially in an office-based practice or even an ambulatory surgery center. One could justify the use of such a device if looking at a study or working in a hospital with access to a scanner. Most scanners are used daily for diagnostic workups but not for pain management procedures. They allow for excellent needle placement and biopsies that are performed.

CT may be the best method to accurately place a needle at small individual sites laden with blood vessels, nerves, and organs that should not be violated. Many studies have compared results of guidance with ultrasound (US) to CT, which is commonly accepted as the gold standard. However the use of CT is rising dramatically, and there are more significant risks.

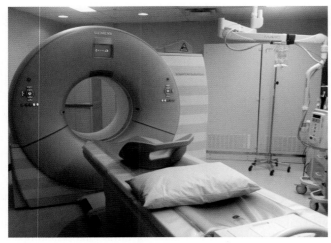

Fig. 3-2 Ultra-fast computed tomography scanner Helicoil GE.

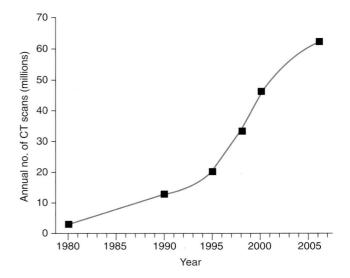

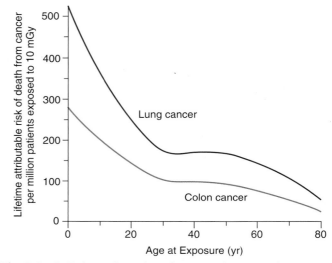

Fig. 3-3 **A,** Estimated number of computed tomography scans performed annually in the United States. **B,** Estimated dependence of lifetime radiation-induced risk of cancer on age at exposure for two of the most common radiogenic cancers. (Modified from Brenner DJ, Hall EJ: Computed tomography—an increasing source of radiation exposure, *N Engl J Med* 357:2277-2284, 2007.)

Safety Concerns

The individual risk from radiation associated with a CT scan is quite small compared with the benefits that accurate diagnosis and treatment can provide. Still, unnecessary radiation exposure during medical procedures should be avoided. This is particularly important when the patient is a child because children exposed to radiation are at a relatively greater risk than adults. The American College of Radiology has noted, "Because they have more rapidly dividing cells than adults and longer life expectancy, the odds that children will develop cancers from x-ray radiation may be significantly higher than adults"[3] (**Fig. 3-3**). Unnecessary radiation may be delivered when CT scanner parameters are not appropriately adjusted for patient size. When a CT scan is performed on a child or small adult with the same technique factors used for a typically sized adult, the small patient receives a significantly larger effective dose than the full-sized patient.

The absorbed dose is the energy absorbed per unit of mass and is measured in grays (Gy). One gray equals 1 joule of radiation energy absorbed per kilogram. The organ dose (or the distribution of dose in the organ) largely determines the level of risk to that organ from the radiation. The effective dose, expressed in sieverts (Sv), is used for dose distributions that are not homogeneous (which is always the case with CT); it is designed to be proportional to a generic estimate of the overall harm to the patient caused by the radiation exposure. The effective dose allows for a rough comparison between different CT scenarios but provides only an approximate estimate of the true risk. For risk estimation, the organ dose is the preferred quantity.

A recent study by *Academic Emergency Medicine*[4] confirms what many doctors already believed; people may be receiving doses of radiation, sometimes unnecessarily, that puts them at a heightened risk for cancer. Researchers found that a typical patient who visited the emergency department received a cumulative radiation dose of 40 mSv over a 5-year period. Ten percent of patients ended up with a staggering 100 or more mSv. Both levels are well above the safety threshold for lifetime radiation exposure. Exposure above the threshold leaves patients vulnerable to increased long-term risk of cancer. As a point of comparison, one chest CT is around 10 mSv of radiation, and a traditional chest radiograph is only 0.02 mSv (**Table 3-1**).

Organ doses from CT scanning are considerably larger than those from corresponding conventional radiography (**Table 3-2**). For example, a conventional anterior-posterior abdominal radiographic examination results in a dose to the stomach of approximately 0.25 mGy, which is at least 50 times smaller than the corresponding stomach dose from an abdominal CT scan.

Radiation doses vary by operator, radiology technician, and even the radiologist who may request additional images to verify areas of concern. Because there is no universal policy as to how many images should be used per examination, concerns among radiologists are on the rise. Precautions for radiation safety are presented in **Box 3-2**.

The use of a CT-guided image to perform most interventional pain procedures does expose a patient and staff to small doses of radiation. Very few procedures actually require a CT scanner to be able to correctly place needles in clinically difficult areas.[5] Waldman[5] notes that celiac plexus blockade and sacroiliac joint blocks have been performed with CT guidance, but each of these procedures can be performed with fluoroscopy guidance.

Table 3-1 Typical Organ Radiation Doses from Various Radiologic Studies

Relevant Organ Dose*	Study Type	Organ (mGy or mSv)
Dental radiography	Brain	0.005
Posterior-anterior chest radiography	Lung	0.01
Lateral chest radiography	Lung	0.15
Screening mammography	Breast	3
Adult abdominal CT	Stomach	10
Barium enema	Colon	15
Neonatal abdominal CT	Stomach	20

*The radiation dose, a measure of ionizing energy absorbed per unit of mass, is expressed in grays (Gy) or milligrays (mGy); 1 Gy = 1 joule per kilogram. The radiation dose is often expressed as an equivalent dose in sieverts (Sv) or millisieverts (mSv). For x-ray radiation, which is the type used in computed tomography (CT) scanners, 1 mSv = 1 mGy.

Table 3-2 Total Radiation for Body Parts

Body Part	Dose
Whole body, critical organs	5 rems in any year
Gonads, lens of eye	(Prospective annual limit) 10-15 rems in a year
Bone marrow	10-15 rems in any 1 year (Retrospective annual limit) (N-18) × 5 rems (long-term accumulation)
Skin	15 rems in any 1 year
Hands	75 rems in any 1 year (25/qtr)
Forearms	30 rems in any 1 year (10/qtr)
Other organs, tissues, and organ systems	15 rems in any 1 year

qtr, Quarter; rem, roentgen-equivalent-man.

Box 3-2 Basic Radiation Safety

By using the ALARA (as low as reasonably achieved) technique, any radiation dose, no matter how small, can have some adverse effects. Therefore, radiation exposure can be minimized in the following ways.

- Time: The shorter the exposure, the less radiation received.
- Distance: Doubling the distance from the exposure means reducing the dose by one-fourth; tripling the distance means only one-ninth the dose.
- Shielding: Lead barriers, aprons, sliding walls, and eyewear, along with hand and arm protectors, all add improved safety and reduce the total dose of radiation exposure.
  - A skirt can be applied to a carbon fiber imaging table that will help prevent scatter from irradiating the user that is particularly close to the patient being treated.
  - Thyroid shielding also is imperative to help reduce excess exposure of the user's thyroid.
  - When females are to be imaged, a small, lightweight apron can be placed over female reproductive organs to add extra protection.

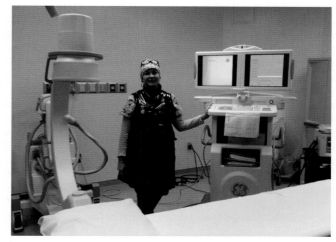

Fig. 3-4 Portable fluoroscope (OEC 9900 GE) at the Space Coast Pain Institute.

Fluoroscopy

The beginning of fluoroscopy can be traced back to November 8, 1895, when Wilhelm Röntgen noticed a barium platinocyanide screen fluorescing as a result of exposure to what he would later call x-rays.[6] Within months of this discovery, the first fluoroscopes were created. Early fluoroscopes were simply cardboard funnels, open at the narrow end for the eyes of the observer. The wide end was closed with a thin cardboard piece that had been coated on the inside with a layer of fluorescent metal salt. The fluoroscopic image obtained in this way was rather faint. Thomas Edison quickly discovered that calcium tungstate screens produced brighter images, and he is credited with designing and producing the first commercially available fluoroscope.

Over the past several years, the use of fluoroscopy has allowed interventional pain physicians to accurately perform injections with precision guidance. What was once considered the gold standard (performing injections blind) is now taboo. A typical injection is performed with either a local anesthetic to confirm the cause of a pain source or in combination with a corticosteroid to help reduce the inflammatory effect caused by an injury or a chronic condition. Confirmation of a painful etiology is necessary to aid in the diagnosis of suspected painful areas. (**Fig. 3-4**).

To be able to clearly visualize critical structures such as nerves and blood vessels or unwanted intrathecal spread of an agent that may lead to a subarachnoid block is a major reason to perform fluoroscopically-guided procedures. The use of a fluoroscope permits the precise targeting of injections. The performance of a selective nerve root injection, for example, requires the placement of a predetermined anesthetic to carefully anesthetize a spinal nerve deemed to be the pain generator. By visualizing the anatomical spread of the contrast material being injected, the enhancement of the suspected painful area can be evaluated for pain relief. Fluoroscopy also is a very good predictor of how difficult the placement of complex devices such as spinal cord stimulator leads may be. With the use of the fluoroscope, the evaluation of spinal segments for optimal needle entry points can be studied prior to the performance of the procedure. Examination under fluoroscopy (visualizing the spine prior to performing the procedure coupled with physical examination) may also be possible. Fluoroscopy also allows one to see the pitfalls that might have been encountered if only surface landmarks had been used.

Disadvantages of Fluoroscopy

Fluoroscopy has several disadvantages. Acquisition and maintenance costs are a huge factor to physicians in private practice. The cost of the device may take several years to recoup. Availability of space in an office is another disadvantage, as the unit requires a large footprint.

Safety Concerns

Radiation safety is a major concern, and in some cases imaging rooms may need to have special construction, including lead shielding. The daily use of fluoroscopy requires a skilled technician to aid in proper device function and positioning of patients in order not to overexpose either the patient or other personnel in the room. Regular and routine maintenance is required for the machine's warranty procedures and to adequately ensure safe delivery of radiation.

As fluoroscopy became increasingly useful as an interventional imaging tool, concerns about increasing exposure times increased scrutiny regarding radiation safety for patients and radiology professionals.[7,8] In 1994, the U.S. Food and Drug Administration entered the picture, issuing public health advisories dealing with serious radiation-related skin injuries resulting from some fluoroscopic procedures.[9] Today's newer techniques and equipment have contributed to lower dose rates, but fluoroscopy procedures still produce the greatest radiation exposures in diagnostic radiology. Investigators continue to study methods to further reduce exposure rates.[7,10]

A key point with the use of the fluoroscope is distance, protection, and exposure. Distance is the main factor at reducing the amount of radiation exposure. The use of a continuous mode of radiation vs. pulsed emission is also a way to reduce exposure. The use of key protective gear is mandatory to ensure that eyes, thyroid, reproductive organs, and extremities are properly protected. The use of a standard dosimeter is also a key safety factor to quantify the amount of radiation one receives. Some physicians will also wear a "ring" dosimeter to measure radiation exposure of hands. There are various shields and safety garments that can be used for almost full body protection.

Pulsed Fluoroscopy Imaging

Some modern fluoroscopes have the capability of pulsed fluoroscopy, whereby the x-ray beam is emitted as a series of short pulses rather than continuously. At reduced frame rates, pulsed fluoroscopy can provide substantial dose savings. Images may be acquired at 15 frames per second rather than the usual 30 frames per second. Each image is displayed multiple times in sequence to provide a 30-frames-per-second display. Pulsed fluoroscopy can also be performed at even lower frame rates (e.g., 7.5 or 3 frames per second), but the display appears choppy when imaging rapidly moving regions such as the heart. This is because simply reducing the number of pulses results in an increase in image noise. Manufacturers may increase the milliamperage setting to achieve a similar visual appearance.

Image Storage

A typical portable fluoroscope used today is versatile and mobile and occupies less space in confined quarters than fixed units (**Fig. 3-5**). These units also allow one to store and archive images for scanning, reprinting, or illustrating details as to where needle placements are located. PACS (picture archiving and communication system) is a combination of hardware and software dedicated to the short- and long-term storage, retrieval, management,

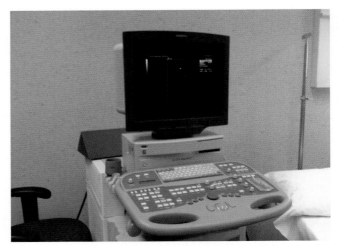

Fig. 3-5 The very safe and effective diagnostic tool, the ultrasound system, at the Space Coast Pain Institute.

distribution, and presentation of images. Electronic images and reports are transmitted digitally via PACS; this eliminates the need to manually file, retrieve, or transport film jackets. The universal format for PACS image storage and transfer is DICOM (digital imaging and communication in medicine). Non-image data, such as scanned documents, may be incorporated using consumer industry standard formats such as PDF (portable document format) after being encapsulated in DICOM.

PACS consists of four major components: the imaging modalities such as CT and magnetic resonance imaging; a secured network for the transmission of patient information; workstations for interpreting and reviewing images; and archives for the storage and retrieval of images and reports. Combined with available and emerging Internet technology, PACS has the ability to deliver timely and efficient access to images, interpretations, and related data. PACS breaks down the physical and time barriers associated with traditional film-based image retrieval, distribution, and display. Placing images of procedures on a template or CD allows for data storage, review, and proof of what was performed. This then confirms the intended procedure.

Conclusion

All imaging techniques may allow exposure to harmful radiation or heat. Although ultrasound appears to be extremely safe, some of its effects are unknown. The safety of the patients and the staff and physician performing these procedures is critical. This is why lead barriers, shields, and distance are major measures to ensure that patients and health care professionals are not exposed to excessive radiation. With all of the image-guided techniques at our disposal, safe use of the devices remains imperative for the patient, staff, and physician team. Adherence to strict principles will allow physicians to continue to provide injection therapy at a reduced risk to all.

References

1. National Council on Radiation Protection and Measurements: *Basic radiation protection*, NCRP Report No. 39, Washington, DC, 1971, The Council, p 106.
2. GF Health Products: Material Safety Data Sheet, Rev No: A. August 2003, accessed from http://www.grahamfield.com/pdfs/MSDS%20 Aerosil%20(AQ106-12)%2007.19.06.pdf.

3. Feigal DW, Jr: Letter regarding CT scan safety.
4. Dill CE, Uraneck K: Radiation Screening. *Acad Emerg Med* 18(1):105, 2011.
5. Waldman S: *Interventional pain management*, ed 2, Leawood, KS, 2011, Headache and Pain Center.
6. Hall EJ: *Radiobiology for the radiologist*, ed 5, Philadelphia, 2002, Lippincott Williams & Wilkins.
7. Mahesh M: The AAPM/RSNA physics tutorial for residents. Fluoroscopy: patient radiation exposure issues. *Radiographics* 21:1033-1045, 2001.
8. King JN, Champlin, AM, Kelsey CA, Tripp DA: Using a sterile disposable protective drape for reduction of radiation exposure to interventionalists. *AJR Am J Roentgenol* 178:153-157, 2002.
9. Fajardo LF, Berthrong M, Anderson RE: *Radiation pathology*, New York, 2001, Oxford University Press.
10. Curry TS, Dowdey JE, Murry RC: Christensen's physics of diagnostic radiology, ed 2, Malvern, PA, 1990, Lea & Febiger.

II Peripheral Nerve Blocks

Chapter 4 Differential Diagnostic Nerve Blocks

Chapter 5 Head and Neck Blocks

Chapter 6 Upper Extremity Peripheral Nerve Blockade

Chapter 7 Lower Limb Blocks

Chapter 8 Cervical and Lumbar Sympathetic Blocks

Chapter 9 Nerve Destruction for the Alleviation of Visceral Pain

Chapter 10 Peripheral Applications of Ultrasonography for Chronic Pain

4 Differential Diagnostic Nerve Blocks

Jerald Garcia, I. Elias Veizi, and Salim M. Hayek

CHAPTER OVERVIEW

Chapter Synopsis: Diagnostic differential neural block (DDNB) is a tool that can help identify the source and nature of pain, particularly in patients for whom a diagnosis has been elusive. A better understanding of the pain can improve the chances of successful treatment. Many forms of DDNB have emerged since the "classic approach" was first used in 1964. Regardless of the specific mechanism of action, DDNB can help differentiate between several types of pain, including placebo-responsive, sympathetic, somatic, visceral, and central pain. Identification of pain as one of these types can in itself clarify a treatment path because it points to a specific source of dysfunction. The DDNB technique is based on the concept that nerve axon fibers vary in their susceptibility to anesthetics and other drugs. This susceptibility arises from the variation in axon fiber diameter, which has been used as a major classification of nerve types. A-fibers are the largest, myelinated fibers and are further classified into subcategories of A-α, A-β, A-γ, and A-δ fibers. Of these, A-δ fibers are most relevant to consideration of nociception; they convey sensations of temperature and sharp pain. B fibers subserve the autonomic nervous system. Unmyelinated C fibers are slowly-conducting sensory nerves that convey many pain sensations, usually with a dull aching or burning quality. The chemical properties of the various blockers used in DDMB are considered here, as are the factors that underlie susceptibility to block. Each approach to the procedure carries its own technical and interpretive considerations as well.

Important Points:
- Despite its limitations, DDNBs can aid in distinguishing, in broader terms, pain with significant peripheral component versus pain with predominant central component.
- When integrated with other clinical findings, DDNBs can guide the physician into understanding predominant pain mechanisms, especially of patients whose pain diagnoses have been elusive and largely untreated.
- DDNBs have the potential ability to prognosticate successful response to interventions such as surgery or neurolysis before its implementation.
- The levels of the block achieved does not imply with certainty conduction block of all nerve fibers.
- Variability exists in the rate of recovery among sympathetic, visceral, and somatic fibers after the blocks wears off.
- The role of local anesthetic properties on the nerve fiber susceptibility is not well defined.
- Local anesthetic formulation (pH, lipophilicity, baricity) could significantly affect the results of the DDNB.
- Pain cannot be characterized as only central even in the event of a negative DDNB result because peripheral mechanisms can still be present.

Clinical Pearls:
- The level of the block and its assessment is important, particularly for abdominal visceral pain, where fibers from visceral organs could synapse over several spinal cord segments.
- DDNBs may help to distinguish, in broad terms, an organic versus non-organic cause for pain.
- DDNBs, together with clinical, radiological, laboratory, history, physical examination, and psychosocial findings, need to be integrated together as parts of a complex puzzle in order to effectively diagnose and meaningfully treat the totality of a patient's pain presentation.

Clinical Pitfalls:
- Neurophysiological data have undermined some of the basic assumptions associated with DDNBs, and in doing so also limit the validity of its interpretation.
- Blocking the action potentials of nociceptive peripheral nerves close to the site of initial injury may not necessarily stop the spontaneous firing of the dorsal root ganglia (DRG), and the patient's perception of pain still remains.
- Interindividual variations in neural anatomy and local anesthetic response need to be taken into account when performing DDNBs.

Introduction

Differential neural blockade has been used to obtain diagnostic information for ill-defined pain conditions that elude specific diagnoses. The technique, although deemed controversial by some,[1] can have the potential to aid pain physicians with a more objective assessment of a patient's pain and in doing so aid in developing a better approach to treatment.[2,3] The International Association for the Study of Pain defines pain as an "unpleasant sensory and emotional experience associated with actual or potential tissue damage, or described in terms of such damage."[4] One aspect of pain is nociception, which entails a complex series of electrochemical events that entail transduction of nociceptive stimuli from receptive nerve endings, transmission of impulses, modulation, and translation of subjective sensory and emotional experiences of pain.[5] Other factors either unrelated or reinforced by this processes contribute to the pain experience. Thus, one of the greatest challenges that face many pain physicians today is identifying the relative contributions of psychosocial, cognitive, visceral, and somatic contributions involved in a patient's perception of pain. The rationale for performing diagnostic differential neural blocks (DDNBs) is based on the selective blockade of specific neurological pathways and/or modalities while sparing others. In doing so, DDNBs have the potential to do the following[6]: (1) help to determine whether a patient has predominantly a physical or psychological component contributing to the experience of pain, (2) aid in assessing whether pain is mediated via sympathetic or somatic fibers, (3) identify potential response to placebo, and (4) predict a patient's likelihood for success from interventions such as surgery or neurolysis.

The approach to DDNB is varied and may have evolved over the years. The "classic approach," as described in 1964 by McCollum and Stephen,[7] proposes varying concentrations of local anesthetic to be injected intrathecally. This approach mainly relies on the relative susceptibilities of the different types of nerve fibers to create a concentration-dependent response differential that enables the selective blockade of specific neuronal pathways while sparing others. The "modified approach" was introduced as a more time-efficient and practical alternative to its classic counterpart.[3,8,9] Subsequently, clinicians used the "epidural approach" in the hopes of minimizing post–lumbar puncture cephalgia associated with spinal injections.[2] Other approaches that have also been introduced include the "anatomical approach" and the "opioid approach." The "anatomical approach" relies on the sequential blockade of specific nerve fibers based on its anatomical locations as opposed to differential susceptibility to varying concentrations of local anesthetic.[3] The "opioid approach," introduced in 1985, suggests the use of epidural opioid in lieu of local anesthetics to eliminate a potential source of bias (i.e., cues of numbness and warmth that the local anesthetic may give to patients undergoing the test).[6] The latter two approaches do not necessarily provide better diagnostic value than the classic or modified approaches. On the contrary, critics have pointed out that they may be less effective in differentiating specific pain pathways as will be discussed further below.[1,10-12]

Whatever the approach, a DDNB's utility should lie in its ability to potentially identify a specific neural pathway or pain syndrome for which a diagnosis has not yet been clearly established, especially when an extensive medical workup fails to identify a cause for the pain.

Historical Perspective

The concept of differential nerve blockade is largely based on the early studies of Gasser and Erlanger in 1929.[13,14] These two American scientists who studied the effects of cocaine on canine peripheral nerves suggested that small-diameter nerve fibers were more susceptible to the blocking actions of local anesthetics compared with larger nerve fibers because the former possess greater surface to volume ratio, thus rendering the axoplasm more readily infiltrated by local anesthetics.[14] This early model of differential neural blockade has come to be known as the "size principle" and has also served as an explanation for the differential loss of function observed clinically during spinal and epidural anesthesia.[15,16] These findings subsequently led to the use of differential spinal blocks as a diagnostic tool for pain.[7,13] However, neurophysiological evidence has since disproven Gasser and Erlanger's concept of nerve

conduction, and over time, their "size principle" has also been challenged.[17-19] In 1989, Fink[20] proposed the "length principle" as an alternative explanation. This principle suggests that for nerve fiber conduction to be blocked, three consecutive nodes of Ranvier must be exposed to the local anesthetic.[21] The "length principle" has been considered an extension rather than a renunciation of the original "size principle" because axonal diameter does correlate with internodal distance.[22] The thicker the diameter of an axon, the further the internodal distance and the less amount of nodes likely exposed to a given amount of local anesthetic. However, the "size principle," which has influenced most of the work on differential blocks, could be misleading because given a sufficient length of nerve, there is no apparent difference in the concentration of local anesthetics required for a conduction nerve block in all fibers.[23] To proponents of DDNBs, Fink's "length principle" provides a valid explanation that links stepwise loss of function observed clinically with neuraxial anesthesia to the concept of differential nerve fiber susceptibility and thus justifies, to a certain extent, its use as a diagnostic tool for pain.[3]

Classification of Five Types of Pain

DDNBs, as classically described, involve injecting saline and then local anesthetic in gradually increasing strengths into the spinal space.[7] The goal is to delineate the underlying pain mechanism that could fall under one of five types:

Placebo-Responsive Pain

Pain is considered to be placebo responsive if relief occurs after the injection of saline. It has been shown that up to 35% of patients with true organic pain actually respond to placebo; however, this is short lived and self-limiting.[24] If pain relief after placebo persists for an extended period of time, an underlying psychogenic pain mechanism may be considered.

Sympathetic Pain

Pain mediated by sympathetic fibers is inferred if the patient experiences relief after sympathetic fibers are blocked with sympatholytic concentrations of anesthetic, which are thought to be lower anesthetic concentrations sufficient enough to block sympathetic preganglionic B fibers while sparing other fiber types.[25,26] Pain relief should occur concomitantly with signs of sympathetic blockade such as temperature changes and sympathogalvanic response (SGR; the activation of sweat glands by postganglionic sympathetic fibers) but without signs of sensory block.

Somatic Pain

Somatic pain is considered if the patient experiences relief only after a higher concentration of anesthetic is injected and cutaneous sensation to pinprick or temperature is abolished. This type of pain is subserved by Aδ fibers, C fibers, or both.

Visceral Pain

Visceral pain is pain originating from internal organs. Stimuli required to elicit pain in visceral organs vary between structures (e.g., the myocardium is sensitive to ischemia but not to mechanical stimulation). The quality of visceral pain is often different from somatic pain. Although somatic pain is initially sharp followed by localized burning or throbbing, visceral pain tends to be poorly localized, presenting as dull, aching sensations. Although this type of pain is conducted by Aδ and C fibers, the ratio of Aδ to C fibers is 1:10 in viscera as opposed to 1:2 in cutaneous afferents.[27]

Furthermore, visceral nociceptive fibers have extensive overlap among their receptive fields.[28,29]

Central Pain

If the patient does not gain any relief from any of the injections despite achieving surgical levels of anesthesia of nerves that cover the target organ, then a central mechanism or pain generator should be suspected. Central pain can be attributed to one of four possible causes, including central lesions, true psychogenic pain, malingering, or encephalization.[2] Central lesions involve damage to or dysfunction of the central nervous system (CNS) above the level of the differential nerve block. Examples include poststroke thalamic pain and multiple sclerosis. Pain with psychogenic features refers to physical pain perpetuated by an underlying psychological disorder such as depression or anxiety. Encephalization is a poorly understood phenomenon that has been proposed to explain central pain[3] whereby chronic, severe pain of peripheral origin becomes self-sustaining at a central level and remains persistent despite removal of the original peripheral triggering mechanism. Malingering is the deliberate feigning or exaggeration of pain or illness in anticipation of some benefit such as financial compensation or avoidance of responsibility. There are no valid clinical methods for its assessment and thus can be difficult to prove or disprove.[30]

Classification of Nerve Fibers

Gasser and Erlanger[14] earlier developed the classification system for peripheral nerve fibers mainly based on axonal diameter, conduction velocity (in meters per second), and myelination. This system is still in use today and basically categorizes nerve fibers into three types: A, B, and C.

A Fibers

A fibers are myelinated fibers and are further classified into four subtypes. A-α fibers, the largest, are about 15 to 20 micrometers in diameter and subserve large motor function and proprioception; A-β fibers are about 8 to 15 μm in diameter, subserving small motor movements, touch, and pressure sensations; A-γ fibers are 4 to 8 μm in diameter and subserve muscle tone and reflex; and A-δ fibers are 3 to 4 μm in diameter, are thinly myelinated, and are responsible for the transmission of temperature and sharp pain.

B Fibers

B fibers are also myelinated and have a diameter of about 3 to 4 μm. These fibers subserve the preganglionic autonomic system.

C Fibers

C fibers are unmyelinated and are only about 1 to 2 μm in diameter. They transmit dull pain and temperature.

Fiber diameter is a function of how heavily myelinated the axons are. Larger A fibers are heavily myelinated and have greater conduction velocities measured as the distance an action potential travels through an axon over time in meters per second. On the other hand, C fibers are unmyelinated and small in size and have the slowest conduction velocity.[31,32] Properties of nociceptive compared with non-nociceptive somatic afferent neurons include a longer action potential duration and a slower maximum rate of fiber firing. These properties appear to be graded according to the conduction velocity group with the slowest fibers having the longest action potential and least rate of fiber firing (C > Aδ > A-α/β).[33]

The Role of Local Anesthetics

Local anesthetics block the propagation of nerve impulses such as those for pain by inhibiting the formation and propagation of action potentials. Several mechanisms have been proposed, but most evidence suggest that the sodium channel is the key target.[34] By diffusing through the axonal membrane, local anesthetics bind to the cytoplasmic side of a sodium channel, thereby inhibiting conformational changes that would have otherwise resulted in the channel's opening for sodium influx and activation. Local anesthetics do not only block inward sodium channels but also the outward potassium channels, which might be an important effect because potassium channels are responsible for repolarization and maintenance of resting membrane potential, which affects excitability.[35,36] Clinical onset depends on the rate of diffusion through the neuronal membrane. Thus, amide-based local anesthetics such as bupivacaine that happen to be more lipophilic are thought to produce nerve blockade more readily than the less lipid soluble ester-based local anesthetics such as procaine. Lipophilicity allows the anesthetic to penetrate a nerve fiber more readily and exert its effect before being removed into the circulation. In theory, a less lipophilic local anesthetic would be the more ideal agent for DDNBs because they produce blockade of smaller fibers (e.g., C fibers) more readily but are then removed by the circulation before they can penetrate the diffusion barriers of larger fibers. As such, greater concentrations of ester-based anesthetics would be needed to create blockade of larger fibers and the differential is more easily established. In vivo studies, however, have found that regardless of type of local anesthetic, a differential in susceptibility exists based on fiber type with A-α fibers consistently less sensitive to local anesthetic, regardless of type, versus the smaller C or A-δ fibers.[37] The order of susceptibility to blockade by local anesthetic is as follows: (most susceptible to least susceptible) B < C < A-δ < A-γ < A-β < A-α.[2,3,20,38]

Proposed Mechanisms of Differential Neural Blockade

DDNBs are based on the premise that a given concentration of local anesthetic can selectively block a specific nerve fiber type while sparing others.[1] The mechanism of this differential effect is not clearly understood.[20,39] Several explanations have been offered.

Bathed Length Principle

For local anesthetics to effectively block a nerve fiber, at least three nodes of Ranvier need to be bathed in the anesthetic because conduction can leap two consecutive blocked nodes but not three.[40] Fink's "bathed length principle" suggests that a functional relationship between local anesthetic susceptibility and fiber length (and therefore size) exists.[20] That is, smaller diameter fibers are more easily blocked than larger diameter fibers, which tend to have greater internodal distance and thus tend to require more anesthetic for three consecutive nodes to be bathed. After the three-node requirement is met, there is a minimum concentration of local anesthetic required for each fiber type to have all of its sodium channels occupied before conduction can be blocked. This is known as the minimum blocking concentration (Cm). Smaller fibers are thought to have smaller Cms than larger fibers, enabling different types of fibers to respond to different concentrations of anesthetic.[19,41]

Sodium Channel Packing

Sodium channel density at the nodes of Ranvier are thought to be increased as fiber size increases.[42] This increased distribution of sodium channels on larger fibers is referred to as "sodium channel packing" and has been proposed as one possible mechanism that explains why larger fibers require a higher Cm than do smaller fibers.[3]

Decremental Conduction

Given an impulse conducting along an axon, there is thought to be a cumulative decrease in the currents excited with successive nodes of Ranvier.[20] For local anesthetic concentrations below the Cm, not enough sodium channels within a node are blocked such that at each node, the action potential undergoes a progressive reduction in amplitude and conduction until succeeding nodes are rendered vulnerable to even suboptimal doses of anesthetic. This phenomenon, referred to as "decremental conduction," has mainly been demonstrated in myelinated axons.[20,43] Thus, for anesthetic concentrations below the Cm, impulse blockade is more likely to occur in fibers in which a greater number of nodes are exposed. Larger fibers are therefore less vulnerable because even if conduction is decrementally slowed, not enough nodes are exposed to the lower anesthetic dose, enabling the impulse to again resume full conduction speed after the conducting membrane is again reached.

Frequency-Dependent Block

This phenomenon occurs when repetitive firing of a nerve effects a cumulative depression of sodium currents such that suboptimal doses of local anesthetic then become sufficient to establish blockade. This explains why preganglionic sympathetic B fibers, which convey repetitive, tonic vasoconstrictive impulses, are most susceptible to local anesthetic.[39,44] It has been proposed that both phenomena, frequency-dependent block and decremental conduction, may superimpose on each other and even further enhance the blocking effect of considerably low concentrations of local anesthetic.[3]

Diagnostic Differential Nerve Block: Classic Approach

The classic DDNB as described below is largely based on the works of Arrowood and Sarnoff in 1948[13] and McCollum and Stephen in 1964.[7] The technique involves injecting local anesthetic into the subarachnoid space to obtain diagnostic information from patients with lower extremity or lower trunk pain. This serves as the prototype diagnostic differential block from which subsequent versions are based.[3]

Description

The physician prepares four solutions of injectate in identical volumes. "Solution A" is labeled on the syringe containing normal saline, "Solution B" is labeled on the syringe containing procaine 0.25%, "Solution C" is labeled in the syringe containing procaine 0.5%, and "Solution D" is labeled on the syringe containing procaine 5%. After informed consent is obtained, the patient is prehydrated with a crystalloid solution via a peripheral intravenous (IV) line. The patient is then positioned laterally with the painful side down. Vital signs, including blood pressure and heart rate, and electrocardiography (ECG) are monitored throughout the procedure. The patient's baseline blood pressure, heart rate, and pain score are recorded. The low back is prepped and draped in the usual sterile fashion. A 25- to 27-gauge spinal needle is inserted at the L2-L3 or L3-L4 interspace and advanced into the subarachnoid

space, which is confirmed by the presence of cerebrospinal fluid (CSF) at the proximal end of the needle. The patient, who is blinded to the type of solution being injected, is asked to inform the physician which, if any, of the four solutions provides relief. The solutions are to be injected in 10- to 15-minute increments starting with Solution A followed by Solution B and then Solution C. If no relief is reported, Solution D is injected last. However, if the patient does report relief, maneuvers that typically reproduce the patient's pain are performed. During this time, the patient is asked to report any recurrence or increase in pain. After each injection, the patient's blood pressure, heart rate, and pain score are noted. Along with this, the physician is required to observe for and record signs of sympathetic blockade (e.g., temperature changes, SGRs), sensory blockade (e.g., no response to pinprick, temperature), and motor blockade (e.g., inability to wiggle the toes) after each and every injection.

Interpretation

If the patient reports relief of pain after the injection of Solution A (normal saline), his or her pain is thought to be placebo responsive. Psychologic facilitatory mechanisms may even be suggested if relief is long lasting because true placebo responses are usually short lived and self-limiting.[3] As such, a repeat procedure or psychological referral may be of value. If pain relief occurs after the injection of Solution B (procaine 0.25%), the inference is that sympathetic preganglionic B fiber activity is mainly involved. This is confirmed by clinical signs of a sympathectomy, which can include an increase in temperature and a SGR without concurrent signs of cutaneous or sensory involvement. These types of patients may respond beneficially to sympathetic blocks. If pain relief occurs after Solution C (procaine 0.5%) is injected and there is clinical evidence of sensory involvement such as diminished cutaneous sensation to pinprick covering the distribution of pain, then the implication is that A-δ fibers, C fibers, or both are involved. If relief is achieved only after Solution D (procaine 5%) is injected, the mechanism remains to be considered somatic in origin, taking into account the potential for interindividual variability with the presumption that some patients may have higher Cms.[3] If the patient does not obtain any relief despite evidence of complete sympathetic, somatic, and even motor blockade, the underlying pain mechanism is thought to be central in origin, which could point to any one of the four possible causes described earlier: CNS lesion, psychogenic pain, malingering, or encephalization.

Limitations

The classic approach can be a time-consuming process that may prove inconvenient to patients and inefficient to physicians who have to continuously monitor the patient to full recovery. When complete blockade is achieved, the time to full recovery can take several hours, which is not quite practical during times when reimbursements and time efficiency go hand in hand. Moreover, patients are required to remain in the lateral decubitus position throughout the procedure itself, limiting their ability to achieve other positions that would have otherwise reproduced the pain. This can thus compromise the reliability of their pain report. The other drawback is that injecting different concentrations of local anesthetic into the intrathecal space does not reliably predict the type of fiber that will be blocked among different individuals who, theoretically, can have different Cms. Finally, because the needle has to remain intrathecally during the length of the procedure, there is an increased theoretical risk for a postdural puncture headache (PDPH) or nerve root and even cord damage compared with the subsequent approaches later developed.

Diagnostic Differential Nerve Block: Modified Approach

The modified approach was developed as a more practical and expeditious alternative to its classic counterpart.[3,8,9] This approach uses only two of the four solutions. The goal is to block all types of fibers immediately. The patient is then observed in reverse order as fibers recover sequentially starting with the larger diameter fibers. Thus, instead of correlating pain relief with onset of fiber blockade, the modified approach correlates the return of pain with the return of fiber function.

Description

The physician prepares two solutions of injectate in identical volumes (≈ 2 mL). "Solution A" is labeled on the syringe containing normal saline, and "Solution B" is labeled on the syringe containing procaine 5%. After informed consent is obtained, the patient is prehydrated with a crystalloid solution via a peripheral IV line. The patient is positioned lateral with the painful side down. Vital signs, including blood pressure and heart rate, and ECG are monitored throughout the procedure. The patient's baseline blood pressure, heart rate, and pain score are noted. The low back is then prepped and draped in the usual sterile fashion. A 25- to 27-gauge spinal needle is then inserted at the L2-L3 or L3-L4 interspace and advanced into the subarachnoid space, which can be confirmed by the presence of CSF at the proximal end of the needle. The patient, who is blinded to the type of solution being injected, is asked to inform the physician which, if either, of the two solutions provides pain relief. The solutions are to be injected in 10- to 15-minute increments starting with Solution A. If there is no relief reported, Solution B is then injected. The patient is then placed in the supine position. If the patient reports relief, maneuvers that typically reproduce the patient's pain are performed, and the patient is told to report any recurrence or increase in pain. After each injection, the patient's blood pressure, heart rate, and pain score are noted. Along with this, the physician should also observe and record signs of sympathetic blockade (e.g., temperature changes, SGRs), sensory blockade (e.g., no response to pinprick, temperature), and motor blockade (e.g., inability to wiggle the toes) after each injection.

Interpretation

If the patient reports relief of pain after the injection of Solution A (normal saline), his or her pain is thought to be placebo responsive. As described previously, long-lasting relief after placebo may suggest an underlying psychogenic mechanism. If pain relief does not occur after injection of Solution B (procaine 5%) and there is evidence of anesthetic blockade, the underlying pain mechanism is thought to be central in origin, which could point to any one of four possible causes: CNS lesions, true psychogenic pain, malingering, or encephalization. If pain relief occurs after the injection of Solution B (procaine 5%), the mechanism is still considered organic with either sympathetic or somatic involvement. At this point, it is assumed that the patient likely will be insensate to pinprick and temperature and may or may not have a motor block. If pinprick or temperature sensation returns and relief continues, the underlying mechanism is then considered sympathetic. If pain returns upon return of pinprick or temperature sensation, the mechanism is likely somatic with A-δ and C fiber involvement.

Limitations

Given that only two solutions are used, this procedure is less time consuming. It also allows for faster recovery time mainly because a lesser amount of local anesthetic is injected. Additionally, the patient does not have to be positioned laterally for the duration of the procedure, and this not only allows for patient comfort but also for the appropriate evaluation of the patient's interpretation of pain relief as other positions that normally reproduce pain can be achieved. Finally, because this technique correlates the return of pain with the return of fiber function after the injection of one highly concentrated local anesthetic, there is less reliance on varying concentrations of local anesthetic and its effects on different fiber types, which could have varied and inconsistent results in different patients with different Cms.

Diagnostic Differential Nerve Block: Epidural Approach

To avoid a spinal puncture and thus diminish the chances of a spinal headache, the epidural approach has been proposed as an alternative to the spinal injections.[6] This epidural approach is procedurally similar to its spinal counterpart with the following exception: instead of the subarachnoid space, the epidural space is accessed for the injection of solutions. Thus, the epidural approach can also be done in two ways, mirroring the classic and modified versions described above.

Description

The epidural approach mirroring the classic procedure was introduced by Raj in 1977.[45] The epidural space is accessed using the loss-of-resistance technique via an epidural needle, and the solutions injected sequentially into the epidural space are as follows: "Solution A" containing normal saline; "Solution B" containing lidocaine 0.5%, considered the mean sympatholytic epidural concentration; "Solution C" containing lidocaine 1%, considered the mean sensory-blocking epidural concentration; and "Solution D" containing lidocaine 2%, considered the mean epidural concentration to block all modalities.

The epidural approach mirroring the modified procedure also involves two solutions of injectate in identical volumes. "Solution A" contains normal saline. "Solution B" contains lidocaine 2%. Alternatively, chloroprocaine may be used. After informed consent is obtained, the patient is prehydrated. The patient is placed in either the sitting or lateral position. Vital signs, including blood pressure and heart rate, and ECG are monitored throughout the procedure. The patient's baseline blood pressure, heart rate, and pain score are noted. The low back is then prepped and draped in the usual sterile fashion. An epidural needle is then inserted and advanced into the epidural space using the loss-of-resistance technique. An epidural catheter may be inserted through the needle that would allow additional injections of Solution B to achieve appropriate levels of anesthesia. The patient, who is blinded to the type of solution being injected, is asked to inform the physician which, if either, of the two solutions provides pain relief. The solutions are to be injected in 15- to 20-minute increments starting with Solution A. If there is no relief reported, Solution B is then injected. The patient is then placed in the supine position. If the patient does report relief, maneuvers that typically reproduce the patient's pain are performed, and the patient is told to report any recurrence or increase in pain. After each injection, the patient's blood pressure, heart rate, and pain score are noted. Along with this, the physician should also observe and record signs of sympathetic blockade (e.g., temperature changes, psychogalvanic reflexes), sensory blockade (e.g., no response to pinprick, temperature), and motor blockade (e.g., inability to the wiggle toes) after each injection.

Interpretation

Interpretation of the results of the epidural approach is similar to that for its subarachnoid counterparts. For the epidural approach mirroring the classic procedure, pain relief after Solution A (normal saline) is thought to be placebo responsive or psychogenic, after Solution B (lidocaine 0.5%) is sympathetic, and after Solution C (lidocaine 1%) or Solution D (lidocaine 2%) is somatic. If no relief is achieved, the underlying pain mechanism is thought to be central in origin.

For the epidural approach mirroring the modified procedure, relief after the injection of Solution A (normal saline) points to placebo-responsive or pain with psychogenic features. If pain relief does not occur after injection of Solution B (lidocaine 2%) and there is evidence of complete anesthetic blockade, the underlying pain mechanism is thought to be central in origin. If relief occurs after the injection of Solution B (lidocaine 2%), the mechanism is considered to be organic with either sympathetic or somatic involvement. If pinprick or temperature sensation returns and relief continues, the underlying mechanism is sympathetic. If pain returns upon return of pinprick or temperature sensation, the mechanism likely involves A-δ and C fibers. This modified epidural approach is less time consuming compared with the classic epidural approach.

Limitations

Local anesthetic, when injected into the epidural space versus the spinal space, can take longer for blockade to occur. Thus, the process can even be more time consuming. As with its spinal counterpart, injecting different concentrations of local anesthetic into the epidural space does not reliably predict the type of modality blocked, given that different people may have different Cms. The epidural approach mirroring the modified procedure addresses some of the limitations set forth by the epidural approach mirroring the classic procedure because not only is it less time consuming but there is also less reliance on the potentially variable and thus confounding effects of different concentrations of local anesthetic to the different types of nerve fibers. This main advantage of the epidural approach is that the intrathecal space is avoided; thus the risk of a having a PDPH, high spinal, or even a spinal cord injury is conceptually diminished.

Diagnostic Differential Nerve Block: Opioid Approach

One criticism of neuraxial DDNBs as previously described is that local anesthetics can provide patients with cues of numbness or warmth in the area of blockade,[1,3,46] especially if they have had previous experience with local anesthetics (e.g., from a laboring epidural or at a dentist office).[6] This cue could potentially or subconsciously alert the patient to the presumed onset of pain relief, which could potentially cast doubt on the interpretation of the patient's subjective response.[1,6,46] Thus, using epidural opioids have been suggested as an alternative to local anesthetics.[6,47] Opioid effects are thought to be more specific and do not provide the cues of numbness or warmth to trigger placebo responses.[1]

Description

The epidural space is accessed using the loss-of-resistance technique via an epidural needle. An epidural catheter is then inserted. A peripheral IV line is also started. Two solutions are injected via the epidural catheter sequentially in 20-minute intervals: "Solution A" contains 5 mL of normal saline; "Solution B" contains 1 µg/kg of fentanyl in 5 mL of normal saline. Forty minutes later, 0.4 mg

of naloxone is injected intravenously with the patient made unaware. If no relief is reported, 15 to 20 mL of lidocaine 2% is injected in the epidural catheter to provide sensory blockade to a level of T4 bilaterally as assessed by pinprick sensation.

Interpretation

Analgesia reported by the patient after the injection of fentanyl indicates a predominantly nociceptive mechanism for the pain versus a predominantly psychologic one. Reversal of analgesia after injection of naloxone by the unaware patient further confirms the primarily nociceptive mechanism. No response to any of the above injections, including lidocaine, implicates predominantly psychologic or social factors.[6]

Limitations

Epidural opioids may not be effective in relieving nonpsychogenic, neuropathic, or visceral pain.[1,11,12] Additionally, IV naloxone does not necessarily reverse the analgesic effects of epidural opioids completely.[48] There have been no formal studies comparing the opioid approach versus the other nonopioid approaches described.[1,6] Therefore, further studies are needed.

Diagnostic Differential Nerve Block: Anatomical Approach

The anatomical approach allows for the assessment of neck, upper extremity, thoracic, abdominal, pelvic, and lower extremity pain.[3] It relies on the anatomical separation of the types of fibers and as such involves the sequential performance of three blocks for each assessment: the placebo block, the sympathetic block, and the somatic block. The anatomical approach allows for the injection of local anesthetic to block only one type of fiber at a time. Additionally, it is thought to obviate the problems associated with a high spinal or epidural block and may be more appropriate to use for assessment of pain in the upper part of the body.[3]

Description

For upper extremity, head, and neck pain, using the anatomical approach begins with the injection of normal saline, usually at the site where the subsequent sympathetic or somatic block is performed. Relief after this injection indicates placebo or psychogenic features as previously described. If the placebo injection fails to provide relief, the practitioner then proceeds to perform a stellate ganglion block with a short-acting local anesthetic. Response to this usually suggests a sympathetic mechanism, as seen in complex regional pain syndrome (CRPS) of the upper extremity. If no relief is obtained, a block of the somatic nerves subserving the painful area is then carried out: trigeminal nerve or C2 blocks assess somatic pain involving the head or face, cervical plexus block for the neck, and brachial plexus block for the upper extremity pain.

For thoracic pain, the anatomical approach can be used, especially in cases in which an epidural DDNB is contraindicated. After the injection of placebo, a thoracic paravertebral sympathetic block is performed. This is followed by either a paravertebral somatic block or intercostal nerve block. Interpretation of results based on pain relief is similar to that previously described for head, neck, and upper extremity pain. The main caveat to using the anatomical approach in this region of the body is the associated increased risk for developing a pneumothorax.[3] For this reason, the epidural approach is considered to be the safer block for the assessment of thoracic pain.

For abdominal pain, as above, placebo is injected first. However, in this location, it is suggested that the somatic block is performed before sympathetic block.[31] The reason for this is that visceral pain, which largely courses via sympathetic fibers, can be more difficult to localize and characterize. Therefore, somatic or chest wall pain in the abdomen needs to be ruled out first.[3] Thus, if a paravertebral or intercostal block produces complete anesthesia of the body wall pain distribution yet the patient's and pain still persists, a celiac plexus or splanchnic nerve block is then performed to confirm if the pain is truly visceral in origin.

There is limited evidence for the use of DDNB as a diagnostic procedure for abdominal visceral pain, especially using an anatomical approach. In a study by Conwell et al,[49] differential neuraxial blockade was used to determine the source of chronic abdominal pain in patients diagnosed with chronic pancreatitis. The modified epidural approach was used, and saline or 2% lidocaine was injected in a stepwise fashion to achieve surgical anesthesia. Patients were evaluated for recovery of motor and sensory function every 10 minutes. On the basis of the response to local anesthetic, pain was characterized as visceral, somatic (nonvisceral), or central in origin. Based on their results, the authors found that the majority of patients had nonvisceral chronic pain (only four of 22 had a positive visceral responses to DDNB) despite a pre-DDNB diagnosis of chronic pancreatitis. While recognizing the limitations of the technique, the authors concluded that DDNB is a useful procedure in attempting to diagnose visceral origin of pain, which could dictate further treatment plans.

For pelvic pain, the sequence is similar to that of abdominal pain. Thus, if there is no response to placebo, an intercostal or paravertebral somatic block is done. This is then followed by a superior hypogastric plexus block, which is subserved by sympathetic fibers. Pain relief only after a superior hypogastric plexus block establishes a high likelihood of true visceral pain.

For lower extremity pain, if a placebo block results in no response, a lumbar sympathetic block is performed at the L2-L4 level followed by a lumbosacral plexus block for somatic blockade. Response after the lumbar sympathetic block signifies a sympathetic mechanism as one sees with lower extremity CRPS. Response only after the lumbosacral plexus block indicates a somatic mechanism.

Interpretation

The anatomical approach is interpreted similar to the classic approach previously described. That is, pain relieved after the placebo block is deemed either placebo responsive or psychogenic. Pain relieved after any of the sympathetic blocks is thought to be sympathetically mediated or visceral if the thorax, abdomen, or pelvis is involved. Pain relieved after any of the peripheral blocks is interpreted as somatic and therefore subserved by A-δ and C fibers. Failure to obtain relief after the three types of blockade is considered to be consistent with an underlying central mechanism as previously discussed.

Limitations

The anatomical approach, when compared with other approaches, can be more painful and less precise.[3] It can involve three separate injections per patient. Additionally, because pain involving visceral structures can be subserved by a combination of sympathetic and somatic fibers,[10] delineating a sympathetic versus a somatic mechanism for thoracic, abdominal, or pelvic pain may not always be as clear cut. Furthermore, there is potential for placebo response after each injection, whether sympathetic or somatic. Finally, because of the increased risk for a pneumothorax when performing

paravertebral sympathetic blocks, the anatomical approach is considered less than ideal for the evaluation of thoracic pain.[3]

Discussion

The concept of differential neural blockade has been described since the 1920s. Yet many decades later, its validity and utility as a diagnostic measure remains under a cloud of controversy and scrutiny.[1,46] The interaction between local anesthetic and nerve fiber is dynamic and influenced by multiple factors such as location of nerve fibers in the nerve bundle, the length exposed to the local anesthetic, the degree of activity of the nerve, and the local tissue factors (e.g., pH).

The basic premise that certain concentrations of local anesthetic block specific fibers in sequential fashion while sparing others is not a widely accepted concept. Hogan and Abram,[1] for example, point to the "impossibility of complete block of one fiber type without at least a partial block of others." In addition, although the sympathetic fibers are thought to be blocked first and recover last, some have argued that there may not be a size-related differential in fiber susceptibility, citing that the larger A-β fibers can be blocked by a concentration that spares the smaller C fibers.[41] It has been demonstrated and confirmed that conduction block in myelinated nerve fibers are not linearly correlated with fiber conduction velocity/fiber size.[50] Evidence that large-diameter fibers are more readily susceptible to local anesthetic is contrary to the notion of DDNB.[19] These findings tend to suggest the absence of a true differential (i.e., sympathetic versus somatic pain may not be as easy to delineate as once thought).

Neurophysiological data have undermined some of the basic assumptions associated with DDNBs and in doing so, also limit the validity of its interpretation.[1,46] For example, one premise of DDNBs is that pain is generated from a single peripheral source, and its impulses then travel via "unique and consistent" neural pathways.[1] However, this may not always be the case. In chronic neuropathic pain states, the dorsal root ganglia (DRG) of injured nerves can spontaneously generate pain impulses with or without peripheral nerve or nociceptor activation. Thus, blocking nociceptor or peripheral nerves close to the site of initial injury but distal to the DRG may not stop the spontaneous firing of the DRG. Therefore, the patient's perception of pain remains. This would then lead to the mistaken assumption that the injured nerve is not responsible for the patient's pain. Pain does not necessarily involve one specific peripheral source, pathway, or mechanism as a simplistic interpretation of a DDNB would suggest. There can be complex and possibly multiple neurophysiological processes that play a role in the generation, propagation, and maintenance of pain, each contributing its own unique dimension and adding to the complexity of the experience of pain. These are factors that need to be taken into consideration by the clinician when interpreting the results of a DDNB.

DDNB is not a one size fits all phenomenon. Interindividual variations in neural anatomy and local anesthetic response need to be taken into account.[1] For example, the Cm can differ among different patients and different patient conditions. Lidocaine 0.25% that is thought to selectively block predominantly sympathetic fibers for some individuals may be enough of a concentration to block all types of sensory fibers for others.[1,6] Actively firing afferent fibers such as those from injured peripheral nerves may be more sensitive to local anesthetic and thus tend to have lower than normal Cms such that very low concentrations of anesthetics can reduce maximum firing rates of the axons and produce pain relief without necessarily diminishing skin sensation to temperature or pinprick.[1] Thus, pain relief may be erroneously attributed to sympathetic blockade when nociceptive fibers were actually blocked. Nerve fiber sensitivity to local anesthetics varies. This is demonstrated by the differential ability of bupivacaine at a given concentration to block sensory fibers, but not motor fibers, to the same extent as lidocaine.[51] The different structure of sodium channels, their distribution throughout the nervous system, and the affinity of different local anesthetics for the various channels could account for variability in the results of the DDNB.

The level of the block and its assessment is important, particularly for the abdominal visceral pain, where fibers from visceral organs could synapse over several spinal cord segments. The sensory modalities used are cold pinprick and touch representing signals carried by different classes of nerve fibers. Differential block has been assessed using cutaneous current perception thresholds (CPTs).[52] This methodology uses an electrical stimulus to enable a direct quantitative assessment of A-β, A-δ, and C fibers. The authors demonstrated that after a spinal block, the return of the CPTs to baseline occurred sequentially: first, the A-β fiber CPTs returned to baseline, and this correlated with the return of touch sensation; then the return of A-δ fiber CPTs to baseline occurred, and this correlated with the return of sharp pinprick sensation; and, finally, the return of C fiber CPTs to baseline occurred, correlated with the return of cold sensation. They also demonstrated that loss of tolerance to a painful stimulus correlated with the recovery of A-β fiber CPTs to baseline at a time when A-δ and C fiber CPTs were still significantly elevated. Because A-β fibers are not considered to carry nociceptive information, the authors concluded that pain can occur when there is partial recovery of A-δ and C fibers and that "assessing the dermatomal level to touch rather than pinprick may be a more useful predictor of the dermatomal level of the block."[52] These variances, if not recognized, can degrade the accuracy of information that DDNBs provide.

Potentially confounding factors exist such as the improper use of pain scales, problems associated with placebo effects, bias from patient expectations, and observer error. These are thought by some to limit the usefulness of the interpretation of DDNBs.[1,6,46] Finally, our concept of pain (especially chronic pain) is constantly evolving as scientific research continues to provide us with new insight. Pain is currently regarded as a predominantly subjective phenomenon with complex physiologic, anatomical, and psychosocial facets that contribute to its totality.[3,46] A patient undergoing a DDNB may be motivated by external factors that enter into his or her reporting. Examples cited are reassurance or confirmation of suspicions to persuade doubting family members or the patients themselves or certification of disability for legal or financial gain.[46] As such, pain can be difficult to measure from a purely quantitative standpoint. Thus, physicians need to use caution and recognize the potential for misinterpretation of DDNBs to avoid inappropriate therapy.[46]

Conclusion

Despite their shortcomings, DDNBs continue to be used in clinical practice today.[3] A retrospective review of 100 patients with chronic pain who underwent a DDNB after all other diagnostic measures had failed to establish a cause has shown that DDNBs are effective in diagnosing the underlying pain mechanism.[53] This same study reports that 74% of the patients studied were unexpectedly found to have an underlying sympathetic mechanism. Had these differential blocks not been performed, it is likely that their pain would have been attributed to a psychogenic mechanism[3] and erroneously treated as such. This is true especially because for many of these

patients, their chronic pain syndrome have come to manifest as "bizarre" signs and symptoms seemingly "unrelated" to the true underlying cause.[3] It is also plausible that had a diagnosis been established and sympathetic blocks performed early on, a more positive outcome would have resulted for these patients.[3] Furthermore, recent studies might enhance the role for DDNB in chronic visceral pain.[49] However, there remains to be a scarcity of controlled studies supporting or negating the use of DDNBs.[46] Additionally, there have been no outcome studies to support any claims that differential blocks lead to the selection of appropriate treatment.[1] Thus, it is difficult to make a definitive conclusion given that further studies are needed.

Regardless, it is our belief that DDNBs do and will continue to have a role in the diagnosis of pain, especially when the underlying cause has remained elusive and prior treatments have not been effective. The utility of DDNBs lie in their ability to distinguish, in broader terms, an organic versus a non-organic cause for pain. To emphasize an earlier point, it is important for physicians to know that DDNB is by no means the gold standard for the diagnosis and management of pain. It has its limitations that need to be recognized and taken into account. Its results need to be interpreted merely as one piece of a complex puzzle. Other clinical, radiological, laboratory, history, and physical examination findings, as well as psychosocial factors, represent the other pieces. All of these pieces need to be integrated together to effectively diagnose and meaningfully treat the totality of a patient's pain presentation.

References

1. Hogan QH, Abram SE: Neural blockade for diagnosis and prognosis. A review. *Anesthesiology* 86:216-241, 1997.
2. Molloy RE, Candido KD: Diagnostic nerve blocks. In Benzon H, Raja SN, Molloy R, Liu S, Fishman SM, editors: *Essentials of pain medicine and regional anesthesia*, ed 2, Philadelphia, 2005, Elsevier, pp 181-189.
3. Winnie AP, Candido KD: Differential neural blockade for the diagnosis of pain. In Waldman SD, editor: *Pain management*, Philadelphia, 2007, Saunders, pp 155-166.
4. Pain terms: a list with definitions and notes on usage. Recommended by the IASP Subcommittee on Taxonomy. *Pain* 6:249, 1979.
5. Heinricher MM, Cheng ZF, Fields HL: Evidence for two classes of nociceptive modulating neurons in the periaqueductal gray. *J Neurosci* 7:271-278, 1987.
6. Cherry DA, Gourlay GK, McLachlan M, Cousins MJ: Diagnostic epidural opioid blockade and chronic pain: preliminary report. *Pain* 21:143-152, 1985.
7. McCollum DE, Stephen CR: The use of graduated spinal anesthesia in the differential diagnosis of pain of the back and lower extremities. *South Med J* 57:410-416, 1964.
8. Ahlgren EW, Stephen CR, Lloyd EA, McCollum DE: Diagnosis of pain with a graduated spinal block technique. *JAMA* 195:813-816, 1966.
9. Ramamurthy S, Winnie AP: Diagnostic maneuvers in painful syndromes. *Int Anesthesiol Clin* 21:47-59, 1983.
10. Al-Chaer ED, Traub RJ: Biological basis of visceral pain: recent developments. *Pain* 96:221-225, 2002.
11. Arner S, Arner B: Differential effects of epidural morphine in the treatment of cancer-related pain. *Acta Anaesthesiol Scand* 29:32-36, 1985.
12. Hogan Q, Haddox JD, Abram S, et al: Epidural opiates and local anesthetics for the management of cancer pain. *Pain* 46:271-279, 1991.
13. Arrowood JG, Sarnoff SJ: Differential spinal block; use in the investigation of pain following amputation. *Anesthesiology* 9:614-622, 1948.
14. Gasser HS, Erlanger J: The role of fiber size in the establishment of a nerve block by pressure or cocaine. *Am J Physiol* 88:581-591, 1929.
15. Bromage PR: An evaluation of bupivacaine in epidural analgesia for obstetrics. *Can Anaesth Soc J* 16:46-56, 1969.

16. Greene NM: Area of differential block in spinal anesthesia with hyperbaric tetracaine. *Anesthesiology* 19:45-50, 1958.

17. Fink BR, Cairns AM: Differential slowing and block of conduction by lidocaine in individual afferent myelinated and unmyelinated axons. *Anesthesiology* 60: 111-120, 1984.

18. Franz DN, Perry RS: Mechanisms for differential block among single myelinated and non-myelinated axons by procaine. *J Physiol* 236:193-210, 1974.

19. Gissen AJ, Covino BG, Gregus J: Differential sensitivities of mammalian nerve fibers to local anesthetic agents. *Anesthesiology* 53:467-474, 1980.

20. Fink BR: Mechanisms of differential axial blockade in epidural and subarachnoid anesthesia. *Anesthesiology* 70:851-858, 1989.

21. Fink BR, Cairns AM: Lack of size-related differential sensitivity to equilibrium conduction block among mammalian myelinated axons exposed to lidocaine. *Anesth Analg* 66:948-953, 1987.

22. Raymond SA, Strichartz GR: The long and short of differential block. *Anesthesiology* 70:725-728, 1989.

23. Fink BR, Cairns AM: Lack of size-related differential sensitivity to equilibrium conduction block among mammalian myelinated axons exposed to lidocaine. *Anesth Analg* 66:948-953, 1987.

24. Beecher HK: The powerful placebo. *JAMA* 159:1602-1606, 1955.

25. Fink BR, Cairns AM: Differential use-dependent (frequency-dependent) effects in single mammalian axons: data and clinical considerations. *Anesthesiology* 67:477-484, 1987.

26. Heavner JE, de Jong RH: Lidocaine blocking concentrations for B- and C-nerve fibers. *Anesthesiology* 40:228-233, 1974.

27. Janig W, Morrison JF: Functional properties of spinal visceral afferents supplying abdominal and pelvic organs, with special emphasis on visceral nociception. *Prog Brain Res* 67:87-114, 1986.

28. Cervero F: Visceral versus somatic pain: similarities and differences. *Dig Dis* 27(suppl 1):3-10, 2009.

29. Cervero F: Sensory innervation of the viscera: peripheral basis of visceral pain. *Physiol Rev* 74:95-138, 1994.

30. Mendelson G, Mendelson D: Malingering pain in the medicolegal context. *Clin J Pain* 20(6):423-432, 2004.

31. Djouhri L, Lawson SN: Abeta-fiber nociceptive primary afferent neurons: a review of incidence and properties in relation to other afferent A-fiber neurons in mammals. *Brain Res Rev* 46:131-145, 2004.

32. Djouhri L, Lawson SN: Differences in the size of the somatic action potential overshoot between nociceptive and non-nociceptive dorsal root ganglion neurones in the guinea-pig. *Neuroscience* 108:479-491, 2001.

33. Lawson SN: Phenotype and function of somatic primary afferent nociceptive neurones with C-, Adelta- or Aalpha/beta-fibres. *Exp Physiol* 87:239-244, 2002.

34. Liu SS: Local anesthetics: clinical aspects. In Benzon H, Raja SN, Molloy R, Liu S, Fishman SM, editors: *Essentials of pain medicine and regional anesthesia*, ed 2, Philadelphia, 2005, Elsevier, pp 558-565.

35. Brau ME, Vogel W, Hempelmann G: Fundamental properties of local anesthetics: half-maximal blocking concentrations for tonic block of $Na+$ and $K+$ channels in peripheral nerve. *Anesth Analg* 87:885-889, 1998.

36. Olschewski A, Hempelmann G, Vogel W, Safronov BV: Blockade of $Na+$ and $K+$ currents by local anesthetics in the dorsal horn neurons of the spinal cord. *Anesthesiology* 88:172-179, 1998.

37. Ford DJ, Raj PP, Singh P, et al: Differential peripheral nerve block by local anesthetics in the cat. *Anesthesiology* 60:28-33, 1984.

38. Rosenberg PH, Heinonen E, Jansson SE, Gripenberg J: Differential nerve block by bupivacaine and 2-chloroprocaine. An experimental study. *Br J Anaesth* 52:1183-1189, 1980.

39. Fink BR: Mechanism of differential epidural block. *Anesth Analg* 65:325-329, 1986.

40. Tasaki I: *Nervous transmission*, Springfield, IL, 1953, CC Thomas, p 164.

41. Fink BR, Cairns AM: Lack of size-related differential sensitivity to equilibrium conduction block among mammalian myelinated axons exposed to lidocaine. *Anesth Analg* 66:948-953, 1987.

42. de Jong RH: Differential nerve block. In *Local Anesthetics*. St. Louis, 1994, Mosby, p 84.

43. Lorente de No R, Condouris GA: Decremental conduction in peripheral nerve. Integration of stimuli in the neuron. *Proc Natl Acad Sci U S A* 45:592-617, 1959.

44. Folkow B: Impulse frequency in sympathetic vasomotor fibres correlated to the release and elimination of the transmitter. *Acta Physiol Scand* 25:49-76, 1952.

45. Raj PP: Sympathetic pain mechanisms and management. Second Annual Meeting of the American Society of Regional Anesthesia, Hollywood, FA 10-11 March 1977.

46. Raja SN: Nerve blocks in the evaluation of chronic pain. *Anesthesiology* 86:4-6, 1997.

47. Cousins MJ, Glynn CJ: New horizons. In Cousins MJ, Bridenbaugh PO, editors: *Neural blockade in clinical anesthesia and management of pain*, Philadelphia, 1980, Lippincott, pp 699-719.

48. Rawal N, Schott U, Dahlstrom B, et al: Influence of naloxone infusion on analgesia and respiratory depression following epidural morphine. *Anesthesiology* 64:194-201, 1986.

49. Conwell DL, Vargo JJ, Zuccaro G, et al: Role of differential neuroaxial blockade in the evaluation and management of pain in chronic pancreatitis. *Am J Gastroenterol* 96:431-436, 2001.

50. Fink BR, Cairns AM: Lack of size-related differential sensitivity to equilibrium conduction block among mammalian myelinated axons exposed to lidocaine. *Anesth Analg* 66:948-953, 1987.

51. Scholz A, Kuboyama N, Hempelmann G, Vogel W: Complex blockade of TTX-resistant $Na+$ currents by lidocaine and bupivacaine reduce firing frequency in DRG neurons. *J Neurophysiol* 79:1746-1754, 1998.

52. Liu S, Kopacz DJ, Carpenter RL: Quantitative assessment of differential sensory nerve block after lidocaine spinal anesthesia. *Anesthesiology* 82:60-63, 1995.

53. Winnie AP, Collins VJ: The pain clinic. I. Differential neural blockade in pain syndromes of questionable etiology. *Med Clin North Am* 52:123-129, 1968.

5 Head and Neck Blocks

Samer Narouze

Chapter Synopsis: This chapter deals with various cephalic nerve and ganglia block procedures. Difficult pain conditions, including cluster headache, other trigeminal autonomic cephalalgias, and persistent idiopathic facial pain, can be treated with block or radiofrequency ablation (RFA) of the sphenopalatine ganglion (SPG). This extracranial structure represents a confluence of autonomic nerve fibers, both sympathetic and parasympathetic. The details of its anatomy and physiology are considered here, which have ramifications for the treatment of these disorders. Potential complications of the procedure stem mainly from disruption of autonomic fibers or the nearby maxillary nerve. Block and neurolytic procedures at the trigeminal nerve and Gasserian ganglion can be used to treat patients with intractable trigeminal neuralgia as well as some orofacial pain syndromes. Although radiofrequency thermocoagulation seems to produce the best outcomes among similar techniques, it also carries a significant risk of complications. Maxillary and mandibular nerve block procedures are used primarily as diagnostic tools, but atlanto-axial and atlanto-occipital joint injections can be used for diagnostic, therapeutic, or prognostic procedures.

Important Points:
- SPG block and RFA are very useful in the management of patients with intractable cluster headaches, migraine, trigeminal autonomic cephalalgias, and persistent idiopathic facial pain ("atypical facial pain").
- Temporary diplopia is very common after SPG block because of spread of the injectate to the abducent nerve in the inferior orbital fissure. Diplopia may be used as a surrogate for a successful needle placement inside the pterygopalatine fossa (PPF).
- Practitioners should be familiar with the possible stimulation scenarios during SPG RFA to avoid lesioning the nearby maxillary nerve or branches. The optimal stimulation paresthesias should be behind the root of the nose.
- Percutaneous radiofrequency thermocoagulation of the Gasserian ganglion is very successful in the management of patients with intractable trigeminal neuralgia when the pharmacological treatment is either ineffective or intolerable.
- Percutaneous radiofrequency thermocoagulation of the Gasserian ganglion is usually considered for elderly patients at high risk for surgical microvascular decompression (MVD). The outcome may be less favorable than MVD, but it is less invasive with lower morbidity and mortality rates.
- The maxillary nerve exits through the foramen rotundum, which is located at the roof of the PPF. Hence, its block is essentially a modified SPG block.
- The mandibular nerve exits through the foramen ovale. The mandibular division (V3) is the most caudad and lateral part of the Gasserian ganglion.
- The mandibular nerve can be blocked with either the lateral pterygoid approach or the foramen oval approach.

Clinical Pearls:
- When performing SPG RFA, first look for inducing paresthesia at the root of the nose only to avoid injuring the maxillary nerve.
- When performing Gasserian ganglion RFA, try to be as selective as possible to the division affected to minimize potential adverse events.
- The approach to maxillary nerve block is essentially the same approach to SPG block; however, the needle is advanced more cephalad towards the foramen rotundum.

Clinical Pitfalls:
- Cranial nerves and ganglia blocks are advanced techniques that may be associated with considerable adverse events. One must be very familiar with the relevant anatomy to ensure a good outcome.
- Atlanto-axial and atlanto-occipital joint injections carry the risk of injuring the nearby vertebral artery. Use only when it is necessary. Always use contrast fluoroscopy. Adjuvant ultrasound may help delineate vertebral artery anatomy (normal or abnormal) before placing the needle.

Introduction

Head and neck blocks are essential in the diagnosis and management of various orofacial pain and headache syndromes. Sometimes the clinical presentation is not specific and has a low positive predictive value. In these cases, the only way to make a definitive diagnosis is by abolition of the headache or pain after blocking the nerve or joint in question.

Sphenopalatine Ganglion Block and Radiofrequency Ablation

Indications

Cluster headache involves activation of the parasympathetic outflow from the superior salivary nucleus of the facial nerve, predominantly through the sphenopalatine ganglion (SPG).[1] The SPG is a large extracranial structure that has rich autonomic innervation (both sympathetic and parasympathetic), which explains the autonomic features associated with cluster headache. SPG block and radiofrequency ablation (RFA) are indicated in the management of intractable medically-resistant cluster headaches, migraines, and other trigeminal autonomic cephalalgias, and intractable orofacial pain syndromes after exhausting other conservative treatment options (e.g., persistent idiopathic facial pain, "atypical facial pain").

Sphenopalatine Ganglion Neuroanatomy

The SPG has rich parasympathetic (preganglionic axons and postganglionic cell bodies and axons) and sympathetic (postganglionic axons) components. The parasympathetic preganglionic cell bodies projecting to the SPG originate in the superior salivatory nucleus (SSN) of the facial nerve in the pons.

The efferent fibers of the SSN travel in the nervus intermedius and divide at the geniculate ganglion to become the greater petrosal nerve and chorda tympani nerve. The first-order parasympathetic neurons in the greater petrosal nerve are joined by the postganglionic sympathetic fibers from the deep petrosal nerve, forming the nerve to the pterygoid canal (vidian nerve). The preganglionic parasympathetic neurons then synapse with the second-order parasympathetic neuronal cell bodies located in the SPG.

The postganglionic parasympathetic fibers then run with branches of the maxillary nerve (V2) to reach their targets. Therefore, the only cell bodies located within the SPG are those of the second-order postganglionic parasympathetic neurons, which may explain the clinical observation that patients after RFA of the SPG usually notice improvement of the autonomic parasympathetic symptoms either earlier or even without improvement of the headache pain.

The sympathetic cell bodies projecting to the SPG originate in the upper thoracic spinal cord (T1-T2). The preganglionic sympathetic neurons then synapse in the cervical sympathetic ganglia, mainly the superior cervical ganglion. The postganglionic second-order sympathetic neurons form the carotid sympathetic plexus and reach the pterygoid canal through the deep petrosal nerve, where it joins the first-order parasympathetic neurons in the greater petrosal nerve, forming the nerve to the pterygoid canal (vidian nerve). Postganglionic sympathetic fibers pass through the SPG without synapsing and innervate mainly blood vessels.

Sphenopalatine Ganglion Anatomy

The SPG is located in the pterygopalatine fossa (PPF), which is a small, upside-down pyramidal space 2 cm high and 1 cm wide. The PPF is located behind the posterior wall of the maxillary sinus and is bordered posteriorly by the medial plate of the pterygoid process, superiorly by the sphenoid sinus, and medially by the perpendicular plate of the palatine bone; laterally, it communicates with the infratemporal fossa. Superolaterally lies the foramen rotundum with the exiting maxillary nerve, and inferomedially, there is the vidian nerve (greater petrosal and deep petrosal nerves) within the pterygoid canal. The PPF contains the internal maxillary artery and its branches, the maxillary nerve, and the SPG and its afferent and efferent branches. The SPG is located posterior to the middle turbinate and is a few millimeters deep to the lateral nasal mucosa. It is suspended from the maxillary nerve by the pterygopalatine nerves; inferiorly, it is connected to the greater and lesser palatine nerves; and posteriorly, it is connected to the vidian nerve. Efferent

branches of the SPG form the posterior lateral nasal and pharyngeal nerves.[2,3]

Approaches to the Sphenopalatine Ganglion

The unique location of the SPG within the PPF, just posterior to the middle turbinate, makes it accessible transnasally as well as with the infrazygomatic approach.

Transnasal Approach   Because the SPG is located a couple of millimeters deep to the lateral nasal mucosa, topical application of local anesthetic solution to the posterior wall of the nasopharynx in the region of the middle turbinate can diffuse across the nasal mucosa to block the SPG.

Transnasal blockade of the SPG was first reported using topical cocaine.[4] Currently, lidocaine 4% is usually used.

The patient is placed in the supine position with the neck extended into a sniffing position. A 10-cm cotton tipped applicator soaked with 4% lidocaine is slowly advanced along the superior border of the middle turbinate until it reaches the posterior wall of the nasopharynx. The applicator is usually left in place for approximately 20 to 30 minutes to allow the local anesthetic to diffuse across the mucosa and reach the SPG.

Transnasal Endoscopic Approach   This endoscopic technique for transnasal injection and blockade of the SPG was first described by Prasanna and Murthy in 1993.[5] This technique allows a needle to be inserted transnasally under vision through the sphenopalatine foramen into the PPF.

Transoral Approach   The PPF can also be accessed transorally by placing a 27-gauge needle inside the greater palatine foramen. This approach is usually used by dentists to block the palatine nerves.[6]

Infrazygomatic Approach   Neuroablation techniques are only feasible with this infrazygomatic approach. Needle placement is usually guided by fluoroscopy; however, computed tomography guidance is reported as well.[7]

The infrazygomatic approach could be either anterior to the mandible or through the coronoid notch of the mandible.

Anterior Approach   The needle entry is inferior to the zygomatic arch, just anterior to the mandible, between the mandibular ramus and the posterior border of the zygomatic bone. The author prefers this approach because the needle can be advanced in a target view toward the PPF without the need to walk the needle off the lateral pterygoid plate (which is usually very painful) (**Fig. 5-1**). Also, it is much easier to steer the needle (cephalad–caudad or anterior–posterior) within the fossa to selectively target different structures within the fossa. However, this approach is not feasible in all patients because there might not be enough room between the mandible and the zygoma to insert the needle.

Coronoid Approach   The needle entry is through the coronoid notch of the mandible. The needle is usually advanced to target the lateral pterygoid plate first and then walked off the bone interiorly to enter the PPF. By that time, the needle usually acquires certain direction, and it is hard to manipulate the needle after it is inside the fossa (**Fig. 5-2**).

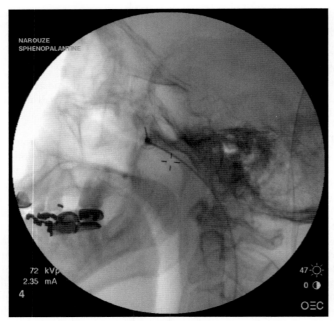

Fig. 5-1 Sphenopalatine ganglion block with the anterior approach. (Reproduced with permission from the Ohio Pain and Headache Institute.)

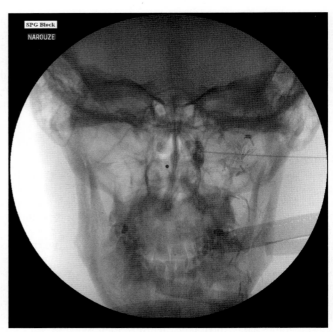

Fig. 5-3 Anteroposterior view showing the needle tip just lateral to the nasal wall. The contrast agent is delineating the pterygopalatine fossa. (Reproduced with permission from the Ohio Pain and Headache Institute.)

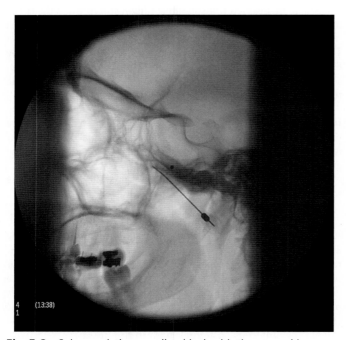

Fig. 5-2 Sphenopalatine ganglion block with the coronoid approach. (Reproduced with permission from the Ohio Pain and Headache Institute.)

Technique of Sphenopalatine Ganglion Block (Infrazygomatic Approach)

With the patient in the supine position and the head inside the C-arm, a lateral view is obtained and either the C-arm or the head of the patient is rotated until both pterygoid plates are superimposed on each other to better visualize the PPF. The skin entry site overlying the fossa is marked just inferior to the zygomatic arch either anterior to the mandible or through the coronoid notch. A 22-gauge, 3.5-inch blunt needle with a slight bend at the tip is used. The needle is first introduced in the lateral view and advanced medially and superiorly toward the PPF using real-time fluoroscopy. When in a proper direction, an anteroposterior (AP) view is obtained, and the tip of the needle is advanced to be just lateral to the nasal wall (**Fig. 5-3**). If the lateral pterygoid plate is encountered, the needle should be walked off the bone anteriorly and cephalad to slip into the fossa (the curved tip will help to guide the needle). A total of 0.1 to 0.2 mL of contrast agent is injected under real-time fluoroscopy to rule out intravascular spread because the PPF contains the maxillary artery and its branches (mainly the sphenopalatine artery). After negative aspiration of blood or air (the needle tip is too advanced into the nasal cavity or the maxillary sinus), 1 to 2 mL of 0.5% bupivacaine with or without steroids is injected slowly.

Radiofrequency Ablation Technique

With the patient in the supine position and the head inside the C-arm, a lateral view is obtained and either the C-arm or the head of the patient is rotated until both pterygoid plates are superimposed on each other to better visualize the PPF. The skin entry site overlying the fossa is marked just inferior to the zygomatic arch either anterior to the mandible or through the coronoid notch. A 22-gauge, 10-cm, blunt RFA needle with a 2- or 5-mm active tip with a slight bend at the tip is used (**Fig. 5-4**). The needle is first introduced in the lateral view and advanced medially and superiorly toward the PPF using real-time fluoroscopy. When in a proper direction, an AP view is obtained, and the tip of the needle is advanced to be just lateral to the nasal wall. If the lateral pterygoid plate is encountered, the needle should be walked off the bone anteriorly and cephalad to slip into the fossa (the curved tip will help to guide the needle). Sensory stimulation is obtained with

Table 5-1 Possible Scenarios of Stimulation before Attempting Radiofrequency Thermocoagulation of the Sphenopalatine Ganglion

Location of Paresthesia	Nerves Stimulated	Location of Needle Tip	Action Needed
Upper teeth and gums	Maxillary branches	Superolateral	Redirect the needle caudally and medially
Hard palate	Greater and lesser palatine nerves	Anterior, lateral, caudal	Redirect the needle posteromedially and cephalad
Root of the nose	SPG efferents; posterior lateral nasal nerves	Correct needle placement	None

SPG, sphenopalatine ganglion.
Adapted from Narouze S: Complications of head and neck procedures, *Tech Reg Anesth Pain Manag* 11:171-177, 2007.

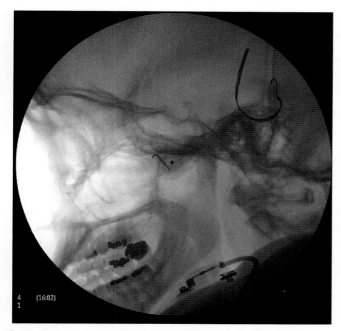

Fig. 5-4 Lateral view showing the RFA needle inside the pterygopalatine fossa (PPF). Note that the tip is curved downward to avoid lesioning of the maxillary nerve, which runs at the roof of the PPF. (Reproduced with permission from the Ohio Pain and Headache Institute.)

50 Hz to look for deep paresthesias behind the root of the nose at less than 0.5 V (**Table 5-1**). After proper stimulation is achieved and before lesioning, 0.1 to 0.2 mL of contrast agent is injected under real-time fluoroscopy to rule out intravascular spread. Then 0.5 mL of lidocaine 2% is injected, and two radiofrequency lesions are carried out at 80° C for 60 seconds each. After lesioning, 0.5 mL of bupivacaine 0.5% and 5 mg of triamcinolone is injected with the aim of preventing postprocedure neuritis.[8]

Efficacy of Sphenopalatine Ganglion Radiofrequency Ablation

In a retrospective analysis of patients with refractory cluster headache treated by RFA of the SPG, 56 patients with episodic cluster headache and 10 patients with chronic cluster headache were followed over a period of 12 to 70 months.[5] In the episodic cluster headache group, 60.7% experienced complete pain relief, but only three of 10 patients with chronic cluster headache had the same

result. This report showed that RFA of the PPG may improve episodic cluster headache but not chronic cluster headache. Recently, however, Narouze and colleagues[8] reported a favorable outcome after intractable chronic cluster headache as well. They reported significant improvement in both mean attack intensity and mean attack frequency for up to 18 months in 15 patients. Of these patients, 20% (three of 15) reported no change or increase in the headache intensity or frequency during the first few postprocedure weeks before noticing improvements in their headache pattern. However, 46.7% (seven of 15) of the patients reported a change in the headache pattern with return to the episodic form of cluster headache at a mean follow-up period of 18 months. Three patients remained headache free and off medications for the duration of the follow-up (18 to 24 months).

Two patients reported complete relief of their usual unilateral headache symptoms, and instead they developed episodic cluster headache on the contralateral side.[8]

Complications of Radiofrequency Ablation

Epistaxis is more frequent after the traditional intranasal topical application of local anesthetic; however, it can occur with this infrazygomatic approach if the needle is advanced too far medially through the lateral nasal wall.[9]

Intravascular injection and hematoma formation can occur after maxillary artery injury, which lies within the PPF (**Fig. 5-5**). Cheek hematoma is the most common complication. Infection is always a possibility, especially if the oral or nasal mucosa was accidentally penetrated.[9]

Reflex bradycardia was reported during radiofrequency lesioning, which could be explained by the rich parasympathetic connections to the SPG.[10] Radiofrequency lesioning of the SPG may result in permanent or, more commonly, temporary hypesthesia or dysesthesia in the palate, maxilla, or posterior pharynx.[2,3,8] Pulsed radiofrequency would seem to be safer; however, there are limited data for its efficacy.[11]

Dryness of the eye as a result of interruption of the parasympathetic supply is also common; however, it is usually only temporary. Temporary diplopia is more common after local anesthetic injections rather than RFA and can be explained by the spread of the injectate from the PPF to the inferior orbital fissure containing the abducent nerve.[12] The author has noticed that most of the patients develop temporary diplopia if the needle tip is really inside the PPF, which is why the volume should be limited to only 1 to 2 mL (**Fig. 5-6**).

A thorough understanding of the anatomy allows the clinician to predict correct needle placement during RFA according to the result of the stimulation and hence can reduce the incidence of complications (**Table 5-1**).[9]

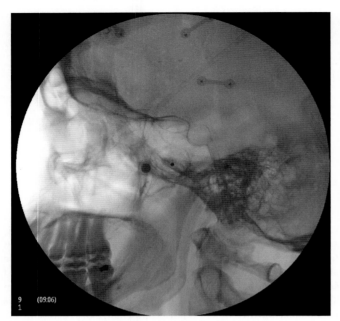

Fig. 5-5 Sphenopalatine ganglion block with the anterior approach showing intravascular spread. (Reproduced with permission from the Ohio Pain and Headache Institute.)

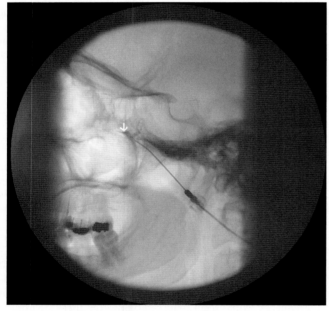

Fig. 5-6 Sphenopalatine ganglion block with the coronoid approach. The contrast is spreading into the inferior orbital fissure (*arrow*). (Reproduced with permission from the Ohio Pain and Headache Institute.)

Trigeminal Nerve and Gasserian Ganglion Block and Neurolytic Procedures

Trigeminal Nerve Block

Indications This is indicated for the diagnosis and management of intractable trigeminal neuralgia, both idiopathic and symptomatic (secondary) trigeminal neuralgia after failure of pharmacological management. It is also indicated before neuroablative or surgical procedures on the Gasserian ganglion to predict the prognosis after such neurodestructive procedures. It is also used for the diagnosis and management of various orofacial pain syndromes.

Percutaneous Gasserian Ganglion Neurolytic Procedures

Indications These are used for the management of intractable trigeminal neuralgia when the pharmacological treatment is either ineffective or intolerable. These procedures are usually used after a favorable response to a diagnostic trigeminal nerve block.

Gamma Knife and Stereotactic Radiation Therapy This is a noninvasive treatment that allows high-dose irradiation of a small section of the trigeminal nerve. This leads to nonselective damage of the Gasserian ganglion.[13]

Percutaneous Balloon Microcompression The Gasserian ganglion is compressed by a small balloon, which is percutaneously introduced through a needle into Meckel's cavity. This leads to ischemic damage of the ganglion cells. The technique may be more suitable for treatment of V1 trigeminal neuralgia of the first branch because the corneal reflex tends to remain intact.[14]

Percutaneous Glycerol Rhizolysis Under fluoroscopy in a sitting position with a flexed head, the needle is introduced into the trigeminal cistern visualized by radiography. Contrast agent is then injected to determine the size of the cistern before an equal volume of glycerol is injected after aspiration of the contrast agent.[15]

Percutaneous Radiofrequency Thermocoagulation of the Gasserian Ganglion This is usually considered for elderly patients at high risk for surgical microvascular decompression (MVD). The outcome may be less favorable than MVD, but it is less invasive with lower morbidity and mortality rates.[16]

Pulsed Radiofrequency Ablation of the Gasserian Ganglion Although it would seem a safer alternative than the commonly used thermal RFA, its efficacy is questioned in a randomized controlled study.[17]

Choice of Percutaneous Gasserian Ganglion Neurolytic Treatment

Few systematic reviews have compared the various treatment approaches for trigeminal neuralgia.[16,18,19] The first choice of treatment should be always conservative management. For those who fail pharmacological treatment, interventional management may be considered (**Fig. 5-7**).

Gasserian Ganglion Anatomy

The Gasserian ganglion lies within Meckel's cavity in the middle cranial fossa close to the petrous bone. It is surrounded medially by the cavernous sinus, superiorly by the inferior surface of the temporal lobe, and posteriorly by the brainstem.[20] Gasserian ganglion has three divisions with a characteristic somatotopic arrangement, in that the ophthalmic division (V1) is the most craniomedial and the mandibular division (V3) is the most caudolateral. The maxillary branch (V2) lies in between. The ophthalmic nerve exits through the superior orbital fissure, the maxillary nerve through the foramen rotundum, and the mandibular nerve through the foramen ovale.

The Technique of Gasserian Ganglion Block The procedure is usually performed with intravenous conscious sedation.

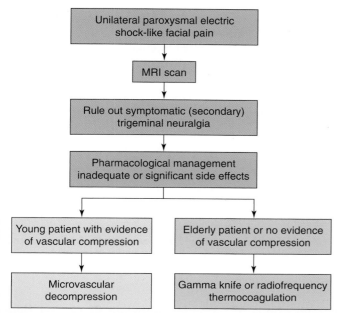

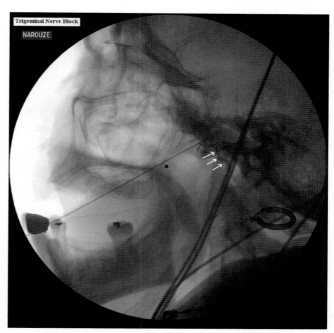

Fig. 5-7 Algorithm for the management of trigeminal neuralgia. MRI, magnetic resonance image.

Fig. 5-9 Gasserian ganglion block. Lateral view showing intravascular spread (*arrows*). (Reproduced with permission from the Ohio Pain and Headache Institute.)

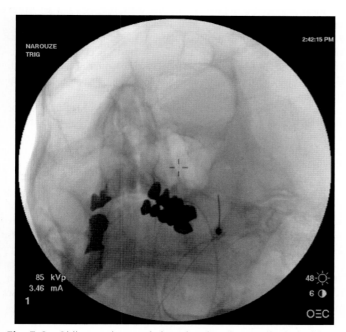

Fig. 5-8 Oblique submental view showing the needle tip inside the foramen ovale. (Reproduced with permission from the Ohio Pain and Headache Institute.)

The patient is in the supine position with the head inside the C-arm. After rotating the C-arm to obtain a submental view, the C-arm is slightly tilted to the affected side (oblique submental view) until the foramen ovale is best visualized (**Fig. 5-8**). It usually projects medially to the mandibular process. The point of the needle is about 2 cm lateral to the corner of the mouth on the ipsilateral side. A 3.5-inch, 22- to 25-gauge blunt nerve-stimulating needle is then advanced toward the foramen ovale under real-time fluoroscopy first in the AP submental view and then in the lateral view.

It is important to place a finger in the mouth to prevent or detect oral mucosa penetration. After the needle is inside the foramen ovale, motor stimulation is started, and muscle twitches should be observed in the mastication muscles (V3). There is no need to advance the needle farther inside the foramen ovale unless cerebrospinal fluid (CSF) will be aspirated from the needle. A total of 0.5 to 1 mL of contrast should be injected under real time fluoroscopy with digital subtraction, if available, to rule out intravascular spread (**Fig. 5-9**). After negative aspiration for CFS and blood, 1 to 2 mL of bupivacaine 0.5% with or without steroids can be injected slowly with close observation of the patient's hemodynamics and vital signs.

The Technique of Gasserian Ganglion Radiofrequency Thermocoagulation The procedure is usually performed under monitored anesthesia care with propofol or dexmedetomidine. The patient is in the supine position with the head inside the C-arm. After the C-arm is rotated so a submental view can be obtained, the C-arm is slightly tilted to the affected side (oblique submental view) until the foramen ovale is best visualized (**Fig. 5-8**). It usually projects medially to the mandibular process. The point of the needle is about 2 cm lateral to the corner of the mouth on the ipsilateral side. A 100-mm 22-gauge radiofrequency needle with a 2-mm active tip is then advanced toward the foramen under real-time fluoroscopy first in the AP submental view and then in the lateral view.

It is important to place a finger in the mouth to prevent or detect oral mucosa penetration. After the needle is inside the foramen ovale, testing stimulation is started. When motor stimulation (masseter muscle, V3) is encountered, the needle needs to be slightly advanced into the foramen carefully about 2 mm to stimulate V2. V1 is even deeper. In the lateral view, the needle tip should be deep into the foramen, overlying the petrous bone (**Fig. 5-10**). Some practitioners advocate that the patient should be covered with a broad-spectrum antibiotic if CSF is aspirated from the

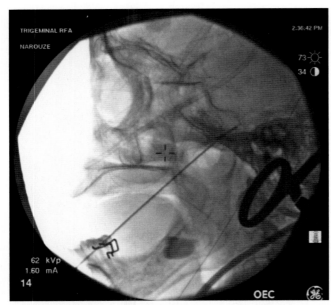

Fig. 5-10 Trigeminal ganglion thermal radiofrequency ablation. Lateral view showing the needle going through the foramen ovale with the needle tip overlying the petrous bone. (Reproduced with permission from the Ohio Pain and Headache Institute.)

Table 5-2 Complications of Percutaneous Gasserian Ganglion Neuroablative Procedures

	Radiofrequency Thermocoagulation	Glycerol Rhizolysis
Complications rate (%)	29.2	24.8
Masticatory weakness (%)	11.9	3.1
Dysesthesia (severe) (%)	3.7	8.7
Anesthesia dolorosa	1.6	2.3
Corneal numbness	9.6	8.1
Keratitis	1.3	2.1
Cranial nerve deficits	0.9	0.2
Meningitis	0.2	0.7

Modified from Lopez BC, Hamlyn PJ, Zakrzewska JM: Systematic review of ablative neurosurgical techniques for the treatment of trigeminal neuralgia, *Neurosurgery* 54:973-982; discussion 982-983, 2004.

needle. The patient is then allowed to wake up, and sensory stimulation can be carried out with 50 Hz. Paresthesia should be felt between 0.05 and 0.1 V in the painful areas. V3 stimulation is encountered superficial and lateral in the foramen, then V2, and V1 is the deepest toward the pons and more medially. After appropriate paresthesia is obtained at the desired sites, a 60° C thermo lesion is carried out for 60 seconds. The corneal reflex and the treated dermatome may be tested for hypoesthesia. If intact, a second lesion is made at 65° C for 60 seconds, and if there is still no hypoesthesia, then a third lesion can be made at 70° C for another 60 seconds.

Efficacy of Radiofrequency Thermocoagulation of the Gasserian Ganglion The first application of radiofrequency in pain medicine was for the treatment of trigeminal neuralgia with reported excellent results. Kanpolat et al[21] evaluated the effectiveness of percutaneous radiofrequency trigeminal rhizotomy in 1600 patients with idiopathic trigeminal neuralgia with a follow-up period of 1 to 25 years. Acute pain relief was accomplished in 97.6% of patients. Pain relief was reported in 92% of patients with a single procedure or with multiple procedures 5 years later. At 10-year follow-up, 52.3% of the patients who underwent a single procedure and 94.2% of the patients who underwent multiple procedures had experienced pain relief. At 20-year follow-up, 41% and 100% of these patients, respectively, had experienced pain relief. After the first procedure was performed, early pain recurrence (<6 mo) was observed in 123 patients (7.7%), and late pain recurrence was observed in 278 patients (17.4%). The authors concluded that percutaneous radiofrequency trigeminal rhizotomy is a minimally invasive, low-risk technique with a high rate of efficacy and the procedure may safely be repeated if pain recurs.

Wu et al[22] also reported their results in 1860 patients with refractory trigeminal neuralgia. The outcome was excellent in 78.8%, good in 17.5%, and poor in 3.7% of cases. Pain recurrence was reported in 11.1% of cases during the first 12 months and 24.8% after 24 months.

Complications of Gasserian Ganglion Block and Neurolysis The Gasserian (trigeminal) ganglion lies within Meckel's cave, which is formed by a dura mater fold that surrounds the posterior two-thirds of the ganglion. Meckel's cave contains CSF, so local anesthetic deposited in this area may spread to other cranial nerves and can potentially cause brainstem anesthesia.[20] Meticulous attention should be paid to avoid intravascular injection.[17] Negative aspiration is unreliable, and injection of the contrast agent should be performed under real-time fluoroscopy with digital subtraction, if available, before injection of the local anesthetic.

In a systematic review of ablative neurosurgical techniques for the treatment of trigeminal neuralgia, Lopez et al[16] concluded that although radiofrequency thermocoagulation (RFT) seems to provide the highest rates of sustained complete pain relief, it is the technique that is associated with the greatest number of complications.

A total of 29.2% of the patients in the analyzed series developed some complications, mostly transient, with RFT, and the rate of complications from glycerol rhizolysis was 24.8%. Stereotactic radiosurgery was the safest technique; only 12.1% of the patients experienced complications, mostly dysesthesias (**Table 5-2**).

Postoperative trigeminal sensory loss affects virtually all patients treated with RFT, and it is considered a side effect rather than a complication. However, in a prospective study, 30% of these patients may experience permanent sensory loss.[23]

Maxillary Nerve Block and Mandibular Nerve Block

Blockade of the maxillary and mandibular nerves or their branches is usually performed as a diagnostic block when more selective nerve block is needed for the diagnosis of various orofacial pain syndromes.

Maxillary Nerve Block

The maxillary nerve exits through the foramen rotundum, which is located at the roof of the PPF.

Technique of Maxillary Nerve Block This uses the same approach as in SPG block; however, the needle is directed more cephalad toward the roof of the PPF to target the maxillary nerve

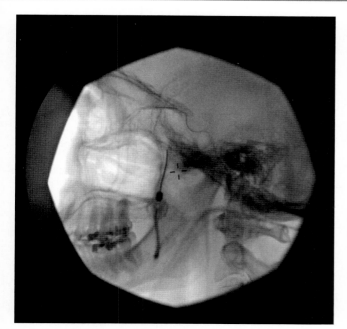

Fig, 5-11 Maxillary nerve block. The needle is directed toward the roof of the pterygopalatine fossa where the foramen rotundum exits. (Reproduced with permission from the Ohio Pain and Headache Institute.)

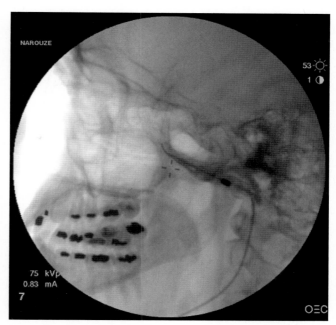

Fig. 5-13 Maxillary nerve block. The curved tip facilitates directing the needle is toward the foramen rotundum. (Reproduced with permission from the Ohio Pain and Headache Institute.)

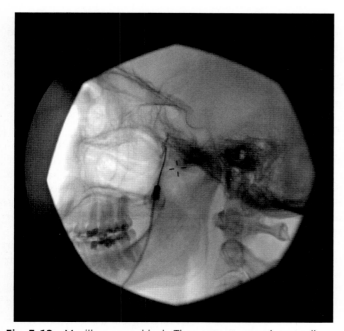

Fig. 5-12 Maxillary nerve block. The contrast agent is spreading cephalad through the foramen rotundum. (Reproduced with permission from the Ohio Pain and Headache Institute.)

as it exits the foramen rotundum on its way to enter the inferior orbital fissure (**Figs. 5-11** to **5-13**).

A nerve-stimulating needle can be used to obtain paresthesia in the maxillary distribution (cheek, upper teeth, and gum). A total of 0.5 mL of contrast agent is injected under real-time fluoroscopy to rule out intravascular spread. After negative aspiration, 1 to 2 mL of bupivacaine 0.5% with or without steroids may be injected slowly.

Mandibular Nerve Block

The mandibular nerve exits through the foramen ovale. The mandibular division (V3) is the most caudad and lateral part of the Gasserian ganglion.

Technique of Mandibular Nerve Block There are two approaches for blockade of the mandibular nerve.

Lateral "Pterygoid Plate" Approach This uses the same approach as in SPG block; however, after the needle approaches the lateral pterygoid plate, it is then walked off posteriorly (contrary to SPG block) and advanced a couple of millimeters medially and cephalad to target the mandibular nerve as it exits the foramen ovale (**Fig. 5-14**).

A nerve-stimulating needle can be used to motor twitches in the masticatory muscles. A total of 0.5 mL of contrast agent is injected under real-time fluoroscopy to rule out intravascular spread. After negative aspiration, 2 mL of bupivacaine 0.5% with or without steroids may be injected slowly.

Anterior "Foramen Oval" Approach This uses the same approach as in Gasserian ganglion block. The author prefers this approach because it is less painful than the lateral approach because walking the needle off the lateral pterygoid plate is usually very painful.

The mandibular division (V3) is the most caudad and lateral part of the Gasserian ganglion. Accordingly, the target is the most lateral part of the foramen ovale, and the needle tip has to stay just outside the foramen oval to avoid contamination of the maxillary division (to make the block as specific as possible). Also, only 1 to 2 mL of local anesthetic should be used. For more technique details, refer to the technique for Gasserian ganglion block above.

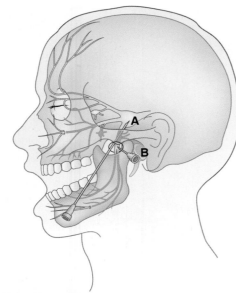

A Gasserian ganglion block through foramen ovale

B Lateral access to mandibular branch

Fig. 5-14 Mandibular nerve block. **A,** Foramen ovale approach. **B,** Lateral approach.

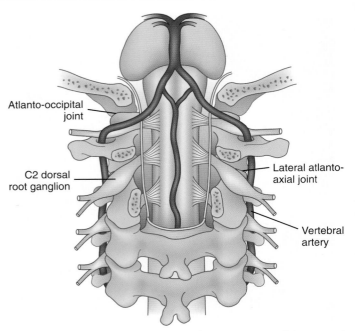

Atlanto-occipital joint

C2 dorsal root ganglion

Lateral atlanto-axial joint

Vertebral artery

Fig. 5-15 Illustration showing the relevant anatomy of the atlanto-occipital and atlanto-axial joints.

Atlanto-Axial and Atlanto-Occipital Joint Injections

Atlanto-Axial Joint Injection

The lateral atlanto-axial joint (AAJ) may account for up to 16% of patients with occipital headache.[24] Clinical presentations suggestive of pain originating from the lateral AAJ include occipital or suboccipital pain, focal tenderness over the suboccipital area, restricted painful rotation of C1 on C2, and pain provocation by passive rotation of C1. These clinical presentations are not specific and therefore cannot be used alone to establish the diagnosis.[25] The only means of establishing a likely diagnosis is a diagnostic block with intraarticular injection of local anesthetic.[24]

Indications The indications are as follows:

- Diagnostic: AAJ injection with local anesthetic is the only way to make a definitive diagnosis of pain stemming from the AAJ.
- Therapeutic: AAJ injection with local anesthetic and steroids may be indicated in the management of AAJ pain. Intraarticular steroids are effective in short-term pain relief originating from the lateral AAJ.[26,27]
- Prognostic: AAJ injection with local anesthetic and steroids may be used as a prognostic tool before AAJ radiofrequency lesioning or AAJ arthrodesis for intractable cases. One report showed favorable long-term outcome after both pulsed and thermal radiofrequency lesioning of the AAJ.[28] In intractable cases not responsive to more conservative management, arthrodesis of the lateral AAJ may be indicated.[29]

Anatomy of the Atlanto-Axial and Atlanto-Occipital Joints AAJ and atlanto-occipital joint (AOJ) intraarticular injections have the potential for serious complications, so it is crucial to be familiar with the anatomy of the joint in relation to the surrounding vascular and neural structures (**Fig. 5-15**). The vertebral artery is lateral to the AAJ as it courses through the C2 and C1 foramina. Then it curves medially to go through the foramen magnum, crossing the medial posterior aspect of the AOJ. The C2 dorsal root ganglion and nerve root with its surrounding dural sleeve crosses the posterior aspect of the middle of the joint. Therefore, during AAJ injection, the needle should be directed toward the posterolateral aspect of the joint. This will avoid injury to the C2 nerve root medially and the vertebral artery laterally (**Fig. 5-15**).[24,27] On the other hand, the AOJ should be accessed from the most superior posterior lateral aspect to avoid the vertebral artery medially.

Technique of Atlanto-Axial Joint Injections

Every effort should be made to make the injection a true intraarticular and not periarticular injection. Those procedures are mainly used in the diagnosis of pain stemming from the joints, and periarticular injection is not target specific because the local anesthetic may contaminate the C2 nerve root, which crosses the posterior aspect of the AAJ. Intraarticular injection is more target specific because it selectively anesthetizes the joint.

The patient is placed in the prone position with a pillow under the chest to allow for slight neck flexion. The fluoroscopy C-arm is brought to the head of the table in an AP direction. Under fluoroscopic guidance, the C-arm is rotated in the sagittal plane until the lateral atlanto-axial joint is better visualized. Using a marking pen, the needle insertion site is marked on the skin overlying the lateral third of the atlanto-axial joint. The skin is prepped and draped in the usual sterile fashion and a skin wheel is raised with local anesthetic at the insertion site. Then a 22- to 25-gauge, 3.5-inch blunt needle is advanced in anterior and medial direction toward the posterolateral aspect of the inferior margin of the inferior articular process of the atlas. This will avoid contact with the C2 nerve root and dorsal ganglion, which crosses the posterior aspect of the middle of the joint (**Fig. 5-15**). After touching the bone to safely establish the correct depth, the needle is withdrawn slightly; directed toward the posterolateral aspect of the lateral atlanto-axial joint; and advanced for couple of millimeters and usually a distinctive pop is felt, signaling entering the joint cavity.

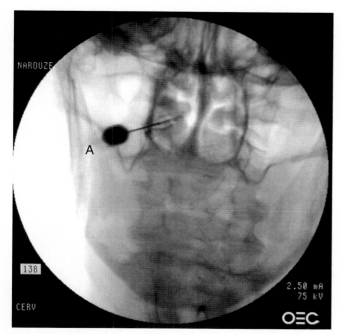

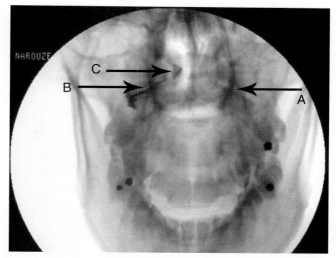

Fig. 5-18 Lateral atlanto-axial joint (AAJ) injection. Lateral AAJ (A), contrast agent within the AAJ (B), and contrast spreading to the median AAJ (C). (Reproduced with permission from the Ohio Pain and Headache Institute.)

Fig. 5-16 Lateral atlanto-axial joint injection. Anteroposterior view showing the needle (A) targeting the lateral third of the joint; the contrast is contained within the joint space. (Reproduced with permission from the Ohio Pain and Headache Institute.)

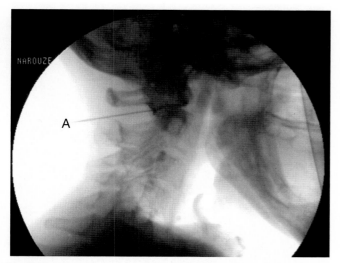

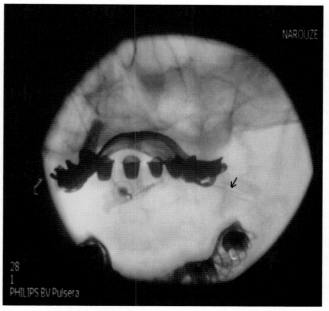

Fig. 5-17 Lateral atlanto-axial joint injection. Lateral view showing that the contrast is contained within the joint space. *A*, needle. (Reproduced with permission from the Ohio Pain and Headache Institute.)

Fig. 5-19 Lateral antanto-axial joint (AAJ) injection. Needle inside the left AAJ with the contrast spreading to the right AAJ (*arrow*). (Reproduced with permission from the Ohio Pain and Headache Institute.)

At this point, a lateral view is obtained, which shows the tip of the needle in the middle of the joint anterior to the posterior margin of the joint. Careful attention should be paid to avoid the vertebral artery that lies lateral to the lateral atlanto-axial joint as it courses through the C1 and C2 foramina. After careful negative aspiration for blood or cerebrospinal fluid, 0.2 mL of water-soluble nonionic contrast agent (Omnipaque 240) is injected to verify intraarticular placement of the tip of the needle.

Injection of the contrast agent is done under direct real-time fluoroscopy to check for inadvertent intraarterial injection, which is manifest by rapid clearance of the contrast agent. AP and lateral views are obtained to ensure that the contrast agent remained confined to the joint cavity without escape to the surrounding structures, especially the epidural space or posteriorly to the C2 ganglion, which will adversely affects the specificity of the block (**Figs. 5-16** and **5-17**). The AP view usually demonstrates the bilateral concavity of the joint with the contrast material inside the joint space (**Fig. 5-16**), and sometimes it shows that the lateral AAJ space may communicate with that of the median AAJ space (**Fig. 5-18**) and the contralateral AAJ space (**Fig. 5-19**). After careful negative aspiration, 1.0 mL of a mixture of bupivacaine 0.5% and 10 mg of triamcinolone is injected.[27]

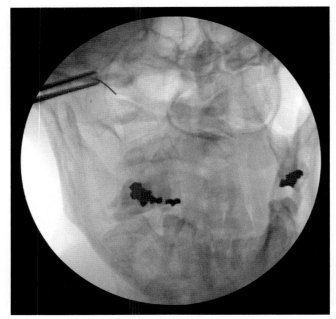

Fig. 5-20 Atlanto-occipital joint injection, anteroposterior view. (Reproduced with permission from the Ohio Pain and Headache Institute.)

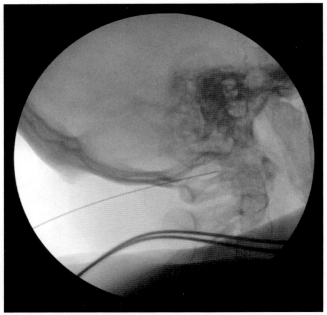

Fig. 5-21 Atlanto-occipital joint injection, lateral view. (Reproduced with permission from the Ohio Pain and Headache Institute.)

Technique of Atlanto-Occipital Joint Injections

This procedure is rarely performed for few reasons. Isolated pain stemming from the AOJ is very rare, and the patient usually has localized occipital pain that is aggravated mainly by head nodding. Therefore, activity modification and conservative management are usually all that is needed. Also, the vertebral artery curves from lateral to medial, crossing the posterior aspect of the C1 body, which makes it vulnerable to injury while the needle is advanced toward the AOJ, especially with improper positioning of the patient.

The positioning and approach are similar to those for AAJ injection. The patient needs to flex his or her head over the neck as much as possible (chin on chest) to open the suboccipital space posteriorly. The AOJ should be accessed from the most superior posterior lateral aspect to avoid the vertebral artery (**Figs. 5-20** and **5-21**).

More recently, ultrasound-assisted AOJ injection in conjunction with fluoroscopy was described. With real-time sonography, the vertebral artery is identified as it curves medially behind the C1 body and accordingly can be avoided from the needle path, and then the procedure can be continued with fluoroscopy to confirm intraarticular placement of the needle (**Fig. 5-22**).[30]

Efficacy of Atlanto-Axial and Atlanto-Occipital Joint Injections

Narouze and colleagues[27] studied 115 patients with cervicogenic headache. Thirty-two patients had a clinical picture suggestive of AAJ pain, and the diagnosis was confirmed in 15 patients with complete abolition of the headache (pain score of 0) after AAJ injection. The prevalence of AAJ pain among patients with cervicogenic headache was 13% (15 of 115 patients). At 1, 3, and 6 months after AAJ intraarticular steroid injection, the mean pain scores dropped from a baseline of 6.8 to 1.9, 3.6, and 3.7 respectively. The authors concluded that intraarticular steroid injection is effective for short-term relief of pain originating from the lateral AAJ.

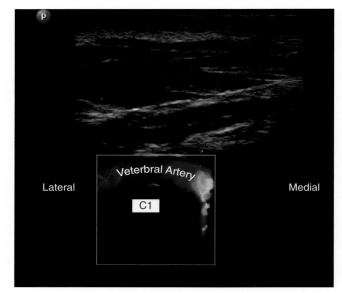

Fig. 5-22 Atlanto-occipital joint injection. Sonogram showing the vertebral artery as it curves medially posterior to C1. (Reproduced with permission from the Ohio Pain and Headache Institute.)

No data are available to demonstrate the efficacy of AOJ intraarticular steroid injections.

Complications of Atlanto-Axial and Atlanto-Occipital Joint Injections

One possible complication is vertebral artery injection or injury. Injection of a contrast agent should be performed under real-time fluoroscopy, preferably with digital subtraction, if available, before the injection of the local anesthetic because negative aspiration is unreliable.[31] Meticulous attention should be paid to avoid

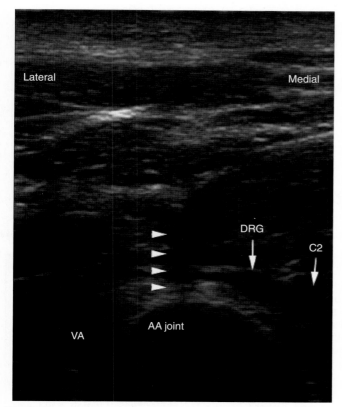

Fig. 5-23 Atlanto-axial joint (AAJ) injection. Sonogram showing the needle targeting the AAJ (*arrows*). C2, C2 nerve root; DRG, dorsal root ganglion; VA, vertebral artery. (Reproduced with permission from the Ohio Pain and Headache Institute.)

intravascular injection because vertebral artery anatomy may be variable. Recently, ultrasound-assisted AAJ injection was reported in an effort to add more safety to the procedure because ultrasonography can identify the relevant soft tissue structures nearby the joint (e.g., vertebral artery and C2 dorsal root ganglion) (**Fig. 5-23**).[30]

Inadvertent puncture of the C2 dural sleeve with CSF leak or high spinal spread of the local anesthetic may occur with AAJ injection if the needle is directed a few millimeters medially.

Spinal cord injury and syringomyelia are potential serious complications if the needle is directed further medially.[9]

References

1. Goadsby P: Pathophysiology of cluster headache: a trigeminal autonomic cephalgia. *Lancet Neurol* 1:251-257, 2002.
2. Salar G, Ori C, Iob I, et al: Percutaneous thermocoagulation for sphenopalatine ganglion neuralgia. *Acta Neurochir (Wien)* 84:24-28, 1987.
3. Sanders M, Zuurmond W: Efficacy of sphenopalatine ganglion blockade in 66 patients suffering from cluster headaches: a 12- to17-month follow-up evaluation. *J Neurosurg* 87:876-880, 1997.
4. Sluder G: The role of the sphenopalatine ganglion in nasal headache. *NY State J Med* 27:8-13, 1908.
5. Prasanna A, Murthy PS: Sphenopalatine ganglion block under vision using rigid nasal sinuscope. *Reg Anesth* 18:139-140, 1993.
6. Ruskin SL: Techniques of sphenopalatine therapy. *Eye Ear Nose Throat Mon* 30:28-31, 1951.
7. Vallejo R, Benyamin R, Yousuf N, et al: Computed tomography-enhanced sphenopalatine ganglion blockade. *Pain Pract* 7(1):44-46, 2007.
8. Narouze S, Kapural L, Casanova J, et al: Sphenopalatine ganglion radiofrequency ablation for the management of chronic cluster headache. *Headache* 49:571-577, 2009.
9. Narouze S: Complications of head and neck procedures. *Tech Reg Anesth Pain Manag* 11:171-177, 2007.
10. Konen A: Unexpected effects due to radiofrequency thermocoagulation of the sphenopalatine ganglion: two case reports. *Pain Digest* 10:30-33, 2000.
11. Bayer E, Racz GB, Miles D, et al: Sphenopalatine ganglion pulsed radiofrequency treatment in 30 patients suffering from chronic face and head pain. *Pain Pract* 5:223-227, 2005.
12. Narouze SN: Role of sphenopalatine ganglion neuroablation in the management of cluster headache, *Curr Pain Headache Rep* 14:160-163, 2010.
13. Young RF, Vermulen S, Posewitz A: Gamma knife radiosurgery for the treatment of trigeminal neuralgia. *Stereotact Funct Neurosurg* 70(suppl 1):192-199, 1998.
14. Belber CJ, Rak RA: Balloon compression rhizolysis in the surgical management of trigeminal neuralgia. *Neurosurgery* 20:908-913, 1987.
15. Hakanson S: Trigeminal neuralgia treated by the injection of glycerol into the trigeminal cistern. *Neurosurgery* 9:638-646, 1981.
16. Lopez BC, Hamlyn PJ, Zakrzewska JM: Systematic review of ablative neurosurgical techniques for the treatment of trigeminal neuralgia. *Neurosurgery* 54:973-982; discussion 982-983, 2004.
17. Erdine S, Ozyalcin NS, Cimen A, et al: Comparison of pulsed radiofrequency with conventional radiofrequency in the treatment of idiopathic trigeminal neuralgia. *Eur J Pain* 11:309-313, 2007.
18. Spatz AL, Zakrzewska JM, Kay EJ: Decision analysis of medical and surgical treatments for trigeminal neuralgia: how patient evaluations of benefits and risks affect the utility of treatment decisions. *Pain* 131:302-310, 2007.
19. Tatli M, Satici O, Kanpolat Y, et al: Various surgical modalities for trigeminal neuralgia: Literature study of respective long-term outcomes. *Acta Neurochir (Wien)* 150:243-255, 2008.
20. Murphy T: Somatic blockade of head and neck. In Cousins M, Bridenbaugh P, editors: *Clinical anesthesia and management of pain*, ed 3, Philadelphia, 1998, Lippincott-Raven, pp 489-514.
21. Kanpolat Y, Savas A, Bekar A, et al: Percutaneous controlled radiofrequency trigeminal rhizotomy for the treatment of idiopathic trigeminal neuralgia: 25-year experience with 1,600 patients. *Neurosurgery* 48:524-532; discussion 532-534, 2001.
22. Wu CY, Meng FG, Xu SJ, et al: Selective percutaneous radiofrequency thermocoagulation in the treatment of trigeminal neuralgia: report on 1860 cases. *Chin Med J* 117:467-470, 2004.
23. Zakrzewska JM, Jassmin S, Bulman JS: A prospective, longitudinal study on patients with trigeminal neuralgia who underwent radiofrequency thermocoagulation of the Gasserian ganglion. *Pain* 79:51-58, 1999.
24. Aprill C, Axinn MJ, Bogduk N: Occipital headaches stemming from the lateral atlanto-axial (C1-2) joint. *Cephalalgia* 22(1):15-22, 2002.
25. Bogduk N: The neck and headache. *Neurol Clin* 22(1):151-171, 2004.
26. Narouze SN, Casanova J: The efficacy of lateral atlanto-axial intra-articular steroid injection in the management of cervicogenic headache. *Anesthesiology* 101(suppl A):A1005, 2004.
27. Narouze SN, Casanova J, Mekhail N: The longitudinal effectiveness of lateral atlanto-axial intra-articular steroid injection in the management of cervicogenic headache. *Pain Med* 8:184-188, 2007.
28. Narouze SN, Gutenberg L: Radiofrequency denervation of the lateral atlantoaxial joint for the treatment of cervicogenic headache. *Reg Anesth Pain Med* 32(suppl A):A-8, 2007.
29. Ghanayem AJ, Leventhal M, Bohlman HH: Osteoarthrosis of the atlantoaxial joints: long term follow up after treatment with arthrodesis. *J Bone Joint Surg (Am)* 78:1300-1307, 1996.
30. Narouze S: Ultrasonography in pain medicine: future directions. *Tech Reg Anesth Pain Manage* 13(3):198-202, 2009.
31. Edlow BL, Wainger BJ, Frosch MP, et al: Posterior circulation stroke after C1-C2 intraarticular facet steroid injection: evidence for diffuse microvascular injury. *Anesthesiology* 112:1532-1535, 2010.

6 Upper Extremity Peripheral Nerve Blockade

Hugh M. Smith and Christopher M. Duncan

CHAPTER OVERVIEW

Chapter Synopsis: This chapter considers the various techniques and indications for upper extremity peripheral nerve blockade. These techniques may be used for pain therapy, regional anesthesia, and diagnostic applications. Although today's image-guided technology provides a valuable tool in carrying out these procedures, a detailed knowledge of the underlying anatomy of the brachial plexus is key to success. These anatomical details and specific technical details of the procedures are described. Blockade of upper extremity nerves is generally very effective, but similar to any nerve block, the procedure carries complication risks. These can be minimized by making strategic treatment decisions before the procedure and by using the safest possible technique for the situation; often, these considerations are unique to each patient.

Important Points:
- Upper extremity blockade may be performed for therapeutic, diagnostic, prophylactic, and prognostic indications.
- Ultrasound-based techniques result in faster onset, shorter procedure time, higher success rates, longer block duration, and fewer vascular punctures than alternative techniques.
- Ultrasonography is not a substitute for thorough understanding of brachial plexus anatomy.

Clinical Pearls:
- Foreknowledge of brachial plexus anatomy and desired site of action is critical to selection of appropriate location of brachial plexus blockade.
- In ultrasound-guided techniques, the deepest and most distal structures from the needle insertion site should be blocked first.
- Successful blockade is associated with nerve stimulation amplitudes of less than 0.7 mA.

Clinical Pitfalls:
- Failure to evoke a motor response during nerve stimulation may occur despite needle-to-nerve contact.
- The risk of nerve injury is multifactorial and may include patient, procedure, and technical factors.

Introduction

Upper extremity peripheral nerve blockade, in one form or another, has been performed since ancient Egypt as evidenced by 5000-year-old pictographs illustrating nerve compression anesthesia for hand surgery.[1] Today, the development of image-guidance technology and efficacious injectable drugs have made upper extremity peripheral nerve blockade an increasingly useful tool in pain physicians' and regional anesthesiologists' diagnostic and therapeutic arsenal. Peripheral nerve blockade is a growing and dynamic field with diverse approaches, technological equipment, and a variety of local anesthetics and adjuvant therapies.

Upper extremity blockade may be performed for a variety of clinical reasons. Treatment of painful conditions and avoiding general anesthesia are among the most common therapeutic indications. However, diagnostic, prognostic, or preemptive nerve blocks also possess tangible value for patients and physicians. Determining the specific neurological distribution of pain, evaluating the potential benefit of blocking specific nerve activity, or attempting to prevent a long-term pain state (e.g., phantom limb pain) are equally important indications for peripheral nerve blockade.

Because of the relatively shallow depth and accessibility of the brachial plexus, multiple classical sites of blockade have been described. These locations or approaches (e.g., interscalene, supraclavicular, axillary) are determined by the specific distal nerves and nerve distributions to be blocked. A fundamental requirement of successful sensory blockade, regardless of the anatomical location, is interruption of afferent nerve conduction at a more proximal contiguous location along the brachial plexus than the stimulus. Even new imaging technologies, such as ultrasonography, which have freed providers from the classical approaches by allowing effective blockade wherever adequate nerve visualization exists, must meet this basic requirement for the block to be effective. Thus modern technology does not obviate the need for a thorough understanding of the various distributions of the brachial plexus.

Brachial Plexus Anatomy

Familiarity with brachial plexus anatomy is critical to optimal and safe performance of peripheral nerve techniques. The most proximal portion of the brachial plexus is located in the posterior triangle of the neck, bordered by the clavicle inferiorly, the trapezius muscle posteriorly, and the sternocleidomastoid muscle anteriorly. There, the plexus is deep to the skin, subcutaneous tissue, deep fascia, and platysma muscle and is formed by the union of the

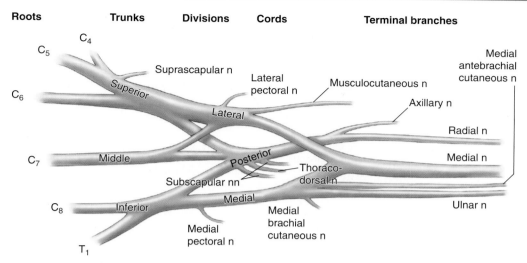

Roots   **Trunks**   **Divisions**   **Cords**   **Terminal branches**

Fig. 6-1   Brachial plexus anatomy. (Reprinted with permission from Torsher L, Smith H, Jacob A: Interscalene blockade. In Hebl JR, Lennon RL, editors: *Mayo Clinic atlas of regional anesthesia and ultrasound-guided nerve blockade*, New York, 2010, Oxford University Press, p 192.)

anterior (ventral) primary rami of cervical nerves five through eight (C5-C8) and the greater part of the first thoracic nerve (T1). In some patients, the fourth cervical (C4) and second thoracic (T2) nerves also contribute to the brachial plexus. At its most proximal, the C5-T1 nerve roots conjoin to form the superior (C5-C6), middle (C7), and inferior trunks (C8-T1) (**Fig. 6-1**).

A superficial landmark, the interscalene groove, overlies the trunks and is palpable as an indentation between the anterior and middle scalene muscles. This groove, at the level of the cricoid cartilage, is the needle entry site used most frequently for interscalene brachial plexus blockade. The phrenic nerve, derived from the C3-C5 nerve roots, runs parallel to the vertebral artery at this location as it passes through the neck on the ventral surface of the anterior scalene muscle. Sonographic study has revealed that the phrenic nerve is visible as a hypoechoic structure in 93% of subjects.[2] The phrenic nerve is immediately adjacent to the superior trunk at the C6 level, thus explaining the uniform deactivation of this nerve during interscalene blockade.[3]

As the three trunks descend toward the first rib, the brachial plexus differentiates into anterior and posterior divisions, corresponding to the ventral and dorsal aspects of the upper extremity. Located posterolateral to the subclavian artery, the divisions pass below the middle third of the clavicle and above the first rib before fusing into medial, lateral, and posterior cords. Approaches to the brachial plexus immediately above and below the clavicle are the so-named supraclavicular and infraclavicular blocks. At the lateral border of the pectoralis minor muscle, the axillary artery is surrounded by the lateral, posterior, and medial cords of the brachial plexus. As the cords enter the axilla, they give rise to the sensorimotor branches of the plexus, the radial, median, ulnar, and musculocutaneous nerves. These peripheral nerves consist of individual myelinated nerve fibers embedded within an endoneurial connective tissue layer and grouped into discrete bundles or fascicles. Nerve fascicles are interlaced by connective tissue and surrounded by an outer epineurial membrane.[4]

Indications and Contraindications

Because several nerves join or diverge from the brachial plexus between its central origins and its most distal peripheral branches,

no single location suffices to produce complete blockade of the upper extremity. Thus, proximal block locations are selected based on foreknowledge of the current or future pain distribution. **Table 6-1** lists the more common indications and techniques for blockade of various elements of the brachial plexus.

Equipment

Blockade of the brachial plexus can be accomplished through a variety of methods based on block location, equipment availability, and the experience of the practitioner. Traditional methods of nerve localization include paresthesia-seeking, nerve stimulation, or transarterial approaches.[5-7] Ultrasonography is increasingly the most common tool for visualizing the neuroanatomy and surrounding structures.[8]

Paresthesia   Paresthesia techniques for nerve identification rely on patient reporting of sensory paresthesia as a needle comes into immediate contact with the nerve. Patients must not be overly sedated, and a long bevel needle is preferred.

Nerve Stimulator   Nerve stimulation uses small electrical currents to induce nerve depolarization and subsequent motor responses. Nerve stimulators generate a square wave, typically one or two times per second and 0.1 seconds in duration. The amplitude is initially set around 1.0 to 1.5 mA and decreased after a motor response is identified. High degrees of block success are obtained when a motor response is maintained below 0.7 mA. Motor response with amplitude less then 0.3 may be associated with an intraneural needle position. Of note, two recent studies[9,10] have demonstrated that needle-to-nerve contact fails to provide a motor response at amplitudes of 0.7 mA up to 15% of the time, a phenomenon that has yet to be adequately explained.

Ultrasound   The superficial depth of the brachial plexus makes it ideal for visualization with ultrasonography. Except for significant patient obesity and infraclavicular blockade, a high-frequency (10- to 15-MHz) linear probe is used to obtain optimal images. Although high frequencies provide high-resolution images, penetration depth is functionally limited to about 1 to 3 cm. To image

Table 6-1: Regional Anesthetic Techniques for Upper Extremity

Brachial Plexus Technique	Level of Blockade	Peripheral Nerves Blocked	Indications	Comments and Contraindications
Interscalene	Upper and middle trunks	Entire brachial plexus, although the inferior trunk (ulnar nerve) is inconsistently blocked	Blockade of the shoulder and proximal and mid humerus	• Phrenic nerve paresis in 100% of patients for duration of the block • Unsuitable for patients unable to tolerate a 30% reduction in pulmonary function
Supraclavicular	Distal trunk and proximal cord	Radial, ulnar, median, musculocutaneous, axillary	Blockade of the mid humerus, elbow, forearm, and hand; inconsistent blockade of shoulder	• "Spinal of the arm" • Risk of pneumothorax requires caution in ambulatory patients • Phrenic nerve paresis in 30% of cases • Possible sympathetic blockade with Horner syndrome
Infraclavicular	Cords	Radial, ulnar, median, musculocutaneous, axillary	Blockade of the elbow, forearm, hand	• Minimal risk of hemothorax or pneumothorax • Relatively rapid onset • Catheter site is easy to maintain • Deep block; contraindicated in anticoagulated patients
Axillary	Peripheral nerves	Radial, ulnar, median; musculocutaneous unreliably blocked	Blockade of the forearm and hand; less often used for procedures near the elbow	• Unsuitable for proximal humerus or shoulder surgery • Requires the patient to abduct the arm
Nerves at the elbow	Peripheral nerves	Radial, ulnar, median	Blockade of the individual nerves of the hand and wrist	• Used to supplement incomplete blocks • Potentially blocking partially anesthetized nerve

deeper structures, lower frequencies (8 to 10 MHz) must be used for better penetration but at the expense of reduced image resolution. Current ultrasonography models include Doppler color-flow features, which facilitate identification of relevant vascular structures.

Techniques

Interscalene

Traditional interscalene blockade of the trunks of the brachial plexus is achieved by inserting a needle between the anterior and middle scalene muscles at the level of the cricoid cartilage in the posterior cervical triangle of the neck (**Fig. 6-2**).

With the needle directed toward the sternal notch, the trunks are encountered at a depth of 1 to 2 cm. This modified technique, described by Winnie in 1970,[11] uses either nerve stimulation or paresthesia to identify the trunks of the brachial plexus. A response in the deltoid or distal arm is acceptable. When sonographic identification of the supraclavicular brachial plexus is performed, the divisions of the brachial plexus are traced cephalad from the clavicle to the interscalene location. In-plane or out-of-plane needle approaches for interscalene blockade have been described. In-plane needle insertion is performed from posterior to anterior to avoid needle trauma to the phrenic nerve. The out-of-plane insertion is performed from the caudal side of the probe.

Supraclavicular

Before the development of ultrasonography, supraclavicular blockade was performed using paresthesia or nerve stimulation. These techniques were associated with a 0.5% to 6.1% risk of

pneumothorax.[4] The use of ultrasonography has renewed interest in the supraclavicular approach to brachial plexus blockade because most providers believe that direct observation allows them to avoid this complication.[8,12,13] It should be noted, however, that case reports of pneumothorax during ultrasound-guided supraclavicular and infraclavicular blockade have been reported. To perform this technique, the ultrasound probe is placed in the supraclavicular fossa angled toward the first rib. An image should be acquired that includes a longitudinal view of the first rib along with a cross-sectional view of the subclavian artery and brachial plexus (**Fig. 6-3**).

An in-plane lateral to medial ultrasound-guided needle approach is used to allow needle visualization throughout the procedure. The needle tip is advanced within the sheath of the brachial plexus using a hydrodissection technique to avoid direct needle trauma to the nerves. Local anesthetic is administered immediately superficial to the first rib and lateral to the artery to ensure blockade of C8-T1 nerve fibers and throughout the rest of the sheath containing the plexus.

Infraclavicular

A touted benefit of the infraclavicular approach to the brachial plexus is that it can be performed with the patient's arm in an adducted position. Two of the most frequently used traditional approaches were initially reported by Wilson et al[14] and Raj et al,[15] which are performed using nerve stimulation or paresthesia nerve localization techniques. In the Raj approach, a needle is inserted at the midpoint of the inferior border of the clavicle. The needle is directed lateral toward the axilla. In the Wilson ("coracoid") approach, the needle is inserted perpendicular to the skin 2 cm

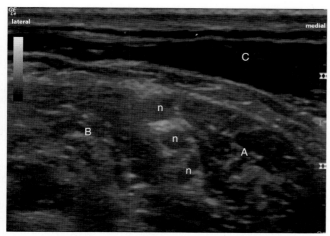

Fig. 6-2 Ultrasound image of the interscalene brachial plexus at the level of the trunks. *A*, anterior scalene muscle; *B*, middle scalene muscle; *C*, sternocleidomastoid muscle; *n*, nerve trunks.

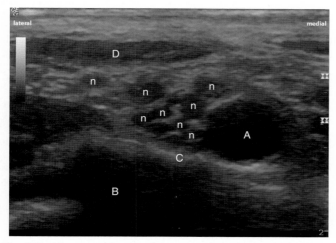

Fig. 6-3 Ultrasound image of the supraclavicular brachial plexus at the level of the divisions. *A*, subclavian artery; *B*, lung; *C*, first rib; *D*, middle scalene; *n*, nerve divsions.

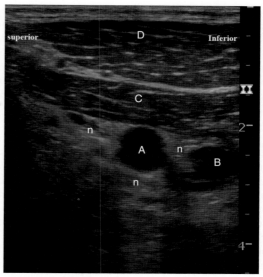

Fig. 6-4 Ultrasound image of the infraclavicular brachial plexus at the level of the cords. *A*, axillary artery; *B*, axillary vein; *C*, pectoralis minor muscle; *D*, pectoralis major muscle; *n*, nerve cords.

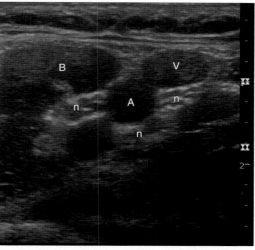

Fig. 6-5 Ultrasound image of the axillary brachial plexus at the level of the branches. *A*, axillary artery; *B*, biceps muscle; *V*, axillary vein; *n*, peripheral nerve branches.

medial and 2 cm inferior to the tip of the coracoid process. A motor or sensory response in the hand is ideal, and biceps or deltoid responses may signify inadequate distal blockade. The deep location of the nerve cords makes this location the most challenging ultrasound-guided block compared with other approaches to the brachial plexus. In-plane or out-of-plane ultrasound-guided approaches can be used.[16-18] The probe is placed perpendicular to the inferior border of the middle of the clavicle, where the subclavian artery and the cords of the brachial plexus can be seen in cross section (**Fig. 6-4**).

In-plane needle insertion should occur in a caudal to rostral direction. Out-of-plane needle insertion should occur in a medial to lateral direction.

Axillary

Multiple techniques have been described for brachial plexus blockade in the axilla. All techniques require a 90-degree abduction of the arm at the shoulder. Common techniques include transarterial, nerve stimulation, paresthesia, and ultrasound guidance. All techniques take advantage of the close proximity of the terminal nerves to the axillary artery. Transarterial techniques rely on blood

aspiration to identify the anterior and posterior walls of the artery to achieve perivascular local anesthetic spread. Nerve stimulation and paresthesia techniques try to avoid vascular puncture and instead rely on individual nerve localization. Injection of local anesthetic around two separate terminal nerve branches is recommended for successful blockade. For ultrasound techniques, the axillary artery remains the most prominent landmark for identifying the neuroanatomical structures (**Fig. 6-5**).

The probe is placed near the axilla perpendicular to the long axis of the arm so the axillary artery can be seen in cross section. The nerves viewed in short axis may be seen in a variety of positions around the artery because anatomical variation in the axilla is significant.[19] In-plane needle guidance is recommended, with deeper and more distal nerves blocked first. In each approach, the musculocutaneous nerve must be blocked separately. The musculocutaneous nerve is highly visible under ultrasonography, typically occupying the fascial interface between the biceps and coracobrachialis muscles. Alternatively, the musculocutaneous nerve may be blocked by subcutaneous injection at the elbow.

Blockade of isolated upper extremity peripheral nerves, either for supplementation of inadequate surgical block or producing selective nerve distribution blockade, is easily performed at a supracondylar location. From medial to lateral, the ulnar, median, and radial nerves are visualized by cross-sectional ultrasonography by scanning with the probe just above the elbow.[20]

Outcomes Evidence

Upper extremity blockade, whether it is for primary anesthesia, postoperative analgesia, or acute pain intervention, is generally highly successful. Block success rates, depending on the anatomical location and end points measured, range from 85% to 100%. Recent evidence has shown that block outcomes using ultrasonography exceed other nerve localization techniques. Specific advantages of ultrasonography in upper extremity blockade include fewer needle passes, faster onset, shorter procedure time, higher success rates, longer block duration, and fewer vascular punctures.[21] Improvements in patient safety related to ultrasonography use, however, are yet to be proven. In fact, pneumothorax, local anesthetic toxicity (seizures and cardiac arrest), and peripheral nerve injury have all been reported during ultrasound-guided upper extremity blockade.[22]

Risk and Complication Avoidance

Peripheral nerve blockade may be associated with a unique set of complications, and care must be taken to minimize relevant risks. Complications may be classified as neurological, vascular, infectious, or related to local anesthetic toxicity. Although rare, peripheral nerve injuries are potentially catastrophic complications that may lead to long-term neuropathic pain or limb disability. Patient, procedure, and technical risk factors have all been identified as potential etiologies. Expert opinion suggests that multiple factors commonly play a role and that patients with several concomitant risks may have a higher incidence of neurological complications. Avoidance, or risk management, is complex but hinges primarily on appropriate preventive decision-making strategies and use of safe techniques. Neurological history and examination may reveal underlying patient neuropathic or degenerative processes that may preclude nerve blockade. Maintenance of sterile technique, use of minimal effective drug doses and concentrations, use of incremental aspiration and injection practices, and avoidance of intraneural or intrafascicular injection are all prudent measures to facilitate patient safety. Thus, use of imaging technology and other methods of nerve localization that allow needle and nerve distinction may help clinicians minimize risk of neurological complication. Recent evidence suggests that disruption of the perineurial membrane, which surrounds and regulates the microenvironment of nerve fascicles, with saline or local anesthetic injection produces histologic changes consistent with nerve injury.[23]

References

1. Barash PG, Cullen BF, Stoelting RK, et al: *Clinical anesthesia*, ed 6, Philadelphia, 2009, Lippincott Williams & Wilkins.
2. Kessler J, Schafhalter-Zoppoth I, Gray AT: An ultrasound study of the phrenic nerve in the posterior cervical triangle: implications for the interscalene brachial plexus block. *Reg Anesth Pain Med* 33(6):545-550, 2008.
3. Urmey WF, Talts KH, Sharrock NE: One hundred percent incidence of hemidiaphragmatic paresis associated with interscalene brachial plexus anesthesia as diagnosed by ultrasonography. *Anesth Analg* 72(4):498-503, 1991.
4. Neal JM, Gerancher JC, Hebl JR, et al: Upper extremity regional anesthesia: essentials of our current understanding, 2008. *Reg Anesth Pain Med* 34(2):134-170, 2009.
5. Aantaa R, Kirvela O, Lahdenpera A, et al: Transarterial brachial plexus anesthesia for hand surgery: a retrospective analysis of 346 cases. *J Clin Anesth* 6(3):189-192, 1994.
6. Selander D, Edshage S, Wolff T: Paresthesiae or no paresthesiae? Nerve lesions after axillary blocks. *Acta Anaesthesiol Scand* 23(1):27-33, 1979.
7. Sia S, Bartoli M, Lepri A, et al: Multiple-injection axillary brachial plexus block: a comparison of two methods of nerve localization-nerve stimulation versus paresthesia. *Anesth Analg* 91(3):647-651, 2000.
8. Kapral S, Krafft P, Eibenberger K, et al: Ultrasound-guided supraclavicular approach for regional anesthesia of the brachial plexus. *Anesth Analg* 78(3):507-513, 1994.
9. Beach ML, Sites BD, Gallagher JD: Use of a nerve stimulator does not improve the efficacy of ultrasound-guided supraclavicular nerve blocks. *J Clin Anesth* 18(8):580-584, 2006.
10. Perlas A, Chan VW, Simons M: Brachial plexus examination and localization using ultrasound and electrical stimulation: a volunteer study. *Anesthesiology* 99(2):429-435, 2003.
11. Winnie AP: Interscalene brachial plexus block. *Anesth Analg* 49(3):455-466, 1970.
12. Franco CD, Gloss FJ, Voronov G, et al: Supraclavicular block in the obese population: an analysis of 2020 blocks. *Anesth Analg* 102(4):1252-1254, 2006.
13. Chan VW, Perlas A, Rawson R, et al: Ultrasound-guided supraclavicular brachial plexus block. *Anesth Analg* 97(5):1514-1517, 2003.
14. Wilson JL, Brown DL, Wong GY, et al: Infraclavicular brachial plexus block: parasagittal anatomy important to the coracoid technique. *Anesth Analg* 87(4):870-873, 1998.
15. Raj PP, Montgomery SJ, Nettles D, et al: Infraclavicular brachial plexus block—a new approach. *Anesth Analg* 52(6):897-904, 1973.
16. Bigeleisen P, Wilson M: A comparison of two techniques for ultrasound guided infraclavicular block. *Br J Anaesth* 96(4):502-507, 2006.
17. Sandhu NS, Capan LM: Ultrasound-guided infraclavicular brachial plexus block. *Br J Anaesth* 89(2):254-259, 2002.
18. Ootaki C, Hayashi H, Amano M: Ultrasound-guided infraclavicular brachial plexus block: an alternative technique to anatomical landmark-guided approaches. *Reg Anesth Pain Med* 25(6):600-604, 2000.
19. Retzl G, Kapral S, Greher M, et al: Ultrasonographic findings of the axillary part of the brachial plexus. *Anesth Analg* 92(5):1271-1275, 2001.
20. Rettke SR, Smith HM: Elbow blockade. In Hebl JR, Lennon RL, editors: *Mayo Clinic atlas of regional anesthesia and ultrasound-guided nerve blockade*, New York, 2010, Oxford University Press, p 467.
21. McCartney CJ, Lin L, Shastri U: Evidence basis for the use of ultrasound for upper-extremity blocks. *Reg Anesth Pain Med* 35(2 suppl):S10-S15, 2010.
22. Neal JM, Brull R, Chan VW, et al: The ASRA evidence-based medicine assessment of ultrasound-guided regional anesthesia and pain medicine: executive summary. *Reg Anesth Pain Med* 35(2 suppl):S1-S9, 2010.
23. Sala-Blanch X, Ribalta T, Rivas E, et al: Structural injury to the human sciatic nerve after intraneural needle insertion. *Reg Anesth Pain Med* 34(3):201-205, 2009.

7 Lower Limb Blocks

Padraig Mahon and Colin J.L. McCartney

CHAPTER OVERVIEW

Chapter Synopsis: Perhaps because spinal and epidural nerve block procedures for both analgesia and anesthesia have been so efficient, peripheral nerve blocks have not been used to their greatest potential. Recent information, however, suggests that the incidence of risk and side effects is lower than these neuraxial procedures for orthopedic surgery of the lower limbs. This chapter recounts the advances in the field of the past 15 years, including the addition of ultrasound guidance. As with any nerve block procedure, the anatomical details of the target structures are of key importance in the technique's success. The neuroanatomy of the lumbar plexus, for example, is particularly complex because it is embedded within the psoas muscle. Methods are also described for block of the femoral nerve, obturator nerve, sciatic nerve, saphenous nerve, ankle, and iliacus fascia block, a sort of three-in-one technique. Both landmark- and ultrasound-guided approaches are considered.

Important Points:

- Unlike the upper extremity, the entire lower extremity cannot be anesthetized with a single injection.
- The lumbosacral plexus from a functional point of view comprises two distinct entities: the lumbar plexus and the sacral plexus.
- This functional distinction frequently requires the performance of two separate blocks, increasing the requirement for local anesthetic and hence the likelihood of systemic toxicity.
- Because of overlying muscle and connective tissue, injections are generally deeper than those required for the upper limb.
- Not surprisingly, ultrasonography has helped increase block success rates, performance times, and onset times for lower limb blocks.
- Ultrasonography helps identify anatomical variation in individual patients and reduces the incidence of vascular puncture.
- Nerve imaging can be technically challenging in the lower limb; low-frequency ultrasound probes are needed for deep structures.
- Stimulating catheters for continuous femoral nerve block are associated with decreased postoperative visual analog scale (VAS) scores.
- Lower limb blocks may impair the patient's ability to mobilize safely, increasing the likelihood of falls and injuries. Patient suitability, type of surgery, and day case or overnight stay all impact the choice of block (or not) to be performed.
- Lower limb surgeries frequently require the use of tourniquets; the combination of direct local anesthetic neurotoxicity, tourniquet-induced ischemia, or crush injury, together with patient factors such as diabetes, must be considered on an individual patient basis with regard to the potential for neurological injury.

Clinical Pearls:

- The estimated distance from the skin to the lumbar plexus is 8.35 cm (range, 6.1–10.1) in men and 7.1 cm (range, 5.7–9.3) in women.[4]
- The distance from the transverse process to lumbar plexus is consistently less than 2 cm in studies.[4]
- Low-pressure injection is more likely to result in unilateral block.[8]
- The femoral nerve frequently divides in the proximal thigh; the practitioner should scan more cephalad if it is difficult to identify.
- The anterior division of the femoral nerve supplies a motor branch to sartorius muscle. Medial and intermediate cutaneous branches supply the skin of the medial and anterior surfaces of the thigh.
- The anterior division is most likely to be stimulated first, so the needle should be moved lateral and slightly deeper to stimulate the posterior division.
- The minimum local anesthetic volume to produce successful block in 50% of patients is 14 to 16 mL of 0.5% bupivacaine and ropivacaine, respectively.
- The use of ultrasonography dramatically reduces the risk of vascular puncture.
- The distance from the anterior superior iliac spine to the pubic tubercle is consistently 12 to 15 cm.
- There is a low chance of vascular injury given block anatomy even with the double-pop or "blind" technique.
- Asking the patient to cough increases intraabdominal pressure, resulting in retrograde expulsion of local anesthetic from the needle hub and confirming correct fascial plane location.
- The use of ultrasonography has made the obturator block more accessible and easier to perform.
- Deposition of local anesthetic in interfascial planes results in a greater than 90% success rate without the need for muscle stimulation as an end point.
- Obturator block reduces opioid consumption and pain scores in patients undergoing major knee surgery.
- The posterior approach described by di Benedetto et al[38] is associated with a low degree of patient discomfort during block performance for sciatic nerve block in the thigh.
- More proximal approaches to the sciatic nerve are more likely to result in blockade of the posterior cutaneous nerve of the thigh, providing an advantage for procedures above the knee.
- Popliteal fossa block anesthetizes the entire leg below the tibial plateau except the skin on the medial aspect of the foot and calf (saphenous nerve).
- If using a blind technique, saphenous paravascular injection greatly increases the chances of a successful block.

Continued

CHAPTER OVERVIEW—cont'd

- The saphenous nerve provides sensation to the medial aspect of the ankle and leg and may need to be blocked separately.
- Systemic toxicity has rarely been reported even with bilateral ankle blocks.
- Patients can mobilize after an ankle block because foot drop does not occur.
- If the saphenous nerve cannot be identified using ultrasonography, perivenous ultrasound-guided injection of local anesthetic is associated with a higher success rate than blind injection alone.

Clinical Pitfalls:
- Epidural spread of local anesthetic is a common side effect with contralateral spread occurring in 9% to 16% of patients.
- Coagulopathy is a major consideration.
- High volumes of local anesthetics are injected into a vascular compartment. If a supplemental or subsequent lower limb block is added, local anesthetic toxicity can become an issue. This has been reported in older patients.
- It is difficult to produce a consistent three-in-one block with a single injection technique.
- The obturator nerve is less frequently anesthetized than the lateral femoral cutaneous nerve when the classical three-in-one block is attempted.
- The accuracy of catheter placement for continuous techniques is important, stimulating catheters result in consistently higher success rates. Motor responses at 1 mA (using the catheter) or less are associated with lower median VAS scores.
- Intraneural injection commonly occurs when the popliteal block is performed using stimulation only.
- A motor response may be frequently difficult to illicit and often absent; when a response is elicited below 0.5 mA, intraneural needle placement is likely for this block.
- Stimulation-only popliteal fossa blocks are better tolerated although less successful than classical higher approaches to the sciatic nerve.
- The saphenous and in particular the deep peroneal nerve are frequently difficult to identify with ultrasonography.

Introduction

This chapter discusses both landmark- and ultrasound-guided approaches to each of the commonly performed lower limb blocks. Until recently, lower limb peripheral nerve blocks have been relatively underusedtilized for anesthesia and analgesia because of the effectiveness and relative simplicity of both spinal and continuous epidural techniques. However, in the past 10 to 15 years, several studies have demonstrated that for major orthopedic surgery, peripheral nerve blocks provide very effective analgesia but with reduced adverse effects compared with central neuraxial blocks. This combined with the ability to perform effective continuous techniques has created a change in practice toward greater use of lower limb blocks, especially in expert hands. More recently, the addition of ultrasound guidance has further improved our efficacy for lower limb techniques.

Lumbar Plexus Block

The anterior rami of T12-L4 form the lumbar plexus. The lumbar nerve roots emerge from the intervertebral foramina and immediately enter the body of the psoas muscle; divide into anterior and posterior divisions; and reunite as they course through the muscle to form the ilioinguinal, genitofemoral, lateral femoral cutaneous, femoral, and obturator nerves. The psoas muscle is enclosed in a fascial sheath continuous superiorly with the thoracic fascia, limited medially by the bodies of the lumbar vertebrae and posteriorly by the transverse processes, ligaments, and quadratus lumborum. Many approaches to the psoas compartment have been described, but probably the best known are those of Winnie and Capdevila. Both have an inferior (L4, L5) needle entry point and both result in spread of local anesthetic within the psoas compartment superiorly to L1 (**Fig. 7-1**).[1]

Winnie (1974) described the first posterior approach to the lumbar plexus and its subsequent modification with the use of nerve stimulation.[2] Bilateral blockade, however, and concurrent epidural and spinal anesthesia occurring with the block led to concerns about its use.[3] Capdevila, among others, proposed a number of modifications to the original description, designed to

reduce the incidence of bilateral block (reportedly 10% to 20%).[4] Capdevila reported a reduction in the incidence of bilateral block to 2%. Mannion et al[5] compared both the Winnie and Capdevila approaches and randomized 60 elderly patients having lower limb arthroplasty to either technique for postoperative analgesia. Twelve patients in the Winnie group (40%) and 10 patients in the Capdevila group developed contralateral spread with many having evidence of bilateral thoracic and lumbar dermatomal spread (eight and five, respectively). Postulated reasons for bilateral spread have included (1) puncture of the epidural sleeve of the femoral nerve,[6] (2) medial needle orientation leading to direct epidural or subarachnoid spread,[4] and (3) spread occurring anterior to the vertebral bodies via areolar connective tissue within the subserous

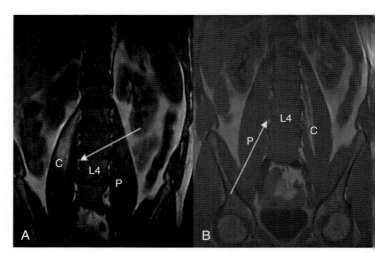

Fig. 7-1 MRI study demonstrating contrast spread within the psoas compartment—the "psoas stripe." **A,** Contrast spread achieved following Capdevila's approach (right psoas muscle). **B,** Contrast spread within the left psoas muscle using Winnie's approach in the same volunteer (1 week apart.) Psoas muscle (*P*), contrast (*C*). (Reproduced from Mannion S, Barrett J, Kelly D, et al: A description of the spread of injectate after psoas compartment block using magnetic resonance imaging, *Reg Anesth Pain Med* 30:567-571, 2005.)

fascial layer as has been previously described to occur in the thorax.[7] Gadsden et al[8] recently demonstrated evidence of bilateral femoral nerve block or neuraxial anesthesia in six and five of 10 study patients, respectively, when injection pressure exceeded 20 psi. Neither effect occurred in 10 other patients randomized to injection pressure less than 15 psi when 35 mL of mepivacaine was injected. This appears to support the hypothesis that local anesthetic administered under high pressure causes extensive cleaving of tissue planes within the psoas muscle. Presumably, this opens up channels through which local anesthetic approaches the intervertebral foramina.

Clinical Utility

Perhaps more so than any other lower limb block, the clinical utility of a psoas compartment block in an individual patient must be weighed against the potential for the complications already discussed. A retrospective study by Macaire et al[9] offers an insight into the incidence of such complications in clinical practice. The study itself involved 42 teams from the United States, Canada, France, Belgium, and Switzerland. In all, 4319 posterior lumbar plexus blocks were reported. Teams declared a 1% to 10% incidence of epidural spread, 11 total spinal anesthetics with one resulting death, 13 intravascular injections with three resulting seizures and one cardiac arrest, four delayed toxic reactions, and 13 incorrect catheter paths. Given the retrospective nature of this report, these figures may well be underestimated.[9] A recent meta-analysis evaluated psoas compartment anesthesia for lower extremity surgery.[10] Thirty studies were included, and the authors concluded that although psoas compartment block was superior to opioids for postoperative analgesia (providing 13 hours of analgesia after a single-shot block), there was insufficient data to recommend this approach as the sole anesthetic for hip or major knee surgery.[10] Conversion rates to general anesthesia were typically in the order of 20% to 25%.

Landmark Technique for Psoas Compartment Block

The Capdevila approach to the psoas compartment block is outlined here because studies in general report lower incidence of bilateral spread. Venous access and standard monitoring (oxygen saturation, electrocardiography, and noninvasive blood pressure monitors) are secured. Because this is a deep block, patient discomfort can be a problem. It is our practice to administer fentanyl 0.5 to 1 µg/kg and 1 to 2 mg of midazolam if required. The patient is positioned in the lateral decubitus position with a slight forward tilt. The side to be blocked is uppermost. Both thighs are flexed, though the foot of the uppermost leg should be positioned over the dependent leg for ease of visibility. The spinous process of L4 is identified as the point at which the intercristal (Tuffier's) line intersects the vertebral column. The posterior superior iliac spine is identified by palpation. From this point, the practitioner draws a line parallel to the spinous process extending cephalad. The practitioner draws out the intercristal line; this intersects with the line originating at the posterior superior iliac spines. The needle puncture point is at the junction of the lateral one third and medial two thirds of the line joining L4 and the line passing through the posterior superior iliac spine. At a minimum, an 80- to 100-mm insulated stimulating needle is needed for this block, and the stimulating current is set at 1.0 mA, 2 Hz, and 0.1 msec. The needle is oriented perpendicular to the skin and advanced until the transverse process of L4 is encountered. The needle is then directed caudally and advanced no more than 20 mm until a quadriceps muscle twitch is seen.[11]

Ultrasound-Guided Technique of Psoas Compartment Block

The patient is positioned similar to that used for the landmark approach. A low-frequency 2- to 5-MHz curved array transducer is used. It is our practice to begin by identifying the sacrum and turning the probe through 90 degrees to image the facet joints of the lumbar vertebrae: L3, L4, and L5. The transducer (with the long axis of the probe parallel to the lumbar spine) is moved laterally to identify the transverse processes of L3, L4, and L5. The hyperechoic transverse processes with the resulting acoustic shadow produce a characteristic "trident sign" shown in **Fig. 7-2**.[12] The ultrasound machine settings (focal zones, depth of the scanning plane, and far-field gain) are now optimized. The psoas muscle has a striated appearance; although the lumbar plexus can be identified with ultrasonography, we have found this difficult to achieve in our adult practice.[11] Local anesthetic (lidocaine 2%) is used to infiltrate the skin and deeper structures. The stimulating needle is introduced along the long axis of the probe in plane from cephalad to caudad (**Fig. 7-3**). We believe this approach is less likely to result in damage to structures such as the lower pole of the kidney (**Fig. 7-4**). The needle tip is angled away from the intervertebral foramina. In performing this block, it is frequently difficult to identify the needle shaft because of the curved array and angle of needle approach. Its position can often only be inferred from tissue movement around the needle when it is rocked side to side or gently probed forward. Entry of the needle into the posterior part of the

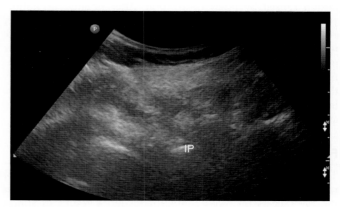

Fig. 7-2 Longitudinal sonogram of the lumbar paravertebral region. The transverse processes (*TPs*) are easily identified and produce acoustic shadowing, L5 is on the left-hand side of the image. The psoas muscle lies inferior to the transverse processes.

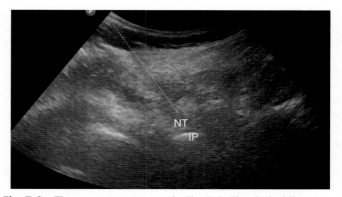

Fig. 7-3 The same sonogram as in Fig. 7-2. The *dashed line* shows the current needle trajectory and needle tip position (*NT*) as it approaches the transverse processes (*TP*) of L4.

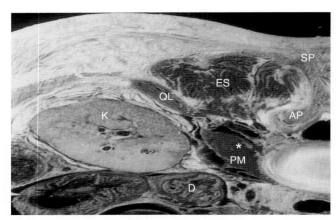

Fig. 7-4 Cross sectional preparation at L3-L4. A branch of the lumbar plexus (*asterisk*) is shown within the posterior part of the psoas muscle (*PM*). The quadratus lumborum muscle (*QL*), erector spinae (*ES*), kidney (*K*), duodenum (*D*), spinous process (*SP*), and articular process (*AP*) are shown. (Reproduced from Kirchmair L, et al: Kirchmair L, Entner T, Wissel J, et al: A study of the paravertebral anatomy for ultrasound-guided posterior lumbar plexus block, *Anesth Analg* 93:477-481, 2001.)

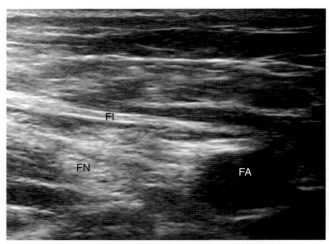

Fig. 7-5 Ultrasound image showing the relationship between femoral nerve (*FN*) and artery (*FA*). *FI*, fascia iliaca.

psoas muscle results in contraction of the psoas muscle seen on the ultrasound screen. The needle is advance slowly to elicit femoral nerve stimulation (patellar twitch) not to be mistaken with hip flexion caused by psoas contraction. After negative aspiration, 10 mL of the local anesthetic solution is slowly injected. Further aspiration after each 10 mL is injected is advisable. It is our practice to use 20 to 30 mL of 0.5% ropivacaine solution. It should be pointed out that in obese patients, because of the technical limitations of ultrasonography, it can be frequently difficult to identify the psoas muscle and associated anatomy.[13] It is thus up to the individual practitioner whether to abandon the procedure or attempt to perform it using stimulation alone.

Femoral Nerve

The femoral nerve is formed by the dorsal divisions of the anterior rami of the spinal nerves L2 to L4 as they condense within the psoas muscle. (Successful psoas compartment block results in almost 100% incidence of femoral nerve block.) The femoral nerve emerges from the lateral aspect of the psoas muscle at the junction of the middle and lower thirds and courses in the gutter between the psoas and the iliacus muscle lying inferior to the fascia iliaca. It enters the thigh when it passes inferior to the inguinal ligament. It lies deep to fascia lata and iliaca, lateral and at times somewhat posterior to the femoral artery (**Fig. 7-5**). At this level, the femoral nerve is rarely a single structure; rather, the nerve has rapidly divided into major anterior and posterior divisions. Other branches include the articular branch to the hip joint and branches to the rectus femoris, sartorius, and pectineus muscles. The anterior branches pierce fascia iliaca and supply sensory innervation to the anterior and medial aspects of the thigh. The posterior branches remain deep to fascia iliaca and innervate the quadriceps and the knee joint and terminate as the saphenous nerve, which supplies sensation to the medial aspect of the leg.

Winnie et al[14] (1973) proposed the inguinal paravascular approach to the lumbar plexus (i.e., the three-in-one block), eliciting femoral nerve paresthesia at the level of the inguinal crease and using larger volumes of local anesthetic combined with pressure distal to the needle entry point. They described successful blockade

of the femoral, ilioinguinal, and lateral cutaneous nerves simultaneously. Recent work has failed to demonstrate consistent block of all three nerves with high-volume local anesthetic injections. At least partial sensory blockade of the lateral femoral cutaneous nerve is achieved in almost all patients; the obturator nerve, however, is least likely to be blocked. In some series, the incidence of successful block is less than 10% irrespective of volume injected.[15,16] This may be because of the medial location of that nerve at the inguinal crease level. Cephalad spread of local anesthetic to the lumbar plexus is limited on magnetic resonance imaging studies and does not appear to consistently occur to the extent postulated earlier by Winnie et al.[14] Rather, the injectate spreads lateral, caudal, and slightly medial (**Fig. 7-6**).[17]

Ultrasound-guided femoral nerve block results in significantly faster sensory onset times over nerve stimulation alone (onset time, 16 minutes vs. 27 minutes using 20 mL bupivacaine 0.5%).[18] Ultrasound guidance also significantly reduces the minimum effective anesthetic volume required for successful nerve block.[19] A recent meta-analysis of 13 studies confirmed that regional blocks performed with ultrasonography were more likely to be successful, had faster onset, had on average a 25% longer duration of action, and took marginally less time to perform (1 minute). Perhaps of most importance, ultrasound guidance reduced the risk of vascular puncture by 80% in real terms (relative risk, 0.16; 95% confidence interval 0.05–0.47; P = .001).[20] At our institution, we continue to use 20 mL of ropivacaine 0.5% as the standard bolus dose for ultrasound-guided analgesic blocks.

Landmark Technique

The patient is positioned in the supine position. In overweight patients, the lower abdomen may have to be retracted and held out of the field using tape. Venous access and standard monitoring are secured. The site of needle insertion is below the level of the inguinal ligament at the level of the groin crease (easily identified by asking the patient to raise his or her leg 15 degrees or so).[22] The femoral pulse is palpated and marked. The insertion point is 1 to 2 cm lateral to the arterial pulsation; the skin is infiltrated with local anesthetic at this point. A 50-mm insulated stimulating needle is used for this block with the stimulating current set at 1.0 mA, 2 Hz, and 0.1 msec. The stimulating needle is advanced at 45 to 60 degrees to the skin in the cephalad direction. Insertion at this level produces the highest rate of needle–femoral nerve contact in

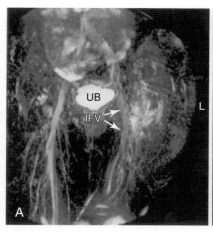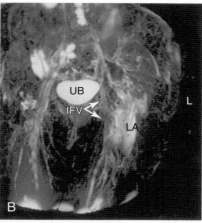

Fig. 7-6 Paracoronal T2-weighted MRI. **A,** Before injection. **B,** Distribution pattern of 30 mL of local anesthetic solution. LA, local anesthetic; LFV, left femoral vein; UB, urinary bladder. (Reproduced from Marhofer P, Schrogendorfer K, Koinig H, et al: Ultrasonographic guidance improves sensory block and onset time of three-in-one blocks, *Anesth Analg* 85:854-857, 1997.)

cadaver studies.[20,21] A distinct loss of resistance is usually felt each time the blunt stimulating needle traverses the fascia layers. A sartorius twitch is frequently the first twitch elicited; the quadriceps twitch (patella dance) is usually elicited by advancing the needle in a more lateral direction and 2 mm deep to the point of original sartorius twitch.[22] The current intensity is then reduced; the needle tip position is adequate when quadriceps contraction persists when the current is 0.2 to 0.5 mA. Many believe that a quadriceps twitch is a prerequisite to successful block (New York Society of Regional Anesthesia), but recent evidence appears to contradict this view.[23]

Ultrasound Technique

A systematic anatomical survey should first be undertaken. With the patient supine, the leg to be blocked is allowed to rotate slightly lateral. A high-frequency linear ultrasound probe scan is used from medial to lateral and then superficial to deep (at the groin crease). The ultrasound transducer is held perpendicular to the imagined path of the femoral nerve at all times (even a tilt of 10 to 15 degrees can render the femoral nerve isoechoic with the iliopsoas muscle).[24] Because of its size in this area, the femoral nerve is often easy to identify and located lateral to the femoral artery (**Figs. 7-5 and 7-7**). Both lie anterior to the iliopsoas muscle. The femoral nerve is often identified as a triangular or wedge-shaped hyperechoic region lateral to the artery. This wedge is bounded superiorly by fascia iliaca, inferiorly by the iliopsoas fascia, and medially by the artery itself. If the nerve has split into anterior and posterior branches at this point, the posterior division that supplies the quadriceps lies most lateral within the triangle. Often, the femoral artery and profunda femoris artery are visible in the same image; we recommend scanning more cephalad, where imaging of the femoral nerve is often easier when the femoral artery alone is imaged. Despite its size, if the femoral nerve is flat or splits very proximal in the thigh, it can be difficult to image.

At our institution, we use a stimulating needle to confirm that the target structure is the femoral nerve. The stimulating needle can be positioned using an in-plane or out-of-plane approach. In the out-of-plane approach, the image is centered on the femoral nerve and the stimulating needle is introduced through the skin at an almost perpendicular angle parallel to the ultrasound beam. The needle tip is visualized as a white dot. A distinct loss of resistance is felt as the needle traverses fascia lata and then fascia iliaca. At this point, caution is needed as the needle tip is directly over the nerve itself. The needle is advanced in millimeter increments until a motor response is elicited if the twitch is sartorius and then orient

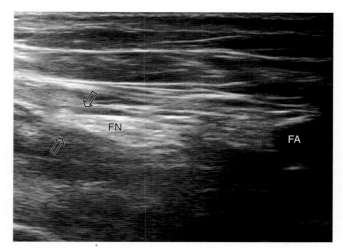

Fig. 7-7 Ultrasound scan at the level of the groin crease after injection of local anesthetic solution (*open arrows*). Note that the local anesthetic solution is deposited mostly underneath or inferior to the nerve. FA, femoral artery; FN, femoral nerve.

the needle more lateral. The local anesthetic solution or injection of dextrose 5% solution (hypoechoic) should bring the nerve (hyperechoic) into better view as the femoral triangle is distended (**Fig. 7-7**). For successful block, the solution must be deposited inferior to the fascia iliaca and not extend superior to and medial to the femoral artery. The appearance of the femoral nerve itself after injection of the local anesthetic exhibits significant variability, depending on patient, body habitus, and imaging equipment (**Figs. 7-7 and 7-8** illustrate this).

Iliacus Fascia Block

Sharrock[25] (1989) described a three-in-one block after an attempted block of the lateral femoral cutaneous nerve of the thigh, sparking interest in other approaches to the three-in-one block outside of those required to stimulate the femoral nerve itself. Medial and lateral spread of local anesthetic beneath the plane of the fascia iliaca is the anatomical basis for this block. Not surprisingly, the obturator nerve (most medial nerve of the lumbar plexus) is less likely to be blocked than if the traditional three-in-one approach is used.[26] Capdevila randomized 100 patients to either block in a prospective randomized controlled trial.[26] Sensory block of the

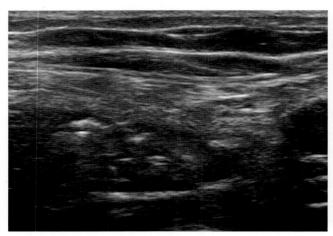

Fig. 7-8 Ultrasound image at the level of the groin crease. The femoral nerve can be clearly seen surrounded by local anesthetic solution and a coiled nerve block catheter. This image is included to demonstrate the variability of the appearance of the femoral nerve space after injection of local anesthetic.

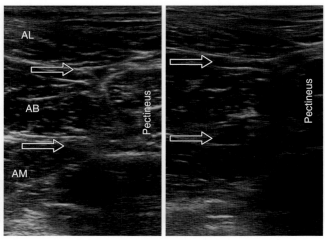

Fig. 7-9 Ultrasound images of medial thigh. **A,** The *upper open arrow* demonstrates anterior obturator branch. The *lower open arrow* shows the plane of posterior branch. **B,** After injection of local anesthetic 3 mL in each plane. The *lower open arrow* shows the plane of the posterior branch of the obturator. The nerve itself can now be seen superior to the pocket of local anesthetic (hyperechoic structure). AB, adductor brevis; AM, adductor medius; L, adductor longus.

femoral, obturator, and lateral cutaneous nerve was achieved in 88%, 38%, and 90%, respectively, of those having fascia iliaca block versus 90%, 52%, and 62%, respectively, of those having three-in-one block.[26] Similar efficacy has been demonstrated in children.[27] Dolan and colleagues[28] compared traditional "blind" fascia iliaca block to ultrasound-guided deposition of local anesthetic beneath the fascia iliaca. Ultrasound-guided block resulted in 82% of patients having complete loss of sensation on the anterior, lateral, and medial aspects of the thigh. Sensory inhibition increased to 95% (versus 60%) of cases on the medial aspect of the thigh when using ultrasonography. It would seem that both femoral and fascia iliaca block are approximately equivalent. Fascia iliaca block has the advantage of reducing the potential for direct needle trauma to the femoral nerve and artery.

Technique of Fascia Iliaca Block

The landmarks for this block are the anterior superior iliac spine, pubic tubercle, and inguinal ligament. The patient is positioned in the supine position. Dalens et al[27] describe drawing a line on the skin connecting the anterior superior iliac spine to pubic tubercle. This line (usually 12 cm in adults) is divided into thirds. At the junction of the lateral and medial two thirds, a second line is drawn perpendicular to and intersecting the line joining anterior superior iliac spine and pubic tubercle. One cm along this line is the insertion point. A blunt needle (an 18-gauge Tuohy needle being a good choice) is inserted perpendicular to the skin at this point. The femoral artery and nerve are 3 to 4 cm medial, so no muscle stimulation end point is sought. A "pop" or give is felt as the needle passes through the fascia lata, and a second loss of resistance is felt as it passes through the fascia iliaca.[27] The local anesthetic should inject easily (similar to injecting into the epidural space), and repeated aspiration should be performed. Asking the patient to cough increases intraabdominal pressure, resulting in retrograde expulsion of local anesthetic from the needle hub. This confirms correct position beneath the fascia iliaca. Because this is a compartment block, a large volume of injectate is important, with most authors using a volume of at least 30 mL.[26,28]

For the ultrasound-guided technique, the anatomical landmarks are the same. A linear 3- to 5-MHz high-frequency probe is used to identify the fascia lata and iliaca together with the iliacus muscle. The needle tip is guided beneath the fascia iliaca, and using transverse short-axis views, the spread of injectate is viewed. Catheters can also be inserted for continuous blocks as for femoral nerve blocks.

Obturator Nerve Block

The obturator nerve enters the leg through the craniomedial part of the obturator foramen. It divides into an anterior branch, which passes between the adductor longus and brevis muscles and a posterior branch between the adductor brevis and magnus muscles, although this is somewhat of an oversimplification (**Fig. 7-9**). The division of the obturator nerve into anterior and posterior divisions within the obturator canal exhibits quite a degree of variability. The anterior branch is initially located in the plane between pectineus and adductor brevis muscles. As it courses down the canal, its course is between adductor longus and brevis muscles.[29] The obturator nerve is motor to the adductor, obturator, and gracilis muscles. The anterior branch provides sensation to a limited area on the medial aspect of the knee. The posterior branch often supplies part of the knee joint. The adductor muscles also receive variable innervation from the femoral and sciatic nerves; thus, successful obturator block does not imply complete absence of adduction. Obturator nerve blocks have been used in patients with cancer and osteoarthritis for pain control. The addition of an obturator nerve block to a femoral three-in-one block for analgesia after total knee arthroplasty is controversial and is currently not recommended for routine use.[30] Studies involving small numbers of participants have produced contradictory results.[31,32] This may reflect interindividual variation in the dermatomal innervation of the anterior branch of the obturator nerve; 32% of patients in one series were reported as having no cutaneous distribution.[33] Small numbers of patients and the omission of ultrasonography make interpreting these studies difficult. It is not our routine practice to include an obturator nerve block as part of the multimodal analgesic regimen used at our institution, but it must be acknowledged that a small number of patients do complain of troublesome medial aspect knee pain following knee arthroplasty.

Technique of Obturator Nerve Block

Selective obturator nerve block has been described as "both difficult and uncomfortable."[34] The use of ultrasonography and published ultrasonographic descriptions have made the process of the block itself easier. Visualizing the branches of the obturator nerve individually can be difficult. Alternatively, deposition of local anesthetic in the fascial planes between the (1) adductor longus and brevis and (2) adductor brevis and magnus will result in a high probability of successful block with minimal time required.[35] Multiple muscle planes are traversed, making this a deep block with the use of sedation advisable. Ten mL of local anesthetic (5 mL in each plane) is sufficient.

The patient is positioned in the supine position with the leg externally rotated 5 to 10 degrees in slight abduction. The medial groin and proximal thigh is exposed. A linear 5- to 10-MHz ultrasound probe is used. A systematic survey is performed, and the femoral artery and vein are identified. The probe is then moved medially along the inguinal crease to identify the fascial planes of the pectineus and adductor muscles. The block needle can be introduced in or out of plane. An 80-mm block needle or 22-gauge spinal needle can be used. The needle tip is first advanced into the plane between the adductor longus and brevis muscles. After negative aspiration, 1 to 2 mL of solution is injected to confirm needle tip position. Interfascial spread should result in separation of the target muscles; 5 mL in total is deposited (**Fig. 7-9**). The needle is then further advanced into the plane between adductor brevis and magnus, and the procedure is repeated. Sinha and colleagues[35] have recently reported a 93% success rate with this technique (defined as a 50% reduction in strength of adductor muscle contraction).

Sciatic Nerve Block

The broad, flat sciatic nerve is formed by the union of the lumbar sacral trunk (comprising the ventral rami of the L4 and L5 nerve roots) and the anterior branches of the first, second, and third sacral nerves. These nerves condense on the pelvic surface of the piriformis muscle to form the sciatic nerve that exits the pelvis and enters the gluteal region via the greater sciatic foramen. The nerve remains 10 cm or so lateral to the midline and passes between the greater trochanter and ischial tuberosity. It emerges inferior to the gluteal muscle and becomes superficial as it passes down the posterior thigh. It divides into the common peroneal and tibial nerves usually approximately 8 cm proximal to the popliteal crease.

Multiple approaches to the sciatic nerve have been described. The nerve is commonly blocked at the gluteal, proximal or mid-thigh, and popliteal fossa levels. Historically, lower approaches or those inferior to the gluteus muscle (i.e., in the thigh) were described as "subgluteal." It is our impression that this type of approach (i.e., proximal and mid-thigh) are increasingly referred to as infragluteal approaches. We describe a traditional landmark- and stimulator-only approach and an ultrasound-guided approach at the gluteal level. The ultrasound-guided approach discussed here is more frequently referred to as the "subgluteal" approach in the context of the recent ultrasound-guided literature.[36,37] Distal sciatic nerve block at the popliteal fossa is also described. As with many other ultrasound-guided blocks, ultrasonography has recently been shown to reduce the minimum effective local anesthetic volume required for successful block.[36]

Landmark Approach to the Sciatic Nerve

The first sciatic nerve block was described by Victor Pauchet in 1920. Winnie modified this approach in 1975. Most recently, di Benedetto et al[38] described a posterior approach to the sciatic nerve that resulted in decreased needle to nerve depth, increased patient satisfaction, and success compared with the classic approach described by Pauchet and later Labat.[39] We describe the approach of di Benedetto here as the nerve stimulator–only technique. However, the ultrasound technique described here, which is very much different in terms of needle entry point, results in a final needle tip position conceptually closer to that approach described by Labat[39] and Mansour and Benetts.[40]

The patient is positioned on the side with that to be blocked uppermost. Standard monitoring is established, and intravenous (IV) access is secured. Adequate sedation using midazolam, fentanyl, or both is important for this block. The thigh is flexed 30 degrees or so on the block side, and the dependent leg is kept straight (Sims position). The greater trochanter is identified and marked as the most lateral bony landmark. The ischial tuberosity is identified by palpating inferiorly and medially from the greater trochanter. The position of this bony landmark is also marked. A line is drawn between the two points. At the midpoint of this line, a second line is drawn perpendicularly in a caudad direction. Four cm along this line is the needle insertion point. At this level, the sciatic nerve is more superficial with only the inferior and thinning aspect of the gluteus maximus muscle overlying it. A skin depression can be palpated and usually seen in the groove between biceps femoris laterally and the more medial semitendinosus muscles. In overweight patients, the skin can be depressed at this point using the middle and index fingers of the nondominant hand; this reduces the distance between the skin and nerve. The stimulating needle is inserted at right angles to the skin plane and advanced (1.5 mA, 2 Hz, 0.1 msec). Sciatic nerve stimulation is typically observed at a depth of 45 ± 13 mm in subjects weighing 73 ± 12 kg.[38]

Ultrasound Technique of Sciatic Nerve Block

The patient is positioned on the side with that to be blocked uppermost. The thigh is flexed on the block side, and the dependent leg is kept straight (Sims position).

The lateral border of the greater trochanter is identified by palpation. This landmark is palpable even in patients with high body mass indexes (BMIs); in this lateral position, adipose tissue "sags" inferiorly, helping with palpation and sonographic identification of the structure. A curvilinear low-frequency ultrasound probe is used having first optimized the ultrasound machine for depth (tissue penetration), placing it firstly over the greater trochanter, which is identified as a hyperechoic structure. Having identified the greater trochanter, the practitioner scans inferiorly and medially with the long axis of the ultrasound probe kept perpendicular to the presumed path of the sciatic nerve. The ischial tuberosity (the next bony prominence encountered) is identified. The sciatic nerve usually lies 10 cm lateral to the midline and close to the ischial tuberosity irrespective of the patient's BMI. After these two landmarks have been identified, the probe is positioned so that both structures appear in the image.

The gluteus maximus muscle is identified (**Fig. 7-10**). The sciatic nerve generally lies in a plane inferior to the gluteus maximus muscle or fascia and anterior to the quadratus femoris muscle fascia (**Fig. 7-10**). After the possible location of the target structure is identified, the resolution settings are optimized so that the target image is optimized. The sciatic nerve can be difficult to image both because of the depth and characteristic of the nerve. At this level,

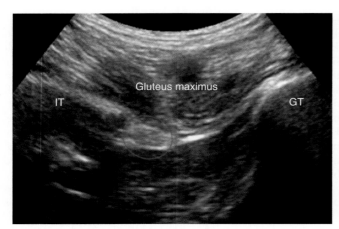

Fig. 7-10 This figure demonstrates the anatomy of the sciatic nerve at the gluteal level. The sciatic nerve (*circle*) is well seen in the fascia between gluteus maximus and quadratus femoris (inferiorly). GT, greater trochanter. IT, ischial tuberosity

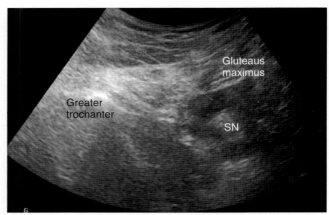

Fig. 7-11 Local anesthetic (20 mL) surrounding the sciatic nerve (SN). The needle trajectory is shown by the *dashed line*.

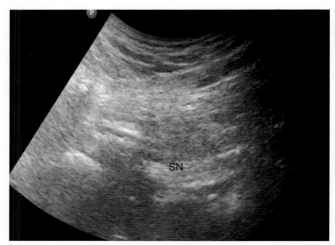

Fig. 7-12 The sciatic nerve (SN) imaged at same level as in Fig. 7-11 (after injection of local anesthetic) with the probe now parallel to the sciatic nerve (i.e., in the long axis orientation rather than transverse as before).

the nerve can often only be definitively identified using stimulation; its ultrasound appearance is a hyperechoic broad, often flat, structure. An 8- to 10-cm stimulating needle is used with the current set at 2.0 mA. The lattermost skin to the probe is anesthetized with local anesthetic, and deeper structures in the needle path (subcutaneous tissue and gluteus maximus muscle) are also infiltrated with local anesthetic. Although this is an in-plane technique, the needle tip can be difficult to identify as the needle approaches the target structure because of the steep angle between the ultrasound beam and needle shaft. If bone is contacted, the needle tip has most likely contacted the ischium; withdraw and angle the stimulating needle more laterally. Often, the first twitches obtained are from the gluteus muscle; twitches of the calf muscles or foot indicate appropriate sciatic stimulation. The stimulating current is decreased and the current intensity noted at which the motor twitch disappears. Recent work demonstrates that an intraneural needle tip position is highly likely in the distal sciatic nerve when an end point for stimulation of a muscle twitch at 0.2 to 0.4 mA is sought (100% intraneural),[41] although this does not imply long-term neurologic damage.[42] Perhaps more worrisome are the results of animal and human sciatic nerve studies; significant subsets demonstrate absent muscle twitches despite intraneural needle tip position and high stimulating currents (>1.0 mA).[41,43] For this reason, we recommend using high stimulating currents to merely identify the target structure. The current intensity is reduced to exclude intraneural needle tip position. Our main end point is the ultrasonographic appearance of injectate pushing away the sciatic nerve from the needle tip and coming to envelop it circumferentially (**Figs. 7-11** and **7-12**).

Sciatic Nerve Block: Popliteal Approach
Distal sciatic nerve block preserves leg flexion and allows reliable anesthesia and analgesia of the calf, tibia, fibula, foot, and ankle. No patient should be allowed to attempt ambulation without crutches after a unilateral popliteal block. The medial aspect of the leg is innervated by the saphenous nerve (distal anterior branch of the femoral nerve), which is described in the next section.

Technique of Popliteal Block The patient is positioned prone or semiprone. Standard monitoring and IV access are secured. If possible, the patient is asked to flex the leg to identify the tendon of biceps femoris laterally and the tendons of semimembranosus and semitendinosus medially. The popliteal crease is easily identified. The level at which the sciatic nerve divides into its two components (the tibial and common peroneal nerves) is variable. Anatomical studies demonstrate this division occurs at a range of 50 to 120 mm proximal to the popliteal crease.[44] At 8 cm proximal to the crease, the nerves typically lie 3 cm medial to the biceps tendon.

As discussed previously, intraneural injection is common when the block is performed by stimulation only. For this reason alone, we recommend the routine use of ultrasonography for this block together with the fact that ultrasound guidance increases the chance of a successful popliteal block over stimulation alone (studies show conflicting results when assessing whether the time taken to perform the block is reduced).[45-47]

A linear 5- to 7-MHz ultrasound probe is used. The probe is placed 8 to 10 cm proximal to the popliteal crease, with the probe perpendicular to the presumed path of the sciatic nerve scan lateral to medial. The popliteal artery is an easily identifiable first landmark. The sciatic nerve usually lies in close proximity and superficial to the artery (**Fig. 7-13, A**). The practitioner scans in a caudad direction following the nerve observing for its bifurcation into the

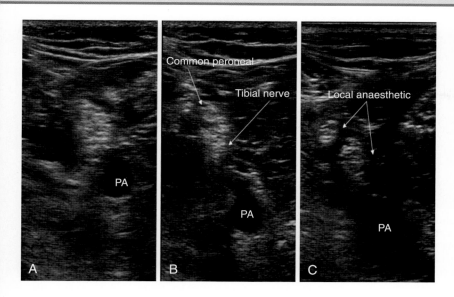

Fig. 7-13   A, The sciatic nerve in close proximity and superficial to the popliteal artery (PA). **B,** Scanning inferiorly to demonstrate the bifurcation. **C,** Local anesthetic solution surrounds both components; in this case, a single injection was sufficient.

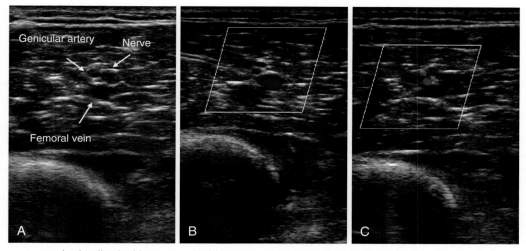

Fig. 7-14   Saphenous nerve in the distal adductor canal with accompanying vascular bundle. Color-flow Doppler is frequently required to distinguish the descending genicular artery from the saphenous nerve. The femoral vein is also seen.

common peroneal (lateral) and tibial nerve (usually larger) component (**Fig. 7-13, B**). After the bifurcation is identified, the direction of scanning is reversed. The injection point is immediately after the bifurcation. A 22-gauge stimulating needle is introduced along the long axis (in plane approach) of the probe. Sala-Blanch et al[48] found that despite clear evidence of needle to nerve proximity, 16 of 37 patients required stimulating currents greater than 1.0 mA to demonstrate any motor response, four of 37 patients had no motor response with current intensity less than 2.0 mA, and only 17 of 37 patients demonstrated a motor response with a current intensity less than 0.5 mA. Robarts et al,[49] reporting on 24 patients, found a motor response could only be elicited at 0.2 to 0.4 mA on intraneural needle placement in 20 patients. In the remaining four, no motor response could be obtained with a stimulating current of 1.5 mA despite intraneural placement. Reassuringly, few patients are reported to develop postoperative neurologic deficits as a result. In view of these findings, it is not our practice to persist in approximating the needle tip to the nerve solely to achieve a motor response. Rather, we carefully inject the first 1 mL of local anesthetic solution, observing for intraneural swelling (>15% increase in nerve diameter) and patient discomfort. In the absence of both, we continue to inject, observing the spread of local anesthetic around the structure. After injection, separation of the two sciatic nerve components should be seen (**Fig. 7-13, C**). A total of 20 to 30 mL of local anesthetic solution is required for adequate block.

Saphenous Nerve Block

The saphenous nerve is the terminal branch of the posterior division of the femoral nerve and provides sensation to the medial aspect of the leg. This includes the anteromedial, posterolateral, and medial aspect of the leg as far distal as the medial malleolus. The recent literature has seen a resurgence of interest in this block.[50-52] The availability of ultrasonography offers the potential of more reproducible and reliable blocks over the older landmark technique, which had a high failure rate.[53] Both are described here.

Contemporary anatomical studies describe the course of the saphenous nerve in the thigh.[51] It separates from the femoral nerve in the proximal thigh and accompanies the femoral artery through the adductor canal. Within the canal and more distal along its course, it accompanies the descending genicular artery (**Fig. 7-14**)

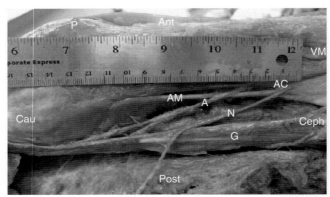

Fig. 7-15 Medial view of a dissected knee. The sartorius muscle is reflected to expose the anatomic structures. The bifurcation of the saphenous nerve (N) can be clearly seen. A, descending genicular artery; AC, adductor canal; Ant, anterior; Cau, caudate; Ceph, cephalad; G, gracilis muscle and tendon; P, patella; Post, posterior; VM, vastus medialis. (Reproduced from Manickam B, Perlas A, Duggan E, et al: Feasibility and efficacy of ultrasound-guided block of the saphenous nerve in the adductor canal, *Reg Anesth Pain Med* 34(6):578-580, 2009.)

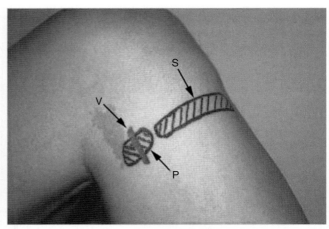

Fig. 7-16 Saphenous nerve block sites, medial aspect of left leg: classical (S) and paravascular (P). Note how the site for paravascular infiltration on the medial side of the tibia lies more lateral to the classic infiltration, explaining the high failure rate associated with the classic technique. V, saphenous vein. (Reproduced from De Mey, Deruyck LJ, Cammu GMD, et al: A paravenous approach for the saphenous nerve block, *Reg Anesth Pain Med* 26:504-506, 2001.)

and emerges alongside it. The descending genicular artery, which supplies the knee itself, arises from the femoral artery just prior to where the femoral artery passes deep to the tendon of adductor magnus (vasoadductor membrane) to enter the popliteal fossa.

The median distance from the proximal patella to the distal end of the adductor canal is 10.25 cm with a range of 7.5 to 11.5 cm in cadaver studies.[51] The saphenous nerve bifurcates into the infrapatellar (which reflects downward) and sartorial branches. This bifurcation occurs at a median distance of 2.7 cm (range, 2.1–3.4) cephalad to the proximal border of the patella and 6.6 cm (range, 5.0–9.0) deep to the medial border of the patella (**Fig. 7-15**).[51]

Landmark Technique of Saphenous Nerve Block

The patient is positioned in the supine position with the knee elevated and leg flexed to 45 degrees. The practitioner palpates for the tibial tuberosity and medial head of gastrocnemius muscle. A blind subcutaneous infiltration is made to raise a "wheal" between both points. The skin may need to be lifted off the tibia, and the needle is inserted parallel to the bone (5 to 7.5 mL of local anesthetic and a 25-gauge needle). Two or three needle insertions may be required. The success rates reported for this classical approach are typically 30% to 40%.[54] De Mey et al[54] report improved success rates (100%) when a modified landmark paravascular technique is used. Cadaveric dissection (*n* = 5) demonstrated a constant relationship between the saphenous vein and nerve. The relationship between nerve and vein was found to be similar in 10 dissections with the nerve being found just medial (within 1 cm) and posterior to the saphenous vein.

De Mey et al[54] performed saphenous nerve block with 100% success rate when local anesthetic was infiltrated or fanned near the vein. A tourniquet around the thigh was used to first identify the vein.[54] **Fig. 7-16** demonstrates the more posterior position of the saphenous injection site. Comfort et al[55] also report 100% successful saphenous nerve block using nerve stimulation at this level, although the time taken to successfully identify the saphenous nerve and perform the block was an average of 11 minutes.[55]

Ultrasound Technique of Saphenous Nerve Block

The patient is positioned in the supine position. Standard monitoring and IV access are secured. A 5- to 7-MHz linear ultrasound probe is used. The ultrasound probe is positioned on the medial surface of the distal thigh 5 to 10 cm proximal to the patella. The probe should be in a transverse orientation with respect to the path of the sartorius muscle. The practitioner scans from lateral to medial to identify the neurovascular bundle. The saphenous nerve may appear hyper- or hypoechoic and is often surrounded by a rim of perineural fat (part of the subsartorial fat pad). Color Doppler ultrasonography is often required to help distinguish the descending genicular artery from the saphenous nerve (**Fig. 7-14**). A 22-gauge needle is introduced in plane from lateral to medial in the fascial plane between the sartorius and vastus medialis muscles. Five to 10 mL of local anesthetic is injected around the nerve.

Ankle Block

The ankle block is easily performed and is a safe, relatively low-risk procedure for both surgical anesthesia and postoperative analgesia. Previously, in the era of the landmark-only approach to the ankle block, many patients required rescue analgesia when the block was used for postoperative analgesia, and yet more anesthetists believed their success rate to be "medium" or "low."[56-58]

The ankle block is useful for forefoot surgery, particularly hallux valgus repair or toe amputation, either as the sole anesthetic or for postoperative analgesia.

The ankle and foot are innervated by five nerves. One of these (the saphenous nerve) is a terminal branch of the femoral nerve. The four remaining nerves are: the tibial, sural, superficial, and deep peroneal nerves (all are branches of the sciatic). Ultrasound and landmark techniques are described. Three to five mL of local anesthetic usually suffices for each block, though this can be reduced when using ultrasound. A block onset time of 20 to 30 minutes when using long-acting local anesthetic solutions should be expected.

Landmark Approach to the Ankle Block

The patient is positioned in the supine position. Standard monitoring and IV access are secured. We do not routinely use nerve stimulation for this block.

We begin by blocking the posterior tibial nerve. The Achilles tendon and medial malleolus are first identified. Along the line between the medial malleolus and the Achilles tendon, the practitioner palpates for the posterior tibial pulse. Posterior to the pulse, a 22-gauge needle is inserted and oriented toward the medial malleolus until bony contact is made. The needle is withdrawn 2 to 3 mm, and 3 to 5 mL of the local anesthetic solution is injected between the Achilles tendon and where the artery is palpated.

An alternative approach is the subsustentacular approach. Again, the medial malleolus is identified; the palpating fingers are moved inferiorly from this point until the lowermost bony prominence of the sustentacular ridge of the calcaneus is palpated. The insertion point is immediately inferior to the ridge. The needle is inserted until bony contact is made. Then it is withdrawn, and 2 to 3 mL of local anesthetic is injected.

Blockade of the sural nerve is similar: the needle is inserted along a line between the lateral malleolus and the Achilles tendon. The Achilles tendon is first palpated, and the needle is inserted anterior to the Achilles tendon and directed toward the lateral malleolus. After bony contact is made, the needle is withdrawn slightly, and 3 to 5 mL of the local anesthetic solution is injected.

The saphenous nerve on the medial aspect of the ankle is blocked by superficial skin injection at the level of the medial malleolus toward the midpoint of the intermalleolar line.

The superficial peroneal nerve is blocked by subcutaneous "fanning" injection of 4 to 5 mL of local anesthetic along a line joining both malleoli, taking care to avoid the saphenous vein.

The deep peroneal nerve can be blocked at the level of the intermalleolar line or more distally along the dorsal aspect of the foot. The landmark is the dorsal artery of the foot (a continuation of the anterior tibial artery), also known as the *dorsalis pedis*. The insertion point is immediately lateral to the pulse. After bony contact is made, 1 to 2 mm of aspirate is withdrawn, and 2 to 3 mL of local anesthetic solution is injected.

Ultrasound Approach to the Ankle Block

We routinely use ultrasonography for both the sural and posterior tibial injections, but we rely on traditional landmark techniques for blockade of the other three nerves. Ultrasonography can be used to identify the dorsalis pedis artery; however, the deep peroneal nerve can be difficult to identify. Antonakakis et al[59] report being unable to identify the nerve in seven of 18 subjects. In the same study, ultrasonography was not shown to improve the success rate of deep peroneal nerve block and led to a longer time to perform the block. However, Benzon et al[60] point out that the nerve is frequently more lateral than expected, emphasizing the need for light pressure when applying the ultrasound probe. This is so as not to compress the artery because it is used as the landmark. They reported very high success rates for combined ultrasonography and stimulator-guided block in volunteers.[60]

Ultrasonography improves the success rate of the sural and tibial nerve block.[61,62] We recommend using a 2.5-cm "hockey stick" high-frequency linear ultrasound probe simply because of the limited size of the scanning surfaces. The sural nerve can frequently be difficult to identify (**Fig. 7-17**). However, the sural nerve is consistently found slightly medial or posterior to the saphenous vein (**Fig. 7-17**).[59] If the structure cannot be definitively identified,

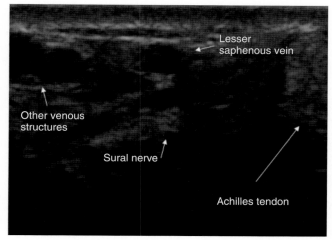

Fig. 7-17 Ultrasound image, lateral aspect of the ankle showing the sural nerve. If the sural nerve is not identified, perivascular injection of local anesthetic near the saphenous vein is likely to result in successful block.

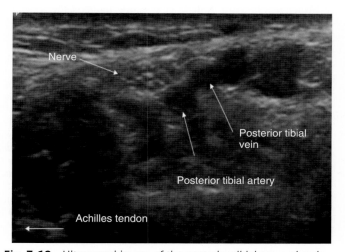

Fig. 7-18 Ultrasound image of the posterior tibial nerve showing its proximity to the tibial artery; in this case, the nerve has a honeycomb appearance.

perivenous ultrasound-guided injection of local anesthetic is associated with a higher success rate and more dense blocks rate than blind injection alone (94% vs. 56%).[61]

The tibial nerve is also best imaged in the short-axis view. The practitioner begins by scanning around the medial malleolus moving toward the Achilles tendon. The area contains several vascular structures, and color Doppler ultrasonography is often required to confirm the nature of anechoic structures (**Fig. 7-18**). The tibial nerve frequently appears as a honeycomb structure and can be differentiated from the flexor hallucis tendon simply by asking the patient to flex the great toe; the tendon should thus move (**Fig. 7-19**). The needle is introduced in plane from lateral to medial, and the practitioner injects circumferentially around the nerve. Although ultrasound-guided tibial nerve block takes longer to perform (159 vs. 79 seconds) and is associated with more needle redirections, its use is associated with a faster onset and more complete blocks at all times.[61]

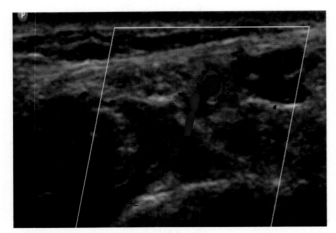

Fig. 7-19 The same image as in Fig. 7-18 is presented here with color-flow Doppler, which can aid in distinguishing vascular from nonvascular structures.

References

1. Mannion S, Barrett J, Kelly D, et al: A description of the spread of injectate after psoas compartment block using magnetic resonance imaging. *Reg Anesth Pain Med* 30:567-571, 2005.
2. Winnie AP, Ramamurthy S, Durani Z, Radonjic R: Plexus blocks for lower surgery: new answers to old problems. *Anesthesiol Rev* 1:11-16, 1974.
3. Auroy Y, Benhamou D, Bargues L, et al: Major complications of regional anesthesia in France: the SOS Regional Anesthesia Hotline Service. *Anesthesiology* 97:1274-1280, 2002.
4. Capdevila X, Macaire P, Dadure C, et al: Continuous psoas compartment block for postoperative analgesia after total hip arthroplasty: new landmarks, technical guidelines and clinical evaluation. *Anesth Analg* 94:1606-1613, 2002.
5. Mannion S, O Callaghan S, Walsh M, et al: Approaches for psoas compartment block. *Anesth Analg* 101:259-264, 2005.
6. Dalens B, Tanguy A, Vanneuville G: Lumbar plexus block in children: a comparison of two procedures in 50 patients. *Anesth Analg* 67:750-758, 1998.
7. Karmakar MK, Kwok WH, Kew J: Thoracic paravertebral block: radiological evidence of contralateral spread anterior to the vertebral bodies. *Br J Anaesth* 84:263-265, 2000.
8. Gadsden JC, Lindenmuth DM, Hadzic A, et al: Lumbar plexus block using a high pressure injection leads to contralateral epidural spread. *Anesthesiology* 109:683-688, 2008.
9. Macarie P, Gaertner E, Choquet O: Le Bloc du Plexus lombaire est-il dangereux? In *Evaluation et traitement de la douleur. SFAR 2002*, Paris, 2002, Elsevier and SFAR, pp 37-50.
10. Touray ST, de Leeeuw MA, Zuurmond WWA, Perez RSGM: Psoas compartment block for lower extremity surgery: a meta-analysis. *Br J Anaesth* 101:750-760, 2008.
11. Awad IT, Duggan EM: Posterior lumbar plexus block. Anatomy, approaches and techniques. *Reg Anesth Pain Med* 30:143-149, 2005.
12. Karmakar MK, Ho AM, Li X, et al: Ultrasound-guided lumbar plexus block through the acoustic window of the lumbar ultrasound trident. *Br J Anaesth* 100:533-537, 2008.
13. Kirchmair L, Entner T, Wissel J, et al: A study of the paravertebral anatomy for ultrasound-guided posterior lumbar plexus block. *Anesth Analg* 93:477-481, 2001.
14. Winnie AP, Ramamurthy S, Durrani Z: The inguinal paravascular technic of lumbar plexus anesthesia: the "3-in-1 block." *Anesth Analg* 52:989-996, 1973.
15. Lang SA, Yip RW, Chang PC, et al: The femoral nerve block revisited. *J Clin Anesth* 5:292-296, 1993.
16. Seegerger MD, Urwyler A: Paravascular lumbar plexus block: block extension after femoral nerve stimulation and injection of 20 vs 40 ml mepivacaine 10 mg/ml. *Acta Anaesthesiol Scand* 39:769-773, 1995.
17. Marhofer P, Nasel C, Sitzwohl C, Kapral S: Magnetic resonance imaging of the distribution of local anesthetic during the three-in-one block. *Anesth Analg* 90:119-124, 2000.
18. Marhofer P, Schrogendorfer K, Koinig H, et al: Ultrasonographic guidance improves sensory block and onset time of three-in-one blocks. *Anesth Analg* 85:854-857, 1997.
19. Casati A, Baciarello M, Di Cianni S, et al: Effects of Ultrasound guidance on the minimum effective anaesthetic volume required to block the femoral nerve. *Br J Anaesth* 98:823-827, 2007.
20. Abrahams MS, Aziz MF, Fu RF, Horn JL: Ultrasound guidance compared with electrical stimulation for peripheral nerve block: a systematic review and meta-analysis of randomized controlled trials. *Br J Anaesth* 102:408-417, 2009.
21. Vloka DJ, Hadzic A, Drobnik L, et al: Anatomical landmarks for femoral nerve block: a comparison of four needle insertion sites. *Anesth Analg* 89:1467-1470, 1999.
22. Nader A, Malik K, Kendall MC, et al: Relationship between ultrasound imaging and eliciting motor response during femoral nerve stimulation. *J Ultrasound Med* 3:345-350, 2009.
23. Anns J, Awad I, McCartney C, et al: An interim analysis of femoral nerve block anatomical insertion point: a prospective, randomised, double-blind controlled trial. *Reg Anesth Pain Med* 33(5):e106, 2008.
24. Soong J, Schafhalter-Zoppoth I, Gray AT: The importance of transducer angle on ultrasound visibility of the femoral nerve. *Reg Anesth Pain Med* 30:505, 2005.
25. Sharrock NE: Inadvertent "3-in-1" block following injection of the lateral femoral cutaneous nerve of the thigh. *Anesth Analg* 59:887-888, 1989.
26. Capdevila X, Biboulet P, Bouregba M, et al: Comparison of the three-in-one and fascia iliaca compartment blocks in adults: clinical and radiographic analysis. *Anesth Analg* 86:1039-1044, 1998.
27. Dalens B, Vanneuville G, Tanguy A: Comparison of the fascia iliaca block with the 3-in-1 block in children. *Anesth Analg* 69:705-713, 1989.
28. Dolan J, Williams A, Murney E, et al: Ultrasound guided fascia iliaca block: a comparison with the loss of resistance technique. *Reg Anesth Pain Med* 33:526-531, 2008.
29. Saranteas T, Paraskeuopoulos T, Alevizou A, et al: Identification of the obturator nerve divisions and subdivisions in the inguinal region: as study with ultrasound. *Acta Anaesthesiol Scand* 51:1404-1406, 2007.
30. Fischer HBJ, Simanski CJP, Sharp C, et al: A procedure-specific systematic review and consensus recommendations for postoperative analgesia following total knee arthroplasty. *Anaesthesia* 63:1105-1223, 2008.
31. Kardash K, Hickey D, Tessler MJ, et al: Obturator versus femoral nerve block for analgesia after total knee arthroplasty. *Anesth Analg* 105:853-858, 2007.
32. Macalou D, Trueck S, Meuret P, et al: Postoperative analgesia after total knee replacement: the effect of an obturator nerve block added to the femoral 3-in-1 nerve block. *Anesth Analg* 99:251-254, 2004.
33. Helayel PE, Da Conceicao DB, Pavei P, et al: Ultrasound-guided obturator nerve block: a preliminary report of case series. *Reg Anesth Pain Med* 32:221-226, 2007.
34. Macrae WA, Coventry DM: Lower limb blocks. In Wildsmith JAW, Armitage EN, McClure JH, editors: *Principles and practice of regional anaesthesia*, London, 1987, Churchill Livingstone, p 219.
35. Sinha SK, Abrams JH, Houle TT, Weller RS: Ultrasound-guided obturator nerve block: an interfascial injection approach without nerve stimulation. *Reg Anesth Pain Med* 34:261-264, 2009.
36. Danelli G, Ghisi D, Fanelli A, et al: The effects of ultrasound guidance and neurostimulation on the minimum effective analgesic volume of mepivacaine 1.5% required to block the Sciatic nerve using the subgluteal approach. *Anesth Analg* 109:1674-1678, 2009.
37. Karmakar MK, Kwok WH, Ho AM, et al: Ultrasound-guided sciatic nerve block: description of a new approach at the subgluteal space. *Br J Anaesth* 98:390-395, 2007.

38. di Benedetto P, Bertini L, Casati A, et al: A new posterior approach to the sciatic nerve block: a prospective, randomized comparison with the classic posterior approach. *Anesth Analg* 93:1040-1044, 2001.

39. Labat G: *Regional anesthesia: its technic and clinical application,* Philadelphia, 1923, WB Saunders.

40. Mansour NY, Benetts FE: An observational study of combined continuous lumbar plexus and single-shot sciatic nerve blocks for post-knee surgery analgesia. *Reg Anesth* 21:287-291, 1996.

41. Robards C, Hadzic A, Somasundaram L, et al: Intraneural injection with low-current stimulation during popliteal sciatic nerve block. *Anesth Analg* 109:673-677, 2009.

42. Sala Blanch X, Lopez AM, Carazo J, et al: Intraneural injection during nerve stimulator-guided sciatic nerve block at the popliteal fossa. *Br J Anaesth* 102:855-861, 2009.

43. Tsai TP, Vuckovic I, Dilberovic F, et al: Intensity of the stimulating current may not be a reliable indicator of intraneural needle placement. *Reg Anesth Pain Med* 33:207-210, 2008.

44. Vlodka JD, Hadzic A, April EW, et al: Division of the sciatic nerve in the popliteal fossa and its possible implications in the popliteal nerve blockade. *Anesth Analg* 92:215-217, 2001.

45. Perlas A, Brull B, Chan VW, et al: Ultrasound guidance improves the success of sciatic nerve block at the popliteal fossa. *Reg Anesth Pain Med* 33:259-265, 2008.

46. Dufour E, Quennesson P, Van Robais Al, et al: Combined ultrasound and neurostimulation guidance for popliteal sciatic nerve block: a prospective randomised comparison with neurostimulation alone. *Anesth Analg* 106:1553-1558, 2008.

47. Danelli G Fanellie A, Ghisi D, et al: Ultrasound Vs nerve stimulation multiple injection technique for posterior popliteal sciatic nerve block. *Anaesthesia* 64:638-642, 2009.

48. Sala Blanch X, Lopez AM, Carazo J, et al: Intraneuronal injection during nerve stimulator-guided sciatic nerve block at the popliteal fossa. *Br J Anaesth* 102:855-861, 2009.

49. Robarts C, Hadzic A, Somasundaram L, et al: Intraneural injection with low-current stimulation during popliteal sciatic nerve block. *Anesth Analg* 109:673-677, 2009.

50. Manickam B, Perlas A, Duggan E, et al: Feasibility and efficacy of ultrasound-guided block of the saphenous nerve in the adductor canal. *Reg Anesth Pain Med* 4(6):578-580, 2009.

51. Horn JL, Pitsch T, Salinas F, Benninger B: Anatomic basis for the ultrasound-guided approach for saphenous nerve blockade. *Reg Anesth Pain Med* 34:486-489, 2009.

52. Krombach J, Gray AT: Sonography for saphenous nerve block near the adductor canal. *Reg Anesth Pain Med* 32:369-370, 2007.

53. Taboada M, Lorenzo D, Oliveira J, et al: Comparison of 4 techniques for internal saphenous nerve block. *Rev Esp Anesthesiol Reamin* 51:509-514, 2004.

54. De Mey JCJ, Deruyck LJ, Cammu GMD, et al: A paravenous approach for the saphenous nerve block. *Reg Anesth Pain Med* 26:504-506, 2001.

55. Comfort V, Lang S, Yip R: Saphenous nerve anaesthesia—a nerve stimulator technique. *Can J Anaesth* 43:852-857, 1996.

56. Rudkin GE, Rudkin HK, Dracopoulos GC: Ankle block success rate: a prospective analysis of 1000 patients. *Can J Anaesth* 52:209-210, 2005.

57. Mc Leod DH, Wong D, Himat V, et al: Lateral popliteal sciatic nerve block compared with ankle block for analgesia following foot surgery. *Can J Anaesth* 42:765-770, 1995.

58. Rudkin GE, Micallef TA: Impediments to the use of ankle block in Australia. *Anaesth Intensive Care* 32:368-371, 2004.

59. Antonakakis JG, Scalzo DC, Jorgenson AS, et al: Ultrasound does not improve the success rate of deep peroneal nerve block at the ankle. *Reg Anesth Pain Med* 35: 217-221, 2010.

60. Benzon HT, Sekhadia M, Benzon HA, et al: Ultrasound-assisted and evoked motor response stimulation of the deep peroneal nerve. *Anesth Analg* 109:2022-2024, 2009.

61. Kirsten R, Sites BD, Chinn CD, et al: Ultrasound improves the success rate of a sural nerve block at the ankle. *Reg Anesth Pain Med* 34:24-28, 2009.

62. Redborg KE, Antonakakis JG, Beach ML, et al: Ultrasound Improves the success rate of tibial nerve block at the ankle. *Reg Anesth Pain Med* 34:256-260, 2009.

8 Cervical and Lumbar Sympathetic Blocks

Samer Narouze and Sean Graham

CHAPTER OVERVIEW

Chapter Synopsis: Many pain syndromes include a sympathetic component, often in the form of output that exacerbates peripheral activation of pain-sensing fibers. Block of these efferent sympathetic nerves can help assess this contribution and in some cases can provide relief. Block of the fibers in these ganglia can also provide a prognosis about subsequent sympathetic denervation treatments. This chapter deals with block of the cervical sympathetic ganglia, which subserve the head, neck, and upper extremities. Interestingly, the population shows some variation in the anatomy of the cervical ganglia, particularly in the inferior of the three, which may be fused with the first thoracic ganglion to form what is known as the stellate ganglion. Some of the most common indications of sympathetically maintained pain include types I and II complex regional pain syndrome, acute herpes zoster and early herpetic neuralgia, phantom limb pain, and other peripheral neuropathies. Conditions that arise primarily from vasoconstrictive conditions can also benefit from stellate ganglion block, and even patients with conditions such as perimenopausal hot flashes and posttraumatic stress disorder have recently seen benefits. The chapter also covers block of lumbar sympathetic ganglia, which is indicated for similar pain disorders of the lower extremities with a component maintained by the sympathetic output. The chapter considers the technical details of the procedure, including various approaches and potential complications.

Important Points:
- Sympathetic blocks provide a valuable diagnostic, prognostic, and therapeutic value to sympathetically maintained pain syndromes.
- Fluoroscopy is a reliable method for identifying bony surfaces, which facilitates identifying C6 and C7 transverse processes; however, this is only a surrogate marker for the cervical sympathetic trunk. It is defined by the fascial plane of the prevertebral fascia, which cannot be visualized with fluoroscopy.
- Ultrasound-guided stellate ganglion block may improve the precision of the procedure by identifying the fascial plane anterolateral to the longus coli muscle.
- When performing lumbar sympathetic block, contrast should be injected with real-time fluoroscopy to minimize the risk of vascular uptake. The sensitivity of the aspiration test and static radiography are very low.

Clinical Pearls:
- Ultrasound-guided stellate ganglion block may improve the safety of the procedure by direct visualization of vascular structures (inferior thyroidal, cervical, vertebral, and carotid arteries) and soft tissue (thyroid, esophagus, nerve roots).
- When performing cervical sympathetic block at C6, the ganglion primarily blocked is the middle cervical ganglion; the cervicothoracic ganglion is blocked if the injectate spreads down to the T1 level.
- There is no safer level for performing stellate ganglion block (C6 level vs. C7 level). However; there may be a safer tool (ultrasound vs. fluoroscopy).

Clinical Pitfalls:
- Stellate ganglion block may be associated with serious complications even in experienced hands. Mastering anatomy is of paramount importance.
- There may be increased risk of pneumothorax and vertebral artery injury with cervical sympathetic blockade at the C7 level, if the block is performed with fluoroscopy or surface landmark techniques. Ultrasound guidance may avoid such complications.
- Neurolytic lumbar sympathetic block carries the risk of genitofemoral neuralgia and lumbar plexus injury with intrapsoas or lateral spread of the neurolytic agent.

Cervical Sympathetic Block

Cervical sympathetic block results in interruption of the sympathetic efferent fibers to the upper extremity, head, and neck. It can provide diagnostic value as to the relative sympathetic contribution to the patient's pain syndrome. It may also provide therapeutic value in patients with a significant sympathetically maintained component to their pain.

Anatomy

The cervical sympathetic chain is composed of superior, middle, and inferior cervical ganglia. However, in approximately 80% of the population, the inferior cervical ganglion is fused with the first thoracic ganglion, forming the cervicothoracic ganglion, also known as the stellate ganglion (**Fig. 8-1**).

The preganglionic sympathetic fibers for the head, neck, and upper extremities have their cell bodies located in the anterolateral

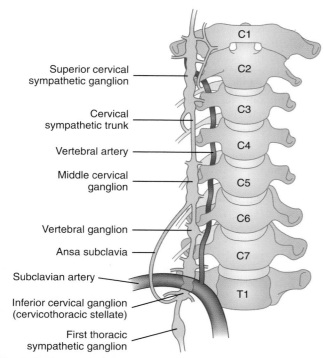

Superior cervical sympathetic ganglion

Cervical sympathetic trunk

Vertebral artery

Middle cervical ganglion

Vertebral ganglion

Ansa subclavia

Subclavian artery

Inferior cervical ganglion (cervicothoracic stellate)

First thoracic sympathetic ganglion

Fig. 8-1 Anatomical representation of the cervical sympathetic chain and stellate ganglion.

horn of the thoracic spinal cord from T1 to T8. Typically, those fibers affecting the head and neck exit with the ventral roots between T1 and T2, and those affecting the upper extremity exit between T2 and T8. After exiting the spinal cord through their respective ventral roots and traveling briefly with the spinal nerves as they exit the spinal canal, the axons continue through the white rami communicantes to ascend sympathetic chain on either side of the vertebral column.

The preganglionic fibers affecting the head and neck region continue cephalad to synapse at the superior, middle, and inferior cervical ganglion. In contrast, the preganglionic neurons affecting the upper extremity synapse at the middle and inferior (stellate) cervical ganglia. Each cervical ganglion then sends postsynaptic branches to various somatic, visceral, and vascular targets.

The superior cervical ganglion sends somatic branches via the gray rami communicantes to the cervical plexus (C1-C4), innervating the structures of the neck. The middle and inferior (stellate) ganglia contribute somatic postganglionics to the brachial plexus (C5-T1), innervating the upper extremities.[1-3] The superior cervical ganglion sends its vascular branches along the internal and external carotid arteries to reach structures in the cranium, orbit, face, nasal and oral cavities, and pharynx. Blockade of efferents to this ganglion is what results in ptosis, miosis, anhydrosis, and enophthalmos, the classic Horner syndrome. The middle ganglion sends vascular branches along the inferior thyroid artery to the larynx, trachea, and upper esophagus. The inferior (stellate) ganglion sends branches to travel along the subclavian and vertebral arteries. All three cervical ganglia are known to provide visceral branches that contribute to the cardiac plexus. The superior ganglion contributes to the superficial cardiac plexus, and the middle and inferior ganglia contribute to the deep cardiac plexus.

Most preganglionic sympathetic efferents innervating the head, neck, and upper extremity either pass through or synapse at the

stellate ganglion. This provides us with an ideal target for blockade of sympathetic efferents to the head, neck, and upper limbs. Occasionally, additional sympathetic innervation to the upper extremity exits the sympathetic chain via gray rami communicantes at T2 and T3 and goes on to the distal upper extremity without ever passing through the stellate ganglion.[4,5] The prevalence of this anomaly is unknown but should be kept in mind when interpreting the results of the block because it could result in failed sympathetic denervation despite adequate blockade of the stellate ganglion.

The stellate ganglion is located medial to the scalene muscles; lateral to the longus colli muscle, esophagus, and trachea along with the recurrent laryngeal nerve (RLN); anterior to the transverse processes and prevertebral fascia; superior to the subclavian artery and the posterior aspect of the pleura; and posterior to the vertebral vessels at the C7 level.[6] This explains why there may be increased risk of pneumothorax and vertebral artery injury with blockade at the C7 level.

The stellate ganglion measures approximately 2.5 cm long, 1 cm wide, and 0.5 cm thick (anteroposterior [AP] diameter). It is usually located posteriorly in the chest in front of the neck of the first rib and may extend to the seventh cervical (C7) vertebral body.[6-8] If the inferior cervical ganglion and first thoracic ganglion are not fused, the inferior cervical ganglion lies in front of the C7 tubercle, and the first thoracic ganglion rests over the neck of the first rib.[6-8] Accordingly, by using the blind technique at C6, the ganglion primarily blocked is the middle cervical ganglion, and the cervicothoracic ganglion is blocked if the injectate spreads down to the T1 level.

Indications

Stellate ganglion blockade is indicated in a variety of disorders related to sympathetic innervation of the head, neck, and upper extremities. It can provide essential diagnostic information about the relative contribution of sympathetic nervous system to a painful disorder. It also provides prognostic information about the probable response to subsequent sympathetic denervation from neurolytic injection, radiofrequency lesioning, or surgical removal. Last, it can frequently be therapeutic in providing analgesia that will permit functional restoration of the affected region.

The most common indication encountered in interventional pain medicine is sympathetically maintained pain (i.e., any painful condition in which there is a significant contribution from the sympathetic nervous system). These include complex regional pain syndrome (CRPS) types I (reflex sympathetic dystrophy) and II (causalgia), acute herpes zoster, early postherpetic neuralgia, atypical facial pain, Bell palsy, postamputation stump pain, phantom limb pain, radiation neuritis, and peripheral neuropathy.

Stellate ganglion blocks are also indicated in conditions associated with limited blood flow within small vessels of the head, neck, and upper extremities. These may include acute peripheral ischemia, vasospasm, atherosclerosis, frostbite, erythromelalgia, scleroderma, Raynaud disease, temporal arteritis, acrocyanosis, and Buerger disease.

Other less commonly encountered indications include hyperhidrosis, Ménière disease, accidental intraarterial injection of intravenous medications, and angina pectoris.[9] More recently, stellate ganglion block has been used for the treatment of patients with hot flashes and posttraumatic stress disorders.[10,11]

Absolute contraindications to stellate ganglion block include coagulopathy, contralateral pneumothorax, and recent myocardial infarction. Glaucoma and atrioventricular block are relative contraindications.

Technique

C6 Anterior Approach The stellate ganglion block is most commonly performed with an anterior approach at C6 transverse process (Chassaignac tubercle).[12-14] The anatomical landmarks allow this block to be performed either with or without fluoroscopic guidance.

The patient is placed in the supine position with support under the shoulders and the head resting flat on the table. This position provides slight extension of the neck and facilitates palpation of the necessary anatomical landmarks. The C6 transverse process can be easily located by first palpating the cricoid cartilage. Chassaignac tubercle is located between the cricoid cartilage and the medial border of the sternocleidomastoid. With the index and middle fingers of the nondominant hand, pressure is applied to compress the subcutaneous tissues and identify the C6 transverse process. The pulsations of the carotid artery should be palpated, and an attempt should be made to retract the carotid artery laterally to keep it out of the path of the needle (**Fig. 8-2**). The cranial and caudal borders of the transverse process are identified with the index and middle fingers, and the block needle is inserted directly between the two fingers to ensure contact with bone.

After antiseptic skin preparation, a 22-gauge 1.5-inch needle should be inserted perpendicular to the skin and advanced until contact is made with Chassaignac tubercle. If bony contact has not been made after advancing to a depth of 1 inch, the needle has likely missed the tubercle and should be withdrawn and redirected using a new cephalocaudad trajectory. Similarly, if a paresthesia is produced with needle advancement, it has contacted a nerve root, and it should be withdrawn and redirected. After contact with bone has been made, the needle should be withdrawn a few millimeters so the tip lies just anterior to the longus colli muscle.

After negative gentle aspiration, an initial test dose of 0.5 to 1.0 mL of local anesthetic should be injected. Intravascular injection of less than 1 mL of local anesthetic has been reported to cause loss of consciousness and seizure activity.[15] If no signs or symptoms of intravascular injection have been observed, a solution of 5 to 10 mL may be injected with re-aspiration after every 3 to 5 mL to help ensure persistent extravascular needle placement.

If using fluoroscopy for the procedure, injection of 1 to 2 mL of nonionic contrast should be injected before injection of local anesthetic. It should be visualized traveling inferiorly with minimal resistance. If the needle tip has been placed medially along the transverse process, contrast spread my have a striated appearance, indicating tip placement within the longus colli muscle (**Fig. 8-3**). If this is the case, the needle should be withdrawn slightly and contrast reinjected to demonstrate the characteristic "honeycomb" appearance indicating that the needle tip is in the appropriate fascial plane anterior to the muscle (**Fig. 8-4**). Real-time fluoroscopy should be used for careful assessment of any sign of intravascular injection.

C7 Anterior Approach The stellate ganglion block can also be performed at C7.[16] The approach is nearly identical to the C6 approach; however, the anatomical landmarks are more difficult to identify because the C7 vertebra has only a vestigial tubercle that is not readily palpable. Hence, the procedure is usually performed with fluoroscopy. When performing the block without fluoroscopic guidance, it is easier to first palpate the C6 tubercle and then move one fingerbreadth inferior as an estimate of the C7 tubercle. At this level, the risk of pneumothorax and vertebral artery injury is higher.[17]

An oblique fluoroscopic approach[18] targeting the junction between the uncinate process and the vertebral body at the C7 level was described in an effort to decrease those risks.

The C7 approach does offer a few advantages, however. Because the needle is closer in proximity to the stellate ganglion, which resides directly anterior to the C7 transverse process, a smaller volume of solution can be injected to produce a more reliable and consistent blockade.[19] This may be of particular value when the patient has failed previous block at the C6 level.

Limitations and Evolution of Current Techniques

Because the stellate ganglion is located in close proximity to various critical structures, its blockade may be associated with a number

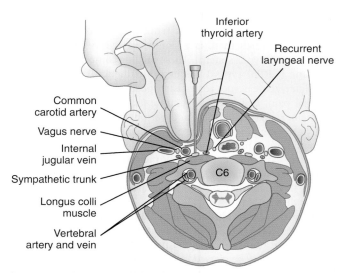

Fig. 8-2 Stellate ganglion block: blind approach at C6. With the index and middle fingers of the nondominant hand, pressure is applied to compress the subcutaneous tissues and identify the C6 transverse process. Note that the carotid artery is retracted laterally to keep it out of the path of the needle.

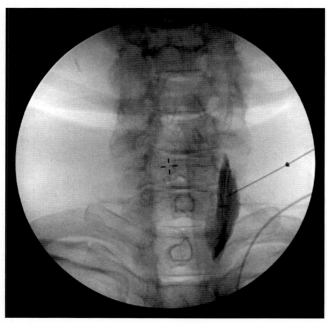

Fig. 8-3 Anteroposterior view showing the spread of the contrast agent within the substance of the longus colli muscle. (Reprinted with permission from the Ohio Pain and Headache Institute.)

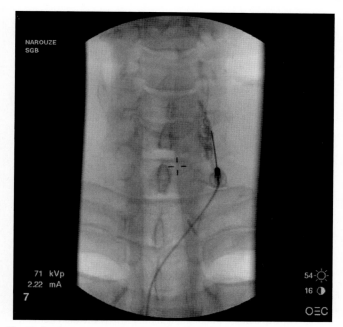

Fig. 8-4 Anteroposterior view showing the correct spread of the contrast agent along the anterior surface of the longus colli muscle; "honeycomb" appearance. (Reprinted with permission from the Ohio Pain and Headache Institute.)

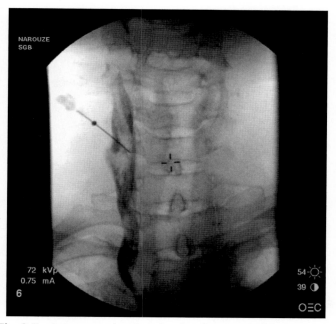

Fig. 8-5 Anteroposterior view showing the spread of the contrast agent along the carotid sheath. (Reprinted with permission from the Ohio Pain and Headache Institute.)

of complications, some of which are life threatening. Accordingly, techniques for blockade have evolved and varied from the use of the standard blind technique to the use of radionuclide tracers,[20] computed tomography,[21] and magnetic resonance imaging.[6,22] However, these techniques are not practical in daily clinical practice because they are time consuming, cost-ineffective, and involve radiation exposure. Fluoroscopy has been suggested as a safer and more effective way to perform stellate ganglion block than the traditional blind approach.[18,23]

Fluoroscopy is a reliable method for identifying bony surfaces, which facilitates identifying C6 and C7 transverse processes; however, this is only a surrogate marker because the location of the cervical sympathetic trunk is defined by the fascial plane of the prevertebral fascia, which cannot be visualized with fluoroscopy.

Vascular structures (inferior thyroidal, cervical, vertebral, and carotid arteries) and soft tissue (thyroid, esophagus, nerve roots) are also not seen with fluoroscopy—contrary to with ultrasonography—and are therefore at risk of injury with fluoroscopy-guided techniques.[24]

Ultrasound-guided stellate ganglion block may improve the safety of the procedure by direct visualization of the related anatomical structures, and accordingly the risk of vascular and soft tissue injury may be minimized. Also, ultrasound guidance allows direct monitoring of the spread of the injectate, so complications such as RLN palsy, intrathecal, epidural, or intravascular spread may be minimized as well. The absence of the spread of local anesthetic during the real-time injection raises the suspicion of intravascular injection.[25]

Ultrasound-Guided Cervical Sympathetic Block

Kapral et al[26] first described ultrasound imaging for stellate ganglion block. In their case series, 12 patients received the classical "blind" stellate ganglion block followed by ultrasound-guided block the next day. The blind technique resulted in "asymptomatic" hematoma formation in three of 12 patients, with no hematoma

occurring with the ultrasound technique. The spread of the local anesthetic was observed under real-time sonography, and the proximity of the local anesthetic to the RLN and nerve root correlated well with complications such as hoarseness and paresthesia. In this study, 5 mL of local anesthetic was administered, and all patients in the ultrasound-guided group developed sympathetic block compared with 10 out of 12 in the blind group.

Shibata et al[27] noted more caudad injectate distribution and better sympathetic blockade with less incidence of hoarseness with ultrasound-guided subfascial injection compared with suprafascial injection.[25] Contrary to the fluoroscopy-guided method, the end point of the needle is not the contact with bone but the prevertebral fascia.[24,27]

With injection anterior to the prevertebral fascia, the solution tends to spread around the carotid sheath (**Fig. 8-5**).[28] In this case, the risk of hoarseness is higher, probably secondary to proximity of the vagus nerve in the carotid sheath and the RLN medial to the carotid and lateral to the trachea.[27,28]

Ultrasonography is very helpful in identifying various arteries (inferior thyroidal, cervical, vertebral, and carotid) in the vicinity of the cervical sympathetic chain. It can even detect vascular anatomical variation.

The vertebral artery runs anteriorly at the C7 level before it enters the foramen of C6 transverse process in about 90% of cases. However, it enters at C5 or higher in the remaining cases.[29] This makes it vulnerable to injury during lower cervical sympathetic block, not only at the C7 level but at C6 as well, a possibility that can be avoided by ultrasound imaging.[24]

The inferior thyroid vessels may be a major source of retropharyngeal hematoma because of their vulnerable and variable anatomy.[30] The inferior thyroid artery originates from the thyrocervical trunk of the subclavian artery and ascends anteriorly to the vertebral artery and the longus colli muscle and then curves medially behind the carotid sheath to enter posteriorly the inferior part of the thyroid lobe. It is vulnerable to injury because it lies

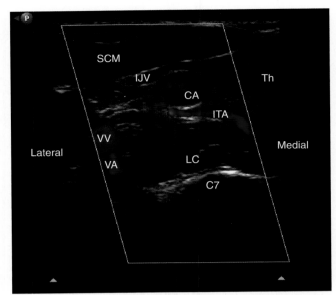

Fig. 8-6   Short-axis sonogram at C7. The vertebral artery (VA) is "exposed" as it is anterior to the transverse process of C7. Also note that the inferior thyroid artery (ITA) can be easily injured in the path of the needle. CA, carotid artery; IJV, internal jugular vein (compressed); LC, longus colli muscle; SCM, sternocleidomastoid muscle; Th, thyroid; VV, vertebral vein. (Reprinted with permission from the Ohio Pain and Headache Institute.)

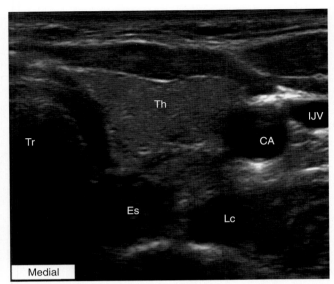

Fig. 8-7   Short-axis sonogram of the anterior neck. CA, carotid artery; Es, esophagus; IJV, internal jugular vein; Lc, longus colli muscle; Th, thyroid; Tr, trachea. (Reprinted with permission from the Ohio Pain and Headache Institute.)

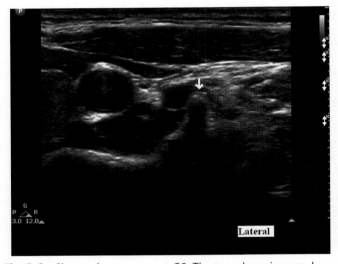

Fig. 8-8   Short-axis sonogram at C6. The transducer is moved slowly laterally and cephalad until the characteristic sharp anterior tubercle of C6 comes into the image (*arrow*). (Reprinted with permission from the Ohio Pain and Headache Institute.)

anterior to the vertebral artery at the C7 level or more commonly when it crosses (at the C6-C7 level) behind the carotid artery from lateral to medial to end in the thyroid gland. This is the most critical portion of the vessel to be injured during performing the procedure with the blind technique or even with fluoroscopic guidance. Because the artery has a variable unpredicted anatomy and has a very tortuous serpentine course, it can be easily injured in the path of the needle. This possibility can be prevented with an ultrasound-guided technique (**Fig. 8-6**).[30]

Also, ultrasound imaging can identify the esophagus, especially on the left (**Fig. 8-7**).[24] The esophagus usually appears as an outpouching behind the trachea and can be better identified by the change in shape and shadowing during swallowing and the presence of a peripheral arc-shaped echogenic line or a boundary hypoechoic zone, which is suggestive of the striated structure of the digestive tract.[31]

This may be even more important in the patient with pharyngoesophageal diverticulum (Zenker diverticulum) as they are usually asymptomatic and detected incidentally by neck sonography.

Placing the needle by ultrasonography closer to the target also minimizes the amount of local anesthetic used and hence improves the patient's safety; Wulf et al[32] reported toxic plasma levels in 30% of patients undergoing stellate ganglion block using 10 mL of bupivacaine 0.5%.

Technique for Ultrasound-Guided Injection

The patient is placed in the supine position with the neck extended in the neutral position. A high-frequency linear transducer (5-12 MHz) is usually used. The transducer is placed horizontally at the root of the neck to obtain a transverse sonogram. Scanning from midline laterally, one can easily identify the trachea, esophagus, thyroid gland, carotid sheath, and longus colli muscle (**Fig. 8-7**). Then the transducer is moved slowly cephalad until the

characteristic sharp anterior tubercle of the transverse process of C6 comes into the image (**Fig. 8-8**). At this point, the C6 and C7 levels are identified, and a careful scanning is performed to identify all of the relevant vessels in the vicinity of the cervical sympathetic chain. The vertebral artery, inferior thyroid artery, and thyrocervical trunk branches should be looked after and identified.[30] A color Doppler scan helps in revealing any variable vascular anatomy. A safe path for the needle should be planned to avoid any puncture to those vital structures. Turning the head to the opposite side usually shifts the carotid sheath more medially, thus creating more room to place the needle lateral to the carotid sheath. The authors usually use an out-of-plane approach, and the ideal placement of the needle tip should be anterolateral to the longus colli muscle and deep to the prevertebral fascia (to avoid spread along the carotid sheath) but superficial to the fascia investing the longus colli muscle (to avoid injecting into the muscle substance). The authors usually use less than 5 mL of local anesthetic, and the injection should be carried out with real-time sonography to monitor the spread of the injectate as above.

Others advocate the use of an in-plane approach with the patient in the lateral position in an effort to minimize the risk of vascular injury.[33]

T2 Anterior Approach

Vallejo et al[34] described the fluoroscopy-guided T2 anterior approach for upper extremity sympathetic blockade. The T2 approach should provide a complete sympathetic block to the upper extremity while using a small volume of local anesthetic because it will allow for blockade of the Kuntz's fibers (see Anatomy section above), thus enhancing the diagnostic accuracy and the therapeutic benefit as compared with traditional stellate ganglion block. Also, the T2 anterior approach may have a lower risk of pneumothorax than the classic posterior paravertebral block approach at T2.

The technique is based on identifying the uncinate process of C7 fluoroscopically as a target for insertion of a catheter through a Touhy needle. Then the catheter can be directed caudally to T2 or T3.

Narouze[35,36] recently described an ultrasound-guided T2 anterior approach. Ultrasonography may improve the safety of the procedure by direct visualization of the related anatomical structures, and accordingly, the risk of vertebral artery or pleura injury may be minimized.

For the T2 anterior approach, the authors prefer to use a high-resolution compact curvilinear array probe (C5-C8) because its small size (however wider footprint) allows room for placing the needle in plane whether in the short- or the long-axis view. The transducer is first applied transversely at the root of the neck to obtain a short-axis view. The C7 can be identified with its characteristic transverse process (lacking the anterior tubercle) as well as its relation to the vertebral artery (**Fig. 8-9**). By moving the probe caudally, T1 will appear in the image, and then afterward with a caudal tilt, one can identify the T2 level.

First, a 22- to 25-gauge blunt needle is inserted out of plane in the short-axis view and advanced with real-time sonography so the

needle tip will lie just lateral to the longus colli muscle. Caution must be exercised to avoid the vertebral artery as it lies anterior to the sympathetic chain at this level. Then a longitudinal axis view is obtained to monitor the tip of the needle as it is advanced caudally along the lateral border of the muscle (**Fig. 8-10**). The final needle position may be checked with real-time fluoroscopy after contrast injection to show the cephalocaudal spread without vascular escape (**Fig. 8-11**).

Complications

Because the anatomy of the stellate ganglion is in close proximity to various critical structures, a number of complications may be

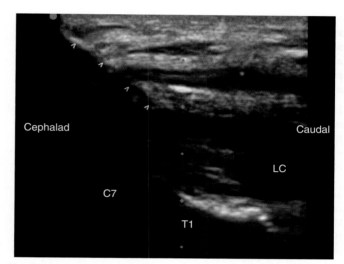

Fig. 8-10 Long-axis sonogram at T1 showing the needle (*arrowheads*) in a caudal direction just anterior to the longus colli muscle (LC). (Reprinted with permission from Ohio Pain and Headache Institute.)

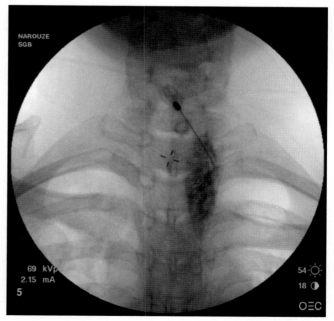

Fig. 8-11 Anteroposterior view showing the caudal spread of the injectate down to T3. (Reprinted with permission from the Ohio Pain and Headache Institute.)

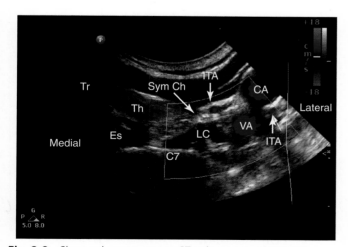

Fig. 8-9 Short-axis sonogram at C7 using a curved (C8-C5) transducer. CA, carotid artery; Es, esophagus; ITA, inferior thyroid artery; LC, longus colli muscle; symp Ch, sympathetic chain; Th, thyroid; Tr, trachea; VA, vertebral artery. (Reprinted with permission from the Ohio Pain and Headache Institute.)

potentially associated with its blockade, some of which are life threatening.[37] Before performing this block, all patients should have a reliable intravenous catheter placed, and full resuscitative equipment should be readily available. When performed properly by an experienced practitioner, the stellate ganglion block has a low incidence of complications.[38] The complications of stellate ganglion block result either from insertion and manipulation of the needle or as a direct result of the injected solution. These complications may include:

- Horner syndrome
- RLN block
- Vagus nerve block
- Phrenic nerve block
- Partial brachial plexus block
- Intravascular injection
- Subarachnoid injection
- Pneumothorax
- Retropharyngeal hematoma
- Esophageal penetration, mediastinal infection, or emphysema
- Discitis

Horner syndrome (ptosis, miosis, anhydrosis, enophthalmos, and nasal congestion) is better classified as a side effect than a complication of stellate ganglion block. It is a result of blockade of the cervical sympathetic chain and is evidence of successful sympathetic blockade.

RLN block is another side effect that occurs frequently secondary to spread of local anesthetic to the RLN. Hardy and Wells[39] reported an incidence of 10% with 10 mL of local anesthetic solution and up to 80% with 20 mL of solution. When unilateral, it results in hoarseness and may cause subjective difficulty breathing. This is rarely of consequence unless the patient has a preexisting contralateral RLN injury, as is common after thyroid surgery. In this circumstance, blockade could produce critical airway obstruction and loss of laryngeal reflexes requiring intubation.

The ultrasound-guided stellate ganglion block approach was associated with much less incidence of RLN block (see earlier discussion).[26,27]

Phrenic nerve block is also common after stellate ganglion block. It results in paralysis of the ipsilateral hemidiaphragm. This is usually only of adverse consequence in patients with preexisting respiratory compromise.

The most serious complications of stellate ganglion block include pneumothorax, subarachnoid injection, intravascular injection, and retropharyngeal hematoma. The proximity of the stellate ganglion to the inferior thyroid, cervical, vertebral, or carotid arteries provides potential for either intravascular injection or vascular trauma with resulting bleeding and hematoma.[30,40] Intravascular injection of even small volumes of local anesthetic may result in loss of consciousness, apnea, and seizure. Retropharyngeal hematoma varies in severity from mild and asymptomatic to severe and causing tracheal compression requiring emergency tracheotomy.[37,41] The frequency of catastrophic retropharyngeal hematoma after stellate ganglion block has been reported to be one in 100,000 cases with resulting airway compromise and obstruction.[37] However, Kapral et al[26] reported a much higher incidence of asymptomatic hematoma with the blind technique.

Lumbar Sympathetic Block

The lumbar sympathetic block results in interruption of the sympathetic efferent fibers to the lower extremities with sparing of the somatic nerves. This provides diagnostic value as to the relative sympathetic contribution to the patient's pain syndrome. It may also provide therapeutic value in those patients with a significant sympathetically maintained component to their pain.

Anatomy

The lumbar sympathetic chain consists of both pre- and postganglionic efferent fibers (**Fig. 8-12**). The preganglionic sympathetic

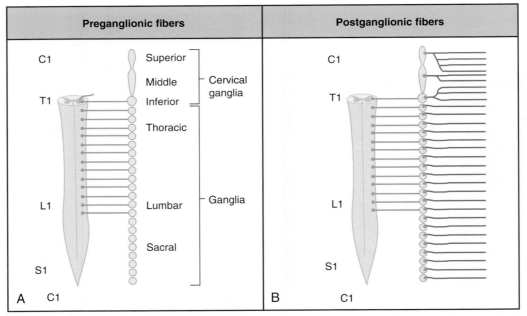

Fig. 8-12 Preganglionic sympathetic fibers leave the ventral rami of mixed spinal nerves (T1-L2) to enter the sympathetic chain ganglia by means of 14 pairs of white rami communicants (**A**), and 31 pairs of gray rami communicants leave the sympathetic chain ganglia (**B**). (Only the left half of the thoracolumbar outflow is illustrated.) (From Bogart BI, Ort VH: *Elsevier's integrated anatomy and embryology*. Philadelphia, 2007, Mosby.)

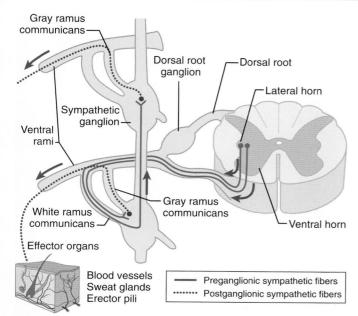

Fig. 8-13 Sympathetic pathway to sweat glands, erector pili muscles, and blood vessels. (From Bogart BI, Ort VH: *Elsevier's integrated anatomy and embryology*. Philadelphia, 2007, Mosby.)

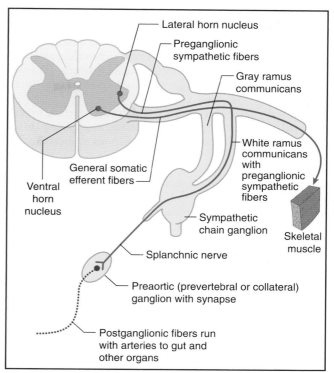

Fig. 8-14 Distribution of the splanchnic (visceral) nerves. Preganglionic sympathetic fibers pass through the sympathetic ganglia to form the lumbar splanchnic nerves that supply visceral structures in the abdomen and pelvis. (From Bogart BI, Ort VH: *Elsevier's integrated anatomy and embryology*. Philadelphia, 2007, Mosby.)

nerves have their cell bodies located within the intermediolateral cell column of the thoracolumbar spinal cord. After exiting the spinal cord through the ventral root and traveling briefly with the spinal nerve as it exits the spinal canal, the axons continue through the white rami communicantes to join the sympathetic chain on either side of the vertebral column (**Fig. 8-13**). Within the sympathetic chain, the efferent fibers take different paths. Some travel up or down the sympathetic chain and synapse with postganglionic neurons within the paravertebral sympathetic ganglia. The postganglionic neurons then exit through the gray rami communicantes and follow somatic nerves or vessels to affect vascular smooth muscle, sudomotor cells, and peripheral nociceptors. Other preganglionic efferents pass on to prevertebral ganglia (aortic plexus and the superior and inferior hypogastric plexuses) before synapsing with postganglionic neurons (**Fig. 8-14**).

The paravertebral ganglia exist along the entire vertebral column. There are considered to be five paired lumbar ganglia that lie along the anterolateral border of either side of the five lumbar vertebrae. Cadaver dissections, however, have shown significant variability in both the number and location of the ganglia.[42] Typically, there are only four ganglia because the L1 and L2 ganglia are commonly fused. The vast majority of sympathetic efferent neurons responsible for vascular tone in the lower extremities pass through the paravertebral ganglia at L2 and L3. Therefore, these ganglia are the targets for lumbar sympathetic blockade. The ganglia at these levels have been most frequently found at the lower third of the L2 vertebra, at the L2-L3 interspace, and at the upper third of the L3 vertebra.[43] Also of note, the lumbar arteries at these levels are known to exit the aorta and travel posteriorly across the middle of the vertebral bodies before branching into radicular or segmental medullary arteries. Hence, the ideal site for blockade of the lumbar sympathetic chain is at the lower third of the L2 vertebral body or the upper third of the L3 vertebral body, both targeting the ganglia and avoiding the segmental lumbar arteries and their branches. Also, lumbar sympathetic block at the L2 level showed the lowest

incidence of psoas muscle injection of contrast in comparison with lumbar sympathetic block at L3 and L4.[44]

The lumbar sympathetic chain is well separated from the lumbar somatic nerves by the psoas major muscle and its fascia. This separation is consistent, and it is what allows selective sympathetic blockade to the lower extremities without affecting sensorimotor function. The only connection between the sympathetic chain and the somatic nerves is via the gray and white rami communicantes. This must be kept in mind, especially when performing neurolytic blocks, because the injectate may track posteriorly along these pathways (or along the path of the needle) and result in somatic nerve injury.

Indications

Lumbar sympathetic blockade is indicated in a variety of disorders related to sympathetic innervation of the lower extremities. It can provide essential diagnostic information about the relative contribution of sympathetic nervous system to a painful disorder. It also provides prognostic information about the probable response to subsequent sympathetic denervation from neurolytic injection, radiofrequency lesioning, or surgical removal. Last, it can frequently be therapeutic in providing analgesia that will permit functional restoration of the affected region.

The most common indication encountered in interventional pain medicine is sympathetically maintained pain (i.e., any painful condition in which there is a significant contribution from the sympathetic nervous system). These include CRPS types I (reflex sympathetic dystrophy) and II (causalgia), acute herpes zoster, early postherpetic neuralgia, postamputation stump pain, phantom limb pain, radiation neuritis, and peripheral neuropathy.

Blockade of the lumbar sympathetics are also indicated in conditions associated with limited blood flow within the small vessels of the lower extremities. These include acute ischemia, atherosclerosis, frostbite, erythromelalgia, Raynaud disease, and Buerger disease.

Other less commonly encountered indications include hyperhidrosis, phlegmasia alba dolens, acrocyanosis, discogenic pain, and accidental intraarterial injection of intravenous medications.[45-47]

Technique

There are essentially two frequently used techniques for performing lumbar sympathetic blockade. The most commonly used technique is the paramedian or "classic" approach that was initially described by Mandle[48] in 1926. A more lateral approach was later developed by Reid and colleagues[49] and published in 1970.

The initial description of the lumbar sympathetic block involved the placement of two separate needles at L2 and L3. Single-needle techniques were described in 1975 by Brown and Kunjappan[50] and in 1985 by Hatangdi and Boas.[51] The single-needle technique is currently the more popular technique when performing blocks with local anesthetic because it saves significant time, produces less postprocedural discomfort, and has similar results.[50,51] One may consider a multiple-needle technique when performing a neurolytic block to minimize the volume of alcohol or phenol injected and decrease the risk of damage to the surrounding tissues.

Classic Approach (Paramedian) The patient is placed in the prone position, and the skin is marked at a site 5 to 6 cm lateral to the spinous process of L3. A skin wheal is raised, and local anesthetic is infiltrated in a path directly perpendicular to the skin down to the transverse process. A 22-gauge needle is then inserted and advanced under fluoroscopic guidance until coming into contact with the inferior border of the transverse process of L3. The needle is withdrawn slightly and redirected in an inferior and medial direction so as to pass underneath the transverse process. It should be advanced until contact is made with the lateral surface of the vertebral body. When bony contact is made, the needle position should be confirmed with AP and lateral fluoroscopic imaging. The needle is then angled in such a way to slip off of the lateral surface of the vertebral body and advanced until the tip lies at the anterolateral edge of L3. Some practitioners use a loss-of-resistance technique using either saline or air to detect the needle exiting anterior to the psoas muscle. Others prefer to simply use lateral fluoroscopic imaging and advance the needle until the tip sits exactly at the most anterior border of the vertebral body.

Lateral Approach The patient is placed in the prone position, and the C-arm is rotated in an oblique direction until the transverse process of L3 is entirely medial to the lateral border of the vertebral body. The advantage of this approach is that it allows advancement of the needle with less risk of hitting the transverse process or the exiting segmental nerve.[5] The skin is marked at what appears on the oblique fluoroscopic image to be the lateral aspect of the L3 vertebral body. Using a 22-gauge, 3.5-inch spinal needle, a skin wheal is raised, and local anesthetic is infiltrated in an oblique path directed toward the L3 vertebral body. A 22-gauge needle is then inserted and advanced under fluoroscopic guidance directly toward the anterolateral border of the vertebral body, taking care not to make bony contact, thereby avoiding patient discomfort (**Fig. 8-15**). It is also reasonable to use lateral

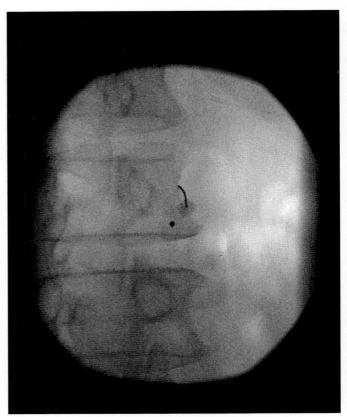

Fig. 8-15 Oblique radiographic view showing the needle just anterior to L3 for lumbar sympathetic block. (Reprinted with permission from the Ohio Pain and Headache Institute.)

fluoroscopic imaging and advance the needle until the tip sits exactly at the most anterior border of the vertebral body (**Fig. 8-16**).

Injection With appropriate needle position confirmed, 1 to 2 mL of contrast is injected and should be visualized tracking in a cephalocaudad direction along the anterolateral surface of L3 and spreading at least one vertebral level above and below the injection site (**Fig. 8-17**). If most of the contrast is noted extending in a caudal and lateral direction tracking along the psoas muscle, the needle should be advanced slightly and contrast reinjected because local anesthetic injected predominantly along the psoas would result in a suboptimal block.[44]

After contrast spread is deemed appropriate, a test dose of 5 mL of a short-acting local anesthetic (2% 3-chloroprocaine or 2% lidocaine) may be injected first to facilitate a rapid onset of the sympathetic block and production of subsequent changes in skin temperature. When skin temperature has begun to increase in the affected lower extremity, a volume of 15 to 20 mL of 0.375% bupivacaine is injected. The patient should be observed in the postblock room for confirmation of sustained increase in lower extremity color and temperature. The skin temperature usually reaches a stable level in approximately 30 minutes.[52]

Temperature Monitoring The most commonly used objective clinical indicator of sympathetic block is skin temperature measurement over the great toe. Skin temperature changes in the lower extremity have been shown to correlate well with increase in

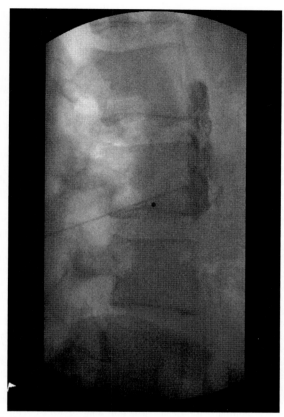

Fig. 8-16 Lateral radiographic view showing the spread of the contrast anterior to the psoas muscle. (Reprinted with permission from the Ohio Pain and Headache Institute.)

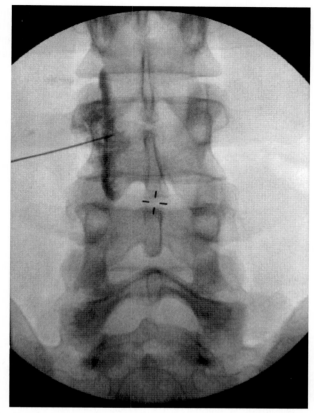

Fig. 8-17 Anteroposterior radiographic view showing the spread of the contrast along the anterolateral surface of L3. (Reprinted with permission from the Ohio Pain and Headache Institute.)

cutaneous blood flow after sympathetic block and may predict the relief of sympathetically maintained pain.[52] Measurements are most commonly made using thermocouple probes applied bilaterally to the great toes of each lower extremity. A more sensitive measurement of temperature may be made using infrared thermography.[53]

The degree of skin temperature changes that signifies adequate sympathetic blockade is not well defined. A mean increase of 3° C has been found to occur after lumbar sympathetic block.[51] In one study, a temperature increase of 2° C higher than the contralateral extremity signified complete sympathetic blockade in most but not all patients.[54] Other investigators have preferred to use a final temperature of 34° C or higher in determining efficacy.[55]

When evaluating a patient's skin temperature changes, some important considerations should be made. One should allow sufficient time before the procedure for the patient's body temperature to settle in response to the room temperature. Otherwise, temperature changes may result from adjustment to the ambient temperature. Also, consider that the increase in temperature may be more pronounced if the initial temperature is lower, as would be seen in someone with late-stage CRPS versus another patient with increased blood flow more typical of early CRPS. Also, patients with occlusive peripheral vascular disease would not be expected to have as significant temperature increase as someone with normal vasculature.

Complications

With careful attention to detail on live fluoroscopic imaging, the incidence of complications related to lumbar sympathetic blockade is minimal.[56,57] The complications result either from insertion and manipulation of the needle or as a direct result of the injected solution. The known complications are as follows:

- Intravascular injection
- Subarachnoid injection
- Renal trauma
- Ureteral stricture
- Lumbar plexus blockade
- Segmental nerve injury
- Infection
- Ejaculatory failure (bilateral lumbar sympathetic block)
- Discitis
- Psoas necrosis
- Genitofemoral neuralgia

When the needle is placed greater than 7 to 8 cm from the midline, there is a risk of penetrating the kidney. This generally only results in insignificant transient hematuria without permanent sequelae. Injection of neurolytic solution could result in ureteral stricture. As the needle passes laterally to the intervertebral foramen, there is risk of injury to the exiting segmental nerve. If the patient begins to complain of paresthesia during advancement, the needle should be withdrawn and a new trajectory taken. Intervertebral disc puncture may occur with the classic and lateral approaches. This carries with it the potential risk of resulting discitis.

Given the close proximity to segmental vessels and their branches, careful attention should be paid to real-time fluoroscopy during injection to minimize the risk of vascular uptake. There is also a small chance of penetrating a dural sleeve with resulting subarachnoid injection. Because of the length and diameter of the sympathectomy needles being used for the block, one should not use aspiration of blood or cerebrospinal fluid as a reliable indicator of vascular or subarachnoid needle placement. The best predictor is real-time fluoroscopic imaging. In one report, the sensitivity of the aspiration test and static radiography were 40.7% and 70.4%, respectively.[44]

Consequences of sympathectomy are more significant when performing neurolytic blockade. When injected into the body of the psoas, muscular necrosis may result. Intrapsoas injection or lateral spread of neurolytic solution may result in genitofemoral neuralgia or injury to the lumbar plexus.[57,58] The symptoms usually resolve within 6 to 12 weeks. A transdiscal technique was reported in an effort to decrease the risk of genitofemoral neuralgia.[59]

References

1. Williams PL: *Gray's anatomy*, ed 38, New York, 1995, Churchill Livingstone.
2. Fitzgerald MJT: *Neuroanatomy: basic and clinical*, ed 3, London, 1996, WB Saunders.
3. Tubbs RS, Loukas M, Remy AC, et al: The vertebral nerve revisited. *Clin Anat* 20:644-647, 2007.
4. Bonica JJ: *Sympathetic nerve blocks for pain diagnosis and therapy*, New York, 1984, Breon Laboratories.
5. Linn CC, Wu HH: Kuntz's fiber: the scapegoat of surgical failure in sympathetic surgery. *Ann Chir Gynael* 90:170-171, 2001.
6. Hogan Q, Erickson SJ: Magnetic resonance imaging of the stellate ganglion: normal appearance. *AJR Am J Roentgenol* 158:655-659, 1992.
7. Raj PP: Stellate ganglion block. In Waldman and Wenner, editors: *Interventional pain management*, Philadelphia, 1996, Saunders.
8. Ellis H, Feldman S: *Anatomy for anesthetists*, ed 3, Oxford, 1979, Blackwell Scientific Publications, pp 256-262.
9. Moore R, Groves D, Hammond C, et al: Temporary sympathectomy in the treatment of chronic refractory angina. *J Pain Symptom Manage* 30(2):183-191, 2005.
10. Lipov EG, Lipov S, Joshi JR, et al: Stellate ganglion block may relieve hot flashes by interrupting the sympathetic nervous system. *Med Hypotheses* 69(4):758-763, 2007.
11. Mulvaney SW, McLean B, de Leeuw J: The use of stellate ganglion block in the treatment of panic/anxiety symptoms with combat-related post-traumatic stress disorder; preliminary results of long-term follow-up: a case series. *Pain Pract* 10(4):359-365, 2010.
12. Bryce-Smith R: Stellate ganglion block. *Anaesthesia* 7:154-156, 1952.
13. Davies RM: Stellate ganglion block, a new approach. *Anaesthesia* 7:151-153, 1952.
14. Carron H, Litwiller R: Stellate ganglion block. *Anesth Analg* 54:567-570, 1975.
15. Raj PP: *Practical management of pain*, ed 3, St Louis, 2000, Mosby.
16. Moore DC, Bridenbaugh LD, Jr: The anterior approach to the stellate ganglion. *JAMA* 160:158-162, 1956.
17. Matsumoto S: Thermographic assessments of the sympathetic blockade by stellate ganglion block (1): comparison between C7-SGB and C6-SGB in 40 patients. *Masui* 40(4):562-569, 1991.
18. Abdi S, Zhou Y, Patel N, et al: A new and easy technique to block the stellate ganglion. *Pain Physician* 7:327-331, 2004.
19. Malmqvist ELA, Bengtsson M, Sorensen J: Efficacy of stellate ganglion block: a clinical study with bupivacaine. *Reg Anesth* 17:340-347, 1992.
20. Baumann JM, Middaugh RE, Cawthon MA, et al: Radionuclide-anesthetic flow study: a new technique for the study of regional anesthesia. *J Nucl Med* 27:1487-1489, 1986.
21. Hogan QH, Erickson SJ, Abram SE: Computerized tomography (CT) guided stellate ganglion blockade. *Anesthesiology* 77:596-599, 1992.
22. Slapppendel F, Thijssen H, Crul BJ, Merx JL: The stellate ganglion in magnetic resonance imaging, a quantification of anatomic variability. *Anesthesiology* 83:424-426, 1995.
23. Elias M: Cervical sympathetic and stellate ganglion blocks. *Pain Physician* 3:294-304, 2000.
24. Narouze S, Vydyanathan A, Patel N: Ultrasound-guided stellate ganglion block successfully prevented esophageal puncture. *Pain Physician* 10:747-752, 2007.
25. Peng P, Narouze S: Ultrasound-guided interventional procedures in pain medicine: a review of anatomy, sonoanatomy and procedures. part I: non-axial structures. *Reg Anesth Pain Med* 34:458-474, 2009.
26. Kapral S, Krafft P, Gosch M, et al: Ultrasound imaging for stellate ganglion block: direct visualization of puncture site and local anesthetic spread. *Reg Anesth* 20:323-328, 1995.
27. Shibata Y, Fujiwara Y, Komatsu T: A new approach of ultrasound-guided stellate ganglion block. *Anesth Analg* 105:550-551, 2007.
28. Christie JM, Martinez CR: Computerized axial tomography to define the distribution of solution after stellate ganglion nerve block. *J Clin Anesth* 7:306-311, 1995.
29. Matula C, Trattnig S, Tschabitscher M, et al: The course of the prevertebral segment of the vertebral artery: anatomy and clinical significance. *Surg Neurol* 48:125-131, 1997.
30. Narouze S: Beware of the "serpentine" inferior thyroid artery while performing stellate ganglion block. *Anesth Analg* 109(1):289-290, 2009.
31. Kwak JY, Kim E: Sonographic findings of Zenker diverticula. *J Ultrasound Med* 25:639-642, 2006.
32. Wulf H, Maier C, Schele H, Wabbel W: Plasma concentration of bupivacaine after stellate ganglion blockade. *Anesth Analg* 72:546-548, 1991.
33. Gofeld M, Bhatia A, Abbas S, et al: Development and validation of a new technique for ultrasound-guided stellate ganglion block. *Reg Anesth Pain Med* 34(5):475-479, 2009.
34. Vallejo R, Plancarte R, Benyamin RM, Santiago-Palma J: Anterior cervical approach for stellate ganglion and T2 to T3 sympathetic blocks: a novel technique. *Pain Pract* 5(3):244-248, 2005.
35. Narouze S: Ultrasound guided percutaneous cervical and upper thoracic sympathetic chain neuroelectrode implant for the treatment of complex regional pain syndrome [abstract]. *Pain Med* 11:298, 2010.
36. Narouze S, El-Sharkawy H: Ultrasound- guided T2 Sympathetic Block with the Anterior Approach [abstract]. *Pain Med* 10:225, 2009.
37. Higa KJ, Hirata K, Hirota K, et al: Retropharyngeal hematoma after stellate ganglion block. *Anesthesiology* 105:1238-1245, 2006.
38. Marples IL, Atkin RE: Stellate ganglion block. *Pain Rev* 8:3-11, 2001.
39. Hardy PAJ, Wells JCD: Extent of sympathetic blockade after stellate ganglion block with bupivacaine. *Pain* 36:193-196, 1989.
40. Huntoon MA: The vertebral artery is unlikely to be the sole source of vascular complications occurring during stellate ganglion block. *Pain Pract* 10(1):25-30, 2010.
41. Okuda Y, Urabe K, Kitajima T: Retropharyngeal or cervicomediastinal hematomas following stellate ganglion block. *Eur J Anaesthesiol* 20:757-759, 2003.
42. Rocco AG, Palombi D, Raeke D: Anatomy of the lumbar sympathetic chain. *Reg Anesth* 20(1):3-19, 1995.
43. Umeda S, Toshiyuki A, Hatano Y: Cadaver anatomic analysis of the best site for chemical lumbar sympathectomy. *Anesth Analg* 66:643-646, 1987.
44. Hong JH, Kim AR, Lee MY, et al: A prospective evaluation of psoas muscle and intravascular injection in lumbar sympathetic ganglion block. *Anesth Analg* 111(3):802-807, 2010.
45. Mekhail N, Malak O: Lumbar sympathetic blockade. *Tech Reg Anesth Pain Manage* 5(3):99-101, 2001.
46. Boas RA: Sympathetic nerve blocks: in search of a role. *Reg Anesth Pain Med* 23(3):292-305, 1998.
47. Kosharskyy B, Rozen D: Lumbar discogenic pain. Disk degeneration and minimally invasive interventional therapies [German]. *Anasthesiol Intensivmed Notfallmed Schmerzther* 42(4):262-267, 2007.
48. Mandle F: *Die Paravertebrale Injektion*, Vienna, 1926, J Springer.
49. Reid W, Watt JK, Gray RG: Phenol injection of the sympathetic chain. *Br J Surg* 57:45-50, 1970.
50. Brown EM, Kunjappan V: Single-needle lateral approach for lumbar sympathetic block. *Anesth Analg* 4:725, 1975.

51. Hatangdi VS, Boas RA: Lumbar sympathectomy: a single needle technique. *Br J Anaesth* 57:285, 1985.

52. Tran KM, Frank SM, Raja SN: Lumbar sympathetic block for sympathetically maintained pain: changes in cutaneous temperatures and pain perception. *Anesth Analg* 90:1396-1401, 2000.

53. Sherman RA, Barja RH, Bruno GM: Thermographic correlates of chronic pain: Analysis of 125 patients incorporating evaluations by a blind panel. *Arch Phys Med Rehab* 68:273-279, 1987.

54. Stevens RA, Stotz A, Kao TC, et al: The relative increase in skin temperature after stellate ganglion block is predictive of a complete sympathectomy of the hand. *Reg Anesth Pain Med* 23:266-270, 1998.

55. Malmqvist ELA, Bengtsson M, Sorensen J: Efficacy of stellate ganglion block: a clinical study with bupivacaine. *Reg Anesth* 17:340-347, 1992.

56. Walsh JA, Glynn CJ, Cousins MJ, Basedow RW: Blood flow, sympathetic activity and pain relief following lumbar sympathetic blockade or surgical sympathectomy. *Anaesth Intensive Care* 13:18, 1984.

57. Cousins MJ, Reeve TS, Glynn CJ, et al: Neurolytic lumbar sympathetic blockade. Duration of denervation and relief of rest pain. *Anaesth Intensive Care* 7:121, 1979.

58. Raskin NH, Levinson SA, Hoffman PM, et al: Post-sympathectomy neuralgia amelioration with diphenylhydantoin and carbamazepine. *Am J Surg* 128:75-78, 1974.

59. Ohno K, Oshita S: Transdiscal lumbar sympathetic block: a new technique for a chemical sympathectomy. *Anesth Analg* 85:1312-1316, 1997.

9 Nerve Destruction for the Alleviation of Visceral Pain

Kacey A. Montgomery and Robert W. Hurley

CHAPTER OVERVIEW

Chapter Synopsis: Visceral pain, which is characteristically diffuse and poorly localized, represents one of the most challenging pain states to treat successfully. Similar to any pain condition, successful treatment rests on proper identification of the cause or at least the pain's anatomical source. This chapter considers the sources and treatment of visceral pain conditions. Organ injury often underlies visceral pain, whether from ischemia, torsion, traction, or contraction. Cancer patients represent a significant component of those who experience visceral pain and are the population most likely to receive neurolytic treatments, the focus of this chapter. Visceral pain that originates in the organs should be distinguished from neuropathic pain with a more central component. Depression and anxiety are often experienced along with visceral pain, perhaps reflective of the cortical sites associated with the pain that underlie their depression. In addition to improving quality of life, control of pain states in cancer patients has the potential to improve survival. The techniques considered include chemical neurolysis using ethyl alcohol or phenol. Celiac plexus neurolysis can produce analgesia in a variety of visceral organs but is indicated only for cancer patients. Other procedures described include neurolysis of the lumbar sympathetic chain, the superior hypogastric plexus, and the ganglion impar plexus. By weighing the significant risks and complications of each patient's circumstances, neurolytic procedures can be used as a successful treatment for visceral pain, often in combination with more conventional opioid drug treatment.

Important Points:
- Visceral pain is commonly more challenging to treat. It is often more diffuse and poorly localizable.
- Visceral organs are rarely innervated by single localizable nerve structures; most organs, especially the perineal and pelvic structures, have dual or more innervation, resulting in only partial treatment when one innervation source is treated in isolation.
- With the development of modern imaging techniques, procedures to provide analgesia to the visceral organs have become low to moderate risk. The majority of catastrophic outcomes associated with neurolytic procedures predated the use of the imaging to visualize the intended structure before administration of neurolytics.
- Patient selection is one of the most important factors in the success of these procedures in the short and long terms. Neurolysis of visceral nerve fibers is controversial in the nonmalignant (noncancer) population because of legitimate concerns regarding deafferentation pain.
- Neurolytic procedures of the visceral nervous system should be considered early in the treatment of cancer patients whose pain is no longer well controlled on moderate doses of analgesics or who are unable to tolerate systemic analgesic medications because of adverse effects.
- Neurolytic procedures for visceral cancer pain are an effective adjunctive treatment that can co-occur with other allopathic and alternative analgesic modalities.

Clinical Pearls:
- Given that there is redundant innervation to many of the visceral organs, it may prove difficult to impossible to alleviate all of a patient's visceral pain with a single intervention; thus a multimodal approach should be taken with these patients.
- Celiac plexus blocks will help to alleviate visceral pain in a multitude of organs from the distal third of the esophagus to the descending colon, including the liver, pancreas, gallbladder, stomach, spleen, kidneys, small intestine, large intestine, and adrenal gland.
- The celiac plexus is approached at the level of T12 to L1.
- The lumbar sympathetic chain is located just anterolateral to the lumbar vertebral bodies, anterior to the origin of the psoas muscle, and is best approached at L2, L3, or L4. This block is performed for visceral pain from the descending colon, upper portion of the sigmoid colon, and kidneys.
- The superior hypogastric block is performed at the level of L5 to S1 for treatment of visceral pain of the lower sigmoid colon, rectum, testicles, ovaries, and uterus.
- A ganglion impar block is performed for pain in the perineal area. The ganglion impar is where the two sympathetic chains join together and is located retroperitoneally at the level of the sacrococcygeal ligament.

Introduction

Visceral pain is a common complaint seen by many different types of physicians, including family medicine, gastroenterologists, oncologists, surgeons, and pain medicine. Visceral pain can be very challenging to diagnose, manage, and treat. This pain can be somatic or visceral in origin, can be related to a malignancy or be noncancer in origin, and is often very diffuse and nonlocalized. Therefore, treatment and management not only depends on the type of pain and its origin but also very often is aimed at the additional factors in the patient's life exacerbating the pain such as stress and anxiety.[1,2]

The history provided by the patient involving the description of pain quality and referral pattern will help elucidate the origin of the pain symptoms. Somatic pain is generally described as well localized and constant in nature with an aching or sharp quality. Somatic pain can often be treated with a combination of nonopioid adjuvant analgesics and local pain interventions. Visceral pain is typically described as vague in origin and of a squeezing, deep, pressure-like quality. Visceral pain is a result of organ injury with resulting transmission of pain via fibers that travel with the sympathetic nervous system.[3] Visceral pain may result from distention, traction, torsion, ischemia, or abnormal contraction of visceral organs and may result in referred somatic complaints.[4] Interventional procedures involving the sympathetic chain may be used to ease the pain of some patients with abdominal malignancies. Finally, neuropathic pain is usually described as a shooting, numbness, tingling, burning type of pain. This type of pain is usually caused by some injury or irritation of the nervous system itself whether it is via direct postsurgical injury or from a tumor encroachment, compression, or invasion of a nerve structure. This type of pain requires a multimodal pharmacological approach, including opioids, tricyclic antidepressants, selective serotonin norepinephrine reuptake inhibitors, and N-methyl-D-aspartate blockers and early aggressive interventional management with spinal cord stimulation; intrathecal medication administration; and, in the case of malignancy-related pain, neurolysis. This chapter focuses on peripheral neurolytic treatment of visceral pain.

Visceral input arrives in the dorsal horn of the spinal cord; lamina I, II and V; and the intermediolateral cell column, sacral parasympathetic nucleus and lamina X.[4] Multiple visceral inputs converge at a single site, thus making exact diagnosis of the location of pain difficult and hence the vague symptoms described by patients.[1] The signal travels from the dorsal horn of the spinal cord to the spinothalamic, spinoreticular, spinomesencephalic, and spinohypothalamic tract.[4] Visceral input terminates in the brain at multiple sites, including the medulla, pons, mesencephalon, hypothalamus, and thalamus,[4] and results in activity of the anterior and midcingulate cortex, frontal cortex, parietal cortex, and cerebellum.[5] The cortical sites associated with visceral pain have involvement in the affective perception of pain and memory and may account for the preponderance of co-morbidities such as anxiety and depression with visceral pain.

The treatment of visceral pain resulting from malignancy is integral to the overall treatment of patients with cancer, the goals being improvement in quality of life and improved functional status.[6] Evidence suggests pain control plays a significant role in cancer survival.[7,8] In treating patients with cancer-related pain, a multimodal and multidisciplinary approach involving medical, interventional, psychological, and social support management produces the highest level of patient satisfaction.

Interventional procedures to treat intractable pain include intrathecal analgesia; epidural analgesia; and the subject of this chapter, neurolytic blocks of the sympathetic chain responsible for the viscera afferent input. One challenge in the treatment of patients with visceral pain with interventional modalities is that total abolition of the pain is nearly impossible secondary to excessive innervations of many of the visceral organs. Unfortunately, in our experience, pain generated outside of the viscera, such as pain secondary to lymphadenopathy, may not be relieved by neurolytic blocks. Therefore, continued supplementation with other sources of pain relief such as opioids and nonopioid adjuvants is needed to control the pain of cancer patients.

Chemical Neurolysis

Chemical neurolysis has been used since the early 1900s when Schloesser used alcohol for the treatment of trigeminal neuralgia.[9] In 1919, Kappis[10] performed the first neurolytic procedure for the relief of visceral pain when he performed a percutaneous celiac plexus block in the treatment of intractable abdominal pain.[9] Many pharmacological agents have been used for neurolysis, including alcohol (ethanol), phenol, glycerol, and hypertonic saline. Nerve destruction depends on the agent, amount, concentration, and rate of injection.[9]

The neurolytic action of alcohol is produced by the extraction of cholesterol, phospholipids, and cerebrosides and the precipitation of mucopeptides from the nerve and supporting myelin sheath.[11] The basal lamina of the Schwann cell sheath remains intact, allowing for new Schwann cell growth, thereby providing the framework for subsequent nerve fiber growth. This framework encourages the regeneration of axons, but only if the cell bodies of these nerves are not completely destroyed.[12] The pathway of degeneration is nonselective and can be observed in peripheral nerves and spinal nerve roots after intrathecal injection and in perineural structures (peritoneum, bowel) after peripheral injections.

Ethyl alcohol in concentrations of 50% to 100% injected perineurally is associated with burning dysesthesias running along the course of the nerve. This sensation is often extremely unpleasant for the patient and can last from a few minutes to a few weeks. To alleviate this, local anesthetic medications are injected before the use of ethyl alcohol. Some physicians will also use this to confirm the correct location of the injectate.

Phenol is a benzene ring with one hydroxyl group substituted for a hydrogen atom. It is usually prepared by the hospital or compounding pharmacy because it is not commercially available in premixed liquid form; however, this practice has ceased in many hospital organizations because of the complexity of sterile compounding. Phenol is poorly soluble in water and, at room temperature, forms only a 6.7% aqueous solution. Consequently, phenol is frequently prepared with contrast dyes and sterile water, saline, or glycerin. When phenol is exposed to room air, it undergoes oxidation and turns a reddish color; however, it has a shelf life of approximately 1 year if refrigerated and shielded from light exposure. When phenol is prepared with glycerin, it has limited spread; hence, injections are well localized. In rats, the aqueous solution of phenol has greater ability to penetrate the perineurium and produce greater endoneurial damage than glycerin preparations, but there is no difference in results after intraneural injection.[13]

Putnam and Hampton[14] first used phenol as a neurolytic agent in 1936, and Mandl used it for a sympathetic ganglion neurolysis in animals in 1947.[15] Originally, it was surmised that phenol had a selective effect on small-diameter, unmyelinated and lightly myelinated nerve fibers, such as C-fiber afferents and A-δ afferents, respectively. Subsequent studies have shown that phenol concentrations determine the type and extent of nerve disruption that also include A-α and A-β fiber damage.[16] At concentrations less than 5%, phenol causes protein denaturation of axons and surrounding blood vessels. At concentrations greater than 5%, phenol can produce protein coagulation and nonselective segmental demyelination.[17]

Unlike alcohol, phenol injection has an initial local anesthetic effect. It is not associated with localized burning but instead creates a sensation of warmth and numbness. Concentrations of 4% to 10% are typically used for neurolysis. Preparations of phenol in glycerin are highly viscous, which may make administration through a small gauge (25-gauge) spinal needle difficult. Careful patient positioning to allow phenol to settle into the desired location is important. When compared with alcohol, phenol seems to facilitate axonal regeneration in a shorter period of time. Electrophysiological studies comparing peripheral nerve destruction in cats showed that those injected with phenol had returned to normal by 2 months; at the end of the same time period, those injected with alcohol still demonstrated depression of compound action potentials.[18] However, another study by Smith[19] suggests regeneration is not completed until approximately 14 weeks after the administration of phenol.

Celiac Plexus Neurolysis

Indication

Neurolysis of the celiac plexus is one of the most commonly performed neurolytic procedures for the treatment of visceral cancer pain. The nerves of the celiac plexus are responsible for the painful sensation of an extremely large anatomical area, innervating the visceral organs from the distal third of the esophagus to the descending colon. This, therefore, includes the liver, pancreas, gallbladder, stomach, spleen, kidneys, small intestines, large intestines (to the descending colon), and adrenal glands; a partial contribution to the bladder; and a small contribution to the testes and epididymis, the ovaries, and the blood vessels surrounding them.[9] Both malignant and nonmalignant pain associated with these organs can be reduced with the neurolytic destruction of the celiac plexus. Although the treatment of nonmalignant pain conditions can be achieved with this technique, it is not recommended for routine use in the treatment of noncancer pain because the procedure is associated with significant and serious complications that may not outweigh the benefits of the procedure. Celiac plexus neurolysis for the treatment of nonmalignant abdominal pain conditions such as chronic pancreatitis has been reported to be more short-lived analgesia than those treated with the same procedure for the treatment of cancer-related pain.[9,20,21] Furthermore, the benefits of the neurolysis are likely to be time limited, and the noncancer patient's life may extend well past the analgesia associated with the procedure. This can leave the patient with their original abdominal pain and partial deafferentation pain, which can be more severe than the initial pain and now with more limited treatment options.

Anatomy

The celiac plexus is located at the level of T12 to L1. It is found in the retroperitoneal space, just anterior and caudad to the crura of the diaphragm (Fig. 9-1). It surrounds the anterior and lateral aspects of the aorta and celiac and superior mesenteric trunks as they divide from the aorta.[22] Most commonly, the celiac plexus ganglia are 0.6 cm and 0.9 cm caudad to the celiac artery on the right and left, respectively.[23] The location of the celiac plexus varies with respect to bony landmarks and can be located anywhere from the T12 to L1 disc space to the middle of the L2 vertebral body.[24] The plexus receives sympathetic fibers from the greater (T9-T10), lesser (T10-T11), and least (T12) splanchnic nerves and parasympathetic fibers from the vagus nerve (**Fig. 9-1**).

Procedure

The celiac plexus may be approached in three different ways: retrocrural, anterocrural, and the splanchnic nerves (**Fig. 9-2**). It can be performed percutaneously in the prone and supine positions using anatomic landmarks, ultrasonography, fluoroscopy, or computed tomography (CT), or through the gastric wall with the assistance of an endoscope.

The most common approach and most thoroughly studied approach is the fluoroscopic or CT-guided posterior percutaneous approach. In this approach, the patient is placed prone, and a 5- to 7-inch small-gauge needle is inserted at the level of the L1 transverse process approximately 5 to 7 cm to the left of midline. This location should coincide with the lateral edge of the L1 vertebral body when viewed in the oblique orientation at approximately 25 to 35 degrees (**Fig. 9-3, A**) depending on the patient's body mass index. After the needle is inserted, it is directed toward the upper third of L1 (**Fig. 9-3, B**) for the retrocrural approach and the lower third of L1 for the anterocrural approach. In performing the retrocrural approach, the needle is advanced just anterior to the anterior border of the body of L1, no more than 0.5 cm. In the anterocrural approach, from the left, the needle is advanced through the aorta (**Fig. 9-3, C**), and the needle is advanced until no more blood is aspirated. At this time, contrast dye should be injected to confirm location in the anteroposterior (AP) and lateral views (**Fig. 9-3, D**). If dye spread appears anterior to the aorta and covers the left and right sides and if the provider is intending anterocrural injection, then a second needle from the right side

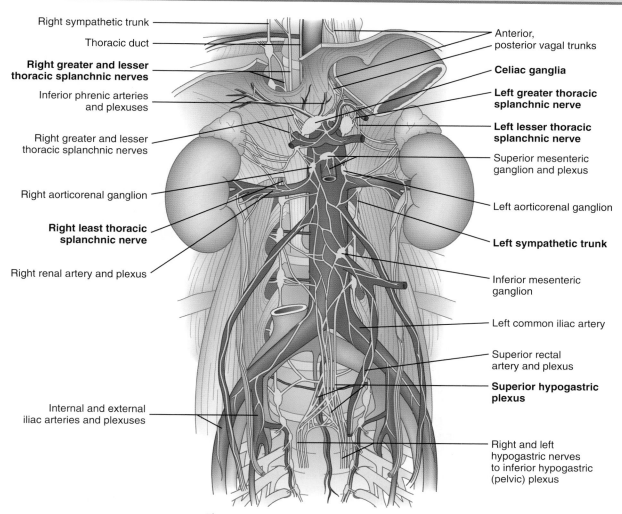

Right sympathetic trunk

Thoracic duct

Right greater and lesser thoracic splanchnic nerves

Inferior phrenic arteries and plexuses

Right greater and lesser thoracic splanchnic nerves

Right aorticorenal ganglion

Right least thoracic splanchnic nerve

Right renal artery and plexus

Internal and external iliac arteries and plexuses

Anterior, posterior vagal trunks

Celiac ganglia

Left greater thoracic splanchnic nerve

Left lesser thoracic splanchnic nerve

Superior mesenteric ganglion and plexus

Left aorticorenal ganglion

Left sympathetic trunk

Inferior mesenteric ganglion

Left common iliac artery

Superior rectal artery and plexus

Superior hypogastric plexus

Right and left hypogastric nerves to inferior hypogastric (pelvic) plexus

Fig. 9-1 Abdominal and visceral ganglia.

need not be placed. In a retrocrural injection, if the dye spread remains in the anterior third of the vertebral body when examined in the lateral view and on both sides when viewed in AP, then a second needle need not be placed. In performing the splanchnic nerve block, the needles are aimed at the body of T12 using a caudocephalad angle (camera cephalad, image intensifier caudad) of 10 to 15 degrees with skin insertion at the L1 level similar to that of the celiac plexus neurolysis to best avoid puncture of the lung pleural or parenchyma. The needle is then directed until it is just short of the anterior border of the T12 vertebral body. After the needle is placed and secure, a local anesthetic agent with epinephrine is injected to test for inadvertent intravascular access. A long-acting local anesthetic is then injected to produce analgesia before ethanol administration (this can be excluded if phenol is the neurolytic).

The volume of neurolytic injected differs for the approaches. Retrocrural celiac plexus neurolysis may require a slightly higher volume of ethanol because it has to spread to the celiac plexus across the crura or envelop the descending splanchnic nerves. Traditionally, these volumes have been in the range of 20 to 25 mL per side. These volumes are often excessive and a total of 15 to 20 mL (7.5-10 cc per side) can be sufficient. The anterocrural approach is similar, and it can require between 15 and 20 mL of the neurolytic drug (divided between the needles if using more than one). The splanchnic neurolysis requires 6 to 8 mL total.[25] The ethanol concentration for these blocks is in the range of 50% to

80% obtained by diluting the neurolytic with contrast to enable visualization of neurolytic medication spread. If the provider has injected 5 to 10 mL of local anesthetic before the administration of the neurolytic, they may take that volume into account for the dilution calculation or preferably wait 5 to 10 minutes between the injections to allow for significant diffusion and absorption of the local anesthetic. If phenol is being used, the concentration most commonly used is in the range of 5% to 10% mixed with contrast, saline, or glycerin.

With advanced imaging, such as CT guidance or ultrasonography, patients who are either unable to lie flat or who have a liver that is too enlarged to allow a posterior entry, a transabdominal radiographic approach can be used but is not recommended unless all other approaches are exhausted because of the high risk of infection secondary to needle entrance into the bowel.[9]

Complications

Complications after a celiac plexus block can be common to all three approaches to the celiac plexus or be unique to that specific approach. Complications include the following:

1. *Orthostatic hypotension* may result after any of the three approaches; however, it is more common with the retrocrural approach (50%) and the splanchnic approach (52%) than the anterocrural approach (10%).[25] Orthostatic hypotension usually lasts up to 5 days after the procedure and should be treated with

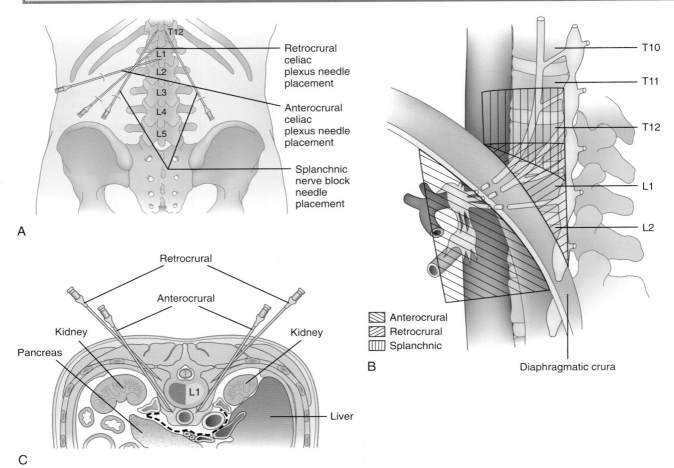

Fig. 9-2 Celiac plexus. **A,** Posterior view: needle approaches to the celiac plexus and splanchnic nerves. **B,** Lateral view: the celiac plexus: *up-down hash marks* represent the medication spread of the splanchnic nerve approach, *hash marks* from the bottom left to the upper right represent retrocrural dye spread, and *hash marks* from the upper left to the lower right represent anterocrural dye spread. **C,** Cross-sectional view of celiac plexus block.

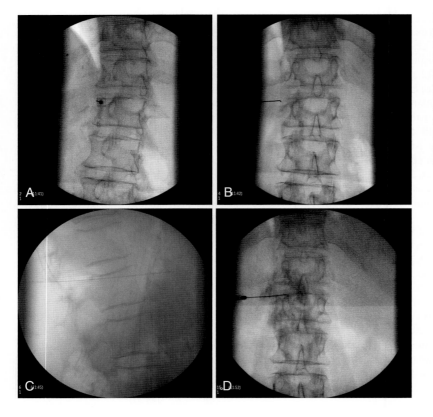

Fig. 9-3 Anterocrural celiac plexus neurolysis performed under fluoroscopy. There was a clinical result of 80% pain relief of abdominal pain 30 minutes after injection of ethanol. **A,** Left oblique view with needle placement at the upper pole of the L1 vertebral body. **B,** Anteroposterior (AP) view. The needle is approaching the lateral border of the vertebral body. **C,** Lateral view: final needle placement anterior to the L1 vertebral body and aorta. There is contrast dye spread anterior to the aorta with no vascular administration. **D,** AP view: final needle placement showing bilateral spread (left > right) of contrast dye.

bed rest, fluid replacement, and care with position changes. To compensate for the venous pooling, wrapping the lower extremities with elastic bandages from the toes to the thighs has been shown to be helpful within the first week after the procedure.

2. *Pneumothorax* may result from an inadvertent puncture during the procedure. It is logical to presume that the highest risk is associated with the splanchnic nerve technique because of the necessary placement of the needle(s) up to T12. However, the only trial comparing the three approaches reported no pneumothoraces.[25] The authors make no mention of radiographic investigation of this complication, although the procedures were performed using fluoroscopic imaging during which a clinically significant pneumothorax could have been appreciated.

3. *Backache* may result after the procedure regardless of the approach. This may simply be the result of local skin trauma with needle placement or secondary to alcohol irritation. A backache should not be taken lightly because it may signal a more serious complication such as a retroperitoneal hematoma. The hematoma may be contained or continuing to enlarge. These patients should be followed with a set of two measurements of hematocrit an hour apart. If a decrease in hematocrit is seen, radiologic imaging is warranted. A retroperitoneal hemorrhage can be devastating, so the combined symptoms of backache with orthostatic hypotension after a procedure should be considered to be a retroperitoneal hemorrhage until proven otherwise. Prompt admission to the hospital should be considered. This could be a result of injury to the aorta or renal, celiac, or superior mesenteric vessels.

4. *Diarrhea* is a common complication after the celiac plexus block with varying rates depending on the approach. Transient diarrhea is a result of sympathetic block of the bowels. The anterocrural approach (65%) was complicated with transient diarrhea more commonly than the splanchnic nerve block (5%) or the retrocrural approach (25%). Diarrhea becomes a major complication in elderly and frail individuals and those who cannot replete their fluids and electrolytes.[26] Treatment includes fluid replacements and antidiarrheal agents such as loperamide. The increase in stool frequency and content can sometimes represent a substantial relief to a large proportion of those patients taking high doses of opioids, resulting in severe refractory constipation.

5. *Abdominal aortic dissection* is a potential complication more common in the anterocrural approach.[27,28] Severe atherosclerotic disease of the aorta may preclude this approach.

6. *Paraplegia* can be a devastating complication of the celiac plexus block, as well as bladder and bowel dysfunction. In one report, paraplegia occurred in one in 683 procedures[29]; however, another report had no such complications.[25] It is a logical belief that the splanchnic or retrocrural approaches would put the patient at higher risk of such complications resulting from vasospasm of the nearby spinal radicular arteries; however, this complication occurs at such a profoundly low rate that it is not possible to state relative risk among the three approaches. Transient motor paralysis can occur secondary to a spasm of the lumbar segmental arteries, which are responsible for perfusion of the spinal cord.[30] In animal models, contraction of these arteries has been shown to occur after exposure to alcohol with no difference based on the concentration used. Thus, patients with atherosclerotic disease with an already compromised perfusion of the spinal cord are at a higher risk of having these complications, especially with use of alcohol as a

neurolytic agent.[30] Although this is a real and devastating complication, the estimate of one in 683 procedures is based on very old studies using techniques that are less commonly performed today.

7. Other *minor complications* from the celiac plexus can include dysesthesia, interscapular back pain, reactive pleurisy, hematuria, and hiccups.

Efficacy

The efficacy of the celiac plexus block has been studied in several trials.[25,30-32] The prospective randomized study by Ischia et al[25] looked at 61 patients with pancreatic cancer pain. Of those, 48% experienced complete pain relief from the neurolytic celiac plexus block. The remaining 52%, or 32 patients, did not experience complete pain relief secondary to either technical failure or the fact that the patient had not just visceral pain but a combination of neuropathic, visceral, and somatic complaints.[25] A second study compared medical therapy with that of the celiac plexus block.[33] The patients who received the neurolytic block used less opioid than those who did not receive the block and thus experienced fewer pharmacologically induced side effects.[33] The presence of lymphadenopathy is a poor prognostic indicator in the success of the neurolytic block; thus, when there is advanced disease outside of the pancreas, a successful outcome is less likely. A meta-analysis looking at 21 retrospective studies showed that pain relief could be achieved in 89% of patients for the first 2 weeks after a block.[34] In patients who were alive at the 3-month interval, 90% of the patients had partial to complete pain relief. Of patients who received the block within the 3-month interval preceding death, 70% to 90% experienced partial to complete pain relief.[34] This meta-analysis did not take into account the approach used or choice and dosage of neurolytic agent used.

There is some controversy regarding the timing of neurolytic treatment in the course of tumor progression. Those who place the neurolytic procedure very early in the cancer progress (early after the onset of pain), such as these authors, believe that the early abolition of pain reduces the likelihood of central or peripheral sensitization and therefore the development of a more challenging pain syndrome latter in the course. Furthermore, early intervention provides an easier target to treat because the tumor growth has not yet physically obstructed access to the plexus. Advanced disease that has spread will usually result in not only visceral pain but also somatic and neuropathic pain.[9] Furthermore, there is evidence showing that high doses of opioids may have a negative effect on immunity.[35] A study by Lillemoe and colleagues[8] showed that patients with nonresectable pancreatic cancer lived longer if they received splanchnic neurolysis. This prospective randomized trial suggested that the patients who had the neurolysis procedure used fewer narcotics and had better-preserved immune functions and also experienced less nausea and vomiting.[8] Others argue that neurolytic blocks should be performed only when patients obtain undesirable side effects from significant dosages of systemic narcotics. Side effects include sedation, constipation, nausea, vomiting, and respiratory depression and may prove to be intolerable to some patients. The ideal time to provide neurolytic treatment has yet to be determined in a rigorous fashion.

Lumbar Sympathetic Neurolysis

Indications

The lumbar sympathetic chain is blocked in cases of visceral pain associated with the descending colon and upper portion of the sigmoid colon, kidney, a partial contribution to the bladder, and ovaries.[36-38] Although this is not the subject of this chapter, blockade of this plexus or chain is also performed in the treatment of lower extremity sympathetically-mediated neuropathic pain syndromes and ischemic pain associated with small vessel peripheral vascular disease. The treatment of the latter pain syndromes with lumbar sympathetic chain neurolysis is very controversial. As discussed in previous sections, neurolysis is most commonly reserved for cancer-related pain secondary to the reduced life expectancy and therefore lower cumulative risk of deafferentation pain. Neurolysis of this plexus for the purpose of relieving visceral pain will result in sympatholysis to the lower extremities as well, and patients will have to provide consent for this known outcome.

Anatomy

The lumbar sympathetic chain is located just anterolateral of the lumbar vertebral bodies anterior to the origin of the psoas muscle.[38] The aorta is anterior and medial to the left sympathetic chain, and the right sympathetic chain approximates the inferior vena cava.[22] The lumbar arteries and veins are present around the sympathetic chain as well.[38]

Procedure

Three approaches are available for the lumbar sympathetic block. Kappis and Mandl developed the classic technique using 3 needles placed 5 to 6 cm from midline at the level of L2, L3, and L4. The needles are angled medially contacting the transverse process of their respective lumbar vertebra. Redirecting and passing inferiorly and medially, the needle is aimed at the vertebral body. The needle is advanced until it is just anterolateral to the respective vertebral body.[38] Reid et al developed the lateral technique in 1970.[39] They initiated their approach 10 to 12 cm lateral to midline, thus avoiding the vertebral body altogether. They designed this approach because they thought that it was difficult to navigate around the vertebral body effectively.[38] A third approach developed by Bryce-Smith[40] took advantage of the tendinous arches at the origin of the psoas muscle. The arches contain lumbar vessels, fat, rami communicantes, and the sympathetic chain anteriorly.[38] This technique uses one insertion point at L3 5 cm lateral to the superior tip of the spinous process directed medially through the psoas muscle, missing the vertebra altogether. Although these are the described standard techniques, with the addition of fluoroscopy and CT, most pain physicians have altered their practice. The most common performed approach is using a fluoroscopic angle of approximately 30 to 35 degrees to allow for the L3 transverse process to just become buried within the vertebral body (**Figs. 9-4, A** and **9-5**). The needle is then inserted at the level of the L3 transverse process and advanced until it contacts the most lateral portion of the vertebral body at which point in lateral view the needle is directed medially and anteriorly until the tip lies in the anterolateral portion of the vertebral body (**Fig. 9-4, B** and **C**). Contrast dye is then injected to confirm the needle tip location. Contrast dye covering the anterolateral aspect of the vertebral body without the appearance of an intramuscular injection confirms appropriate placement (**Fig. 9-4, D** and **E**). After this, a test dose with lidocaine and epinephrine can be performed, although the test is not necessary if real-time fluoroscopy or digital subtraction angiography is performed. A solution of 5 to 8 cc of bupivacaine is then injected to anesthetize the nerves before injection of the neurolytic medication. A range of 5 to 10 cc of 50% to 80% ethanol can be used for neurolysis. If contrast is included in the ethanol, one can guide the volume of injection by the cephalad–caudal and dorsal–ventral spread of the ethanol.

Complications

Complications resulting from performing a lumbar sympathetic block include the following:

1. *Accidental neuraxial injection* may result in a total spinal, as described in two case reports by Gay and Evans,[41] or death.[42] This risk is exceptionally low with the use of imaging techniques.
2. *Genitofemoral neuralgia* is the most common complication after chemical lumbar sympathetic neurolysis.[22,38] The incidence ranges from 6% to 40%.[43-45] The hyperesthesia is usually transient, rarely exceeding 2 to 6 weeks.[38] Neuralgia affecting the lateral aspect of the thigh has also been reported.[39] An increased frequency of occurrence may be related to the use of alcohol compared with phenol, although there is not a conclusive study evaluating this.[43]
3. *Postdural puncture headache* secondary to inadvertent dural puncture has been noted.[38]
4. *Paraplegia* associated with lumbar sympathetic blocks is rare, although it has been described with celiac plexus blocks and thoracic paravertebral blocks.[46-48] Inadvertent intrathecal injection of a chemical neurolytic agent has resulted in paralysis and limb weakness, which are usually transient in nature.[49] However, permanent weakness has been reported.[46]
5. *Aseptic meningitis* from inadvertent breach in septic technique has also been seen.[38]
6. *Renal and ureter penetration.*[39,50,51] Using CT imaging, a study by Weyland et al[52] advised not exceeding midline by 6 cm, 7 cm, and 10 cm at L2, L3, and L4, respectively.
7. *Bleeding* occurs with puncture of the inferior vena cava, aorta, or surrounding vasculature. Intravascular phenol injection may result in seizures or cardiac dysrhythmias if injected in large volumes.[53]
8. *Rare complications* include allergic reactions, Horner syndrome, and the potential inability to ejaculate in men who have received bilateral lumbar sympathetic neurolysis.[39,44,54,55]

Efficacy

A study comparing phenol chemical neurolysis with radiofrequency thermocoagulation for lumbar sympathectomy showed that 89% of patients after neurolysis with phenol had a sympathetic block after 8 weeks, and only 12% had a block after 8 weeks in the radiofrequency group.[22,56]

Superior Hypogastric Plexus Neurolysis

Indications

Patients with pain secondary to cancer invasion or nonmalignant conditions involving the lower portion of the sigmoid colon to the rectum, testicles, ovaries, uterus, fallopian tubes, or a partial sympathetic innervation of the bladder and ureters[36] may benefit from a superior hypogastric block.

Anatomy

The afferent fibers innervating pelvic structures travel in the sympathetic nerves and ganglia. For pain syndromes involving cancer invasion into the pelvic organs, it has been suggested that a superior hypogastric plexus (SHP) neurolytic block should be considered even in advanced stages of disease.[57] The plexus is situated retroperitoneally extending from the lower edge of L5 to the upper third of S1 (**Fig. 9-6, A**).

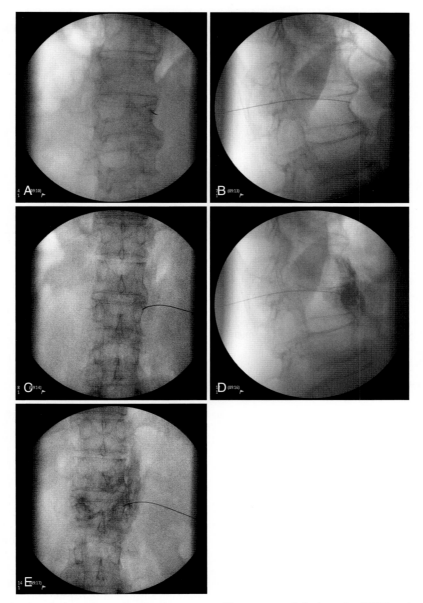

Fig. 9-4 Lumbar sympathetic neurolysis performed under fluoroscopy. There was a clinical result of 50% pain relief of abdominal pain 20 minutes after injection of ethanol. **A,** Right oblique view: right L2 transverse process shadow is within the vertebral body and therefore doe not obstruct needle placement. Needle placement is at the level of the L2 transverse process. **B,** Lateral view: needle placement in the anterolateral aspect of the L2 vertebral body. **C,** Anteroposterior (AP) view: final needle placement without contrast dye (note the thirteenth rib). **D,** Lateral view: final needle placement with contrast dye covering the lumbar sympathetic chain L1 to L3. **E,** AP view: final needle position with predominantly right-sided spread of contrast dye.

Procedure

There are two main approaches to the SHP (**Fig. 9-6,** *B*). Using the two-needle technique, the patient is placed in a prone position with two 7-cm needles directed medially and caudad so that the tip of the needles lay anterolateral to the L5-S1 intervertebral disc space (**Fig. 9-7,** *A* and *B*).[57,58] This approach avoids transgression of the intervertebral disc, but it has a higher rate of neurapraxia related to needle trauma to the L5 nerve roots as they exit the L5-S1 foramen. Avoidance of injection into the iliac vessels is accomplished with aspiration. If blood is aspirated, a transvascular approach can be used. Accurate placement is verified using fluoroscopy with the tip of the needle at the junction of L5 and S1 on an anteroposterior view.

The second approach is the transdiscal technique in which a single needle is placed in a similar manner to a discogram of the L5-S1 intervertebral disc. With the patient positioned prone, a single 7-inch spinal needle is placed through the disc using an oblique angle of approximately 25 to 30 degrees so the needle tip ends in the midline immediately anterior to the L5-S1 disc (**Fig. 9-8,** *A* and *B*). Contrast injection confirms proper placement (**Fig. 9-8,** *C* and *D*). After the needle has been confirmed to be in the correct position, a local anesthetic can be used diagnostically and then ethanol or phenol can be used as a neurolytic solution. The volume of neurolytic is guided by the spread of the agent (when mixed with contrast); common volumes range from 5 to 10 cc.

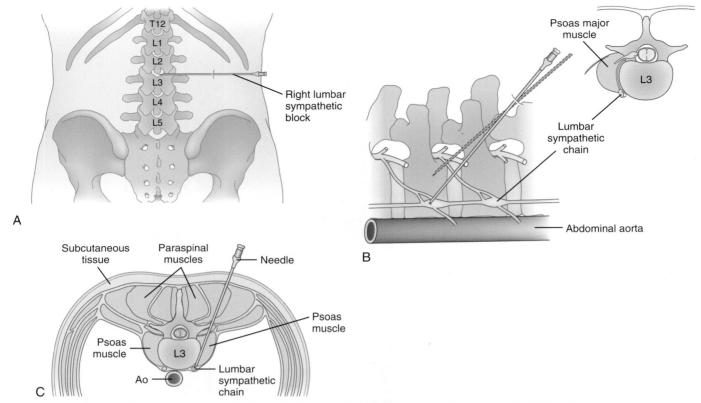

Fig. 9-5 Lumbar sympathetic block. **A,** Posterior view. **B,** Lateral view. **C,** Cross-sectional view. Ao, aorta.

Complications

Complications after this procedure are not as common as with the celiac plexus neurolytic block. If the needle tip is located more lateral than anterolateral of the L5 disc, retrograde spread to the L5 nerve roots may occur; this can be associated with predicted neurologic deficits if a neurolytic agent is used. The transdiscal approach can be associated with discitis, although this has not been reported. The two needle lateral approach can be associated with L5 nerve injury as discussed above. Bleeding and infection associated with any invasive procedure are also potential risks.

Efficacy

In a study composed of 227 patients receiving a diagnostic block for pelvic pain, 79% had a favorable result and thus underwent a SHP block. Of these, 72% had a reduction in pain scores at 3 months and a decrease in opioid requirements.[59]

Ganglion Impar Neurolysis

Indications

Visceral pain can extend into and include the perineal area. Although this is often discussed as neurolysis of the sympathetic nervous system, at this level and the SHP, the organs have significant parasympathetic input that may also account for a portion of nociceptive transmission. Sympathetic input of the distal urethra, vulva, distal rectum, and distal third of the vagina and parasympathetic innervation to the bladder combine at the nerve plexus called the ganglion impar. Patients with visceral pain in these organs usually complain of a burning or urgency type of sensation.

Anatomy

The ganglion impar is located at the end of the two sympathetic chains where they join together. It is located retroperitoneally at the level of the sacrococcygeal junction.

Procedure

Two approaches using fluoroscopy have been described in performing a ganglion impar block (**Fig. 9-9**). A trans-sacrococcygeal joint approach involves placement of a 20- to 22-gauge needle through the sacrococcygeal ligament until it is just anterior to the sacrum, with the patient in a prone position (**Fig. 9-10**). The second approach places the patient in the lateral decubitus position with hips flexed. A 3.5-inch needle is placed through the anococcygeal ligament using fluoroscopy. A finger is placed in the rectum to avoid inadvertent puncture. The needle is guided along the anococcygeal ligament. This latter approach has fallen out of favor because of its complexity and increased risk to the patient and interventionalist of needle puncture. Phenol 6% has been the traditional neurolytic agent of choice, but ethanol provides excellent neurolysis that is comfortable for the patient provided sufficient local anesthetic is first injected. Small volumes are used for this injection; often 1 to 3 mL of 80% ethanol or 6% phenol is sufficient to produce analgesia.

Complications

Complications in performing a ganglion impar block are not well described in the literature. Complications could include rectal puncture, intravascular injection, inadvertent epidural spread, or infection.

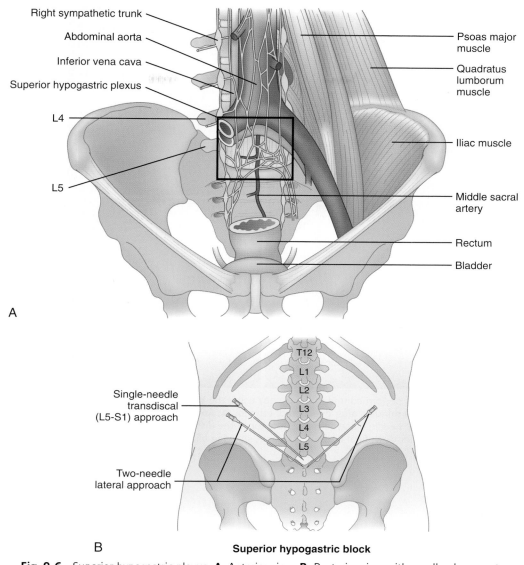

Right sympathetic trunk
Abdominal aorta
Inferior vena cava
Superior hypogastric plexus
L4
L5

Psoas major muscle
Quadratus lumborum muscle
Iliac muscle
Middle sacral artery
Rectum
Bladder

A

T12
L1
L2
L3
L4
L5

Single-needle transdiscal (L5-S1) approach

Two-needle lateral approach

B   **Superior hypogastric block**

Fig. 9-6   Superior hypogastric plexus. **A,** Anterior view. **B,** Posterior view with needle placement.

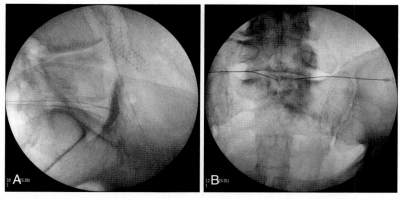

Fig. 9-7   Superior hypogastric neurolysis performed under fluoroscopy using the two-needle posterior–lateral approach. There was a clinical result of 90% pain relief of pelvic pain 30 minutes after injection of ethanol. **A,** Lateral view: bilateral needle position anterior to the L5-S1 intervertebral disc. Note the position of the bilateral iliac vessels (Dacron grafts). **B,** Anteroposterior view: bilateral needle placement anterior to the L5-S1 disc approached with a needle track lateral to the disc.

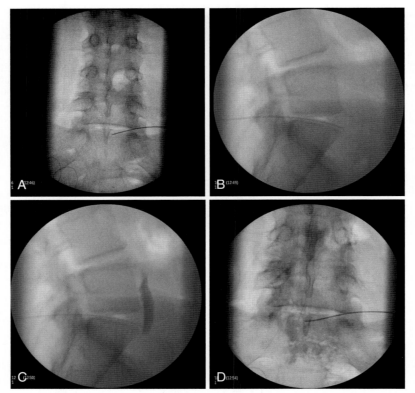

Fig. 9-8 Superior hypogastric neurolysis performed under fluoroscopy using the single-needle transdiscal approach. There was a clinical result of 90% pain relief of pelvic pain 30 minutes after injection of ethanol. **A,** Anteroposterior view: needle placement from the right side traversing the L5-S1 disc. **B,** Lateral view: needle placement just anterior to the disc. **C,** Lateral view: final needle placement showing appropriate dye spread. **D,** Anteroposterior view: final needle placement showing bilateral spread of contrast dye.

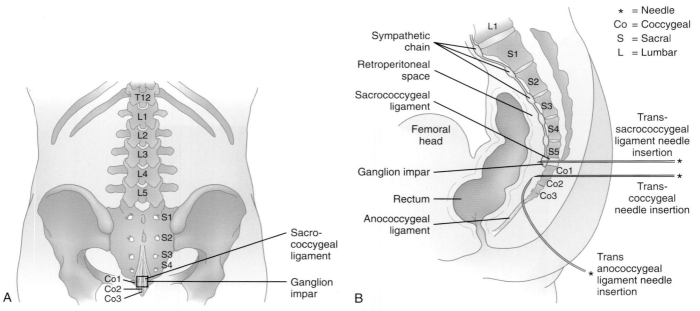

Fig. 9-9 Ganglion impar. **A,** Posterior view. **B,** Lateral view with needle placement.

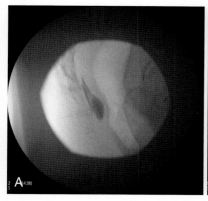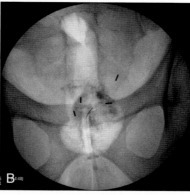

Fig. 9-10 Ganglion impar neurolysis performed under fluoroscopy. There was a clinical result of 60% pain relief of perineal pain 30 minutes after injection of ethanol. **A,** Lateral view: needle placement through the sacrococcygeal ligament with appropriate dye spread. (Note the prominent Co1-Co2 joint space that could also be used for this injection.) **B,** Anteroposterior view: needle placement showing bilateral dye spread.

Efficacy

In a prospective study by Plancarte et al,[60] patients with perineal pain who had failed pharmacologic treatment were evaluated. All of the patients had pain confined to the perineal area. Using a trans-sacrococcygeal approach, eight of 16 patients experienced complete relief with the remaining eight patients experiencing a 60% to 90% reduction in pain.[60] Of note, the ganglion impar block has not been shown to be efficacious in the treatment of patients with coccydynia.[61]

Conclusion

Celiac plexus, lumbar sympathetic, superior hypogastric, and ganglion impar neurolytic blocks are effective therapeutic interventions in the treatment of patients with visceral pain. Each procedure is not without significant risks and complications, and each has a variable efficacy and success rate. In the hands of a skilled practitioner with proper technique and patient selection, these interventional procedures allow for an alternative or supplement to opioid therapy in the treatment of visceral pain without the patient having to endure the side effects of large doses of opioids.

References

1. Ness T: Chronic abdominal, groin, and perineal pain of visceral origin. In Breivik H, Campbell W, Nicholas M, editors: *Textbook of clinical pain management: chronic pain*, London, 2008, Hodder & Stroughton, pp 567-586.
2. Bhatia V, Tandon R: Stress and the gastrointestinal tract. *J Gastroenterol Hepatol* 20:332-339, 2004.
3. Newman PP: Visceral afferent functions of the nervous system. *Monogr Physiol Soc* 1-273, 1974.
4. Ness T: Applied physiology: persistent visceral pain. In Wilson PR, Watson PJ, Haythornthwaite JA, et al, editors: *Clinical pain management: chronic pain*, London, 2008, Oxford University Press, pp 37-47.
5. Athwal BS, Berkley KJ, Hussain I, et al: Brain responses to changes in bladder volume and urge to void in healthy men. *Brain* 124:369-377, 2001.
6. Ferrell BR, Wisdom C, Wenzl C: Quality of life as an outcome variable in the management of cancer pain. *Cancer* 63:2321-2327, 1989.
7. Liebeskind JC: Pain can kill. *Pain* 44:3-4, 1991.
8. Lillemoe KD, Cameron JL, Kaufman HS, et al: Chemical splanchnicectomy in patients with unresectable pancreatic cancer. A prospective randomized trial. *Ann Surg* 217:447-455; discussion 456-457, 1993.
9. Williams J: Nerve blocks—chemical and physical neurolytic agents. I: In Sykes N, Fallon MT, Patt RB, editors: *Clinical pain management: cancer pain*, London, 2003, Arnold, pp 235-244.

10. Kappis, M: Sensibilitat und locale Anasthesia in chirurginchen Gebiet der Bauchhohle mit besonderer Berucksichrigung der Splanchnicus. *Anasthesie Beitr Z Klin Chir* 115:161, 1919.
11. Rumsby MG, Finean JB: The action of organic solvents on the myelin sheath of peripheral nerve tissue. II. Short-chain aliphatic alcohols. *J Neurochem* 13:1509-1511, 1966.
12. Bonica J, Buckley F, Moricca G, et al: Neurolytic blockade and hypophysectomy. In Bonica J, editor: *The management of pain*, Philadelphia, 1990, Lea & Febiger, pp 1980-2039.
13. Westerlund T, Vuorinen V, Kirvela O, et al: The endoneurial response to neurolytic agents is highly dependent on the mode of application. *Reg Anesth Pain Med* 24:294-302, 1999.
14. Putnam TJ, Hampton AO: The technic of injection into the Gasserian ganglion under roentgenographic control. *Arch Neurol Psychiatry* 35:92-98, 1936.
15. Mandl F: Aqueous solution of phenol as a substitute for alcohol in sympathetic block. *J Int Coll Surg* 13:566-568, 1950.
16. Nathan PW, Sears TA, Smith MC: Effects of phenol solutions on the nerve roots of the cat: an electrophysiological and histological study. *J Neurol Sci* 2:7-29, 1965.
17. de Leon-Casasola OA: Drugs commonly used for nerve blocking: neurolytic agents. In Raj PP, editor: *Practical management of pain*, St. Louis, 2000, Mosby, pp 575-578.
18. Gregg RV, Costantini CH, Ford DJ, et al: Electrophysiologic investigation of alcohol as a neurolytic agent. *Anesthesiology* 63(suppl A):A250, 1985.
19. Smith MC: Histological findings following intrathecal injections of phenol solutions for relief of pain. *Br J Anaesth* 36:387-406, 1964.
20. Bell SN, Cole R, Roberts-Thomson IC: Coeliac plexus block for control of pain in chronic pancreatitis. *Br Med J* 281:1604, 1980.
21. Waldman SD: Celiac plexus block. In Weiner RS, editor: *Innovations in pain management*, Orlando, 1990, PMD Press, pp 10-15.
22. Day M: Sympathetic blocks: the evidence. *Pain Pract* 8:98-109, 2008.
23. Romanelli DF, Beckmann CF, Heiss FW: Celiac plexus block: efficacy and safety of the anterior approach. *AJR Am J Roentgenol* 160:497-500, 1993.
24. Buy JN, Moss AA, Singler RC: CT guided celiac plexus and splanchnic nerve neurolysis. *J Comput Assist Tomogr* 6:315-319, 1982.
25. Ischia S, Ischia A, Polati E, et al: Three posterior percutaneous celiac plexus block techniques. A prospective, randomized study in 61 patients with pancreatic cancer pain. *Anesthesiology* 76:534-540, 1992.
26. Matson J, Ghia J, Levy J: A case report of a potentially fatal complication associated with Ischia's transaortic method of celiac plexus block. *Reg Anesth Pain Med* 10:193, 1985.
27. Sett SS, Taylor DC: Aortic pseudoaneurysm secondary to celiac plexus block. *Ann Vasc Surg* 5:88-91, 1991.
28. Kaplan R, Schiff-Keren B, Alt E: Aortic dissection as a complication of celiac plexus block. *Anesthesiology* 83:632-635, 1995.
29. Davies DD: Incidence of major complications of neurolytic coeliac plexus block. *J R Soc Med* 86:264-266, 1993.

30. Brown DL, Rorie DK: Altered reactivity of isolated segmental lumbar arteries of dogs following exposure to ethanol and phenol. *Pain* 56:139-143, 1994.

31. Wong GY, Schroeder DR, Carns PE, et al: Effect of neurolytic celiac plexus block on pain relief, quality of life, and survival in patients with unresectable pancreatic cancer: a randomized controlled trial. *JAMA* 291:1092-1099, 2004.

32. De Cicco M, Matovic M, Bortolussi R, et al: Celiac plexus block: injectate spread and pain relief in patients with regional anatomic distortions. *Anesthesiology* 94:561-565, 2001.

33. Mercadante S: Celiac plexus block versus analgesics in pancreatic cancer pain. *Pain* 52:187-192, 1993.

34. Eisenberg E, Carr DB, Chalmers TC: Neurolytic celiac plexus block for treatment of cancer pain: a meta-analysis. *Anesth Analg* 80:290-295, 1995.

35. Yeager MP, Colacchio TA, Yu CT, et al: Morphine inhibits spontaneous and cytokine-enhanced natural killer cell cytotoxicity in volunteers. *Anesthesiology* 83:500-508, 1995.

36. Mitchell G: The Innervation of the kidney, ureter, testicle and epididymis. *J Anat* 70:10-32, 1935.

37. Aveline C, Gautier JF, Vautier P, et al: Postoperative analgesia and early rehabilitation after total knee replacement: a comparison of continuous low-dose intravenous ketamine versus nefopam. *Eur J Pain* 13:613-619, 2009.

38. Middleton W, Chan V: Lumbar sympathetic block: a review of complications. *Tech Reg Anesthes Pain Manage* 2:137-146, 1998.

39. Reid W, Watt JK, Gray TG: Phenol injection of the sympathetic chain. *Br J Surg* 57:45-50, 1970.

40. Bryce-Smith R: Injection of the Lumbar Sympathetic Chain. *Anaesthesia* 6(3):150-153, 1951.

41. Gay GR, Evans JA: Total spinal anesthesia following lumbar paravertebral block: a potentially lethal complication. *Anesthesth Analg* 50:344, 1971.

42. Bradsher JT, Jr: Complications following paravertebral lumbar sympathetic block with Nupercaine in oil; report of a case. *N Engl J Med* 240:291-293, 1949.

43. Cousins MJ, Reeve TS, Glynn CJ, et al: Neurolytic lumbar sympathetic blockade: duration of denervation and relief of rest pain. *Anaesth Intensive Care* 7:121-135, 1979.

44. Raj P: Sympathetic nerve blocks. In Raj P, editor: *Practical management of pain*, St. Louis, 1992, Mosby, pp 792-812.

45. Boas R, Hatangdi V, Richards E: Lumbar sympathectomy: a percutaneous chemical technique. *Adv Pain Res Ther* 1:685-689, 1976.

46. Smith RC, Davidson NM, Ruckley CV: Hazard of chemical sympathectomy. *Br Med J* 1:552-553, 1978.

47. Parris WC, Kirshner HS: Motor paralysis of the lower extremities following lumbar sympathetic block. *Anesthesiology* 78:981-983, 1993.

48. Echenique Elizondo M, Gurutz Linazasoro C: [Reversible partial paraplegia after sympathetic lumbar block]. *Neurologia* 10:101-103, 1995.

49. Wood KM: The use of phenol as a neurolytic agent: a review. *Pain* 5:205-229, 1978.

50. Brown EM, Kunjappan V: Single-needle lateral approach for lumbar sympathetic block. *Anesth Analg* 54:725-729, 1975.

51. Wheatley JK, Motamedi F, Hammonds WD: Page kidney resulting from massive subcapsular hematoma. Complication of lumbar sympathetic nerve block. *Urology* 24:361-363, 1984.

52. Weyland A, Weyland W, Carduck H, et al: Optimization of the image intensifier-assisted technique of lumbar sympathetic block. Computed tomographic simulation of a paravertebral puncture access. *Der Anaesthesist* 42:710, 1993.

53. Benzon HT: Convulsions secondary to intravascular phenol: a hazard of celiac plexus block. *Anesth Analg* 58:150-151, 1979.

54. Egbert LD: Horner's syndrome; complication of lumbar sympathetic block. *Anesthesiology* 16:811-812, 1955.

55. Stanton-Hicks M: Lumbar sympathetic nerve block and neurolysis. In *Interventional pain management*, ed 2, Philadelphia, 2001, WB Saunders, pp 485-492.

56. Gee W, Ansell J, Bonica J: Pelvic and perineal pain of urologic origin. In Bonica JJ, editor: *The management of pain*, Philadelphia, 1990, Lea & Febiger, pp 1368-1394.

57. de Leon-Casasola OA, Kent E, Lema MJ: Neurolytic superior hypogastric plexus block for chronic pelvic pain associated with cancer. *Pain* 54:145-151, 1993.

58. Plancarte R, Amescua C, Patt RB, et al: Superior hypogastric plexus block for pelvic cancer pain. *Anesthesiology* 73:236-239, 1990.

59. Plancarte R, de Leon-Casasola OA, El-Helaly M, et al: Neurolytic superior hypogastric plexus block for chronic pelvic pain associated with cancer. *Reg Anesth* 22:562-568, 1997.

60. Plancarte R, Amescua C, Patt R, et al: Presacral blockade of the ganglion of Walther (ganglion impar). *Anesthesiology* 73(suppl A):A751, 1990.

61. Patijn J, Janssen M, Hayek S, et al: Coccygodynia. *Pain Pract* 10(6):554-559, 2010. doi: 10.1111/j.1533-2500.2010.00404.x. Epub 2010.

10 Peripheral Applications of Ultrasonography for Chronic Pain

Philip Peng

CHAPTER OVERVIEW

Chapter Synopsis: Ultrasonic imaging has provided a relatively new tool in the management of patients with pain disorders, primarily in guiding injection procedures. Ultrasonography may provide some advantages over more traditional landmark-guided approaches or in situations in which fluoroscopy or computed tomography (CT) scans are not optimal. This chapter considers the contributions of ultrasound technology to injection of peripheral structures. Suprascapular nerve (SSN) block may be indicated in a variety of painful conditions that affect the shoulder. The intercostal nerve supplies the skin and musculature of the chest and abdominal wall; a block may be used to affect postsurgical and chronic pain conditions affecting these areas. The so-called border nerves—the ilioinguinal (IL), iliohypogastric (IH), and genitofemoral (GF) nerves—subserve sensations of the skin between the thigh and abdomen. Damage to these nerves, which may occur during surgery, can result in neuropathy with pain in the groin areas. The lateral femoral cutaneous nerve carries sensations from the skin of the upper leg and is also susceptible to neuropathic conditions. Block of the pudendal nerve can be used for diagnostic and therapeutic purposes for various painful conditions of the pelvis. The piriformis muscle is the target of injection for piriformis syndrome, an unusual but underdiagnosed cause of buttock and leg pain. The anatomical and technical considerations connected with each of these procedures are discussed here with an emphasis on the use of ultrasound guidance.

Important Points:

- Applying ultrasonography for injection of peripheral structures in chronic pain is a very useful technique because it offers an affordable and portable device that provides visualization of the target structures.
- In contrast, fluoroscopy is not designed to visualize various soft tissues in the injection of the peripheral structures.
- Ultrasound-guided injections of peripheral structures have mostly been validated in the literature, showing with high accuracy in reaching the target structures, in contrast to the poor location of target structures with conventional landmark-based techniques.
- The ideal injection site for the SSN is along the course of the nerve between the suprascapular and spinoglenoid notches, where the nerve is contained in a compartment.
- The risk of pneumothorax with intercostal nerve injection is real because the distance between the intercostal nerve and pleura is usually less than 0.5 cm. The ideal injection site is at the costal angle where the nerve is in between two layers of muscle in the subcostal groove.
- Although it is abundantly clear that the course of the IL and IH nerves is highly variable medial to anterior superior iliac spine (ASIS) and is very constant lateral to ASIS, all landmark-based techniques proposed the needle insertion site medial to ASIS with a high failure rate. Ultrasonography allows accurate injection of the IL and IH nerves lateral to the ASIS.
- The course of GF nerve is highly variable, but the genital branch consistently transverses the inguinal canal. Ultrasonography can accurately locate the inguinal canal and the spermatic cord, allowing blockade of the genital branch of GF nerve.
- The lateral femoral cutaneous nerve is a small peripheral nerve with a variable course in the infrainguinal region. Experience is required to locate this nerve with ultrasonography.
- Pudendal nerve blockade at the ischial spine level can be achieved either by CT scan or ultrasonography with the visualization of the interligamentous plane; a fluoroscopy-guided technique relies on the surrogate landmark, the ischial spine.
- Ultrasonography can accurately locate the piriformis muscle and confirm the location of injectate in the muscle, but a fluoroscopy-guided technique coupled with contrast injection can misguide the needle location in 70% of injection in a validation study.

Introduction

Application of ultrasonography in pain medicine (USPM) is a rapidly growing medical field in interventional pain management. It is evidenced by the remarkable increase in the publication of literature on ultrasound-guided injection[1] and the remarkable increase in the number of USPM workshops held in the past 3 years in North America, Europe, and Asia.

Traditionally, interventional procedures for pain management are performed either by a landmark-based technique or with imaging guidance such as fluoroscopy and computed tomography (CT) scanning. A comparison of the advantages and disadvantages of various imaging equipment is summarized in **Table 10-1**. Based on the target structures, the application of USPM can be classified into three areas: peripheral, axial, and musculoskeletal (**Table 10-2**). Applying ultrasonography for the injection of peripheral

Table 10-1: Advantages and Disadvantages of Various Imaging Equipment

	Fluoroscopy	Computed Tomography	Ultrasonography
Soft tissue visualization	None to poor	Excellent	Good
Radiation risk	+-++[a]	++	—
Cost[b]	+++-++++	+++++	++-+++
Portability	+	—	++-+++
Infrastructure	++	++++	—
Real-time guidance	+	—	+
Bone imaging	Excellent	Excellent	Poor to good
Deep structures imaging	Fairly reliable	Reliable	Unreliable

[a]The radiation risk depends on the clinician usage and increases with the use of multiple images, real-time fluoroscopy, and digital subtraction angiography.
[b]The cost varies with the models of the fluoroscopy and ultrasound machine chosen, but in general, fluoroscopy is more costly than ultrasonography.
Reproduced with permission from USRA, Toronto Western Hospital, Toronto [www.usra.ca].

Table 10-2: Comparison Among Three Major Areas of Applications of Ultrasound in Pain Medicine

	Peripheral	Axial	Musculoskeletal
Target structures visualization	Soft tissue (++)	Spine (poor to +)	Bursa or joint (+-++)
Conventional technique	Mostly blind	Image guided	Mostly blind
Level of difficulty	I-II	II-III	I

Reproduced with permission from USRA, Toronto Western Hospital, Toronto [www.usra.ca].

structures is particularly useful because it allows the visualization of various soft tissues (nerve, muscle, tendon, or vessels), and most of the interventional pain procedures for peripheral structures are performed without imaging guidance. This chapter reviews the relevant anatomy, sonoanatomy, and the injection techniques of a few peripheral structures.

Suprascapular Nerve

First described in 1941,[2] suprascapular nerve (SSN) block has been performed over the years by anesthesiologists, rheumatologists, and pain specialists to manage the pain that follows trauma[3] or shoulder surgery,[4,5] to ameliorate the pain associated with various chronic shoulder pain syndromes (adhesive capsulitis, frozen shoulder, rotator cuff tear, and glenohumeral arthritis),[6-9] and to aid in the diagnosis of suprascapular neuropathy.[10]

Anatomy and Sonoanatomy

The SSN originates from the superior trunk of the brachial plexus (formed by the union of the fifth and sixth cervical nerves). It then runs parallel to the omohyoid muscle and courses under the trapezius before it passes under the transverse scapular ligament in the suprascapular notch (**Fig. 10-1**). Entering the suprascapular fossa, the SSN passes beneath the supraspinatus and curves around the lateral border of the spine of the scapula (spinoglenoid notch) to the infraspinatus fossa (**Fig. 10-2**). In the supraspinatus fossa, it gives off two branches: one to the supraspinatus muscle and another as an articular branch to the shoulder joint; and in the infraspinatus fossa, it gives off branches to the infraspinatus muscle and to the shoulder joint and scapula. The sensory component of the SSN provides fibers to about 70% of the shoulder joint. There is no significant cutaneous branch of this nerve.

The suprascapular notch is located on the superior margin of the scapula and medial to the coracoid process. The size and shape of the notch are highly variable and even absent in up to 8% of

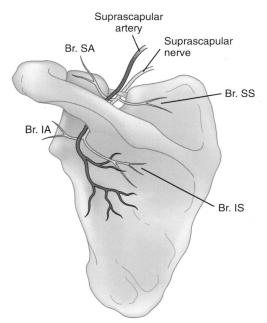

Fig. 10-1 Suprascapular nerve and its branches of the left shoulder. The superior articular branch (Br. SA) supplies the coracohumeral ligament, subacromial bursa, and posterior aspect of the acromioclavicular joint capsule. The inferior articular branch (Br. IA) supplies the posterior joint capsule. Br. IS, branch to the infraspinatus muscle; Br. SS, branch to the supraspinatus muscle. (Modified with permission from USRA, Toronto Western Hospital, Toronto [www.usra.ca].)

cadavers.[11] Above the transverse scapular ligament run the suprascapular artery and vein, although rarely, the artery travels along with the SSN through the notch. The suprascapular fossa is bordered by the spine of the scapula dorsally, by the plate of the scapula ventrally, and by the supraspinatus fascia superiorly, forming a classic compartment, the only exit through which is the suprascapular notch.

The ideal site to perform the SSN injection is at the floor of the scapular spine between the suprascapular notch and spinoglenoid notch (**Fig. 10-2**).[12] First, this technique is independent of the notch as a target. Thus, it avoids the risk of pneumothorax if one considers the direction of the needle. This technique is also feasible in individuals without a suprascapular notch (8% of the population). Second, the suprascapular fossa forms a compartment and retains the local anesthetic around the nerve with a small volume.[13] In contrast, depositing local anesthetic at the notch level will potentially result in the spread of local anesthetic to the brachial plexus.[13] Third, although imaging the suprascapular notch is possible, advancing the needle perfectly in plane in this orientation is very challenging (**Fig. 10-3**). A slight deviation in the anterior direction will direct the needle toward the thorax.

When imaging the suprascapular fossa with ultrasonography, the two key muscles in the scan are trapezius and supraspinatus

muscles (**Fig. 10-4**). The SSN is often seen accompanied by the suprascapular artery on the floor of the scapular spine between the suprascapular notch and spinoglenoid notch (**Fig. 10-5**). The scapula spine forms an angle (39.5 degrees ± 5.8 degrees) to the axis of the scapula blade,[14] so the orientation of the ultrasonography probe should be closer to the coronal plane to visualize the contents of the suprascapular fossa (**Fig. 10-6**).

Existing Techniques

Various approaches have been described. In general, the targets for the SSN are either at the suprascapular notch itself or in the suprascapular fossa.[1] To direct the needle to these targets, various methods have been used, including a "blind" insertion using various landmarks,[2] a peripheral nerve stimulator[3] or electromyography,[7] and a direct insertion using fluoroscopic[15] or CT scan guidance.[16]

There are a few disadvantages to targeting the SSN at the notch using the blind or landmark-guided approach, including the risk of pneumothorax, intravascular injection, and nerve injury.[17] In an attempt to evaluate needle tip placement radiologically following a "blind" needle placement, Brown et al[18] demonstrated that the

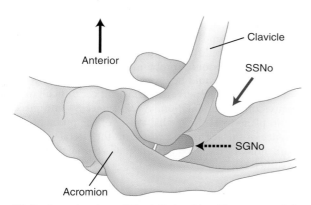

Fig. 10-2 Superior view of the left shoulder. The course of the suprascapular nerve enters the suprascapular fossa through the suprascapular notch (SSNo) and then enters the infrascapular fossa through the spinoglenoid notch (SGNo). (Modified with permission from USRA, Toronto Western Hospital, Toronto [www.usra.ca].)

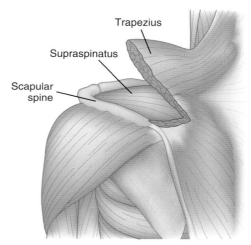

Fig. 10-4 Left shoulder showing the muscle layers in the suprascapular fossa. (Modified with permission from USRA, Toronto Western Hospital, Toronto [www.usra.ca].)

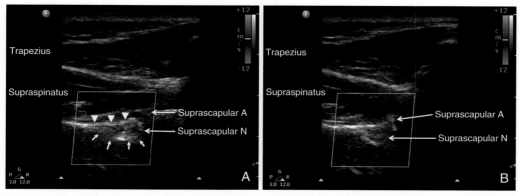

Fig. 10-3 **A,** Ultrasonographic image of suprascapular nerve in the suprascapular notch (*arrows*). Note that at this level, the suprascapular artery is above the transverse scapular ligament (*arrowheads*). **B,** Ultrasonographic image of the suprascapular nerve slightly posterior to the plane obtained in **A.** The suprascapular artery can be seen running toward the floor of the scapular spine. By the same token, a slight deviation anteriorly will direct the needle toward the thorax. A, artery; N, nerve. (Reprinted with permission from USRA Toronto Western Hospital, Toronto, [www.usra.ca].)

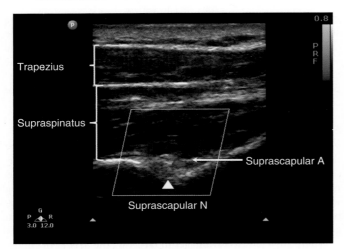

Fig. 10-5 Ultrasonographic image of the suprascapular nerve on the floor of the scapular spine between the suprascapular notch and spinoglenoid notch. Both suprascapular nerve (N) and artery (A) run underneath the fascia of supraspinatus muscle. (Reprinted with permission from USRA, Toronto Western Hospital, Toronto [www.usra.ca].)

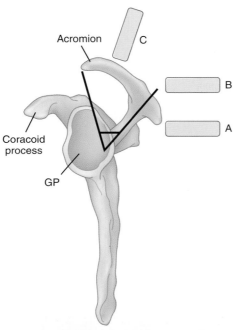

Fig. 10-6 Lateral view of the scapula. The scapula spine forms an angle (39.5 degrees ± 5.8 degrees) to the axis of the scapula blade. The content of the suprascapular fossa cannot be revealed when scanning from the ultrasound probe A, which is behind the dorsal border of the scapular spine, because of the obstruction of view from the scapular spine. By moving the ultrasound probe position to B, the content of the suprascapular fossa cannot be revealed either. The optimal ultrasound probe position is at C when the probe is almost at the coronal plane with a slight anterior tilt. (Modified with permission from USRA, Toronto Western Hospital, Toronto [www.usra.ca].)

proximity of the "needle tip-to-notch" was poor. The precision of the needle tip location can be improved by fluoroscopy or CT scan guidance. Placing the needle into the suprascapular fossa is a popular alternative.[13] The technique is easy to perform and further minimizes the risk of pneumothorax because of the direction of

the needle. To ensure that the SSN is blocked, an adequate volume of solution is injected into the suprascapular fossa compartment. A recent CT scan study showed that 10-mL injectate spread to the brachial plexus in the axilla in three of 33 cadavers.[13] They also showed that blind injection could lead to placement of the needle in or even above the supraspinatus muscle.

Four articles described the sonoanatomy of the SSN relevant to the nerve injection.[12,19-21] Most of them[19-21] described the visualization of the suprascapular notch, transverse scapular ligament, and suprascapular artery and nerve. The ultrasound probe was placed in the suprascapular fossa in the long axis of supraspinatus muscle. According to some authors[19,20] the ultrasound image showed the suprascapular notch (as a curved continuous hyperechoic line), transverse scapular ligament, and SSN. A correlation study with fluoroscopy and cadaver dissection suggested the site of injection was actually at the suprascapular fossa between the suprascapular notch and spinoglenoid notch (**Fig. 10-2**).[12]

Ultrasound-Guided Injection Technique

With the patient in sitting or prone position, ultrasound scanning is performed with a linear ultrasound probe (7-13 MHz) placed in a coronal plane over the suprascapular fossa with a slight anterior tilt. The probe is place in an orientation such that it is in the short axis to the line joining medial aspect of the coracoid process (approximating the suprascapular notch) and posterior aspect of the acromion (reflecting the position of the spinoglenoid notch). The supraspinatus and trapezius muscles and the bony fossa underneath them should come into view (**Fig. 10-5**). By adjusting the angle of the ultrasound probe in a cephalocaudad direction, the SSN and artery should be brought into view in the trough of the floor (**Fig. 10-5**). The nerve can sometimes be difficult to visualize because of the orientation. A 22-gauge, 80-mm needle is inserted in plane from the medial aspect of the probe because of the presence of the acromion process on the lateral side. Because of the proximity of the nerve, an injectate volume of 5 to 8 mL is usually sufficient.

> **Clinical Pearls and Pitfalls:**
> - The SSN is a medium-sized nerve (approximately 2.5 mm in size).
> - One should avoid scanning the SSN at the suprascapular notch because (1) it is challenging to obtain the narrow plane of the suprascapular notch and to guide the needle to this target and (2) there is the risk that injectate will spill outside the notch to the brachial plexus.
> - Knowing the oblique course of this is important because two common mistakes in scanning the SSN are (1) scanning along the orientation of the scapular spine or supraspinatus muscle and (2) probe orientation too close to the transverse plane instead of close to the coronal plane (**Fig. 10-6**).

Intercostal Nerve

The intercostal nerves (ICNs) supply skin and musculature of chest and abdominal wall. Blockade of ICNs has been in clinical use for decades for treatment of acute and chronic pain conditions affecting the thorax and upper abdomen.[22] ICN blockade provides excellent analgesia for pain from rib fractures[23] and from chest and upper abdominal surgery.[24] Neuroablation of ICN may be used to manage chronic pain conditions such as postmastectomy and postthoracotomy pain.[25-28]

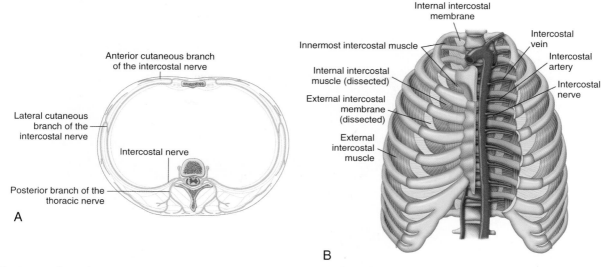

Fig. 10-7 **A**, Branches of the typical intercostal nerves. **B**, Intercostal muscles in the chest wall. (Reprinted with permission from USRA, Toronto Western Hospital, Toronto [www.usra.ca].)

Anatomy and Sonoanatomy

The ICNs are the ventral rami of the 12 thoracic nerves (**Fig. 10-7, A**). After exiting from the spine, the ICNs are located between the pleura and the internal intercostal membrane and subsequently traverse the membrane. Between costal tubercles and costal angles, the ICNs lie between the external intercostal muscle and internal intercostal membrane, which are immediately adjacent to the parietal pleura. The course of ICNs for that distance really deserves their name "intercostal" nerve (or "in between ribs"). From the costal angle onward, the ICNs run deep to the subcostal groove within the internal intercostal muscles, thus creating an innermost muscular layer known as the innermost intercostals muscle (**Fig. 10-7, B**).[29,30] Readers should be aware that in some anatomy textbooks, the ICNs are described to situate in between the two layers of internal intercostal muscle. The ICNs travel in the costal groove accompanied by intercostal vein and artery and the neurovascular bundle is arranged from above downwards in the manner: "V-A-N" (**Fig. 10-8**). At a distance about 5 to 8 cm anterior to the angle of the rib, the groove ends and blends into the surface of the lower edge of the rib. The lateral cutaneous branch of the ICN, which supplies the skin of the chest, branches off and pierces the external intercostal muscle in the region between the posterior and midaxillary line. As the ICN approaches the midline anteriorly, it pierces the overlying muscles and skin to terminate as the anterior cutaneous branch (**Fig. 10-7, A**).

Under ultrasound scanning, different layers of the intercostal muscles and the pleura can be visualized (**Fig. 10-9**). The pleura appear as a definite hyperechogenic line that glides with respiratory movement. Normally, two types of artifacts can be visualized: reverberation artifacts appearing as a series of horizontal lines parallel to the pleural interface and vertical comet tail artifacts. The neurovascular bundle cannot be visualized under normal circumstances because it is covered by the rib except in the region between costal tubercles to costal angle. However, the location of the ICN can be estimated by directing the needle in between the internal and innermost intercostal muscle.

Existing Techniques

The classic landmark-based technique is performed with the patient in the sitting position. The ICN block is usually performed

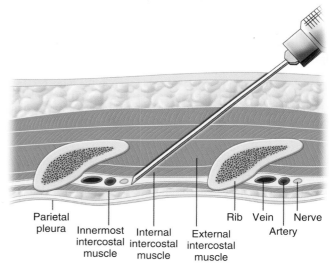

Fig 10-8 Cross section of chest wall showing intercostal muscles and neurovascular bundles. (Reprinted with permission from USRA, Toronto Western Hospital, Toronto [www.usra.ca].)

at the angle of the rib to ensure that the tissues innervated by the lateral cutaneous nerve are blocked. The most feared complication with the existing "blind" technique is pneumothorax. The distance between the neurovascular bundles to the pleura in thin patients is usually within 0.5 cm.[26] The injection is performed after negative aspiration for air and blood, but this maneuver cannot reliably prevent pneumothorax or hemothorax . The incidence of pneumothorax ranges anywhere from 0.09% to 8.7%.[22,31,32]

The fluoroscopic technique is performed with the patient in the prone position. The appropriate rib is identified under fluoroscopic anteroposterior (AP) view, and the needle is introduced in the inferior margin of the rib. After negative aspiration, a contrast injection is performed to ensure appropriate spread before injection.[27] This technique does not theoretically minimize the risk of pneumothorax because the pleura cannot be visualized with fluoroscopy.

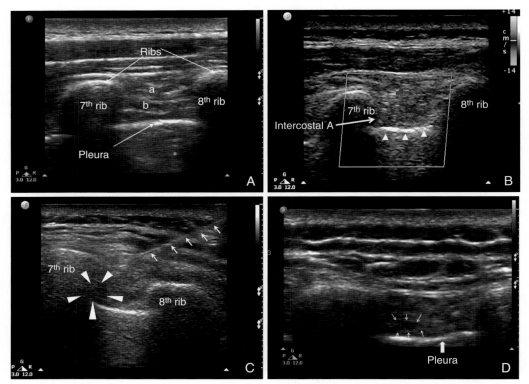

Fig. 10-9 A, Ultrasonographic image showing the intercostal muscles and pleura at the angle of rib between seventh and eighth rib. The *asterisk* shows a reverberation artifact. a, external intercostal muscle; b, internal intercostal muscle. **B,** A similar image taken 2 cm medial to the angle of rib. The intercostal artery is seen in the intercostal space. The pleura appears as a hyperechoic line and is indicated by the *arrowheads*. **C,** Intercostal space after injection. The needle is indicated by the *arrows* and the local anesthetic by the *arrowheads*. **D,** Ultrasonographic image after injection. The *small arrows* outline the collection of local anesthetic. (Reprinted with permission from USRA, Toronto Western Hospital, Toronto [www.usra.ca].)

The use of ultrasound guidance for intercostal block was recommended from the personal experiences in two reviews.[1,33] Either the in-plane or out-of-plane technique was recommended. However, both reviews emphasized hydrodissection to ensure the visualization of the needle tip. A small case series also confirmed the feasibility and technical advantages of ultrasound-guided cryoablation of the ICNs in four patients with postthoracotomy pain syndrome.[26]

Ultrasound-Guided Injection Technique

The patient is in the prone position, and a linear probe (7-13 MHz) is ideal for the superficial structures. The site is at the costal angle (≈7 cm from the midline). Both the in-plane and out-of-plane technique can be used. The authors prefer the in-plane technique because the direction of the needle is similar to the classical technique described for ICN block, and the complete needle path can be traced.[1] The needle entry site is the upper margin of the rib one level caudal to the targeted ICNs. After the needle penetrates the skin, the ultrasound probe can be rolled over the needle, which is advanced deep to the internal intercostal muscle. One of the drawbacks for the in-plane technique is that when the probe is not perfectly in line with the needle, the practitioner may have a false impression of the location of the needle tip. Because the distance between the costal groove and the pleura is in the dimension of 0.5 cm, it is advisable to inject a small amount of injectate when the needle is in the external intercostal muscle to confirm the needle tip position. Under real-time injection, intravascular injection should be suspected if the spread of the medication is not visualized. After the needle tip is confirmed deep to the internal

intercostal muscle, the local anesthetic can be injected, and spread of medication can be seen.

Clinical Pearls and Pitfalls:
- The course of ICNs is "intercostal" from the costal tubercle to costal angle (i.e., between the ribs). Although one can locate the intercostal artery and thus the neurovascular bundle, the ICNs are adjacent to the parietal pleura. Injection at this site is recommended only for very experienced practitioners. The author recommends the injection site at the costal angle.
- The neurovascular bundle at the level of costal angle cannot be visualized by ultrasound scanning because it is already hidden by the rib. The estimation of this space is judged by the muscle layers.

Ilioinguinal, Iliohypogastric, and Genitofemoral Nerves (Border Nerves)

The ilioinguinal (IL), iliohypogastric (IH), and genitofemoral (GF) nerves are the primary nerves providing sensory innervation to the skin bordering between the thigh and abdomen. Therefore, they are also called border nerves collectively.[1] Injury to the IL and IH nerves is a known risk in open appendectomy incisions, postinguinal herniorrhaphy, low transverse incisions (e.g., Pfannenstiel incision), and during trocar insertion for laparoscopic surgery of the abdomen and pelvis.[34-38] Patients with neuropathy after injury to these nerves present with groin pain that may extend to the scrotum or the testicle in men, the labia majora in women, and the medial aspect of the thigh. Accurate diagnostic block of those nerves is important in understanding the etiology of the clinical problem.

Anatomy and Sonoanatomy

The IL and IH nerves originate from the T12 and L1 nerve roots. Emerging near the lateral border of the psoas major muscle, the nerves extend diagonally toward the crest of the ilium (**Fig. 10-10**).

The IH nerve pierces the transversus abdominis muscle above the iliac crest midway between the iliac crest and the twelfth rib. The IL nerve runs caudally and parallel to the IH nerve. Here, both nerves can be found consistently (90%) between the transversus abdominis and internal oblique muscles.[39] Terminal branches of the IH nerve perforate the external oblique muscle aponeurosis 4 cm lateral to the midline to supply the skin over the lower portion of the rectus abdominis.[40] The IH nerve also provides sensory innervation to the skin above the tensor fasciae lata through a lateral cutaneous branch. Terminal branches of the IL nerve enter the inguinal canal through the deep inguinal ring and may lie upon the cremasteric muscle and fascial layer of the spermatic cord in men or round ligament in women.[41,42] This terminal branch is often accompanied by the genital branch of the GF nerve, and wide variations in the course of these nerves within the inguinal canal have been documented.[4,8,10,12-14] The terminal sensory branches may innervate the skin of the mons pubis, inner thigh, inguinal crease, and anterior surface of the scrotum or anterior third of the labia.

The GF nerve originates from the first and second lumbar nerve roots (**Fig. 10-10**). It emerges on the anterior surface of the psoas muscle either a single trunk or separate genital and femoral branches.[43] The femoral branch passes laterally over the external iliac artery and then penetrates the fascia lata to enter the femoral sheath. Terminal branches provide cutaneous innervation to the femoral triangle.[44] The genital branch also crosses in front of the external iliac artery but then passes through the ventral aspect of the internal ring of the inguinal canal. Anatomical studies describe this branch running between the cremaster and internal spermatic fascia, incorporating with the cremasteric fascia, or lying outside of the spermatic cord.[42,44,45] Terminal sensory branches may innervate the scrotum and possibly the upper, inner, and medial thigh.[42]

Anatomical studies highlight the variability of the IL, IH, and GF nerves. Variations from conventional descriptions have been reported with respect to communication among nerves, penetration of fascial layers, branching patterns, and dominance patterns.[1] The most consistent anatomical location for the IL and IH nerves to perforate the abdominal muscular layers is lateral and superior to the anterior superior iliac spine (ASIS), where they run between the transversus abdominis and internal oblique muscular layers.

The recommended area for ultrasound scanning of IL and IH nerves is lateral and superior to the ASIS (**Fig. 10-11**). At this position, the iliac crest appears as a hyperechoic structure adjacent to which appear the three muscular layers of the abdominal wall (**Fig. 10-12**). Below the transversus abdominis, peristaltic movements of the bowel may be detected. After the muscular layers have been identified, the II and IH nerves will be found in the split fascial plane between the internal oblique and transversus abdominis muscle layers. Both nerves should be within 1.5 cm of the iliac crest at this site, with the II nerve closer to the iliac crest.[46] The nerves are usually in close proximity to each other[47] and located on the "upsloping" split fascia close to the iliac crest. In some cases, the nerves may run approximately 1 cm apart. The deep circumflex iliac artery that is close to the two nerves in the same fascial layer can be revealed with the use of color-flow Doppler (**Fig. 10-13**). A neural structure within the fascial split may also be seen medial and on the flat part of the internal oblique and transversus abdominis muscle junction. This is the subcostal nerve, and if mistaken for the IL and IH nerves, the nerve blockade will result in aberrant distribution of anesthesia.

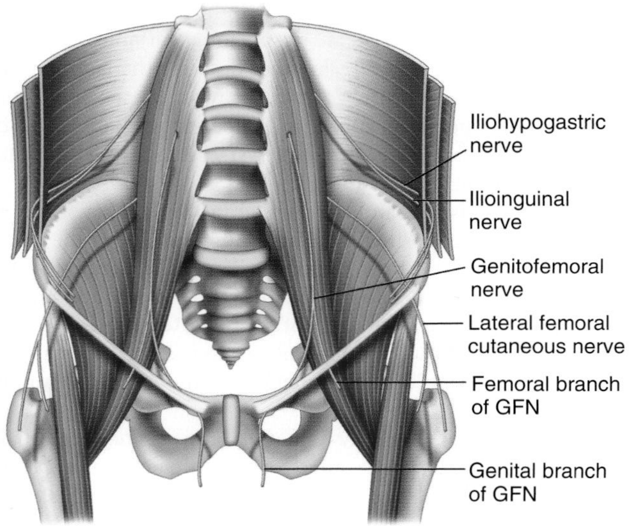

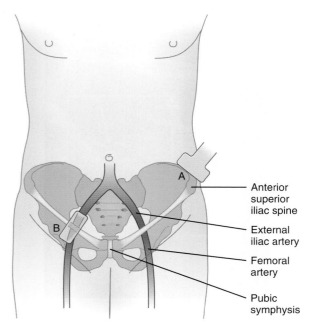

Fig. 10-11 Schematic diagram showing the position of the ultrasound probe. Probe A is placed above and three fingerbreadths lateral to the anterior superior iliac spine and is in the short axis of the course of ilioinguinal nerve (i.e., at right angle to the iliac crest). Probe B is placed in the inguinal line in long axis of femoral and external iliac artery. (Modified with permission from USRA, Toronto Western Hospital, Toronto [www.usra.ca].)

Fig. 10-10 Schematic diagram showing the pathway of ilioinguinal, iliohypogastric, and genitofemoral nerve (GFN). (Reprinted with permission from USRA, Toronto Western Hospital, Toronto [www.usra.ca].)

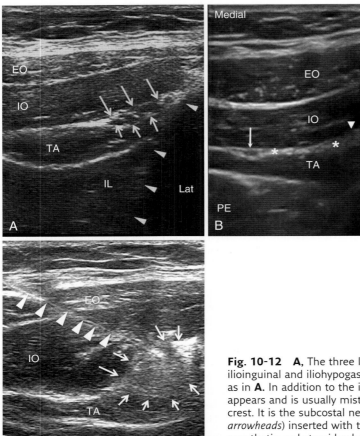

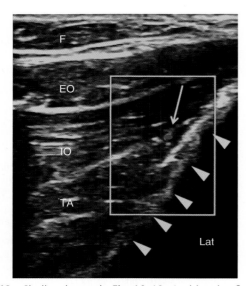

Fig. 10-12 **A,** The three layers of muscles and the fascia split (*white arrows*) with the ilioinguinal and iliohypogastric nerves inside. *Arrowheads* outline the iliac crest. **B,** Similar view as in **A.** In addition to the ilioinguinal (*arrow*) and iliohypogastric (*asterisk*) nerves, a third nerve appears and is usually mistaken as the ilioinguinal nerve but is much farther from the iliac crest. It is the subcostal nerve (twelfth intercostal nerve). **C,** The needle (outlined by *arrowheads*) inserted with the in-plane technique; the *arrows* outline the spread of the local anesthetic and steroid solution. EO, external oblique muscle; IL, iliacus; IO, internal oblique muscle; Lat, lateral; PE, peritoneum; TA, transverse abdominis muscle. (Reprinted with permission from USRA, Toronto Western Hospital, Toronto [www.usra.ca].)

Fig. 10-13 Similar view as in Fig. 10-12, *A* with color-flow Doppler. A branch of the deep circumflex iliac artery is shown in red. *Solid arrows* outline the iliac crest. EO, external oblique muscle; F, subcutaneous fat; IO, internal oblique muscle; Lat, lateral; TA, transverse abdominis muscle. (Reprinted with permission from USRA, Toronto Western Hospital, Toronto [www.usra.ca].)

Existing Technique

As discussed previously, there is a high degree of anatomical variability in not only the course of the nerves but also their branching patterns, areas of penetration of the fascial layers, and dominance patterns.[1] The sites at which the IL and IH nerves pierce the abdominal wall muscle layers are significantly variable.[36] Unfortunately, virtually all injection techniques describe the landmark for injection medial to the ASIS.[1,48] By far the most consistent location of the II and IH nerves is lateral and superior to the ASIS where the nerves are found between the transverses abdominis and internal oblique muscular layers (90%).[39,40]

Because the existing landmark-based techniques rely on blind infiltration of local anesthetic through different layers, the risk of complications are well understandable. These include inadvertent femoral nerve block,[49,50] colonic puncture,[51,52] and vascular injury.[53] More importantly, the failure rate of the blind technique lies in the range of 10% to 40%.[54,55] This failure rate is attributed to the potential for injecting local anesthetic into the wrong abdominal plane.[55]

The use of ultrasonography in IL and IH nerves has been evaluated in clinical practice in adults and validated in a cadaver study.[46,56-58] All three clinical studies or reports used ASIS as landmark, and the position of the probe was above ASIS and moved along the line joining the ASIS and umbilicus. When the probe is placed too near to ASIS, the external oblique muscle layer may be missed. When the probe is too far away from the ASIS (the "bone shadow of iliac crest" not in the scan), the nerve seen in between the transverses abdominis and internal oblique muscular layers is likely the twelfth intercostal nerve instead.

The description of a GF nerve block is mainly a "blind" technique[59,60] and relies on the pubic tubercle, inguinal ligament, inguinal crease, and femoral artery as landmarks. One involves infiltration of local anesthetic immediately lateral to the pubic tubercle caudad to the inguinal ligament.[60] In another method, a needle is inserted into the inguinal canal to block the genital branch.[59] The blind techniques described are essentially infiltration techniques and rely on high volumes of local anesthetic for consistent results. Although the basis of this landmark is not clear, the needle is likely directed toward the spermatic cord, and important structures of the spermatic cord (testicular artery and vas deferens) or the peritoneum are at risk.

Ultrasound-guided blockade of the genital branch of the GF nerve has been described in several review articles.[1,48,61] The genital nerve is difficult to visualize, and blockade is achieved by identification of the inguinal canal. In males, the GF nerve may travel within or outside the spermatic cord. Thus, the local anesthetic and steroid is deposited both outside and within the spermatic cord. Ultrasound-guided blockade of the femoral branch of the GF nerve has also been described, and cryoanalgesia of the femoral branch of GF nerve was performed.[62]

Ultrasound-Guided Injection Technique

The IH and IL nerves are superficial nerves that are best viewed with a linear probe of high frequency (6-13 MHz). In very obese patients, a linear medium frequency probe may be useful. The probe is placed cranial and three fingerbreadths lateral to the ASIS with the transducer perpendicular to the inguinal ligament and its lateral end in contact with the iliac crest (**Fig. 10-11**). The hyperechoic shadow of the iliac crest can be visualized, and the probe is then tilted until all three layers of the muscles are brought into view. The peritoneum can be seen as the fascia layer underneath the transversus abdominis. Between the layers of the transversus abdominis and the internal oblique muscles, the IL and IH nerves can be visualized within the splitting of the fascia layer (**Fig. 10-12**). With Doppler ultrasonography, branches of the deep circumflex iliac artery can be identified within this fascia split (**Fig. 10-13**). In some patients (those with previous surgery or multiple childbirth), either the IIH and IIN or the fascia split is difficult to visualize; the target will be the fascia plane between the internal oblique and transverse abdominal muscles. Both the out-of-plane and in-plane technique can be used, and the volume of injectate is between 6 and 8 mL.

The genital branch is difficult to visualize directly unless a high-frequency probe (≤18 MHz) is used. Furthermore, the GF nerve can be found within or outside the spermatic cord. Thus, the most reliable method is to infiltrate the inguinal canal and deposit the injectate both inside and outside the spermatic cord.[1] The patient is placed in a supine position, and the surface anatomy of the ASIS, inguinal ligament, and femoral artery is established. A linear ultrasound transducer of high frequency (6-13 MHz) is placed over the femoral artery along its long axis (**Fig. 10-11**). The transducer is moved cephalad over the artery, which starts to descend at a steep angle toward the inguinal ligament. At this point, the femoral artery transitions to become the external iliac artery and runs in a retroperitoneal plane (**Fig. 10-14**). After the external iliac artery is identified, the inguinal canal can be viewed superficial to the vessel as an oval soft tissue structure (**Fig. 10-14**). This contains the

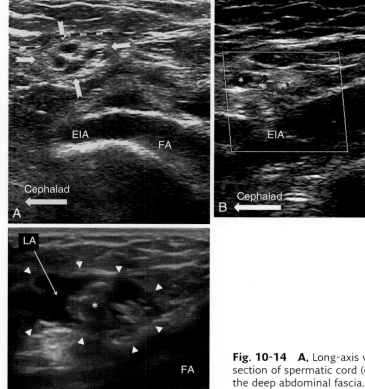

Fig. 10-14   A, Long-axis view of the femoral and external iliac arteries showing the cross section of spermatic cord (outlined by *arrows*) in a male patient. The *red dashed line* outlines the deep abdominal fascia. **B,** Similar view as **A** with color Doppler showing the vessels inside the spermatic cord. **C,** After injection, the inguinal canal can be well visualized (outlined by *arrows*) filled with local anesthetic (LA). The spermatic cord is indicated by the *asterisk.* (Reprinted with permission from USRA, Toronto Western Hospital, Toronto [www.usra.ca].)

spermatic cord in men and the round ligament in women. The canal is then scanned medially so the final ultrasound probe position is approximately one fingerbreadth away from the pubic tubercle. In males, testicular arteries may be identified in the spermatic cord as pulsatile structures and confirmed with the use of color-flow Doppler (**Fig. 10-14**). Vessels may be accentuated by asking the patient to cough or perform a Valsalva maneuver, which increases blood flow through the pampiniform plexus. The vas deferens may also be identified as a thick, tubular structure.

An in-plane or out-of-plane technique may be used. With an out-of-plane technique, the needle approaches the inguinal canal from the lateral aspect of the probe. This helps to avoid arterial puncture because the needle tip will be directed away from the artery. Given the anatomical variability of the genital branch of the GFN, 4 mL of local anesthetic is injected within and 4 mL outside of the spermatic cord in men. In women, 5 mL of local anesthetic is injected around the round ligament only. In males, the local anesthetic should not contain epinephrine so as to avoid vasoconstriction of the testicular arteries. Steroid can be added for the management of patients with chronic pain syndromes.

Clinical Pearls and Pitfalls:
- The IL and IH nerves should always be located two to three fingerbreadths lateral to the ASIS. In patients who are obese, with a history of ventral hernia, multiple childbirths, or abdominal surgeries, the nerves may even be impossible to visualize. However, identification of the three layers of muscles is always possible.
- The practitioner should avoid scanning to medial to the ASIS because the external oblique may be missed.
- Sometimes a fascia appears in the subcutaneous fat that creates an illusion of two layers with the deeper layer mistaken as the external oblique muscle. Therefore, the practitioner should scan medially and laterally to trace the layer. The fascia in the subcutaneous fat is inconsistent, but the external oblique muscle gets thicker when traced laterally.
- When a nerve is discovered along with an artery in the plane between the internal oblique and the transversus abdominis muscles, it is not necessarily the IL or IH nerve. Both nerves should be within 1.5 inches from the iliac crest. A nerve discovered in a scan farther away from the iliac crest is likely the twelfth ICN or subcostal nerve.
- The technique for the scanning of the genital branch of GFN is essentially the scanning of the inguinal canal, and some other methods have been described in the radiology literature.
- Epinephrine-containing solutions should not be used in the GFN injection in males because it is close to the spermatic cord.

Lateral Femoral Cutaneous Nerve

The lateral femoral cutaneous nerve (LFCN) provides sensory innervation to the skin of the anterior and lateral parts of the thigh as far as the knee. Regional block of the LFCN is performed for acute pain relief after surgical procedures and for the diagnosis and treatment of meralgia paresthetica.[1] The latter condition is a painful mononeuropathy of the LFCN, which presents with unpleasant paresthesia, pain, and numbness in the anterolateral aspect of the thigh.[63] The incidence in a primary care setting was estimated at 4.3 per 10,000 person-years.[64] Anesthesiologists are commonly involved in the management of this group of patients because of their expertise in the interventional procedures.[1,65]

Anatomy and Sonoanatomy

The LFCN is a purely sensory nerve that arises from branches of dorsal divisions of the second and third lumbar nerves (**Fig. 10-15**). It emerges from the lateral border of the psoas major and crosses the iliacus muscle obliquely toward the ASIS.[66] The nerve then passes under the inguinal ligament medial and close to the ASIS (at a distance of 3.6 ± 2.0 cm). Entering the thigh, the LFCN turns laterally and downward, where it typically divides into the anterior and posterior branches (**Fig. 10-15**).[67] The course and location of the LFCN as it crosses the inguinal ligament has been found to be quite variable, such as far medial to ASIS, over the iliac crest, or through the sartorius muscle. Although the nerve courses medial to the ASIS most of the time, it can pass over or even posterior to the ASIS in up to 25% of patients.[66-68] Although the LFCN commonly enters the thigh superficial to the sartorius muscle beneath the fascia lata, the LFCN passes through the muscle itself in 22% of cases.[69] The LFCN has been shown to cross under the inguinal ligament as far as 4.6 to 7.3 cm medial to the ASIS.[67,70,71] The LFCN divides into an anterior and a posterior branch in the thigh. The anterior branch becomes superficial at a variable distance below the inguinal ligament and divides into branches that are distributed to the skin of the anterior and lateral parts of the thigh as far as the knee. The posterior branch pierces the fascia lata and subdivides into filaments that pass backward across the lateral and posterior surfaces of the thigh, supplying the skin from the level of the greater trochanter to the middle of the thigh.

The LFCN is a small peripheral nerve, and its course is highly variable. To locate the nerve successfully with ultrasound scanning, one needs to be aware of a few important principles:

1. A sound knowledge of anatomy of the course and direction of the LFCN as well as the structures around LFCN helps to appreciate location of the nerve (**Figs. 10-15** and **10-16**).[72]
2. The nerve is better appreciated with dynamic scanning or sweeping view because of the size of the nerve and its proximity with fascia layer.[72,73]

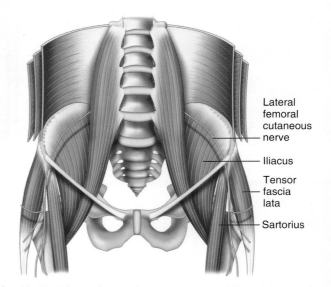

Lateral femoral cutaneous nerve

Iliacus

Tensor fascia lata

Sartorius

Fig. 10-15 The pathway of a typical course of lateral femoral cutaneous nerve. Note that the nerve courses beneath the inguinal ligament and runs superficially to the sartorius muscle and then in between this muscle and tensor fascia lata muscle. (Reprinted with permission from USRA, Toronto Western Hospital, Toronto [www.usra.ca].)

3. The LFCN nerve may appear as hyperechoic, hypoechoic, or mixed structure (**Fig. 10-17**), depending on the course of the nerve itself (under or through the inguinal ligament or over the iliac crest), the special tissue architecture in the corresponding area (surrounded by fatty tissue in the plane between the sartorius and tensor fascia lata), and the frequency of the transducer used (the higher-frequency probe is likely to produce artifacts).[72-75]

4. The LFCN in patients with severe or advanced symptoms of meralgia paresthetica is likely to be swollen or enlarged (pseudoneuroma) and likely to be picked up ultrasonography.[69]

5. The LFCN can commonly be found in the infrainguinal region, either superficial to the sartorius muscle or between sartorius and tensor of fascia lata muscles. In the latter case, it is a fat-filled space (Professor B. Moriggl, personal communication).

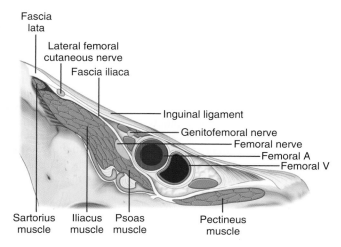

Fig. 10-16   Nerves at the inguinal area. A, artery; V, vein.
(Reprinted with permission from USRA, Toronto Western Hospital, Toronto [www.usra.ca].)

Ultrasound-Guided Injection Technique

With the patient in the supine position, the ASIS and the inguinal ligament are marked on the skin. Using a high-frequency linear array transducer (6-13 MHz), the ASIS is visualized as a hyperechoic structure with posterior acoustic shadowing (**Fig. 10-17**). The ultrasound probe is placed over the ASIS initially with the long-axis view of inguinal ligament and is then moved distally. The sartorius muscle will be seen as an inverted triangular-shape structure. Attention is paid to the orientation of the probe to the course of the nerve. The LFCN will appear as one or more hyperechoic or hypoechoic structures in the short-axis view. If the nerve cannot be identified, the alternative is to look for the LFCN in the plane between the tensor of the fascia lata and the sartorius muscle. After the LFCN has been identified, a needle is advanced in plane with the ultrasound probe. Alternatively, the needle can be advanced out of plane using a nerve-stimulating needle to confirm placement.

When the LFCN cannot be identified by the above methods, two methods can be tried. One is to inject dextrose 5% solution to hydrodissect the plane between fascia lata and fascia over the iliacus muscle. The other is to locate the proximity of the nerve with a transdermal nerve stimulator to locate the nerve percutaneously.[74]

Clinical Pearls and Pitfalls:

■ One common practice for an inexperienced practitioner is to scan close to the ASIS at the inguinal line. Knowing the highly variable course, it may be easier to scan at either (1) two to three fingerbreadths below the ASIS and look for the LFCN in the anterior surface of the sartorius muscle or (2) the fat-containing plane between the sartorius and tensor fascia lata muscle.

■ The LFCN can appear as hyperechoic or hypoechoic structures and as one nerve or two or multiple small nerves.

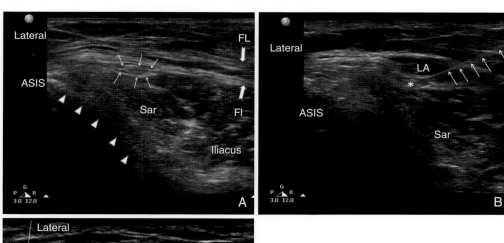

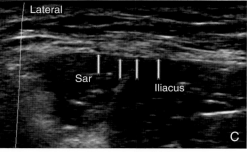

Fig. 10-17   A, Ultrasonographic picture showing the lateral femoral cutaneous nerve (LFCN). The LFCN is indicated by *line arrows*. The fascia is indicated by *bold arrows*, and the ilium is indicated by *solid arrowheads*. ASIS, anterior superior iliac spine; FI, fascia iliaca; L, fascia lata; Sar, sartorius muscle. **B,** Postinjection ultrasonographic picture; the needle is indicated by *arrows*. The *asterisk* shows the LFCN. LA, local anesthetic. **C,** The LFCN has already branched into smaller nerves and appears as hypoechoic structures (*solid line arrows*). (Reprinted with permission from USRA, Toronto Western Hospital, Toronto [www.usra.ca].)

Pudendal Nerve

The pudendal nerve supplies the anterior and posterior urogenital areas (clitoris, penis, vulva, and perianal area). Chronic pelvic pain involving the sensory distribution of the pudendal nerve is termed *pudendal neuralgia*.[2] The classical presentation includes pain that is worse with sitting and relieved or diminished on standing, lying on the nonpainful side, or sitting on a toilet seat.[2] A pudendal nerve block serves both diagnostic and therapeutic purposes.[48]

Anatomy and Sonoanatomy

The pudendal nerve is formed from the anterior rami of the second, third, and fourth sacral nerves (S2, S3, and S4). Exiting the pelvis through the greater sciatic notch, the pudendal nerve is accompanied by the internal pudendal artery on its medial side and travels dorsal to the sacrospinous ligament abutting the attachment of the latter to the ischial spine (**Fig. 10-18**). At this level, the nerve is situated between the sacrospinous and sacrotuberous ligaments (interligamentous plane).[76-78] The nerve then swings ventrally to enter the lesser sciatic foramen and then Alcock's canal,[78,79] which is the fascial tunnel formed by the duplication of the obturator internus muscle under the plane of the levator ani muscle on the lateral wall of ischiorectal fossa (**Fig. 10-18**).[80] The pudendal nerve subsequently gives off three terminal branches: the dorsal nerve of the penis (or clitoris); the inferior rectal nerve; and the perineal nerve, providing the sensory branches to the skin of penis (or clitoris), perianal area, and posterior surface of the scrotum or labia majora. They also innervate the external anal sphincter (inferior rectal nerve) and deep muscles of the urogenital triangle (perineal nerve).

The path of the pudendal nerve either in between the sacrotuberous and the sacrospinous ligaments or through Alcock's canal makes it susceptible to entrapment.[81] In Alcock's canal, possible cause of entrapment can be the falciform process of the sacrotuberous ligament or fascia of the obturator internus muscle.

To date, the best imaging technique for Alcock's canal is CT scan. Ultrasonography is useful in imaging the interligamentous plane at the ischial spine level. The pudendal nerve is a thin nerve, measuring 4 to 6 mm at the level of the ischial spine.[82] Nerves of this size can be difficult to detect with ultrasonography at the ischial spine, which is on average 5 cm deep to the skin.[82] These circumstances may account for why the pudendal nerve is visualized with ultrasonography as little as 47.2% of the time.[82]

To reveal the structures at this level, the key is the recognition of the ischial spine (**Fig. 10-19**, probe position C). A few hints can be very helpful in identifying the ischial spine: (1) the spine appears as a straight hyperechoic line, and the ischium cephalad is seen as a curved line because it forms the posterior aspect of the acetabulum (**Fig. 10-20**); (2) the sacrospinous ligament appears as a hyperechoic line in continuity with the medial end of the ischial spine, with lower echogenicity than bone; (3) the sacrotuberous ligament is seen as a light hyperechoic line ventral to the gluteus maximus muscle overlapping the fascia ventral to this muscle and appears parallel and dorsal to the sacrospinous ligament; and (4) the internal pudendal artery can be localized with the use of color-flow Doppler in close proximity to the ischial spine (**Fig. 10-20**). Another arterial pulsation is often seen lateral to the tip of the ischial spine and is accompanied by the sciatic nerve. This is the descending

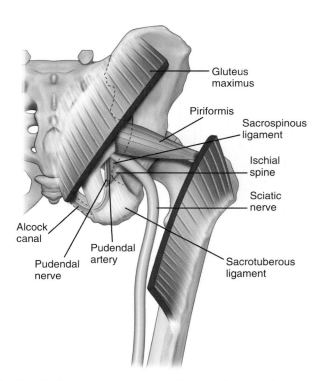

Fig. 10-18 Posterior view of pelvis showing the pudendal neurovascular bundle and piriformis muscle. The gluteus maximus muscle was cut to show the deeper structures. Note that the pudendal nerve and artery run in the interligamentous plane between the sacrospinous and sacrotuberous ligament and subsequently into Alcock's canal. (Reprinted with permission from USRA, Toronto Western Hospital, Toronto [www.usra.ca].)

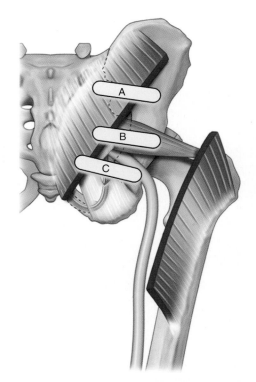

Fig. 10-19 Three different positions of ultrasound probe: the ilium at the level of the posterior superior iliac spine (A), at the level of the greater sciatic notch (B), and at the level of the ischial spine (C). (Reprinted with permission from USRA, Toronto Western Hospital, Toronto [www.usra.ca].)

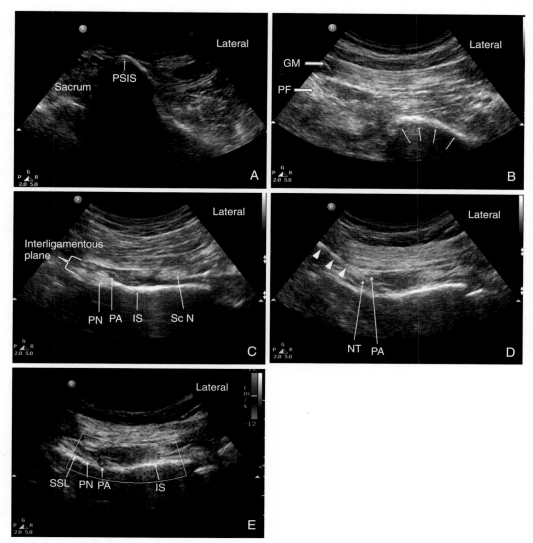

Fig. 10-20   A, Ultrasound image at probe position A. **B,** Ultrasound image at probe position B. *Line arrows* outline the ischium, which is curved as it forms the posterior portion of the acetabulum. **C,** Ultrasound image at probe position C. **D,** Needle insertion with an in-plane technique and the needle tip just medial to the pudendal artery. **E,** Color-flow Doppler to show pudendal artery. GM, gluteus maximus muscle; IS, ischial spine; NT, needle tip; PA, pudendal artery; PF, piriformis muscle; PN, pudendal nerve; PSIS, posterior superior iliac spine; Sc N, sciatic nerve; SSL, sacrospinous ligament. (Reprinted with permission from USRA, Toronto Western Hospital, Toronto [www.usra.ca].)

branch of the inferior gluteal artery. Mistaking this artery for the pudendal artery will result in sciatic nerve block.

Existing Technique

The transgluteal approach is the most popular route of injection for pudendal neuralgia, allowing blockade at the ischial spine and Alcock's canal. At the level of ischial spine, both ultrasonography and CT scan are ideal for visualizing the interligamentous plane because they identify all of the important landmarks, which are the ischial spine, sacrotuberous ligament, sacrospinous ligament, pudendal artery, and pudendal nerve.[1] Traditionally, fluoroscopy has been used to guide needle placement using the ischial spine as a surrogate landmark.[76] The needle is placed medial to the ischial spine, which corresponds to the course of the pudendal nerve at this level.[76] The major limitation of fluoroscopy is that it cannot accurately demonstrate the interligamentous plane.[1,61] At the level of the ischial spine, the pudendal artery lies between the pudendal nerve and the pudendal artery in the majority of cases (76% to 100%). Therefore, injectate may not spread to the pudendal

nerve using this landmark. In addition, the potential proximity of the sciatic nerve at this level makes it susceptible to the anesthetic if spread of the injectate is not visualized in real time. Furthermore, the depth for needle insertion cannot be assessed with fluoroscopy.[83]

Two reports described the ultrasound visualization of the pudendal nerve.[84,85] Validation of the ultrasound-guided procedure in a clinical setting was performed recently. The study demonstrated the reliability of blocking the pudendal nerve in the interligamentous plane at the ischial spine level.[82]

Ultrasound-Guided Injection Technique

The patient is placed in the prone position. A curvilinear probe with a low frequency (2-5 MHz) is required to visualize the structures given its location deep to the gluteus maximus muscle. The ultrasound transducer should be first placed transversely over the posterior superior iliac spine (PSIS) to visualize the sacroiliac joint. After this is seen, the transducer is moved laterally to view the ilium (**Fig. 10-20**). The posterior aspect of the iliac wing should be clearly visualized as a hyperechoic line descending laterally. After the iliac wing has been identified, the angle of the probe is rotated such that it would be in line with the long axis of the piriformis muscle as it runs from the sacrum to the greater trochanter. As scanning continues caudally, the hyperechoic line of the ilium starts to disappear in the medial aspect of the image at the level of the sciatic notch. The lateral aspect of the ultrasound image continues to display a curved hyperechoic line representing the ischium. At this level, two separate muscular layers are identified: the gluteus maximus and the piriformis muscles. Scanning slightly more caudally, the curved line of the ischium becomes straighter as it transitions to the ischial spine. At this point, the sacrospinous ligament should be seen as a slight hyperechoic structure extending from the tip of the ischial spine, projecting toward the sacrum (**Fig. 10-20**). The sacrotuberous ligament may also be seen at this level deep to the gluteus maximus muscle. The piriformis muscle will no longer be visualized. The pudendal artery lies slightly medial to the tip of the ischial spine and the pudendal nerve situated medial to the artery. It may not be clearly visualized under ultrasonography given its small diameter and depth in the gluteal region.

Optimization of the ultrasound image before needle insertion is vital to the success of this block. The image must clearly show the interligamentous plane formed by the sacrotuberous and sacrospinous ligaments as well as the pudendal artery (the pudendal nerve may or may not be seen). The purpose of image optimization is to ensure that the injected solution is well contained between the ligaments where the nerve is potentially compressed. The image quality of these soft tissues should not be compromised

---

Clinical Pearls and Pitfalls:

- Always make sure one can visualize and insert the needle when the sacrospinous ligament is in view and the spread of the injectate is between the sacrospinous and sacrotuberous ligaments. This is important because it ensures that the injection is into the interligamentous plane.
- When the needle is inserted as in-plane technique, the needle is usually poorly visualized because of the steep angle. One can minimize this by having the needle entry point inserted in a far medial location. In some patients, the sacrum may prevent the advancement of the needle. In that situation, the needle should be inserted from lateral to medial.
- The pudendal nerve can be easier to visualize with Doppler ultrasonography because one will appreciate the displacement of the artery by a hyperechoic structure.
- Injection is medial to the pudendal artery, which is usually found medial to the ischial spine. If an artery is seen lateral to the ischial spine, the practitioner should suspect that it is the descending branch of the inferior gluteal artery that accompanies sciatic nerve. A few hints will suggest that is not pudendal artery: (1) scan farther medially and caudally and the pudendal artery will appear on the medial aspect, (2) the visualization of the sciatic nerve adjacent to the artery, and (3) the artery is seen more than 1 cm lateral to the ischial spine. However, the pudendal artery can be found lateral to the ischial spine or in a mistaken scan when the level of scan is above the ischial spine. In the latter case, the sacrospinous ligament cannot be seen.
- The practitioner should always keep an eye where the injectate spreads. In a situation in which the injectate is moving laterally, one should be concerned that it will spill to the sciatic nerve, so the needle should be relocated slightly in the medial direction.

---

by tilting the probe to find the needle. The needle must instead be reinserted or repositioned until it is within the path of the ultrasound beam.

The needle is inserted medial to the probe so the tip comes to lie medial to the pudendal artery. Frequently, the needle must be inserted at a steep angle to reach this target, and it may not be well visualized. To avoid this, the needle entry point may be chosen at a more medial location. As the needle passes through the sacrotuberous ligament, increased resistance against the needle is felt, which quickly gives way as it passes through the ligament. The needle tip should now be between the sacrotuberous and sacrospinous ligaments. Infiltration of 1 to 2 mL of normal saline confirms the position of the needle in this interligamentous plane. A solution containing local anesthetic and steroid (5 mL) is injected when the final needle position is deemed satisfactory. Epinephrine is avoided so that vasoconstriction of the pudendal artery does not occur. If solution spreads laterally past the pudendal artery, sciatic nerve involvement becomes more likely, and the needle should be repositioned more medially.

Piriformis Injection

Piriformis syndrome is an uncommon and often underdiagnosed cause of buttock and leg pain. The clinical presentation of this syndrome has been well described elsewhere in the literature.[86,87] The management of piriformis syndrome includes the injection of the piriformis muscle with local anesthetic and steroids[87] or the injection of botulinum toxin.[88]

Anatomy

The piriformis muscle originates from the anterior surface of the second, third, and fourth sacral vertebrae and the capsule of the sacroiliac joint. Running laterally anterior to the sacroiliac joint, the piriformis muscle exits the pelvis through the greater sciatic foramen (**Fig. 10-18**). At this point, the muscle becomes tendinous, inserting into the upper border of the greater trochanter as a round tendon. The piriformis functions as an external rotator of the lower limb in the erect position, an abductor when supine, and a weak hip flexor when walking.[86]

All neurovascular structures exiting the pelvis to the buttock pass through the greater sciatic foramen, and the sciatic nerve is one of them. There are six possible anatomical relationships between the sciatic nerve and the piriformis muscle. The most common arrangement is found when the undivided nerve passes below the piriformis muscle (78% to 84%).[89,90] The second most common arrangement is found when the divided nerve passes through and below the muscle (12% to 21%). The aberrant course of the sciatic nerve through the piriformis muscle can cause sciatica and may suggest the important role of a nerve stimulator in the injection of the piriformis muscle.

The piriformis muscle is the only muscle passing through the greater sciatic notch. The key sonoanatomy is to locate the muscle in the sciatica notch. At this level, the piriformis muscle is covered by the gluteus maximus muscle on the dorsal aspect. In some circumstances, the border between the two muscles may be difficult to visualize (in very obese patients). The piriformis muscle can be easily differentiated by the gliding movement with the internal and external rotation of the hip.

Existing Techniques

Various image-guided techniques used to inject the piriformis muscle have been described, including fluoroscopy,[91] CT,[92] and magnetic resonance imaging (MRI).[93] Electrophysiological

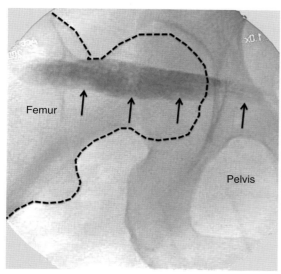

Fig. 10-21 Radiographic contrast (indicated by *arrows*) outlining the piriformis muscle. The *dashed line* outlines the femoral head and neck. (Reprinted with permission from USRA, Toronto Western Hospital, Toronto [www.usra.ca].)

guidance has been used alone and in conjunction with the above modalities.[94] Contrast injection is commonly used in fluoroscopic-guided technique to confirm needle placement within the piriformis muscle (**Fig. 10-21**), which has been shown to be unreliable.[95] A validation study with cadavers suggested that fluoroscopically-guided, contrast-controlled injection was only accurate in guiding an intrapiriformis injection in 30% of the injections.[95] In cases in which the needle was incorrectly placed, the usual final position of the needle was within the gluteus maximus muscle, which overlies the piriformis.

In contrast, ultrasonography is seen as an attractive imaging technique because it provides visualization of the soft tissue and neurovascular structures and allows real-time imaging of the needle insertion toward the target. Furthermore, the success of injection can be assessed by the spread of injectate under ultrasonography.[1] Multiple reports of ultrasound-guided piriformis muscle injection have been published with similar techniques described.[96,97] The accuracy of needle placement with ultrasonography was recently validated in a cadaveric study suggesting an accuracy of 95%.[95]

The use of ultrasonography allows for direct visualization of the piriformis muscle.[45,46] Using this technique, one may see the needle insert within the substance of the muscle and visualize the spread of injectate within or around the muscle. Adjacent anatomical structures such as the sciatic nerve are also visualized. This technique has proven accurate and reproducible.[45,47] Furthermore, the cost is significantly lower than MRI or CT scanning, and ultrasonography is available to a greater number of physicians.

Ultrasound-Guided Injection Technique

The patient is placed in the prone position. A curvilinear probe with a low frequency (2-5 MHz) is required to visualize the muscle given its location deep to the gluteus maximus muscle. Similar to the technique for pudendal nerve injection, the ultrasound transducer should be first placed transversely over the PSIS. After the iliac wing is identified, the angle of the probe is rotated such that it would be in line with the long axis of the piriformis muscle as it runs from the sacrum to the greater trochanter. As scanning continues caudally, the hyperechoic line of the ilium starts to recede

from the medial aspect of the image at the level of the sciatic notch. The lateral aspect of the ultrasound image continues to display a curved hyperechoic line representing the ischium. At this level, two separate muscular layers are identified: the gluteus maximus and the piriformis muscles (**Fig. 10-20, B**). By internal and external rotation of the patient's hip with the knee flexed, the piriformis muscle can be seen gliding underneath the gluteus maximus muscle. The sequence of scanning the PSIS first and then moving the probe caudally is important because the ultrasound image of the lesser sciatic notch may be confused with that of the greater sciatic notch.

After the piriformis muscle is identified, a long 22-gauge stimulating needle is used for injection within or around the piriformis muscle in the sciatic notch. The needle insertion can be made medially or laterally to the ultrasound probe. After the needle has been advanced midway through the gluteus maximus muscle, stimulation of the muscle can be performed at 1.2 mA, which produces a distinctive contraction. Stimulation is paused, and the needle is further advanced to the piriformis muscular layer. If the needle tip is in contact with the piriformis muscle and stimulation is resumed, muscular contraction in the gluteal region is now greatly diminished given the smaller muscle bulk of the piriformis. Ultrasound imaging should show that only the piriformis muscular layer contracts with stimulation. Nerve stimulation is important to identify the proximity of the needle to the sciatic nerve.

Injection may be made around the sheath of the muscle or within the muscle itself. If injection around the sheath is desired, a small amount of normal saline (<0.5 mL) should be injected to confirm the needle tip is in the fascial plane between the gluteus maximus and piriformis muscles. If intramuscular injection is required, the needle is advanced further so that strong piriformis muscle contractions are obtained. A small amount of normal saline (<0.5 mL) is injected to confirm needle tip location.

Clinical Pearls and Pitfalls:
- Although internal and external rotation of the piriformis muscle is a very useful maneuver to differentiate between the gluteus maximus and piriformis muscle, the image can be similar when the probe is scanning the lesser sciatic notch. Therefore, the practitioner needs to make sure the scanning starts from the ilium and the probe is then moved caudally.
- The suggested injection site is at the sciatic notch when the muscle belly is the thickest.

Conclusion

Ultrasonography is a valuable tool for imaging peripheral structures, guiding needle advancement, and confirming the spread of injectate around the target tissue, all without exposing health care providers and patients to the risks of radiation. More studies on the efficacy and safety of ultrasound-guided techniques are required.

References

1. Peng P, Narouze S: Ultrasound-guided interventional procedures in pain Medicine: A review of anatomy, sonoanatomy and procedures. Part I: non-axial structures. *Reg Anesth Pain Med* 34:458-474, 2009.
2. Wertheim HM, Rovenstine EA: Suprascapular nerve block. *Anesthesiology* 2:541-545, 1941.
3. Gleeson AP, Graham CA, Jones I, et al: Comparison of intra-articular lignocaine and a suprascapular nerve block for acute anterior shoulder dislocation. *Injury* 28:141-142, 1997.

4. Ritchie ED, Tong D, Chung F, et al: Suprascapular nerve block for pain relief in arthroscopic shoulder surgery: a new modality? *Anesth Analg* 84:1306-1312, 1997.

5. Neal J, McDonald S, Larkin K et al: Suprascapular nerve block prolongs analgesia after nonarthroscopic shoulder surgery but does not improve outcome. *Anesth Analg* 96:982-986, 2003.

6. Emery P, Bowman S, Wedderburn L, Grahame R: Suprascapular nerve block for chronic shoulder pain in rheumatoid arthritis. *BMJ* 299:1079-1080, 1989.

7. Jones DS, Chattopadhyay C: Suprascapular nerve block for the treatment of frozen shoulder in primary care: a randomized trial. *Br J Gen Pract* 49:39-41, 1999.

8. Karatas GK, Meray J: Suprascapular nerve block for pain relief in adhesive capsulitis: comparison of 2 different techniques. *Arch Phys Med Rehabil* 83:593-597, 2002.

9. Shanahan EM, Ahern M, Smith M, et al: Suprascapular nerve block (using bupivacaine and methylprednisolone acetate) in chronic shoulder pain. *Ann Rheum Diseases* 62:400-406, 2003.

10. Romeo AA, Rotenberg DD, Bach BR, Jr: Suprascapular neuropathy. *J Am Acad Orthop Surg* 7:358-367, 1999.

11. Natsis K, Totlis T, Tsikaras P, et al: Proposal for classification of the suprascapular notch: a study on 423 dried scapulas. *Clin Anat* 20:135-139, 2007.

12. Peng P, Wiley MJ, Liang J, Bellingham G: Ultrasound-guided suprascapular nerve block: a correlation with fluoroscopic and cadaveric findings. *Can J Anesth* 57:143-148, 2010.

13. Feigl GC, Anderhuber F, Dorn C, et al: Modified lateral block of the suprascapular nerve: a safe approach and how much to inject? A morphological study. *Reg Anesth Pain Med* 32:488-494, 2007.

14. Mallon WJ, Brown HR, Vogler JB, Martinez S: Radiographic and geometric anatomy of the scapula. *Clin Orthop Relat Res* 277:142-154, 1992.

15. Shah RV, Racz GB: Pulsed mode radiofrequency lesioning of the suprascapular nerve for the treatment of chronic shoulder pain. A case report. *Pain Physician* 6:503-506, 2003.

16. Schneider-Kolsky ME, Pike J, Connell DA: CT-guided suprascapular nerve blocks: a pilot study. *Skeletal Radiol* 33:277-282, 2004.

17. Moore DC: Block of the suprascapular nerve. In Thomas CC, editor: *Regional nerve block*, ed 4, Springfield, IL, 1979, pp 300-303.

18. Brown DE, James DC, Roy S: Pain relief by suprascapular nerve block in gleno-humeral arthritis. *Scand J Rheumatol* 1988; 17:411-415.

19. Gofeld M: Ultrasonography in pain medicine: a critical review. *Pain Pract* 8:226-240, 2008.

20. Harmon D, Hearty C: Ultrasound-guided suprascapular nerve block technique. *Pain Physician* 10:743-746, 2007.

21. Yucesoy C, Akkaya T, Ozel O, et al: Ultrasonographic evaluation and morphometric measurements of the suprascapular notch. *Surg Radiol Anat* 31:409-414, 2009.

22. Moore DC, Bridenbaugh LD: Intercostal nerve block in 4333 patients: indications, technique and complications. *Anesth Analg* 41:1-10, 1962.

23. Karmakar MK, Ho AMH: Acute pain management of patients with multiple fractured ribs. *J Trauma* 54:612-615, 2003.

24. Kopacz DJ, Thompson GE: Intercostal blocks for thoracic and abdominal surgery. *Tech Reg Anesth Pain Manage* 2:25-29, 1998.

25. Green CR, de Rosayro M, Tait AR: The role of cryoanalgesia for chronic thoracic pain: results of a long-term follow up. *J Natl Med Assoc* 94:716-720, 2002.

26. Byas-Smith MG, Gulati A: Ultrasound-guided intercostal nerve cryoablation. *Anesth Analg* 103:1033-1035, 2006.

27. Cohen SP, Sireci A, Wu CL, et al: Pulsed radiofrequency of the dorsal root ganglia is superior to pharmacotherapy or pulsed radiofrequency of the intercostal nerves in the treatment of chronic postsurgical thoracic pain. *Pain Physician* 9:227-235, 2006.

28. Stolker RJ, Vervest AC, Groen GJ: The treatment of chronic thoracic segmental pain by radiofrequency percutaneous partial rhizotomy. *J Neurosurg* 80:986-992, 1994.

29. Rendina EA, Ciccone AM: The intercostal space. *Thorac Surg Clin* 17:491-501, 2007.

30. Graeber GM, Nazim M: The anatomy of the ribs and the sternum and their relationship to chest wall structure and function. *Thorac Surg Clin* 17:473-489, 2007.

31. Knowles P, Hancox D, Letheren M, et al: An evaluation of intercostal nerve blockade for analgesia following renal transplantation. *Eur J Anaesthesiol* 15:457-461, 1998.

32. Shanti CM, Carlin AM, Tyburski JG: Incidence of pneumothorax from intercostal nerve block for analgesia in rib fractures. *J Trauma* 51:536-539, 2001.

33. Curatolo M, Eichenberger U: Ultrasound-guided blocks for the treatment of chronic pain. *Tech Reg Anesth Pain Manage* 11:95-102, 2007.

34. Cardosi RJ, Cox CS, Hoffman MS: Postoperative neuropathies after major pelvic surgery. *Obstet Gynecol* 100:240-244, 2002.

35. Luijendijk RW, Jekel J, Storm RK, et al: The low transverse Pfannenstiel incision and the prevalence of incisional hernia and nerve entrapment. *Ann Surg* 225:365-369, 1997.

36. Whiteside JL, Barber MD, Walters MD, Falcone T: Anatomy of the ilioinguinal and iliohypogastric nerves in relation to trocar placement and low transverse incisions. *Am J Obstet Gynecol* 189:1574-1578, 2003.

37. Sippo WC, Burghardt A, Gomez AC: Nerve entrapment after Pfannenstiel incision. *Am J Obstet Gynecol* 157:420-421, 1987.

38. Choi PD, Nath R, Mackinnon SE: Iatrogenic injury to the ilioinguinal and iliohypogastric nerves in the groin: case report, diagnosis, and management. *Ann Plast Surg* 37:60-65, 1996.

39. Jamieson RW, Swigart LL, Anson BJ: Points of parietal perforation of the ilioinguinal and iliohypogastric nerves in relation to optimal sites for local anaesthesia. *Q Bull Northwest Univ Med Sch* 26:22-26, 1952.

40. Mandelkow H, Loeweneck H: The iliohypogastric and ilioinguinal nerves. Distribution in the abdominal wall, danger areas in surgical incisions in the inguinal and pubic regions and reflected visceral pain in their dermatomes. *Surg Radiol Anat* 10:145-149, 1988.

41. Oelrich TM, Moosman DA: The aberrant course of the cutaneous component of the ilioinguinal nerve. *Anat Rec* 189: 233-236, 1977.

42. Ducic I, Dellon AL: Testicular pain after inguinal hernia repair: an approach to resection of the genital branch of genitofemoral nerve. *J Am Coll Surg* 198:181-184, 2004.

43. Rab M, Ebmer And J, Dellon AL: Anatomic variability of the ilioinguinal and genitofemoral nerve: implications for the treatment of groin pain. *Plast Reconstr Surg* 108:1618-1623, 2001.

44. Liu WC, Chen TH, Shyu JF, et al: Applied anatomy of the genital branch of the genitofemoral nerve in open inguinal herniorrhaphy. *Eur J Surg* 168:145-149, 2002.

45. Lichtenstein IL, Shulman AG, Amid PK, et al: Cause and prevention of postherniorrhaphy neuralgia: a proposed protocol for treatment. *Am J Surg* 155:786-790, 1988.

46. Eichenberger U, Greher M, Kirchmair L, et al: Ultrasound-guided blocks of the ilioinguinal and iliohypogastric nerve: accuracy of a selective new technique confirmed by anatomical dissection. *Br J Anaesth* 97:238-243, 2006.

47. al-Dabbagh AK: Anatomical variations of the inguinal nerve and risks of injury in 110 hernia repairs. *Surg Radiol Anat* 24:102-107, 2002.

48. Peng PWH, Tumber PS: Ultrasound-guided interventional procedures for patients with chronic pelvic pain—a description of techniques and review of literature. *Pain Physician* 11:215-224, 2008.

49. Rosario DJ, Jacob S, Luntley J, et al: Mechanism of femoral nerve palsy complication percutaneous ilioinguinal field block. *Br J Anaesth* 78:314-316, 1997.

50. Van Schoor AN, Boon JM, Bosenberg AT, et al: Anatomical considerations of the pediatric ilioinguinal/iliohypogastric nerve block. *Paediatr Anaesth* 15:371-377, 2005.

51. Johr M, Sossai R: Colonic puncture during ilioinguinal nerve block in a child. *Anesth Analg* 88:1051-1052, 1999.

52. Amory C, Mariscal A, Guyot E, et al: Is ilioinguinal/iliohypogastric nerve block always totally safe in children? *Pediatr Anaesth* 13:164-166, 2003.

53. Vaisman J: Pelvic hematoma after an ilioinguinal nerve block for orchialgia. *Anesth Analg* 92:1048-1049, 2001.

54. van Schoor AN, Boon JM, Bosenberg AT, et al: Anatomical considerations of the pediatric ilioinguinal/iliohypogastric nerve block. *Paediatr Anaesth* 15:371-377, 2005.

55. Weintraud M, Marhofer P, Bosenberg A, et al: Ilioinguinal/iliohypogastric blocks in children: where do we administer the local anesthetic without direct visualization? *Anesth Analg* 106:89-93, 2008.

56. Hu P, Harmon D, Frizelle H: Ultrasound guidance for ilioinguinal/iliohypogastric nerve block: a pilot study. *Ir J Med Sci* 176:111-115, 2007.

57. Gofeld M, Christakis M: Sonographically guided ilioinguinal nerve block. *J Ultrasound Med* 25:1571-1575, 2006.

58. Gucev G, Yasui GM, Chang TY, Lee J: Bilateral ultrasound-guided continuous ilioinguinal-iliohypogastric block for pain relief after Cesarean delivery. *Anesth Analg* 106:1220-1222, 2008.

59. Broadman L: Ilioinguinal, iliohypogastric, and genitofemoral nerves. In Gay SG, editor: *Regional anesthesia. An atlas of anatomy and techniques*, St. Louis, 1996, Mosby, pp 247-254.

60. Conn D, Nicholls B: Regional anaesthesia. In Wilson IH, Allman KG, editors: *Oxford handbook of anaesthesia*, ed 2, New York, 2006, Oxford University Press, pp 1055-1104.

61. Bellingham GA, Peng PWH: Ultrasound-guided interventional procedures for chronic pelvic pain. *Tech Reg Anesth Pain Manag* 13:171-178, 2009.

62. Campos NA, Chiles JH, Plunkett AR: Ultrasound-guided cryoablation of genitofemoral nerve for chronic inguinal pain. *Pain Physician* 12:997-1000, 2009.

63. Park JW, Kim DH, Hwang M, Bun HR: Meralgia paresthetica caused by hip-huggers in a patient with aberrant course of the lateral femoral cutaneous nerve. *Muscle Nerve* 35:678-680, 2007.

64. van Slobbe AM, Bohnen AM, Bernsen RM, et al: Incidence rates and determinants in meralgia paresthetica in general practice. *J Neurol* 251:294-297, 2004.

65. Grossman MG, Ducey SA, Nadler SS, et al: Meralgia paresthetica: diagnosis and treatment. *J Am Acad Orthop Surg* 9:336-344, 2001.

66. de Ridder VA, de Lange S, Popta J: Anatomical variations of the lateral femoral cutaneous nerve and the consequences for surgery. *J Orthop Trauma* 13:207-211, 1999.

67. Grothaus MC, Holt M, Mekhail AO, et al: Lateral femoral cutaneous nerve: an anatomic study. *Clin Orthop Relat Res* 437:164-168, 2005.

68. Murata Y, Takahashi K, Yamagata M, et al: The anatomy of the lateral femoral cutaneous nerve, with special reference to the harvesting of iliac bone graft. *J Bone Joint Surg Am* 82:746-747, 2000.

69. Dias Filho LC, Valença MM, Guimarães Filho FAV, et al: Lateral femoral cutaneous neuralgia: an anatomical insight. *Clin Anat* 16:309-316, 2003.

70. Hospodar PP, Ashman ES, Traub JA: Anatomic study of the lateral femoral cutaneous nerve with respect to the ilioinguinal surgical dissection. *J Orthop Trauma* 13:17-19, 1999.

71. Ropars M, Morandi X, Huten D, et al: Anatomical study of the lateral femoral cutaneous nerve with special reference to minimally invasive anterior approach for total hip replacement. *Surg Radio Anat* 31:199-204, 2009.

72. Bodner G, Bernathova M, Galiano K, et al: Ultrasound of the lateral femoral cutaneous nerve. Normal findings in a cadaver and in volunteers. *Reg Anesth Pain Med* 34:265-268, 2009.

73. Hurdle MF, Weingarten TN, Crisostomo RA, et al: Ultrasound-guided blockade of the lateral femoral cutaneous nerve: technical description and review of 10 cases. *Arch Phys Med Rehabil* 88:1362-1364, 2007.

74. Ng I, Vaghadia H, Choi PT, Helmy N: Ultrasound imaging accurately identifies the lateral femoral cutaneous nerve. *Anesth Analg* 107:1070-1074, 2008.

75. Damarey B, Demondion X, Boutry N, et al: Sonographic assessment of the lateral femoral cutaneous nerve. *J Clin Ultrasound* 37:89-95, 2009.

76. Robert R, Prat-Pradal D, Labat JJ, et al: Anatomic basis of chronic perineal pain: role of the pudendal nerve. *Surg Radiol Anat* 20:93-98, 1998.

77. Peng PWH, Antolak SJ, Gordon AS: Pudendal Neuralgia. In: Goldstein I, Pukall C, Goldstein A, editors: *Female sexual pain disorders: evaluation and management*, ed 1, Oxford UK, 2009, Wiley-Blackwell Publisher, pp 112-118.

78. Mahakkanukrauh P, Surin P, Vaidhayakarn P: Anatomical study of the pudendal nerve adjacent to the sacrospinous ligament. *Clin Anat* 18:200-205, 2005.

79. Shafik A, Doss SH: Pudendal canal: surgical anatomy and clinical implications. *Am Surg* 65:176-180, 1999.

80. Amareno G, Lanoe Y, Ghnassia RT, et al: Alcock's canal syndrome and perineal neuralgia. *Rev Neurol* 144:523-526, 1988.

81. Warrick R, Williams PL: Myology: fascia of the truck. In Warrick R, Williams PL, editors: *Gray's anatomy*, ed 36, Edinburgh, UK, 1980, Churchill, pp 542-564.

82. Rofaeel A, Peng P, Louis I, et al: Feasibility of real-time ultrasound for pudendal nerve block in patients with chronic perineal pain. *Reg Anesth Pain Med* 33:139-145, 2008.

83. Hough DM, Wittenberg KH, Pawlina W, et al: Chronic perineal pain caused by pudendal nerve entrapment: anatomy and CT-guided perineural injection technique. *Am J Roentgenol* 181:2:561-567, 2003.

84. Kovacs P, Gruber H, Piegger J, Bodner G: New, simple, ultrasound-guided infiltration of the pudendal nerve: ultrasonographic technique. *Dis Colon Rectum* 44:9:1381-1385, 2001.

85. Gruber H, Kovacs P, Piegger J, Brenner E: New, simple, ultrasound-guided infiltration of the pudendal nerve: topographic basics. *Dis Colon Rectum* 44:9:1376-1380, 2001.

86. Papadopoulos EC, Khan SN: Piriformis syndrome and low back pain: a new classification and review of the literature. *Orthop Clin North Am* 35:65-71, 2004.

87. Benzon HT, Katz JA, Benzon HA, Iqbal MS: Piriformis syndrome: anatomic considerations, a new injection technique, and a review of the literature. *Anesthesiology* 98:1442-1448, 2003.

88. Fishman LM, Anderson C, Rosner B: Botox and physical therapy in the treatment of piriformis syndrome. *Am J Phys Med Rehabil* 81:936-942, 2002.

89. Beason LE, Anson BJ: The relation of the sciatic nerve and its subdivisions to the piriformis muscle. *Anat Rec* 70:1-5, 1937.

90. Pecina M: Contribution to the etiological explanation of the piriformis syndrome. *Acta Anat* 105:181-187, 1979.

91. Fishman S, Caneris O, Bandman T, et al: Injection of the piriformis muscle by fluoroscopic and electromyographic guidance. *Reg Anesth Pain Med* 23(6):554-559, 1998.

92. Fanucci E, Masala S, Sodani G, et al: CT-guided injection of botulinic toxin for percutaneous therapy of piriformis muscle syndrome with preliminary MRI results about denervative process. *Eur Radiol* 11:2543-2548, 2001.

93. Filler A, Haynes J, Jordan S, et al: Sciatic pain of non-disc origin and piriformis syndrome: diagnosis by magnetic resonance neurography and interventional magnetic resonance imaging with outcome of resulting treatment. *J Neurosurg Spine* 2:99-115, 2005.

94. Fishman L, Konnoth C, Rozner B: Botulinum neurotoxin type B and physical therapy in the treatment of piriformis syndrome: a dose finding study. *Am J Phys Med* 83:42-50, 2004.

95. Finoff JT, Hurdle MFB, Smith J: Accuracy of ultrasound-guided versus fluoroscopically guided contrast controlled piriformis injections. A cadaveric study. *J Ultrasound Med* 27:8:1157-1163, 2008.

96. Huerto AP, Yeo SN, Ho KY: Piriformis muscle injection using ultrasonography and motor stimulation-report of a technique. *Pain Physician* 10:5:687-690, 2007.

97. Smith J, Hurdle M-F, Locketz AJ, Wisniewski SJ: Ultrasound-guided piriformis injection: technique description and verification. *Arch Phys Med Rehabil* 87:12:1664-1667, 2006.

SECTION

III Injections for Back Pain

Chapter 11 Therapeutic Epidural Injections: Interlaminar and Transforaminal

Chapter 12 Facet (Zygapophyseal) Intraarticular Joint Injections: Cervical, Lumbar, and Thoracic

Chapter 13 Medial Branch Blocks: Cervical, Thoracic, and Lumbar

Chapter 14 Radiofrequency Rhizotomy for Facet Syndrome

Chapter 15 Sacroiliac Joint Injections and Lateral Branch Blocks, Including Water-Cooled Neurotomy

Chapter 16 Pulsed Radiofrequency

Chapter 17 Discogenic Pain and Discography for Spinal Injections

Chapter 18 Minimally Invasive Intradiscal Procedures for the Treatment of Discogenic Lower Back and Leg Pain

Chapter 19 Vertebral Augmentation

Chapter 20 Ultrasound-Guided Lumbar Spine Injections

Chapter 21 Ultrasound-Guided Cervical Spine Injections

Chapter 22 Musculoskeletal Injections: Iliopsoas, Quadratus Lumborum, Piriformis, and Trigger Point Injections

Chapter 23 Ultrasound-Guided and Fluoroscopically Guided Joint Injections

11 Therapeutic Epidural Injections: Interlaminar and Transforaminal

Marc A. Huntoon and Abram H. Burgher

CHAPTER OVERVIEW

Chapter Synopsis: Similar to many spinal injection therapies, epidural injections for the treatment of sciatica have evolved in recent years because of a better understanding of the underlying condition. Initially, injections consisted of a simple anesthetic and later of corticosteroids. This chapter covers more recent findings that have led to refinement of the technique. Radiculopathy is the loss of sensory or motor conduction that can arise from a herniated intervertebral disc. These poorly vascularized structures can be damaged by mechanical impingement, which then may lead to an inflammatory response raised by spinal glia. This inflammatory soup, which contains cytokines and tumor necrosis factor-α, likely mediates the painful component known as radicular pain. When a patient complains of low back pain without leg pain, discogenic pain may be a more likely candidate, which may also be treated with epidural injection. Spinal stenosis can also cause similar radicular pain. These spinal disorders require a combination of imaging results, electrodiagnostic studies, and physical examination for proper diagnosis and treatment. Recent reviews of the literature suggest that some injection procedures can provide short-term relief from radicular pain caused by these conditions. This chapter also describes the technical aspects of the procedures and avoiding risks of complications.

Important Points:
- The natural history of discogenic radicular pain is to improve without any intervention.
- Most trials of epidural steroids suggest short-term benefit with injection via multiple techniques.
- Best practice of nonsurgical radicular pain syndromes is yet to be defined. Few comparative nonsurgical trials have been conducted.
- Because of the rare but catastrophic nature of some of these complications with the favorable natural history of discogenic radicular pain, optimization of safety should be of primary concern.
- Future directions in research could look at alternative pharmacological agents or techniques to address the pathophysiology of radicular pain syndromes.

Clinical Pearls:
- Transforaminal epidural techniques place the medication in the anterior epidural space nearer the putative site of pathology.
- Digital subtraction angiography techniques are a simple and inexpensive addition to conventional fluoroscopy and may be useful in complication reduction from inadvertent vascular injection.
- Infectious risks may be mitigated by strict aseptic technique, including a chlorhexidine-based scrub, mask, hand asepsis (surgical wash), and caution in high-risk patients.
- Imaging should be reviewed when possible before injections, particularly in the cervical region.

Clinical Pitfalls:
- Patient response should be based on outcome of each injection, and proscriptive use of specific numbers of injections (e.g., three epidurals) is not evidence based.
- Because the evidence does not suggest which technique, if any, is superior to another, each patient should be approached individually.

Introduction

The use of therapeutic epidural injections for the treatment of sciatica with back and leg pain dates back approximately 80 years. Initially, therapeutic epidurals were predominately transsacral (caudal) injections of local anesthetics such as procaine.[1] After the introduction of corticosteroids into clinical practice,[2] researchers in Europe were the first to inject corticosteroids into the epidural space.[3,4] The techniques of administration have gradually been modified, with early use of higher volume caudal epidural injections eventually being largely replaced, first by level-specific interlaminar epidural injections and second by transforaminal epidurals performed with fluoroscopic guidance. Despite the increasing sophistication and advances in the techniques of steroid injection, a number of authors still question the role of these injections for the therapy of sciatica. In particular, two physician specialties (neurology and occupational medicine) have published guidelines or reviews suggesting that these injections are performed too often with uncertain results.[5,6] Other authors are beginning to examine the role of alternate compounds such as etanercept for the treatment of sciatica based on the underlying pathophysiology.[7] Finally, a recent head-to-head trial of several conservative treatments (including injections in some) compared with surgical therapies was performed demonstrating the superiority of surgery, at least in the first year.[8] This trial augmented the previous large-scale trials comparing surgical with nonsurgical therapies.[9,10] This chapter discusses the current role of therapeutic epidural injections.

Basic Science

Radiculopathy is most commonly associated with intervertebral disc herniation and likely includes two distinct pathways: mechanical compression and cytokine-mediated radiculitis.[11] Mechanical impingement may induce poor tissue oxygen delivery to the spinal (radicular) nerve, resulting in an inadequate nutritional supply and decreasing the vascular perfusion to critical levels. Interestingly, however, mechanical compression alone may not result in pain.[12,13] *Radiculopathy* describes neurological conduction loss (sensory or motor) occurring secondary to mechanical impingement or compression (e.g., disc protrusion, herniation, or extrusion) pressing on the spinal nerve in the foramina. Other common causes of radiculopathy include spondylosis, vertebral subluxation, and ligamentum flavum hypertrophy or thickening.[14] Abnormal nerve conduction may manifest as sensory loss, depressed spinal reflexes, or motor deficits. *Radicular pain* may occur concomitantly with radiculopathy or separately. The pain is thought to be an inflammatory phenomenon induced by neurochemical products such as cytokines. Cytokines are produced by spinal glia. They include tumor necrosis factor-α (TNF-α) and several interleukins. Herniated nucleus pulposus may induce the release of such inflammatory mediators, leading to a chemical radiculitis. Olmarker et al[15] found that the application of a homogenate of disc material onto porcine cauda equina induced functional and morphologic changes in those nerves. Then Igarashi and colleagues[16] reported that in a rat model, TNF-α applied to the dorsal root ganglia produced functional and morphological changes that were identical to that seen with nucleus pulposus material. Burke et al[17] found increased levels of the inflammatory cytokines interleukin-6 (IL-6) and IL-8 in disc material taken from patients with known disc disease. Finally, further study produced compelling evidence that TNF-α inhibitors could reduce the histological and functional changes caused by nucleus pulposus material. These studies cemented the concept that TNF-α and other cytokines were causative agents in the development of radiculitis and further suggested an entirely new pharmacological treatment strategy for patients with sciatica.[18]

Discogenic pain is another pathological condition for which epidural therapies are occasionally tried. Discogenic pain is unlike radicular pain in that the patient will predominately complain of low back pain without significant leg involvement that is exacerbated by the sitting position, spinal flexion, heavy lifting, or other stresses. The intervertebral disc is a very poorly vascularized structure that receives nutrients primarily by diffusion. Intervertebral disc innervation is complex, arising primarily from nerve ingrowth through the vertebral endplate into the outer third of the disc annulus. Nerve fiber types in the annulus fibrosis are peptidergic, using neurotransmitter substances such as calcitonin gene-related peptide. Nerve fibers are small and follow new blood vessels.[19]

Establishing Diagnosis

Generally, the diagnosis of a condition that may respond to a therapeutic epidural injection is based on a combination of the history, physical examination, imaging results, and electrodiagnostic studies. Evidence of motor weakness, decreased sensation, loss of deep tendon reflexes, tension signs (e.g., straight-leg raise sign), and characteristic dermatomal involvement may indicate spinal nerve impingement is causing the radiculopathy or radicular pain. Likewise, patients with pain from spinal stenosis or postsurgical discogenic pain may be candidates for therapeutic epidural injections. Patients with spinal stenosis may present with pain that is worsened by going down an incline or stairs or progressive neurogenic claudication with walking. Usually, rest promptly improves the claudication symptoms, unlike vascular claudication symptoms. Patients generally walk with their trunks flexed forward pushing a walker or shopping cart, which seems to relieve their symptom exacerbation when in extension. Patients with epidural fibrosis or postsurgical scarring may manifest just a few weeks to months of improvement followed by resumption of similar back and leg pain. In these cases, one must obtain new imaging to ascertain whether there is recurrent disc protrusion, a new protrusion at another level, or evidence of fibrosis.

Indications and Contraindications

Therapeutic epidurals are generally used in three major instances: (1) for the symptomatic treatment of radicular pain secondary to an intervertebral disc herniation, protrusion, or extrusion causing a combination of back and leg pain in a characteristic dermatomal pattern (**Fig. 11-1**); (2) spinal stenosis presenting with symptoms of neurogenic claudication, radicular pain, or mixed pain (**Fig. 11-2**); and (3) postoperative back and leg pain caused by recurrent disc material, granulation tissue or scarring, or other causes (**Fig. 11-3**). In some cases, therapeutic epidural injections may also be performed in cases of discogenic pain or for tumor-related nerve pain when a radicular syndrome is manifested by the tumor growth into the foramen or around the exiting spinal nerve (**Fig. 11-1**). How these therapeutic procedures are applied is also somewhat variable depending on regional variations in the use of initial conservative therapies, the specialty of origin of the managing

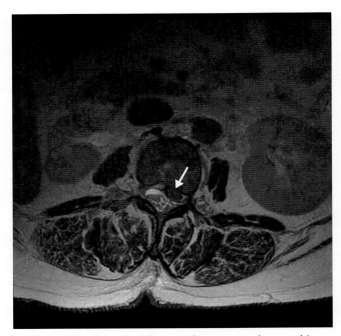

Fig. 11-1 T2-weighted axial magnetic resonance image with L2-L3 left disc extrusion (*arrow*).

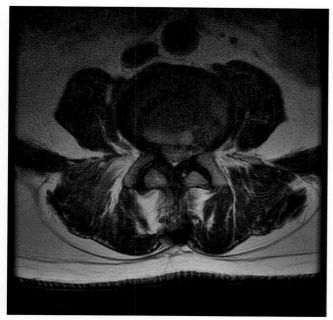

Fig. 11-2 Severe spinal stenosis caused by a combination of broad-based disc bulging, ligamentum flavum hypertrophy, and facet joint hypertrophy.

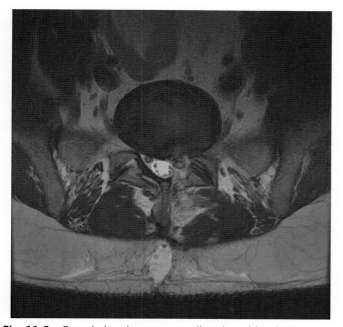

Fig. 11-3 Granulation tissue surrounding the exiting S1 nerve root.

clinician, and the availability of clinicians capable to do therapeutic epidurals. However, population-based examinations of therapeutic epidural injections have not demonstrated any long-term advantage to their use in terms of reduced surgical volumes or enhanced functionality.[20]

Spinal stenosis is most commonly acquired but can be congenital. Large studies are lacking for results of therapeutic epidural injections. The natural history of spinal stenosis is reassuring, however. Johnsson and colleagues[21] demonstrated that older patients with spinal stenosis commonly presented with low back pain (100%), claudication (75%), radicular pain (12.5%), and mixed symptoms (12.5%). Interestingly, the patients with spinal stenosis did not appear to worsen significantly over a 4-year period, with equal numbers showing improvement as progression.

Patients with worse clinical and functional symptoms most often had surgical laminectomy without fusion. At 8 to 10 years, the patients treated with either surgical or nonsurgical approaches had similar rates of satisfaction with current state, back pain incidence, and symptom improvement. Patients with initial surgical treatment had better leg pain and functional status. Overall, the results suggested that patients may be optimally managed in a shared decision model.[22]

Imaging

Numerous studies have demonstrated that a high percentage of patients who are clinically asymptomatic will have significant findings on magnetic resonance imaging (MRI).[23] In most cases, the MRI should be read before proceeding with the injection and is mandatory before cervical epidurals. The size of the spinal canal, presence of intervertebral disc protrusion or extrusion, any neural impingement, presence of degenerative changes, or any possible abnormality in the path of the proposed needle placement will need to be accounted for.

The high rate of false-positive scans mandates an approach to patient evaluation that requires a large degree of concordance among the imaging, electrodiagnostic testing, the history, and the physical examination. In some cases, a diagnostic spinal nerve injection to independently verify which root is involved in pain generation is requested before surgical intervention. Studies performed more than 2 decades ago were the first to suggest that image guidance could significantly improve the accuracy of epidural administration of medication.[24] Johnson et al[25] later published 5489 consecutive injections performed with fluoroscopic guidance with contrast injection. Their results suggested an extremely safe conduct of these outpatient injections could be accomplished with a high degree of accuracy and precision.

Guidelines

A number of exhaustive guidelines have been published in the past several years. Although these rigorous examinations of the literature aim to be fair, balanced, and inclusive of only high-quality studies, they invariably fall short because of specialty biases, differences in interpretation of the evidence, and other inconsistencies. Because the overall quality of the available medical literature is actually quite poor, guideline authors produce documents with nebulous or lukewarm core statements, leaving the readers confused as to their meaning. Many of the diagnostic tests for spinal disorders have uncertain accuracy, so clinicians must rely on a combination of imaging results, electrodiagnostic studies, physical examinations, and sometimes nerve blocks. Thus, treatments for these conditions are equally uncertain.

The American Pain Society Clinical Practice Guideline for Low Back Pain is one of the more recent published guidelines.[26] The authors reviewed randomized controlled trials and systematic reviews that met the following criteria: (1) published in English language or included in an English language review; (2) evaluated adult patients who were not pregnant and had back or leg pain or both; (3) evaluated a targeted interventional therapy; and 4) reported specific outcomes such as back function, health status, work disability, or patient satisfaction. A total of 1331 study citations were reviewed of which 105 met inclusion criteria. In addition, 58 full text reviews yielded 30 that met inclusion criteria. The guideline statements supported fair evidence that epidural steroid injections yielded short-term benefit for radiculopathy caused by disc prolapse but were inferior to surgery. Chymopapain chemonucleolysis injections for radiculopathy were supported by good evidence, but this therapy is no longer used in the United States because of uncommon severe allergic reactions. The guidelines overall conclusions were that few nonsurgical interventions have been shown to be effective.

The American Society of Interventional Pain Physicians also published guidelines regarding the use of interventional techniques in chronic spinal pain.[27] These guidelines also rigorously evaluated available literature using an evidence grading system from the United States Preventative Services Task Force criteria with five levels of evidence. Their findings were supportive of level I for caudal epidural injections for radiculitis or discogenic pain without radiculitis. The level of evidence for cervical thoracic and lumbar epidurals for managing radiculitis was level II-1 or II-2.

The American Society of Anesthesiologists also recently updated its practice guidelines. The purpose of these guidelines is to promote optimized pain control, improved functionality, enhanced quality of life, and minimized adverse effects of therapies. No specific outcomes were warranted by the task force. The guidelines endorse epidural steroids with or without local anesthetic injection for relief of back pain for periods of 2 weeks to 3 months (Category B2 evidence), and neck pain relief for periods of 1 week to 12 months (Category B3 evidence). Image guidance was suggested as representative of current best practice.[28]

Guidelines have been published for cervical radicular pain as well by the World Institute of Pain. A clinical algorithm for management recommends interlaminar epidural corticosteroid injections for subacute radicular pain and pulsed radiofrequency adjacent to the dorsal root ganglion for more chronic pain (**Fig. 11-4**).[29] Cervical transforaminal epidurals are not recommended because of complications and a small negative controlled trial.[30,31]

Outcomes Evidence

A study by Carette and colleagues[32] has been regarded highly by reviewers in several recent guidelines committees. They performed a randomized, placebo-controlled trial examining up to three lumbar interlaminar epidural steroid injections for sciatica. A total of 158 patients received injections for unilateral or bilateral lower extremity pain. Patients had signs of nerve root irritation or compression and computed tomographic (CT) evidence of appropriate level nerve root compression. Patients received either methylprednisolone or saline. Functionality was the primary outcome measure based on Oswestry Disability Index (ODI). Major criticisms of the study were the lack of fluoroscopic guidance and the large injectate volume (8 mL) compared with 1 mL of isotonic saline in the control epidural injection group. The study demonstrated no statistically significant change in functional improvement using ODI scores but did find that leg pain was reduced at 6 weeks in the corticosteroid treatment group (difference in mean change of −0.11; 95% confidence interval, −21.1 to −0.9; P = .03), with a treatment effect no longer present at 3 months.

Karppinen and colleagues[33] performed a randomized, double-blind trial to test the efficacy of periradicular steroid injections for sciatica. A total of 163 patients with unilateral lower extremity pain were studied. Although MRI was recorded, concordant imaging was not a study requirement for inclusion. A total of 80 patients in each group were randomized, and they received either methylprednisolone (80-120 mg) or saline. The primary outcome measure in

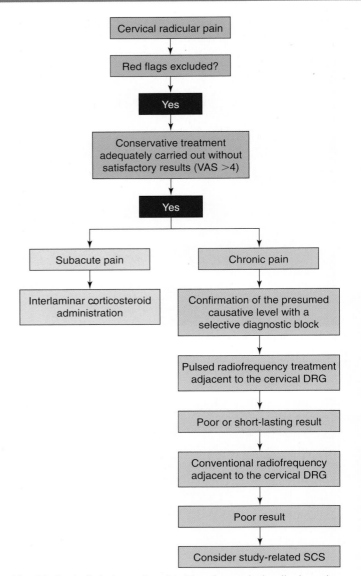

Fig. 11-4 A clinical practice algorithm for cervical radicular pain. DRG, Dorsal root ganglion; SCS, spinal cord stimulation; VAS, visual analog scale. (Adapted from Van Zundert J, Huntoon M, Patijn J, et al: Cervical radicular pain, *Pain Pract* 10:1-17, 2010.)

this study was back and leg pain visual analogue scale. Three patients were not randomized because a contrast outline of the involved spinal nerve could not be obtained. The authors did not comment on contrast spread to the anterior epidural space. The results showed short-term improvement for leg pain in the steroid–bupivacaine group at 2 weeks. Reduced leg pain was 45% versus 24% for the placebo (P <.01) group. Back pain was better in the steroid group at 3 months. No difference between groups was seen at 1 year. Only one injection was evaluated for this study. This has been criticized by some because they theorize that additional injections may have augmented the response.

Riew et al[34] performed a randomized controlled trial of fluoroscopically-guided lumbar transforaminal epidural steroid injections compared with local anesthetic injection. The need for lumbar spine surgery was the primary outcome. The 55 patients studied had lower extremity pain and imaging confirmation foraminal impingement. A total of 28 patients received a betamethasone and bupivacaine injection compared with 27 patients who received bupivacaine transforaminal injection only. Patients treated with betamethasone had a reduction in need for surgery compared with the local anesthetic group. A later review of the same cohort of patients revealed that those who did not have surgery during the original study period were still able to avoid surgery several years later.

Manchikanti et al[35-38] assessed the utility of adding corticosteroid to local anesthetic for caudal epidural injections in a randomized and blinded fashion. Four patient groups were separately studied according to the etiology of their pain: discogenic, radicular, postlaminectomy, or spinal stenosis. More than 200 patients were included in their four studies. Injections were 10 mL total volume containing lidocaine 0.5% and either 6 mg of betamethasone or 40 mg of methylprednisolone. All injections were performed with fluoroscopic guidance. On average, pain and functional status improved in all four groups at 12 months of follow-up regardless of whether they received corticosteroid. Patients could be divided into responders or nonresponders within two injections, generally. Interestingly, patients with spinal stenosis showed similar improvement to a group receiving lumbar spine surgery in a study by Weinstein et al.[39]

Ackerman and Ahmad[40] randomized 90 patients with lumbar radicular pain caused by disc herniation to receive up to three caudal, interlaminar, or transforaminal epidural injections under fluoroscopic guidance. Each injection included 40 mg of triamcinolone in saline (20 mL total for caudal injections and 4 mL total volume for interlaminar or transforaminal injections). At 6 months, three or fewer patients in the caudal or interlaminar groups had complete pain relief versus nine patients in the transforaminal group with complete relief. Patients with no pain relief were less common in the transforaminal group compared with the other groups. The authors concluded that the transforaminal route was superior because it was more likely to result in placement of the steroid in the anterior epidural space, the putative site of pathology.

Two randomized trials of cervical epidural steroid injections have been performed. Anderberg et al[31] compared selective nerve root proven cases of radiculitis that were randomized to either corticosteroid or local anesthetic alone. No significant differences were noted between groups. In an older study of interlaminar epidural corticosteroid administration for cervicobrachial pain, Stav et al[41] demonstrated short-term improvement in a small study of patients receiving lidocaine and steroid epidural injections. Range of motion, work status, and pain relief were superior in the epidural steroid group. Vallee et al[42] performed fluoroscopically-guided transforaminal epidural steroid injection on 34 levels for 32 patients with radicular pain caused by herniated disc or spinal stenosis. After needle placement, aspiration was performed to assist in the identification of vascular or intrathecal placement, but no contrast dye was injected. Prednisone 100 mg without local anesthetic was then injected. No complications were observed, and patients were improved at 2 weeks and 6 months. This technique is more likely to result in complications and should not be replicated (see Complications section).

In summary, the evidence seems to support the use of interlaminar, caudal, and transforaminal corticosteroid injections for radicular pain caused by spinal stenosis or disc pathology for short-term analgesia. Most studies suggest modest benefits for variable periods of 2 weeks to perhaps 3 months. The short-term benefit from epidural injections and the natural history of radicular pain may complement each other in regard to patient clinical improvement. The impact of other aggressive conservative therapies such as medications, exercise, physical therapies, and cognitive behavioral strategies combined with epidural corticosteroids has not been studied. Significant complications of epidural steroid administration can occur (see Complications section). Certain safety measures may reduce these complications, but their impact is unclear and difficult to study given the relative rarity of these serious complications. Limited head-to-head studies have been performed comparing interlaminar with transforaminal with caudal approaches to the epidural space, which may be relevant given the unique risks to the patient with each approach.

Equipment and Technique

Cervical Transforaminal

The patient is placed in the supine position with the head turned slightly opposite to the side being targeted. Depending on the angle of the flat detector or image intensifier of the fluoroscope, the optimal angle of skin entry can vary. One should mark the location of the external jugular vein and both carotid artery and internal jugular veins to avoid transgressing these structures. The surface of the skin should be superficially prepared with chlorhexidine and alcohol solution (superior to iodinated agents) and sterilely draped. Some operators choose blunt needles, some use Quincke beveled needles with the distal tip slightly curved, and others use Whitacre pencil point needles. A newer product that has a needle and catheter system designed to avoid vascular penetration has been recently marketed. No studies to date have compared whether one type of needle or whether a needle and catheter combination is superior to another in terms of the incidence of vascular penetration or catastrophic complications. A subcutaneous skin wheal is raised, and either a 25- or 22-gauge needle is selected for a coaxial fluoroscopic technique. The transverse oblique view of the intervertebral foramina should be adjusted to optimize the maximal circumference of the foramina. One approach targets the equatorial posterior aspect of the foramen, touching the superior articular process (SAP) at the posterior aspect of the foramen. The author generally targets the junction of the posterior middle third and posterior superior third of the foramen. From the SAP, the needle is "walked" into the posterior aspect of the foramen as above, making sure that an anteroposterior (AP) projection does not show the needle tip extending beyond the midsagittal plane of the cervical articular pillar.[4] The ascending and deep cervical arteries seem to enter in the more inferior aspect of the foramen and are larger at the outer aspect of the foramen. When the needle is in position, various safety measures are used, as discussed in the Complications section, including local anesthetic test dosing, real-time fluoroscopic contrast injections, and digital subtraction techniques.

Transforaminal Lumbar Epidural

The patient is placed in the prone position on the fluoroscopy table, and an oblique view is obtained with the SAP bisecting the vertebral body of the level above. The inferior aspect of the pedicle at the sagittal bisector is targeted, at approximately the 6:00 position of the pedicle at the same level. A chlorhexidine/alcohol-based prep solution is applied to sterilize the area, and sterile drapes are applied around the skin entry site. One issue of importance is the length of the needle. The authors usually use a 22- or 25-gauge 3.5-inch Quincke tip needle with a distal bend. However, many patients require a 5-inch or longer needle depending on body habitus. A skin wheal and subcutaneous infiltration, usually 1% lidocaine, allows initial needle entry, with some opting for blunt needles. Nonionic contrast injection of 0.2 to 1.0 cc should demonstrate a

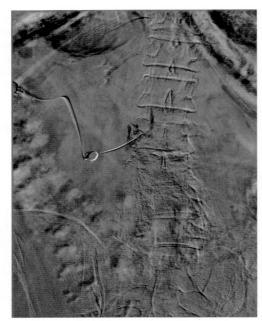

Fig. 11-5 A left L2 transforaminal epidural is shown with digital subtraction technique. Note that contrast flows medial to the pedicle into the epidural space. No vascular uptake is seen in this critical area.

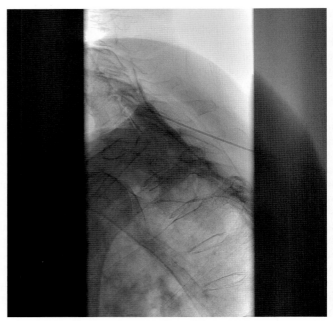

Fig. 11-6 Interlaminar cervical epidural. Note that contrast spread in the lateral view is linear and dorsal. The needle is just anterior to the base of the spinous process, a safe visual landmark.

neurogram as well as epidural spread medially and outlining the pedicle. Digital subtraction is used to substantiate lack of vascular uptake (**Fig. 11-5**). Local anesthetic test dosing with 1 cc of 1% lidocaine is also useful to prevent accidental administration of corticosteroid particulate into a feeder artery to the anterior spinal artery. Nonparticulate steroid may be used to further prevent complications.

Risk and Complication Avoidance

Previous reviews have discussed potential complications from therapeutic epidural injections. Complications are generally from the following causes: (1) needle trauma (dural puncture, spinal cord injury, spinal hematoma), (2) ischemic injury (accidental injection into or injury to an artery causing vasospasm or embolization of particulate corticosteroids [spinal cord or brain infarction]) or laceration, (3) infectious (epidural abscess, meningitis, discitis), 4) drug-related complications (e.g., iatrogenic Cushing's syndrome, steroid myopathy, avascular necrosis, or 5) miscellaneous.

Infectious Complications

In the modern era after the introduction of MRI, the spontaneous risk of epidural abscess has been reported at 0.88 persons per 100,000 per year. Most patients who develop abscesses in the spine are immunocompromised, and *Staphylococcus* species are most prevalent.[43] Gaul et al[44] reported on the cases of meningitis admitted to a neurological intensive care unit over an 8-year span during the years 1992 to 2000. Interestingly, eight of 128 patients had recently received corticosteroid spinal injections. Patients usually present within 2 weeks with worsening axial pain. A high degree of suspicion is warranted, and MRI imaging should be arranged in emergent fashion because surgical exploration and decompression may be necessary. Laboratory findings (erythrocyte sedimentation

rate and C-reactive protein) may be far more helpful than granulocyte counts in the initial evaluation.

Ischemic Complications

It has become apparent over the past decade that some apparent vascular events may be increasing in frequency and that particulate steroids might be involved through embolization of the spinal cord and brainstem, resulting in brain or spinal cord infarction. Scanlon et al[30] performed a survey of members of the American Pain Society in an attempt to glean some idea of how prevalent these complications might be. Several fatalities were reported,[45,46] suggesting that caution in performing transforaminal injections should be extremely high. Previous authors had documented that the blood supply is variable and that segmental medullary vessels in the cervical region might arise from the deep or ascending cervical arteries (or both) in addition to the vertebral arteries.[47] Baker et al[48] were the first to suggest that a sequence of safety measures should be considered, including real-time contrast injection, digital subtraction techniques, and test dosing. A recent case report[49] suggests that these cases are indeed embolic events and that they may not be confined to epidural injections but involve virtually any cervical injection in areas of critical arteries.

Needle Injuries

The most dreaded complications in the cervical spine area may well be a needle stick into the cervical spinal cord. Although these are uncommon, one should routinely examine the MRI imaging before performing an interlaminar injection to make sure that there is adequate area for the needle to enter the epidural space. Case reports of spinal injury[50] suggest that this is a necessary step. The ligamentum flavum is discontinuous above the upper thoracic region, so a characteristic loss of resistance may be absent.[51] A lateral radiograph may be helpful in determining depth of the needle after assuring that the needle is coaxial in the AP image (**Fig. 11-6**).[52]

References

1. Evans W: Intrasacral epidural injection in the treatment of sciatica. *Lancet* 1225-1229, 1930.
2. Hench PS, Kendall EC, Slocumb CH, et al: The effect of a hormone of the adrenal cortex (17-hydroxy-11-dehydrocorticosterone: Compound E) and of pituitary adrenocorticotropic hormone on rheumatoid arthritis. *Proc Staff Meet Mayo Clin* 24:181-197, 1949.
3. Robecchi A, Capra R: idrocortisone (composto F). Prime esperienze cliniche in campo reumatologico. *Minerva Med* 98:1259-1263, 1952.
4. Li'evre JA, Bloch-Michel H, Pean G, et al: hydrocortisone en injection locale. *Rev Rheum* 20:310-311, 1953.
5. Armon C, Argoff CE, Samuels J, Backonja M-M: Assessment: use of epidural steroid injections to treat radicular lumbosacral pain: report of the Therapeutics and Technology Assessment Subcommittee of the American Academy of Neurology. *Neurology* 68:723-729, 2007.
6. American College of Occupational and Environmental Medicine (ACOEM): Low back disorders. In *Occupational medicine practice guidelines: evaluation and management of common health problems and functional recovery of workers*, ed 2, Elk Grove Village, IL, 2007, American College of Occupational and Environmental Medicine.
7. Cohen SP, Bogduk N, Dragovich A, et al: Randomized, double- blind, placebo-controlled, dose- response, and pre-clinical safety study of transforaminal epidural etanercept for the treatment of sciatica. *Anesthesiology* 110:1116-1126, 2009.
8. Weinstein JN, Tosteson TD, Lurie JD, et al: Surgical vs nonoperative treatment for lumbar disk herniation The Spine Patient Outcomes research Trial (SPORT): a randomized trial. *JAMA* 296:2441-2450, 2006.
9. Weber H: Lumbar disc herniation. A controlled, prospective study with ten years of observation. *Spine* 8:131-140, 1983.
10. Atlas S, Keller R, Wu Y, et al: Long-term outcomes of surgical and nonsurgical management of sciatica secondary to lumbar disc herniation: 10 year results from the Maine Lumbar Spine Study. *Spine* 30:927-935, 2005.
11. Rhee JM, Schaufele M, Abdu WA: Radiculopathy and the herniated lumbar disc. Controversies regarding pathophysiology and management. *J Bone Joint Surg Am* 88:363-370, 2006.
12. Kuslich SD, Ulstrom CL, Michael CJ: The tissue origin of low back pain and sciatica: a report of pain response to tissue stimulation during operations on the lumbar spine using local anesthesia. *Orthop Clin North Am* 22:181-187, 1991.
13. Kawakami M, Tamaki T, Hayashi N, et al: Mechanical compression of the lumbar nerve root alters pain related behaviors induced by the nucleus pulposus in the rat. *J Orthop Res* 18:257-264, 2000.
14. Bogduk N: *Clinical anatomy of the lumbar spine and sacrum*, ed 3, Edinburgh, 1997, Churchill Livingstone.
15. Olmarker K, Rydevik B, Nordborg C: Autologous nucleus pulposus induces neurophysiologic and histologic changes in porcine cauda equine nerve roots. *Spine* 18:1425-1432, 1993.
16. Igarashi T, Kiduchi S, Shubayev V, et al: Exogenous tumor necrosis factor-alpha mimics nucleus pulposus-induced neuropathology. Molecular, histologic, and behavioural comparisons in rats. *Spine* 25:2975-2980, 2000.
17. Burke JG, Watson RWG, McCormack D, et al: Intervertebral discs which cause low back pain secrete high levels of proinflammatory mediators. *J Bone Joint Surg* 84:196-201, 2002.
18. Olmarker K, Rydevik B: Selective inhibition of tumor necrosis factor-alpha prevents nucleus induced thrombus formation, intraneural edema, and reduction of nerve conduction velocity: possible implications for future pharmacologic treatment strategy of sciatica. *Spine* 26:863-869, 2001.
19. Brown MF, Hukkanen MVJ, McCarthy ID, et al: Sensory and sympathetic innervation of the vertebral endplate in patients with degenerative disc disease. *J Bone Joint Surgery Br* 79:147-153, 1997.
20. Friedly J, Chan L, Deyo R. Increases in lumbosacral injections in the Medicare population: 1994 to 2001. *Spine* 2007; 32:1754-1760.
21. Johnsson KE, Rosen I, Uden A: The natural course of lumbar spinal stenosis. *Clin J Orthop Rel Res* 279:82-86, 1992.
22. Atlas SJ, Keller RB, Wu YA, et al: Long term outcomes of surgical and non-surgical management of lumbar spinal stenosis: 8 to 10 year results from the Maine lumbar spine study. *Spine* 30:936-943, 2005.
23. Boden SD, Davis DO, Dina TS, et al: Abnormal magnetic resonance scans of the lumbar spine in asymptomatic subjects. A prospective investigation. *J Bone Joint Am* 72:403-408, 1990.
24. el-Khoury GY, Ehara S, Weinstein JN, et al: Epidural steroid injection: a procedure ideally performed with fluoroscopic control. *Radiology* 168:554-557, 1988.
25. Johnson BA, Schellhas KP, Pollei SR: Epidurography and therapeutic epidural injections: technical considerations and experience with 5334 cases. *Am J Neuroradiology* 20:697-705, 1999.
26. Chou R, Atlas SJ, Stanos SP, Rosenquist RW: Nonsurgical interventional therapies for low back pain: a review of the evidence for an American Pain Society Clinical Practice Guideline. *Spine* 34:1078-1093, 2009.
27. Manchikanti L, Boswell MV, Singh V, et al: Comprehensive evidence-based guidelines for interventional techniques in the management of chronic spinal pain. *Pain Physician* 12:699-802, 2009.
28. American Society of Anesthesiologists: Practice guidelines for chronic pain management: an updated report by the American Society of Anesthesiologists Task Force on Chronic Pain Management and the American Society of Regional Anesthesia and Pain Medicine. *Anesthesiology* 112:810-833, 2010.
29. Van Zundert J, Huntoon M, Patijn J, et al: Cervical radicular pain. *Pain Pract* 10:1-17, 2010.
30. Scanlon GC, Moeller-Bertram T, Romanowsky SM, Wallace MS: Cervical transforaminal epidural injections: more dangerous than we think. *Spine* 11:1249-1256, 2007.
31. Anderberg L, Annertz M, Persson L, et al: Transforaminal steroid injections for the treatment of cervical radiculopathy: a prospective and randomized study. *Eur Spine J* 16:321-328, 2007.
32. Carette S, Leclaire R, Marcoux S, et al: Epidural corticosteroid injections for sciatica due to herniated nucleus pulposus. *N Engl J Med* 336:1634-1640, 1997.
33. Karppinen J, Malmivaara A, Kurunlahti M, et al: Periradicular infiltration for sciatica: a randomized controlled trial. *Spine* 26:1059-1067, 2001.
34. Riew KD, Yin Y, Gilula L, et al: The effect of nerve- root injections on the need for operative treatment of lumbar radicular pain: A prospective, randomized, controlled, double-blind study. *J Bone Joint Surgery Am* 82:1589-1593, 2000.
35. Manchikanti L, Cash KA, McManus CD, et al: Preliminary results of randomized equivalence trial of caudal epidural injections in managing chronic low back pain: part 1. Discogenic pain without disc herniation or radiculitis. *Pain Physician* 11:785-800, 2008.
36. Manchikanti L, Singh V, Cash KA, et al: Preliminary results of randomized equivalence trial of caudal epidural injections in managing chronic low back pain; part 2. Disc herniation and radiculitis. *Pain Physician* 11:801-815, 2008.
37. Manchikanti L, Singh VJ, Cash KA, et al: Preliminary results of randomized equivalence trial of caudal epidural injections in managing chronic low back pain: part 3. Post-surgical syndrome. *Pain Physician* 11:817-831, 2008.
38. Manchikanti L, Cash KA, McManus CD, et al: Preliminary results of randomized equivalence trial of fluoroscopic caudal epidural injections in managing chronic low back pain: part 4. Spinal stenosis. *Pain Physician* 11:833-848, 2008.
39. Weinstein JN, Tosteson TD, Lurie JD, et al: Surgical versus nonsurgical therapy for lumbar spinal stenosis. *N Engl J Med* 358:794-810, 2008.
40. Ackerman WE, Ahmad M: The efficacy of lumbar epidural steroid injections in patients with lumbar disc herniations. *Anesth Analg* 104:1217-1222, 2007.
41. Stav A, Ovadia L, Sternberg A, et al: Cervical epidural steroid injection for cervicobrachialgia. *Acta Anaesthesiol Scand* 37:562-566, 1993.
42. Vallee JN, Feydy A, Carlier RY, et al: Chronic cervical radiculopathy: lateral-periradicular corticosteroid injection. *Radiology* 218:886-892, 2001.

43. Ptaszynski AE, Hooten WM, Huntoon MA: The incidence of spontaneous epidural abscess in Olmsted County from 1990-2000: a rare cause of spinal pain. *Pain Med* 8:338-343, 2007.

44. Gaul C, Neundorfer B, Winterholler M: Iatrogenic (para)spinal abscesses and meningitis following injection therapy for low back pain. *Pain* 116:175-176, 2005.

45. Brouwers PJAM, Kottink EJBL, Simon MAM, Prevo RL: A cervical anterior spinal artery syndrome after diagnostic blockade of the right C6 nerve rood. *Pain* 91:397-399, 2001.

46. Rozin L, Rozin R, Koehler SA, et al: Death during transforaminal epidural steroid nerve root block (C7) due to perforation of the left vertebral artery. *Am J Forensic Med Pathol* 24(4):351-355, 2003.

47. Huntoon MA: Anatomy of the cervical intervertebral foramina: vulnerable arteries and ischemic neurologic injuries after transforaminal epidural injections. *Pain* 117:104-111, 2005.

48. Baker R, Dreyfuss P, Mercer S, Bogduk N: Cervical transforaminal injection of corticosteroids into a radicular artery: a possible mechanism for spinal cord injury. *Pain* 103:211-215, 2003.

49. Edlow BL, Wainger BJ, Frosch MP, et al: Posterior circulation stroke after c1-2 intraarticular facet steroid injection: evidence for diffuse microvascular injury. *Anesthesiology* 112:1532-1535, 2010.

50. Field J, Rathmell JP, Stephenson JH, Katz NP: Neuropathic pain following cervical epidural steroid injection. *Anesthesiology* 93:885-888, 2000.

51. Lirk P, Kolbitsch C, Putz G, et al: Cervical and high thoracic ligamentum flavum frequently fails to fuse in midline. *Anesthesiology* 99:87-90, 2003.

52. Huntoon MA: Cervical spine: case presentation, complications and their prevention. *Pain Med* 9(suppl):S35-S40, 2008.

12 Facet (Zygapophyseal) Intraarticular Joint Injections: Cervical, Lumbar, and Thoracic

Jason E. Pope and Jianguo Cheng

CHAPTER OVERVIEW

Chapter Synopsis: It is estimated that nearly half the general population experiences spinal pain. In many cases, this pain arises from the facets, the tiny, paired joints between each vertebra of the spine. Although the facet joints promote stability of the spine, they also prevent spinal injury by limiting the bones' range of motion. Naturally, these structures are richly innervated and therefore subject to painful conditions. This chapter considers the anatomical details of facets at the cervical, thoracic, and lumbar levels, which impact the procedures to inject the joints. Fluoroscopy is generally required to visualize during the injection procedure, but ultrasonography and computed tomography may also be used. Other technical details and risk of complications are also considered.

Important Points:

■ Facet arthropathy is a significant contributor to spinal pain in the cervical, thoracic, and lumbar regions.
■ Intraarticular injection or medial branch block with a small volume of local anesthetic play a critical role in establishing the diagnosis because no radiographic modality, historical, or physical exam finding has proven reliable.
■ Recent guideline statements suggested dual controlled comparative medial branch blocks with subsequent radiofrequency ablation have better evidence for outcomes, although intrarticular joint injections are more appropriate in patients who are not good candidates for radiofrequency procedures.
■ Facet injections are generally safe, but complications have been reported.

Clinical Pearls:

■ Image guidance with fluoroscopy or ultrasound is mandatory for facet injections.
■ The specificity of diagnostic intraarticular facet injection may be increased by limiting the use of intravenous sedatives or opioids and local anesthetics for anesthesia of the needle tracks.
■ The volume of intraarticular injection should be limited to 0.5 mL for cervical and thoracic facets and 1 mL for lumbar facets, as the cervical, thoracic, and lumbar facets can accommodate 0.5 to 1 mL, 0.75 mL, and 1.0 to 1.5 mL volume.
■ A reduction in concordant pain of >50% is as reliable as a >80% pain reduction in predicting therapeutic outcomes.
■ When a steroid is used in the cervical region for therapeutic purpose, a nonparticulate injectate is recommended to avoid vascular embolization.

Clinical Pitfalls:

■ Lateral approach for cervical facet injection in decubitus position is easier to perform and better tolerated by patients. However, caution should be exercised to avoid parallax of fluoroscopy images at the level of injection in order to focus on the appropriate side of injection.
■ For thoracic facet injection, careful, incremental, and measured correction and advancement of the needle should be performed to minimize the risk of pneumothorax and subarachnoid injection.
■ Strict adherence to meticulous aseptic technique is essential to avoid infectious complications.

Introduction

Spinal pain is extremely common. The incidences of pain in the neck, thoracic, and low back are estimated at 44%, 15%, and 56%, respectively, in the general population.[1] Facet arthropathy is an important source of spinal pain, and facet interventions are the second most common procedure performed in the United States by pain physicians, behind epidural steroid injections. This chapter focuses on the intraarticular injections of facet joints between vertebrae C2 through S1 for diagnostic and therapeutic purposes. The injection of the atlanto-axial joint (AAJ) between vertebrae C1-C2 is discussed elsewhere.

Prevalence of Facet Joint Pain

Estimates of lumbar facetogenic pain vary, from 15% of all back pain complaints[2] to 59.6% males and 66.7% females in the community based on a population study.[3] The prevalence of lumbar facetogenic pain, determined by placebo-controlled diagnostic blocks using a criterion of 90% pain reduction, ranges from 27% to 40% in patients with axial low back pain.[4,5] Sedation may increase false-positive rates of diagnostic blocks by 10%, but psychological comorbidity has not been shown to affect the diagnostic accuracy. Aging is positively related to the prevalence of lumbar facet arthropathy, with an occurrence of 89% in individuals 60 to 69 years old. The most common level is at L4-L5.[2]

The prevalence of thoracic facet pain ranges between 33% and 48% with a 95% confidence interval based on responses to comparative controlled diagnostic blocks.[6] The prevalence of cervical facet pain is 30% to 70% of cases[7-9] and is not significantly affected by prior surgery, psychopathology, or age. The most commonly affected facet is C4-C5 (14.62%) followed by C3-C4, C2-C3, C5-C6, and C6-C7, respectively.[10] There is no proven correlation between clinical manifestation of facetogenic pain and facet arthrosis shown by imaging studies or cadaveric observations. Diagnostic block remains the best available tool to identify facetogenic pain despite its high false-positive rates (39% to 53%).

Thus, facet arthropathy accounts for approximately 40% of axial cervical and thoracic pain and approximately 30% of axial lumbar pain. The most commonly affected levels are C4-C5 at the cervical region and L4-L5 at the lumbar region. Whereas lumbar facet pain is more age dependent, predominantly occurring in elderly adults, cervical and thoracic facet pain is not significantly affected by age.

Establishing Diagnosis

Numerous studies have attempted to determine the historical, or physical, and radiographic findings that correlate with pain associated with facet arthropathy. None has been proven specific, sensitive, and reliable.[2] Consequently, diagnosis is primarily based on pain reduction and mobility improvement in response to controlled diagnostic facet blocks.[4,6,11] The diagnosis of facetogenic pain is suggested by controlled comparative (lidocaine/bupivacaine) medial branch blocks. A criterion of 80% pain reduction and the ability to perform maneuvers that were painful before the diagnostic intervention are commonly used. However, a recent study suggests that using 50% pain reduction as a criterion for positive

diagnostic block is just as effective as using 80% pain reduction in predicting the outcomes of medial branch radiofrequency ablation.[12]

Even though facetogenic pain is primarily determined by diagnostic blocks, clinical findings from history and physical examinations usually help physicians decide if diagnostic facet blocks are warranted. For example, pain from the AAJ is typically provoked by head rotation with the neck slightly flexed forward. This information may lead to an AAJ block rather than a cervical facet block. Therefore, taking the patient history and performing a physical examination is still an indispensable step in establishing a diagnosis of facet pain. Pain referral patterns for cervical and thoracic facet pain have been generated,[2,13-15] as shown in **Fig. 12-1**.

Cervical Facet Pain

Restricted range of motion is not pathognomonic for facet pain and can present in a variety of neck disorders, such as whiplash injury. Point tenderness was recently evaluated in 33 patients by assessing pain pressure thresholds in symptomatic and asymptomatic facets joints.[16] Although the pain pressure thresholds are significantly lower in patients with neck pain, this approach is not diagnostic for cervical facet joint pain. Neck point tenderness can be indicative of myofascial pain or associated with tension headache.[17] No provocative tests tend to produce pain in the referral patterns. As a general rule, the upper facet joints may cause headache, and the lower joints may have pain referred to the shoulder in a nondermatomal distribution. Cervical radicular pain is usually absent.

Thoracic Facet Pain

Pain from thoracic facet joints may be provoked by facet capsule distention,[14] such as extension, lateral bending, and twisting or paraspinal pressure overlying the facet joints. Pain is often nonradicular, and there is no associated weakness.

Lumbar Facet Pain

Lumbar facet joint pain is typically described as back pain with or without nondermatomal leg pain above the knee. Paraspinal tenderness overlying the facets produced by pressure is suggestive.[18] Facet pain is typically not confined to a dermatomal distribution (nonradicular). Motor function and reflex assessment are usually intact.

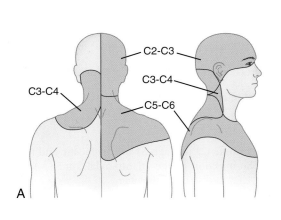
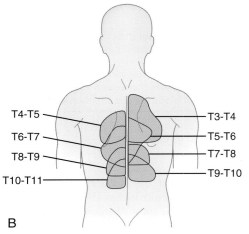

Fig. 12-1 Maps of referred pain from the cervical (**A**) and thoracic (**B**) facets. (Part A adapted from Bogduk N, Marland A: The cervical zygapophysial joints as a source of neck pain, *Spine* 13:610-617, 1988; part B adapted from Dreyfuss P, Tibiletti C, Dreyer SJ: Thoracic zygapophyseal joint pain patterns: a study in normal volunteers, *Spine* 19:807-811, 1994.)

Anatomy of the Facet Joints

The vertebral column most commonly consists of seven cervical, 12 thoracic, and five lumbar vertebrae. Two adjacent vertebrae make joint connections through the intervertebral disc in the front and a pair of facet joints in the back, with the exception of C1-C2 vertebrae. The facet is a true synovial joint between the inferior and superior articular processes composed of a synovial membrane, hyaline cartilage, and fibrous capsule. These joints function to support the stability of the spine and prevent injury by limiting excessive motion in all directions.

The facet joints have rich innervation, including encapsulated, unencapsulated, and free nerve endings.[2] These innervations provide nociception through C and A-δ afferents as well as proprioception through low-threshold, rapidly adapting mechanoreceptors.[19] Immunocytochemistry of facet joints demonstrated the presence of substance P, calcitonin-gene-related peptide, and neuropeptide Y, suggesting pain transmission and sympathetic fibers.[20-22] Facet joint distraction in rats produces spinal astrocyte activation and persistent mechanical allodynia.[23] The expression of a binding protein BiP, also known as growth-related protein 78, is upregulated 2.1-fold in the dorsal root ganglion after painful distraction injury to the rat C6-C7 facet, indicating neuronal stress activation.[24] Cytokines and neurotrophic factors are upregulated in dorsal root ganglion neurons in models of facet joint inflammation.[25-28]

The architecture and orientation of the facet joint vary with function and position along the vertebral column.[29-31] The lumbar facet joint can accommodate an average of 1 to 1.5 mL fluid. The joint is C shaped and is encased posteriorly in a fibrous capsule of approximately 1 mm thick composed of collagenous tissue. The lumbar facet joint is supported posteriorly by multifidus muscle, superiorly and inferiorly by fibroadipose menisci forming subcapsular recesses, and anteriorly by the ligamentum flavum.[31] The inferior portion of the joint is larger than the superior portion. Any given facet joint has dual innervation from two segmental medial branch nerves: one arising at the given level and one from one segment above as shown in **Fig. 12-2**. Consequently, a given medial branch nerve innervates two facet joints, the ascending branch to the caudal portion of the facet above and the descending branch to superior portion of the facet below. For example, the L3 medial branch nerve courses along the junction of the superior articular process and the transverse process of L4 under the mamilloaccessory ligament, supplying the caudal portion of the ipsilateral L3-L4 facet joint, and then courses caudally to supply the ipsilateral superior portion of the L4-L5 facet joint. Conversely, the L3-L4 facet has dual innervation from the L2 and L3 medial branches.

The thoracic facet joint can accommodate no more than 0.75 mL of fluid and is more vertically oriented than the lumbar or cervical facet joints. On average, they are approximately 75 degrees from the sagittal and transverse planes. Similar to the lumbar facets, the thoracic facet joints also have dual innervation. The dorsal ramus arises from the lateral margin of the intervertebral foramen and then courses dorsally, inferiorly, and laterally within the intertransverse space, where it continues over the superolateral portion of the transverse process and runs between the semispinalis thoracis and thoracic multifidus. The dorsal surface of the transverse process is the bony landmark for thoracic medial branch nerve at T1-T4 and T9-T10 levels. The T11-T12 medial branch courses have similar anatomical relationships to the lumbar medial branch nerves as described. It is important to note that the course of the thoracic medial branch differs from lumbar and in some cases does not contact the transverse process. The lack of

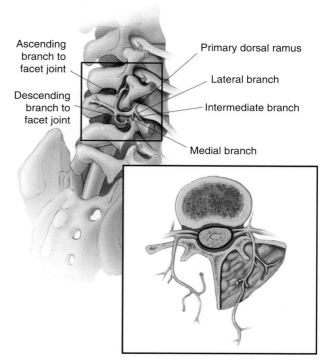

Fig. 12-2 Schematic illustration of lumbar facet innervations. (Adapted from Cohen SP, Raja SN: Pathogenesis, diagnosis, and treatment of lumbar zygapophysial (facet) joint pain, *Anesthesiology* 106:591-614, 2007.)

association with a bony landmark, particularly at T5-T8, makes the thoracic facet medial branch a challenging target for percutaneous interventional procedures.

The cervical facet joints are between the articular pillars of the vertebrae and are oriented approximately 45 degrees from the transverse plain and 80 degrees from the sagittal. The cervical facet joint can accommodate approximately 0.5 to 1.0 mL of fluid. The lateral recess is the target for percutaneous intervention, formed by a thick lateral fibrous capsule and synovial-lined recesses. There is some anatomical variability with the innervation of the cervical facet joints. The medial branch nerve arises from the posterior ramus and passes around the ipsilateral articular pillar, and similar to the thoracic and lumbar facet joints, innervate two joints. Therefore, a given medial branch nerve innervates the inferior portion of the superior facet joint and the superior portion of the inferior facet joint. For example, the C4 medial branch nerve innervates the inferior portion of the C3-C4 facet and the superior portion of the C4-C5 facet. Conversely, each facet joint receives medial branches from above and below. The posterior rami in the cervical region provide little innervation to the paraspinal muscles. Fascia and tendons of the semispinalis capitis muscle ensure the medial branches are adjacent to the periosteum.

Special attention is required for the C2-C3 facet joint and the C1-C2 (atlanto-axial) joint. There are four occipital nerves that may contribute to neck pain and headaches. The suboccipital nerve is the dorsal primary rami of C1. The greater occipital nerve is the medial branch of dorsal primary rami of C2. The lesser occipital nerve is the ventral primary rami of C2 and C3. The least occipital nerve, or third occipital nerve, is the medial sensory branch of dorsal ramus of C3. The C2-C3 facet receives the majority of its innervation from the C3 dorsal ramus. The C1, C2, and C3 nerves have been implicated in the trigeminocervical complex as a source of headaches.

Guidelines for Intervention

The latest published practice guidelines for chronic pain management by the American Society of Anesthesiologists Task Force on Chronic Pain Management and the American Society of Regional Anesthesia and Pain Medicine state:

> *Randomized controlled trials report equivocal findings regarding the efficacy of facet joint steroid injections compared with facet saline injections regarding pain relief for patients with low back pain (Category C2 evidence). However, studies with observational findings for facet joint injections indicate that pain scores are improved over baseline scores for assessment periods of 1-6 months (Category B2 evidence). … Intraarticular facet joint injections may be used for symptomatic relief of facet-mediated pain.*[32]

In addition, a recent prospective study tested intraarticular injection of hylan G-F 20 in patients with painful lumbar facet joint arthropathy and reported significant improvement in pain scores, quality of life, and opioid consumption for 6 months.[33] Studies of injecting nonsteroid agents may represent a new direction of intraarticular facet therapy.

The American Society of Interventional Pain Physicians did not recommend intraarticular injections for either diagnostic or therapeutic benefit.[34] The International Spine Intervention Society described guidelines for thoracic intraarticular facet joint blocks as an emerging procedure and did not comment on intraarticular lumbar or cervical facet joint blocks.[35] Both guidelines suggest better evidence (level I or II) with medial branch blocks for diagnosis and radiofrequency ablation for therapeutic benefit after two positive comparative controlled diagnostic blocks using 80% pain reduction. However, for patients who are not ideal candidates for radiofrequency ablation, such as those with pacemakers, intraarticular facet block with a mixture of local anesthetic and steroid is a viable option.

Indications and Contraindications

Facet interventions are indicated in patients with moderate to severe spinal pain that is somatic and nonradicular (or headache), lasts longer than 3 months in duration, with functional limitation or impairment; failure of more conservative therapies (exercise, physical therapy, simple analgesics); and lack of evidence supporting primarily a discogenic, myofascial, or radicular pain source. Importantly, the patient should have the ability to undergo physical therapy after the intervention.[34,35]

Contraindications include anything that would preclude neuraxial procedures, such as lack of informed consent; hemodynamic instability; coagulopathy or thrombocytopenia; pregnancy; infection overlying the puncture site; inability to see target site secondary to hardware; inability of the patient to lie in the procedure position; or allergy to contrast, steroids, local anesthetics, and so on. Readers are referred to American Society of Regional Anesthesia and Pain Medicine guidelines for regional anesthesia and anticoagulation.[36]

Techniques for Facet Joint Injection

Informed consent is obtained before an intravenous line is placed in a preblock room. The site of the procedure is labeled, and the

---

Equipment

Fluoroscopy setup
Radiolucent table
Anesthesia monitors for ECG, pulse oximetry, and blood pressure
22- or 25-gauge 3.5-inch spinal needle
26-gauge 1-inch needle for subcutaneous infiltration
1% lidocaine for subcutaneous infiltration (methylparaben free)
0.5% bupivacaine (methylparaben free)
Triamcinolone 40 mg or dexamethasone 7.5 mg
Low osmolar nonionic contrast media or iso-osmolar nonionic contrast media 3 mL
Three sterile Luer lock 3-mL syringes
Optional sterile 1-mL tubing
Betadine, alcohol, or Hibiclens prep
Sterile 4 × 4 inch gauze
Sterile drape or sterile towels
Lead apron, thyroid shield, lead glasses
Sterile gloves, mask, surgical cap

ECG, electrocardiography.

---

patient is transported to the procedure room, where the patient is positioned either in the lateral decubitus position with the procedure side up or in a prone position, depending on the level of injections in the spine. Patients are monitored with standard ASA monitors that include three-lead electrocardiography, pulse oximetry, and noninvasive blood pressure measurement at least every 5 minutes. A sign-in process is performed to confirm the patient's identity, allergies, procedure site, body position, and necessary equipment. Light sedation with anxiolytics such as benzodiazepines and fast-acting opioids are sometimes used, although it is often unnecessary. Heavy sedation, with propofol in particular, is not recommended to ensure effective communication with the patient during the procedure.

Cervical Facet

Lateral Approach The patient is self-positioned in the lateral decubitus position with the symptomatic side up. The head is placed in the neutral position or slightly extended to the contralateral side (supporting side) to facilitate needle placement. The site is prepped and draped in sterile fashion. The articular pillars and vertebral endplates are aligned under lateral view of fluoroscopy so there is no parallax at the level of the injection site. After the targeted facet has been identified, a radiopaque marker is placed on the skin to localize the entry point, where 1 mL of 1% lidocaine is injected and a 25-gauge 3.5-inch spinal needle is advanced in plane coaxial approach to contact the targeted facet joint under intermittent fluoroscopy guidance. Nonionic contrast of 0.1 to 0.2 mL is injected under a "live" fluoroscopic view to ensure intraarticular filling without vascular spread as shown in **Fig. 12-3** (compare *A* and *B*, before and after 0.1 mL contrast injection at the C4-C5 facet as indicated by the *arrows*). The joint accommodates between 0.5 to 1 mL of volume. After proper needle position has been confirmed, 0.5 mL of local anesthetic is injected for diagnostic purposes or a combination of 0.5 mL of local anesthetic and steroid is injected for therapeutic purposes. The needle is then slowly removed, the skin is cleaned, and a bandage is applied, and the patient is transported to the postblock recovery area. It is noteworthy that a true lateral view is critically important to avoid inadvertent entry of the needle into the spinal canal. Also, the needle should first contact the articular pillar of the targeted facet joint and then walk off the pillar to enter the joint to avoid overshoot of the needle into the spinal canal.

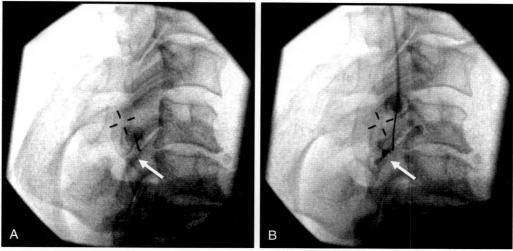

Fig. 12-3 Cervical facet intraarticular injection: lateral approach. **A,** Spinal needle is placed in the C4-C5 facet joint (*arrow*). **B,** Injection of 0.1 mL of contrast partially filled the facet joint (*arrow*).

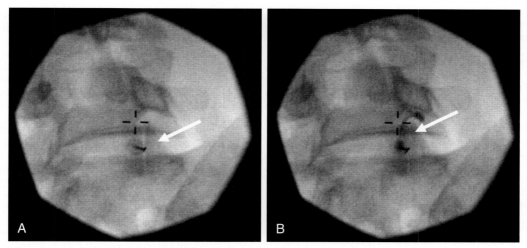

Fig. 12-4 Lumbar facet intraarticular injection. **A,** Spinal needle is placed in the L5-S1 facet joint (*arrow*). **B,** Injection of 0.1 mL contrast partially filled the facet joint (*arrow*).

Posterior Approach The patient is self-positioned prone with the head in neutral position. The skin is prepped and draped in sterile fashion. The C-arm is rotated slightly oblique and then caudad to align the X-ray beam parallel to the surface plane of the facet joint. After the trajectory has been determined, the spinal needle is advanced under intermittent fluoroscopic guidance into the joint, maintaining a coaxial view of the needle. The rest of the injection is the same as for the lateral approach.

Thoracic Facet

The patient is in the prone position with the head in a neutral position. After the targeted vertebral levels have been identified, the skin is prepped and draped in sterile fashion. The endplates of the superior and inferior articular processes are aligned with the fluoroscopy beam. The facet joint is in between the pedicles of the adjacent vertebrae. Using a 25-gauge 3.5-inch spinal needle, the entry site is caudal to the target facet joint along an ipsilateral interpedicular line. Using intermittent anteroposterior fluoroscopy, the needle is advanced in a cephalad, anterior direction along an ipsilateral interpedicular parasagittal plane until osteal laminar

contact is made on the caudal vertebral body. Contralateral oblique lateral fluoroscopic imaging can confirm appropriate needle placement and should be used to enter into the caudal portion of the facet joint. If the needle deviates medially from the ipsilateral interpedicular parasagittal plane, it may risk entering the epidural space; if the needle trajectory is lateral, it may injure the pleura of the lung. The joint accommodates 0.75 mL volume. Under "live" fluoroscopy, 0.1 mL of contrast is injected to ensure nonvascular spread. After proper needle position has been confirmed, for diagnostic and therapeutic purposes, 0.5 mL of local anesthetic or a combination of local anesthetic and steroid is injected. The needle is then slowly removed, a bandage is applied, and the patient is transported to the postblock area.

Lumbar Facet

The patient is self-positioned prone. The skin is prepped and draped in sterile fashion. The targeted facet is identified with fluoroscopy, and the C-arm is rotated ipsilateral oblique (25 to 35 degrees) to "open" the facet joint (**Fig. 12-4**). Sometimes a caudocranial angulation of the C-arm (image intensifier toward the head) is required to better visualize the joint space in between the superior and inferior articular processes. The needle is advanced in a coaxial manner with intermittent fluoroscopy to enter in caudal pole of the facet joint. The lumbar facet joint accommodates 1 to 1.5 mL of volume. After the needle has been engaged, 0.1 mL of contrast may be injected, confirming intraarticular spread as shown in **Fig. 12-4** (compare *A* and *B*, before and after contrast injection at the L5-S1 facet as indicated by the *arrows*). After proper needle position has been confirmed, for diagnostic purposes, 0.5 mL of local anesthetic is injected; for therapeutic purposes, a combination of 0.5 to 1 mL of local anesthetic and steroid is injected. The needle is then slowly removed, a bandage is applied, and the patient is transported to the postblock recovery area.

Imaging

Multidirectional C-arm fluoroscopy is required to perform the blocks using a radiolucent table. Fluoroscopy with film archiving capability is suggested. Ultrasonography is an emerging modality to guide needle placement in the cervical region for intraarticular facet injection and medial branch blocks. Computed tomography has also been used.

Patient Management and Evaluation

The patient should be monitored in the recovery room for at least 15 minutes after the procedure. Relief of concordant pain and increased mobility of provocative movements are assessed before discharge. Written discharge instructions include limiting activities the day of the procedure; resuming all activities the next day; and contacting the physician if there is any weakness, fever, chills, or erythema or induration at the site of the procedure. A pain diary and globally perceived effect are commonly used for evaluation of the outcome.

Outcomes Evidence

There was limited evidence supporting intraarticular anesthetic or steroid injection for diagnostic or therapeutic purposes.[5,6,11] Nevertheless, intraarticular injection can be used in patients who are not ideal candidates for radiofrequency ablation of the facet medial branches, such as those with pacemakers. Furthermore, lumbar facet intraarticular injection of hylan G-F 20 appears effective in pain reduction, improving quality of life, and reducing opioid consumption for 6 months.[33]

Risk and Complication Avoidance

Facet joint injection is generally considered to be a very safe procedure. However, significant complications have been reported, including spinal cord injury associated with cervical facet injection and pneumothorax associated with thoracic facet injections.[37] Vascular injection of local anesthetics or steroids is a concern associated with spinal procedures. The radicular arteries are the main source of blood to the spinal cord and usually enter the spinal canal in the cervical region through the neuroforamen accompanying the C4-C6 nerve roots.[38] Pneumothorax is a concern for any paraspinal thoracic procedure. Other complications reported after facet injections include spondylodiscitis, meningitis and chemical meningism, septic arthritis, and epidural abscess.[37] Postdural puncture headache has also been reported.[39] The effect on the hypothalamic–pituitary–adrenal axis is likely similar to that of epidural steroid injections.[40]

Many of these complications may be prevented by observing strict aseptic techniques and by performing the procedures with clear understanding of the anatomy and the techniques. Adequate monitoring, early detection, aggressive treatment, and accurate documentation are required when complications do occur to minimize the adverse outcomes.[37]

References

1. Linton SJ, Hellsing AL, Hallden K: A population based study of spinal pain among 35-45-year-old individuals. *Spine* 23:1457-1463, 1998.
2. Cohen SP, Raja SN: Pathogenesis, diagnosis, and treatment of lumbar zygapophysial (facet) joint pain. *Anesthesiology* 106:591-614, 2007.
3. Kalichman L, Li L, Kim DH, et al: Facet joint osteoarthritis and low back pain in the community-based population. *Spine* 33:2560-2565, 2008.
4. Datta S, Lee M, Falco FJ, et al: Systematic assessment of diagnostic accuracy and therapeutic utility of lumbar facet joint interventions. *Pain Physician* 12:437-460, 2009.
5. Schwarzer AC, Wang S, Bogduk N, et al: Prevalence and clinical features of lumbar zygapophysial joint pain: a study in an Australian population with chronic low back pain. *Ann Rheum Dis* 54:100-106, 1995.
6. Alturi S, Datta S, Falco FJE, Lee M: Systematic review of diagnostic utility and therapeutic effectiveness of thoracic facet joint interventions. *Pain Physician* 11:611-629, 2008.
7. Manchikanti L, Manchikanti KN, Pampati V, et al: The prevalence of facet-joint-related chronic neck pain in postsurgical and nonpostsurgical patients: a comparative evaluation. *Pain Pract* 8:5-10, 2008.
8. Lord SM, Barnsley L, Wallis BJ, Bogduk N: Chronic zygapophysial joint pain after whiplash: A placebo-controlled prevalence study. *Spine* 21:1737-1744, 1996.
9. Manchukonda R, Manchikanti KN, Cash KA, et al: Facet joint pain in chronic spinal pain: An evaluation of prevalence and false-positive rate of diagnostic blocks. *J Spinal Disord Tech* 20:539-545, 2007.
10. Lee MJ, Riew KD: The prevalence cervical facet arthrosis: an osseous study in a cadaveric population. *Spine J* 9:711-714, 2009.
11. Falco FJ, Erhart S, Wargo BW, et al: Systematic review of diagnostic utility and therapeutic effectiveness of cervical facet joint interventions. *Pain Physician* 12:323-344, 2009.
12. Cohen SP, Stojanovic MP, Crooks M, et al: Lumbar zygapophysial (facet) joint radiofrequency denervation success as a function of pain relief during diagnostic medial branch blocks: a multicenter analysis. *Spine J* 8:498-504, 2008.
13. Bogduk N, Marsland A: The cervical zygapophysial joints as a source of neck pain. *Spine* 13:610-617, 1988.
14. Dreyfuss P, Tibiletti C, Dreyer SJ: Thoracic zygapophyseal joint pain patterns: a study in normal volunteers. *Spine* 19:807-811, 1994.
15. Dwyer A, Aprill C, Bogduk N: Cervical zygapophyseal joint pain patterns: a study in normal volunteers. *Spine* 15:453-457, 1990.
16. Siegenthaler A, Eichenberger U, Schmidlin K, et al: What does local tenderness say about the origin of pain? An investigation of cervical zygapophysial joint pain. *Anesth Analg* 110:923-927, 2010.
17. Headache Classification Subcommittee of the International Headache Society: The International Classification of Headache Disorders: 2nd edition. *Cephalalgia* 24(suppl 1):9-160, 2004.
18. Cohen SP, Hurley RW, Christo PJ, et al: Clinical predictors of success and failure for lumbar facet radiofrequency denervation. *Clin J Pain* 23:45-52, 2007.
19. Cavanaugh JM, Ozaktay AC, Yamashita HT, King AI: Lumbar facet pain: biomechanics, neuroanatomy and neurophysiology. *J Biomech* 29:1117-1119, 1996.
20. Ashton IK, Ashton BA, Gibson SJ et al: Morphological basis for back pain: the demonstration of nerve fibers and neuropeptides in the lumbar facet joint capsule but not in the ligamentum flavum. *J Orthop Res* 10:72-78, 1992.
21. Bucknill AT, Coward K, Plumpton C, et al: Nerve fibers in lumbar spine structures and injured spinal roots express the sensory

neuron-specific sodium channels SNS/PN3 and NaN/SNS2. *Spine* 27:135-140, 2002.

22. Miyagi M, Ohtori S, Ishikawa T, et al: Up-regulation of TNF alpha in DRG satellite cells following lumbar facet joint injury in rats. *Eur Spine J* 15: 953-958, 2006.

23. Dong L, Odeleye A, Jordan-Sciutto KL, Winkelstein BA: Painful facet injury induces neuronal stress activation in the DRG: Implications for cellular mechanism of pain. *Neurosci Lett* 443:90-94, 2008.

24. Fukui S, Ohseto K, Shiotani M: Patterns of pain induced by distending the thoracic zygapophyseal joints. *Reg Anesth* 22:332-336, 1997.

25. Cavanaugh JM, Lu Y, Chen C, Kallakuri S: Pain generation in lumbar and cervical facet joints. *J Bone Joint Surg Am* 88:63-67, 2006.

26. Ohtori S, Takahashi K, Chiba T, et al: Sensory innervation of the cervical facet joints in rats. *Spine* 26:147-150, 2001.

27. Cavanaugh JM, Ozaktay AC, Yamashita HT, King AI: Lumbar facet pain: biomechanics, neuroanatomy and neurophysiology. *J Biomech* 29:1117-1129, 1996.

28. Masharawi, Y, Rothschild B, Dar G, et al: Facet orientation in the thoracolumbar spine: Three dimensional anatomic and biochemical analysis. *Spine* 29:1755-1763, 2004.

29. Punjabi MM, Oxland T, Takata K, et al: Articular facets of the human spine. Quantitative three-dimensional anatomy. *Spine* 18:1298-1310, 1993.

30. Rathmell JP: *Atlas of image-guided intervention in regional anesthesia and pain medicine*, Philadelphia, 2006, Lippincott.

31. Bogduk N: *Clinical anatomy of the lumbar spine and sacrum*, ed 3, Edinburgh, 1997, Churchill Livingstone, pp 33-42.

32. Practice guidelines for chronic pain management: an updated report by the American Society of Anesthesiologists Task Force on Chronic Pain Management and the American Society of Regional Anesthesia and Pain Medicine. *Anesthesiology* 112:810-833, 2010.

33. DePalma MJ, Ketchum JM, Queler ED, Trussell BS: Prospective pilot study of painful lumbar facet joint arthropathy after intra-articular injection of hylan G-F 20. *PM R* 1:908-915, 2009.

34. Manchikanti L, Boswell MV, Singh V, et al: comprehensive evidence-based guidelines for interventional techniques in the management of chronic spinal pain. *Pain Physician* 12:699-802, 2009.

35. Bogduk N, editor: International Spine Intervention Society: *Practice guidelines: spinal diagnostics and treatment procedures*, Kentfield, CA, 2004, Standards Committee of the International Spine Intervention Society.

36. Horlocker TT, Wedel DJ, Rowlingson JC, et al: Regional anesthesia in the patient receiving antithrombotic or thrombolytic therapy: ASRA evidence-based guidelines (third edition). *Reg Anesth Pain Med* 35:64-101, 2010.

37. Cheng J, Abdi S: Complications of joint, tendon and muscle injections. *Tech Reg Anesth Pain Manag* 11:141-147, 2007.

38. Chakravorty BG: Arterial supply of the cervical spinal cord (with special reference to the radicular arteries). *Anat Rec* 170:311-329, 1970.

39. Cohen SP: Postdural puncture headache and treatment following successful lumbar facet block. *Pain Digest* 4:283-284, 1994.

40. Kay J, Findling JW, Raff H: Epidural triamcinolone suppresses the pituitary-adrenal axis in human subjects. *Anesth Analg* 79:501-505, 1994.

13 Medial Branch Blocks: Cervical, Thoracic, and Lumbar

Seth A. Waldman, Vinita Parikh, and Dawood Sayed

CHAPTER OVERVIEW

Chapter Synopsis: Zygapophyseal (facet joints) are a common cause of axial back pain. Blockade of the corresponding medial branches to the corresponding joint can lead to significant reductions in patient pain scores and increase in function.

Important Points:
- Radiographic imaging is nonspecific in the diagnosis of facetogenic mediated back pain.
- Findings on radiographs, computed tomography, and magnetic resonance imaging are often inconclusive.
- Diagnostic local anesthetic nerve blocks of the medial branches are the best way to diagnose facet pain.

Clinical Pearls:
- It is important to know the location of the medial branches at the different levels in the spine.
- Needle placement differs when performing cervical, thoracic, or lumbar medial branch blocks.

Clinical Pitfalls:
- It is vital to realize the innervation of the facet joints as the facet joints receive dual innervation from two spinal nerves.
- The physician must block the medial branches at the appropriate levels.

Establishing a Diagnosis

History and Physical Examination

History and physical examination are important for exclusion of other causes of spinal pain. On reviewing the medical history, several conditions can affect the facet joints. These include osteoarthritis, inflammatory arthritides (rheumatoid arthritis, ankylosing spondylitis, and reactive arthritis), synovial impingement, meniscoid entrapment, chondromalacia facetae, pseudogout, synovial inflammation, and villonodular synovitis.[1-4] Signs on clinical examination that may point to facet pain include tenderness over the facet joints on palpation; pain that is characterized as deep, dull, and aching; pain that is difficult to localize; and stiffness, especially in the morning. Sudden onset of pain noted with twisting, bending, or rotary movements and pain aggravated on extension and lateral bending more than flexion are also consistent with facet joint–mediated pain, although the latter finding is unreliable. Additional physical examination findings may include muscle spasm and either hypalgesia or hyperalgesia over the area of pain. Flexion, extension, and rotation may or may not be decreased. The straight-leg raise results are usually negative. Given all of the above, the clinical criteria for facet joint–mediated pain are generally nonspecific and unreliable.[5-7] Most maneuvers used in physical examinations are likely to stress several structures simultaneously, especially the discs, muscles, and facet joints, thus failing to provide any reasonable diagnostic criteria based on physical examination.

As stated previously, history and physical examination, along with radiologic imaging, cannot reliably be used to diagnose painful zygapophyseal joints. Therefore, medical branch blocks are needed to diagnose facetogenic pain.[8] Numerous studies have tried to predict who will respond to facet joint injections. Revel et al[9] identified seven variables associated with a positive response to facet joint injections: age older than 65 years, pain that was not exacerbated by coughing, pain not worsened by hyperextension, pain not worsened by forward flexion, pain not worsened when rising from flexion, pain not worsened by extension-rotation, and pain well relieved by recumbency. A later study by Revel et al[10] found the presence of five among seven variables distinguished 92% of the patients responding to lidocaine injection and 80% of those not responding to lidocaine. However, further investigations of Revel et al's variables by other investigators have been proven wrong.[5]

Injections in Facilitating the Diagnosis

Facet joint–mediated pain can be diagnosed with placebo-controlled or controlled local anesthetic diagnostic blocks using either facet joint blocks or medial branch blocks. The choice of technique used should be based on evidence of effectiveness of diagnosis and ease of technique. Evidence for diagnostic medial branch blocks using 80% pain relief with controlled diagnosed blocks are noted to be Level I or II-1 based on U.S. Preventive Services Task Force criteria.[11,12] Medial branch blocks are relatively easier to perform and safer than intraarticular blocks because medial branch blocks can be performed even with osteophyte formation, which prevents entry into the facet joint. Additionally, the target area of the medial branch prevents overpenetration of the needle into the spinal canal during placement, therefore decreasing the possibility that the needle will pass through the target and into the spinal canal and cord, which can occur during intraarticular injections. Medial branch blocks also have therapeutic validity, but the therapeutic validity of intraarticular injection is lacking.[11]

False-positive rates of single local anesthetic blocks are high, ranging from 27% to 63% for cervical, 42% to 58% for thoracic, and 21% to 33% for lumbar medial branch blocks.[12-14]

Because of high false-positive rate of single local anesthetic blocks, numerous experts advocate performing diagnostic double blocks with either saline control or two different local anesthetics. Control blocks using normal saline under double-blind conditions is the most rigorous form of control blocks, requiring three blocks of the same joint. The first block would have to be with the local anesthetic to establish prima facie that the joint is symptomatic. To maintain the controlling effect of change and blinding, the second block would have to be either normal saline or inactive agent, and the third block would need to be the reciprocal agent.[8] Despite this evidence, in a systematic study of the cost-effectiveness of using controlled facet blocks, Bogduk and Holmes[15] determined that the use of placebo-controlled injections cannot be justified in the United States based on financial considerations.

In clinical practice, controlled diagnostic blocks with two local anesthetics with different durations are used. A true-positive response is one in which the patient reports complete relief of pain for a shorter duration when short-acting local anesthetic is used and a longer duration when a long-acting agent is used.[16] Lidocaine 1% to 2% commonly used for the first block with a positive response is followed by a later block with bupivacaine 0.25% to 0.5% 2 to 4 weeks later.[11,17] Response patterns of medial branch blocks using bupivacaine and lidocaine were defined by Barnsley et al.[16]

1. **Concordant response:** The patient experiences long-lasting relief after bupivacaine but short-lasting relief after lidocaine with relief in both instances lasting no longer than the expected duration of action of the agent used.
2. **Prolonged concordant response:** The patient experiences a longer lasting relief after bupivacaine than that after lidocaine, but the duration of relief with either or both agents exceeds the expected duration of action of the anesthetic used.
3. **Discordant response:** The patient achieves relief after lidocaine that is longer than that after bupivacaine, but relief in either instance is within the expected duration of action of the agent used.
4. **Discordant prolonged response:** The patient experiences relief after lidocaine that is longer than that after bupivacaine, but relief after either anesthetic is longer than the expected duration of action of the agent used.
5. **Discrepant response:** The patient fails to experience relief when the same nerves are blocked on a second trial.

A concordant response confirms that the joint is the source of pain with confidence of 85%.[18]

Anatomy

The Facet Joint
The basic anatomical unit of the spine is referred to as a three-joint complex that consists of paired zygapophyseal joints and an intervertebral disc (**Fig. 13-1**).[19] This articular triad functions to stabilize and support the spine along with limiting motion of the spine.

The term *zygapophyseal joint* (or facet joint) originated from the Greek root *zygos*, meaning yoke or bridge, and *physis*, meaning outgrowth. Therefore, the facet joints bridge the vertebrae behind the vertebral foramina.[20] Facet joints are paired diarthrodial synovial joints formed by inferior articular process of one vertebra and superior articular process of the subjacent vertebra. Facet joints share the same general characteristics of synovial joints. As true

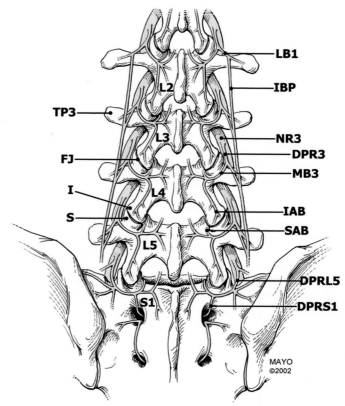

Fig. 13-1 Illustration of the posterior view of the lumbar spine and the posterior neural structures. Laminae of L2 through S1 are labeled. DPRL5, dorsal primary ramus of L5; DPRS1, dorsal primary ramus of S1; DPR3, dorsal primary ramus of L3; FJ, facet (zygapophyseal) joint L3-L4; I, inferior articular process of L4; LB1, lateral branch of dorsal primary ramus of L1; IAB, inferior articular branches from L3 medial branch (supplies L4-L5 facet joint); IBP, intermediate branch plexus; MB3, medial branch of dorsal primary ramus of L3; NR3, third lumbar nerve root; S, superior articular process of L5; SAB, superior articular branches from L4 (supplies L4-5 facet joint also); TP3, transverse process of L3. (Copyright © 2003 by Mayo Foundation for Medical Education and Research.)

synovial joints, each facet joint contains distinct joint space capable of accommodating 1 to 1.5 mL of fluid, a synovial membrane, hyaline cartilage surfaces, and fibrous capsule. The fibrous capsule of the facet joint is composed mostly of collagenous tissue arranged more or less in transverse fashion to provide maximum resistance to flexion. The thick fibrous joint capsule is covered by synovial membrane superiorly, posteriorly, and inferiorly. Anteriorly, the synovial membrane lacks a true fibrous capsule and instead is in direct contact with the ligamentum flavum.[19]

Facet joints are richly innervated with three types of nerve endings: encapsulated (Ruffini-type endings, pacinian corpuscles), unencapsulated, and free nerve endings.[19] The presence of low-threshold, rapidly adapting mechanosensitive neurons lining the facet capsule suggests that in addition to transmitting nociceptive information, the facet capsule also serves proprioceptive function.[21,22]

Facet capsule nerve endings contain substance P, calcitonin gene-related peptide, and neuropeptide Y.[23,24] Inflammatory mediators such as prostaglandins, inflammatory cytokinase, interleukin 1B, interleukin 7, and tumor necrosis factor have also been found in facet joint cartilage and synovial tissue.[25,26]

The orientation of the facet joints varies at the cervical, thoracic, and lumbar regions. Facet joints oriented parallel to the sagittal plane provide substantial resistance to axial rotation but minimal resistance to shearing forces (backward and forward sliding), and facet joints oriented more in a coronal plane tend to protect against flexion and shearing forces but provide minimal protection against rotation. The cervical facets are orientated in a coronal plane, which allows for flexion, extension, and lateral bending. The C2-C3 to C5-C6 facets are angled 35 degrees from the coronal plane, and C7-T1 are angled 22 degrees from the coronal plane. Orientation of the C5-C6 facet joint is between 22 and 35 degrees. All cervical facet joints from C2-C3 to C7-T1 are angled 110 degrees from the midline posterior sagittal plane. In the cervical spine, it is important to remember that the vertebral artery passes through the foramen of the transverse process of C1-C6.[27]

Facet joints in the thoracic spine differ from that of the cervical and lumbar spines in that their orientation is in a more coronal direction, which allows thoracic facet joints to play an important role in stabilization of thoracic spine during flexion loading. The T1-T2 facet joint is angled 66 degrees from a transverse plane, with the cephalad end more anterior than the caudad end. The T3-4 to T11-T12 facet joints are angled 75 degrees from the transverse plane. The T1-T2 to the T11-T12 facet joints are uniformly angled 110 degrees from the midline posterior sagittal plane. The T12-L1 facet joint is 25 degrees oblique to the sagittal plane from the midline posteriorly, which is similar to the lumbar orientation.[28,29]

The upper lumbar facet joints (T12-L2) are oriented closer to the midsagittal plane of the vertebral body, which allows limited rotational movements and favors flexion and extension. The lower facet joints tend to be oriented in a more coronal angle, which allows for greater rotational movements. The lumbar facet joints' cephalad ends are farther anterior than the caudad ends because the facet joints are tipped approximately 10 degrees. In the upper lumbar spine, approximately 80% of the facet joints are curved, and 20% are flat; in the lower lumbar spine, these numbers are reversed.[30,31] The lumbar facet joints transition from a coronal orientation to a sagittal positioning with age. Some studies have shown a positive association between degenerative spondylolisthesis and more sagitally oriented lower lumbar facet joints.[32]

Innervation

Cervical

The facet joints are innervated by the dual nerve supply from the medial branch of the dorsal ramus. Cervical facet joints from C3-C4 to C7-T1 are supplied by medial branches from the same level and the level above. Medial branch nerves arise from the posterior primary rami located in the cervical intertransverse space and then passes dorsally and medially to wrap around the waist of the articular pillar. The location of this nerve on the articular pillar is essentially the same as those of nerves C4-C8. The medial branches are bound to the periosteum by an investing fascia and are held against the articular pillars by tendons of the semispinalis capitis. The C7 medial branch crosses the root of the C7 transverse process and therefore lies higher on the lateral projection of the C7 articular pillar.[33]

The C2-C3 facet joint differs in innervation in that their innervation comes from the third occipital nerve along with C2 and C3 medial branches. Two medial branches usually arise separately from the C3 dorsal ramus. The superior and larger branch is the third occipital nerve (also known as the superficial medial branch), and the inferior branch is the deep medial branch. The third occipital nerve innervates C2-C3 joint. It curves dorsally and medially around the superior articular process of the C3 vertebra and crosses the C2-C3 facet joint either just below or across the joint margin. It also provides cutaneous neural supply for the suboccipital region. The C3 dorsal ramus is the only cervical dorsal ramus below C2 that has a cutaneous distribution.[34,35]

The C8 medial branch runs a course similar to the upper thoracic nerves. It arises from the dorsal ramus within lateral margin of the intervertebral foramen of C7-T1. Because of the C8 medial branch and seven cervical vertebrae, numbering of medial branches is different in the cervical region compared with in the thoracic and lumbar spine. The facet joint is innervated by a cervical medial branch at the same level and level above for C4-C7. For example, the C5-C6 facet joint is innervated by the medial branches of C5 and C6. This numbering applies to the C4 through C7 levels.[34,36]

Medial branches of the cervical posterior rami are different than lumbar medial branches in that they supply mainly the facet joints and have limited innervations of the posterior neck muscles (the multifidus, interspinalis, semispinalis cervicis, and semispinalis capitis).

Thoracic Innervation

Medial branch nerves from two segmental levels innervate each thoracic facet. The medial branch has ascending branches that form when the medial branch passes caudal to the zygapophyseal joint and descending branches form where the medial branch crosses the transverse process to pass to the next joint below. The configuration of the upper thoracic (T1-T3) and lower thoracic (T9-T10) spine are reasonably consistent. Medial branches arise from the dorsal ramus within 5 mm of the lateral margin of the intervertebral foramen, where it passes dorsally, inferiorly, but mostly lateral within the intertransverse space. Opposite the tip of the transverse process, the medial branch curves dorsally through the intertransverse space, aiming for the superolateral corner of the transverse process. It crosses this corner and then travels caudad across the transverse process surface in the cleavage plane between the origins of the multifidus medially and the semispinalis laterally. The nerve than runs inferiorly and medially over the dorsal aspect of the multifidus. Exceptions to this configuration occur at the midthoracic level (T4-T8), where the medial branch does not reliably make bony contact with the transverse process. The nerve at times is suspended in the intertransverse space. The course is separated from the transverse process by the multifidus. There is no relation with contact to bone in these levels.

The course of the medial branches of T11 and T12 also vary because of different osseous anatomy at these levels. The T12 transverse process is shorter compared with other levels. Therefore, the T11 branch runs across the lateral surface of the root of the relatively short T12 transverse process. At the T12 level, the medial branch assumes a course analogous to those of the lumbar medial branches.[28,37,38]

Lumbar Innervation

A given lumbar facet joint is innervated by nerve fibers from medial branch nerves at two levels. The medial branch nerve at a given level innervates the inferior portion of the facet above and the superior portion of the facet below except for L5, which sends an ascending articular branch only to the L5-S1 joint.

The primary dorsal rami divide into three nerves as they approach their respective transverse processes: the medial branch, intermediate branch, and lateral branch. The medial branch is the largest of the dorsal branch nerves. The medial branch has three branches as well. The proximal branch hooks around the articular process to supply the facet above. The medial descending branch passes medially and downward to innervate the superior and medial portions of the facet capsule below, the multifidus and interspinales muscles and ligament, and the periosteum of the neural arch. The ascending branch supplies the facet above. The other two main branches of the dorsal ramus are the intermediate branch and the lateral branch. The intermediate branch sends fibers into the longissimus muscles. The lateral branch innervates the iliocostalis muscle, the thoracolumbar fascia, the skin of the lower back and buttock, and the sacroiliac joint, but does not innervate the facets.[22,39]

The medial branches of L1-L4 rami have a predictable course. These medial branches come off the dorsal ramus and exit from the intervertebral foramen, piercing the intertransverse ligament and crossing the superior border of the transverse process. The branches then travel along the junction of the transverse process and superior articular process. This junction is often referred to as a "groove." The medial branch nerve runs in the groove along the lateral aspect of the neck of the superior articular process, traveling caudally and posteriorly where it is in direct contact with the base of the superior surface of the transverse process, passing under the mamilloaccessory ligament. At L3, L4, and L5 levels, this ligament can become calcified. The medial branch nerve then proceeds inferiorly and posteriorly, where it sends fibers cephalad to innervate the caudad capsular margin of the adjacent superior joint capsule. Then it sends fibers to the next lower level at its cephalad capsular margin.[20,40]

The course of the L5 medial branch is somewhat modified because the transverse process is replaced by the ala of the sacrum. The L5 medial branch is not the medial branch of L5 but rather the dorsal primary ramus of L5, which is longer. The dorsal ramus pierces the intertransverse ligament and runs caudally and posteriorly along the groove formed by the junction of the superior articular process and sacral ala. The L5 dorsal ramus divides into two branches, a medial and lateral branch. The L5 medial branch curves medially around the base of the L5-S1 joint, sending an articular branch to this joint and then supplying the multifidus muscles. There is no mamilloaccessory ligament at this level. However, fibrous tissue fixes the position of the nerve at the base of the superior articular process. The lateral branch of the L5 dorsal ramus runs caudad to communicate with the S1 dorsal ramus lateral branch.[41,42]

The name of the joint blocked is numerically the same as the names of the transverse processes targeted for injection, but the names of the nerves are one segment higher. For example, the L2 medial branch (which courses over the base of the L3 transverse process) innervates both the inferior portion of the L2-L3 facet joint and the superior portion of the L3-L4 facet joint. The superior portion of L2-L3 facet joint is innervated by the L1 medial branch.

Basic Science

Pain Referral Patterns

The distribution of referred pain appears to be related to the innervation of the medial and lateral branches of the dorsal rami. Studies of mapping out referral patterns have used asymptomatic volunteers and pain patients. Referral patterns from cervical zygapophyseal joints were studied by Dwyer et al.[43] In their first study, the facet injections were done in normal volunteers, which showed certain referral patterns. The accuracy of referral patterns were later studied on symptomatic patients. Referral patterns obtained were C2-C3 as pain located in the upper cervical region and extending at least onto the occiput. The C3-C4 pattern is located over the

posterolateral cervical region without substantial extension into the occiput and extending caudally over the posterolateral aspect of the neck without entering the region of the shoulder girdle. The C3-C4 pattern basically covers the area that is coextensive with the underlying levator scapulae muscle. Whereas the C4-C5 pattern is concentrated over the angle formed by the top of the shoulder and side of the neck, the C5-C6 pattern spreads laterally toward the shoulder with the main area draping over the top, front, and back of the shoulder girdle, with a base coinciding with the spine of the scapula. The C6-C7 pattern extends below the spine of the scapula. The typical C7-T1 pain pattern extends into the paravertebral area with coverage over the scapulae.[44]

The thoracic facets may produce middle back pain that is paraspinous with neuralgic characteristics. Thoracic referral patterns were noted by joint distention in normal volunteers. Some overlap was noted in the thoracic area. The pain was usually one to two segments inferior and lateral to the involved joint and unilateral. The T1-T2 joint pain was noted to be below the inferior angle of the scapulae. Despite this, there is a wide overlap in thoracic referral patterns that makes them unreliable.[44-46]

Referred pain from the lumbar zygapophyseal joints and medial branches has been examined in numerous studies showing overlap of referred pain between each level.[47,48] Pain from L1-L3 has been shown to extend into the flank, hip, and upper lateral thighs. Pain from L3-S1 has been shown to extend deeper into the thigh, usually laterally and posteriorly and also into the groin area. Referred pain from the L4-5 and L5-S1 facet joints can also cause pain extending into the lower lateral leg, below the knee, and even to the foot at times.[20,47,49] Referred pain may also assume a pseudoradicular pattern, making the underlying diagnosis difficult to confirm based on pain patterns.[50]

Imaging

Radiologic imaging such as computed tomography (CT) and magnetic resonance imaging (MRI) have shown to be nonspecific in the diagnosis of facetogenic-mediated pain. Studies in asymptomatic volunteers showed a prevalence of facet degeneration of 8% to 14%. Findings on imaging do not correlate well with symptoms.[51,52] Stojanovic et al[53] studied the correlation between MRI pathology and response to diagnostic medial branch blocks and radiofrequency denervation. Their study showed a possible correlation between lumbar facetogenic pain and MRI abnormalities.[53] Schwarzer et al[54] showed that the degree of degenerative changes seen on CT did not correlate well with facet joint–mediated spinal pain. Single-photon emission computed tomography (SPECT) has been shown to identify probable joint inflammation, but its effectiveness in predicting successful medial branch blocks is not well known.[55] The potential of fluorodeoxyglucose positron emission tomography (FDG-PET) has limited value for the diagnosis of facet joint arthropathy and is expensive.[56] In conclusion, accurately diagnosing facet joint–mediated pain via correlation with radiological findings is unreliable.

Indications and Contraindications

Indications

The purpose of medial branch blocks is to test if the patient's pain is relieved by anesthetizing the target nerves. Patients who should be included for diagnostic medial branch blocks may have pain that is somatic or nonradicular pain in the neck, upper back, mid back, lower back, upper or lower extremity, or chest wall, or headaches. Pain should be intermittent or continuous with a visual analog score an average of 6 or more on a scale of 0 to 10 that causes functional disability. Pain should last for at least 3 months or longer. Patients should have spinal pain of unknown origin and lack neurological deficits. Patients should have tried and failed conservative management, which includes oral medications such as nonsteroidal antiinflammatory drugs (NSAIDs), physical therapy, exercise, and bed rest.[11,13]

Contraindications

Contraindications are those for any regional block.

Absolute contraindications are those conditions in which the conduct of a needle procedure under radiographic control could cause potential risk to the patient's health and include:

1. Bacterial infection
   a. Systemic
   b. Localized to site of injection
2. Coagulopathy
   a. International normalized ratio >1.5
   b. Platelets <50,000
3. Severe allergy to medications to be injected
4. Patient refuses procedure or is unable to understand or cooperate with the procedure.
5. Pregnancy

Relative contraindications are conditions that require special consideration because of the risk they pose. They do not preclude the performance of medial branch blocks; however, because of these conditions, the investigator may elect not to perform the procedure. If they do proceed, special precautions are necessary.

Relative contraindications include:

1. Concurrent treatment with non-NSAIDs that could compromise coagulation
2. Allergy to contrast dye: The patient may have to be premedicated with corticosteroid and H_1 and H_2 antagonists.
3. Neurological signs: Neurological disorders should be managed before proceeding with medial branch blocks.

Techniques

Target Identification
Cervical

Positioning   Cervical medial branch blocks can be performed with the patient in the prone, supine, or lateral position. If using the lateral approach, the patient is placed in the lateral decubitus position with the painful side up. A cushion can be placed underneath the patient's head to keep the neck parallel to the table. The patient can use a pillow or device to hug or accommodate the arms if needed. The prone position is also a commonly used approach to the cervical medial branches.

Needle Placement   The target points for cervical medial branch blocks from the third to the sixth medial branches is the "centroid" of the articular pillars with the same segmental number as the target nerve (**Fig. 13-2**). The centroid is found at the intersection of the two diagonals of the diamond-shaped pillar. This target point can be seen with true lateral fluoroscopic imaging in which the silhouettes of the articular pillars on each side at a given segment are superimposed. To confirm superimposition, the x-ray beam should be tilted around the long axis of the patient for splitting of the superimposed articular pillar silhouettes to occur. Therefore, the ipsilateral articular processes are noted. It is important to confirm a true lateral view because it is essential to eliminate

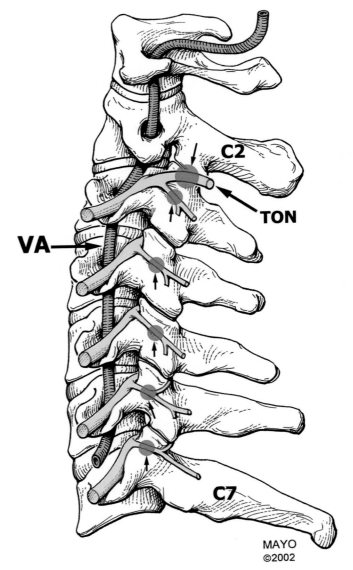

Fig. 13-2 Target zones for cervical medial branch block. Lateral illustration of cervical spine showing target zones (*black arrows pointing to green circles*) located at the midportion of the C2 through C7 articular pillars. The third occipital nerve (TON) is a relatively large nerve branch that may require three separate blocks at the level of the C2 inferior facet or C3 superior facet and where it courses lateral to the C2-C3 facet joint. VA, vertebral artery. (Copyright © 2003 by Mayo Foundation for Medical Education and Research.)

any risk of aiming the needle toward the contralateral side of the neck. It is important to have the target point in the center of the x-ray beam so it appears on the center screen when using fluoroscopy. Keeping the target point in the center avoids parallax errors.

It is important to remember that the vertebral artery from C2 to C7 is located anterior to the facet joint from both a lateral and posterior approach. With a posterolateral approach, the needle should pass through fascia and muscle and remain posterior to the vertebral artery. The puncture point on the skin is selected overlying the target point. The needle tip should be placed at the intended puncture site with the shaft aligned parallel to the x-ray beam, which allows the needle to be directed straight toward the target point. For the patient's comfort, the needle should be quickly inserted through the skin. When going thorough neck musculature, to minimize discomfort, especially at upper cervical levels, the practitioner should avoid piercing the sternocleidomastoid muscle if possible. If the initial puncture site overlies the sternocleidomastoid, then the patient's head should be rotated slightly into the pillow. This maneuver attempts to draw the muscle forward and away from the puncture site. The needle can be advanced under lateral fluoroscopic guidance. Corrections toward the target should be made superficially with only fine corrections made when the tip of the needle enters close to the target point. Periodic checking with fluoroscopy should be done to ensure correct position and orientation as the needle is advanced to the target point. Needle placement is then confirmed after negative aspiration with 0.3 mL of contrast. The pillars should be noted on the lateral view. The interventionalist should see spread of contrast across the lateral surface of the articular pillar, filling the concavity that lodges the targeted medial branch. Excess injectate from this site can also spread in a rostrodorsal direction across the plane located between the semispinalis capitis and multifidus. After proper placement is confirmed with contrast, 0.3 mL of local anesthetic is used to anesthetize the target nerve. The needle should be held against the bone during injection.

The transverse process of C7 tends to displace the medial branch relatively higher than the other typical cervical medial branches. Therefore, the target point for the C7 medial branch block lies higher, at the apex of the superior articular process of C7. If the target point is selected too low for C7, the needle may appear to rest on the superior articular process when it is resting on the transverse process. In the lateral view, the target point for the C7 medial branch block will rest higher than the silhouette of the C7 transverse base superimposed on the superior articular process of C7. Final needle placement should be near the apex of the superior articular process of C7. Needle advancement should be checked frequently to not allow the needle tip to stray outside the triangular silhouette of the C7 superior articular process. If the needle tip strays, it could be advanced into the C8 intervertebral foramen or through the C6-C7 zygapophyseal joint. After contact with the superior articular process is made with the needle tip, a posteroanterior (PA) view should be done to confirm that the needle placement is against the lateral margin of the superior articular process. If the needle is noticed to be located at the C7 transverse process, then lateral views should be used for needle adjustments. After the needle is in the final position, 0.3 mL of contrast is injected to confirm spread over the intended target. After confirmation of the needle as not being epidural or intravascular, 0.3 mL of local anesthetic is injected. The needle is then withdrawn approximately 4 mm, and 0.3 mL of local anesthetic injection should be repeated. The depth of needle withdrawal can be gauged with a lateral view. This step of reinjection is done because of the variation of the C7 medial branch, which is displaced by the semispinalis capitis muscle away from bone rather than running across the surface of the articular process. Another anatomical variation to consider is the height of the C7 superior articular process. When a tall C7 superior articular process is present, an additional block at the junction of the transverse process with the superior articular junction may be needed because of variants in the C7 medial branch course where the nerve crosses the root of the transverse process.

A C8 medial branch block is needed to block the C7-T1 facet. The C8 medial branch block is approached similar to thoracic or lumbar medial blocks. The C8 medial branch courses over the base of the T1 transverse process. The needle tip is placed at the junction of the superior articulating facet and base of the transverse process

of T1. The needle is advanced to this site via a trajectory down the x-ray beam. Contrast (0.3 mL) is injected under continuous "live" anteroposterior (AP) imaging to confirm the position and rule out intravascular uptake. After contrast confirms needle placement, 0.3 mL of local anesthetic is injected.

The third occipital nerve is thicker than the medial branches of the typical cervical dorsal rami; therefore, multiple target points are needed for blocking the nerves involving the C2-C3 facet joint. The target points are located along a vertical line that bisects the articular pillar of C3. There are three target points; the highest target point is immediately above the subchondral plate of the C2 inferior articular process. The lowest point is immediately below the subchondral plate of the C3 superior articular process. The middle point lies midway between these points, usually on the subchondral plate of the superior articular process of C3. Needle advancement is toward the middle of the three target points lateral to the C2-C3 facet joint capsule at the level of the joint. When the needle rests on bone and is in position, the needle is withdrawn slightly (≈3 mm) to ensure the needle has not penetrated the joint capsule. After injection of contrast to rule out venous uptake, injection with 0.3 mL of local anesthetic is done. The needle tip is then readjusted either to the cranial target point (anteroinferior margin of C2 inferior articular facet) or caudad target point (anterosuperior margin of C3 superior articular facet), where 0.3 mL of local anesthetic will also be injected at each spot. If contrast is used, distribution when one has achieved correct needle placement will show spread across the surface of the joint, where the target nerve is held against the joint by the overlying splenius capitis muscle (**Figs. 13-3** to **13-7**).

Thoracic

Positioning   The patient lies in the prone position.

Needle Placement   The target landmarks for thoracic medial branches are the transverse processes. At the upper thoracic levels, the target point is more medial than compared with the lower thoracic levels. For the T1-T4 and T10 medial branch blocks, the target point is the junction of the superolateral corner of the transverse process. The T4-T8 nerves (the target point) do not lie on

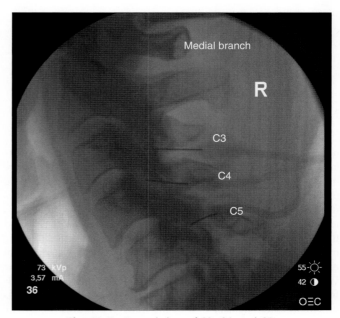

Fig. 13-3   Lateral view of C3, C4, and C5.

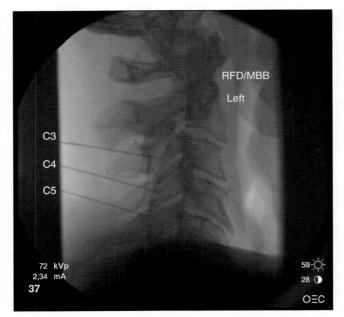

Fig. 13-4 Left lateral view of C3, C4, and C5. MBB, medial branch block; RFD, radiofrequency denervation.

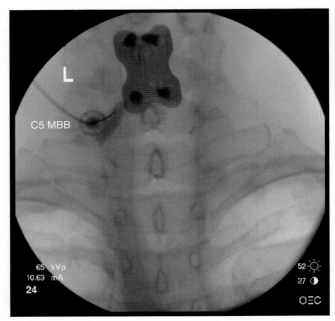

Fig. 13-6 Anteroposterior view of C6. MBB, medial branch block.

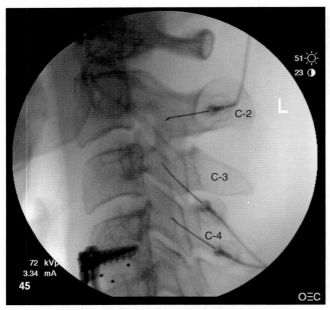

Fig. 13-5 Lateral view of C2, C3, and C4.

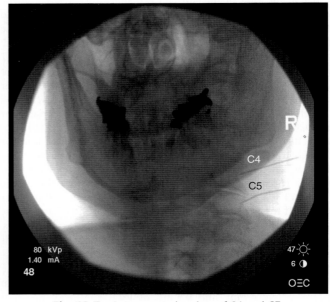

Fig. 13-7 Anteroposterior view of C4 and C5.

bone. The target point is the dorsal surface of the ribs that articulates with the transverse process. For the T11 and T12 medial branches, target points are similar to those for the lumbar medial branches. The target point is the junction of the root of the superior articular process and the root of the transverse process. To identify the target point, the ipsilateral oblique view is used to find the "Scotty dog" view. The radiographic target point for thoracic medial branch blocks is found cephalad to the superomedial margin of the transverse process. Cranial or caudal tilt of the C-arm is needed for optimal separation of the transverse process from the costovertebral junction. If the transverse process is obscured, better visualization of the transverse process occurs by rotating the C-arm to the opposite side of interest.

It is important to remember to name the target joints and target transverse processes appropriately. Their segmental nerves are different from those of the target nerves.

To decrease the risk of pneumothorax, the needle position should be dorsal to the target bone. The needle should be advanced down the beam of the x-ray. The needle is placed on the superior lateral corner of the transverse process at T1-T4 and T9 and T10. The needle is placed on junction of superior articular process and transverse process at T11 and T12.

Contrast is injected to confirm adequate spread covering the target area for the nerve and exclude intravascular uptake. At the midthoracic level (T5-T8), there is no validated technique for blocking the medial branches because of the unusual and variable

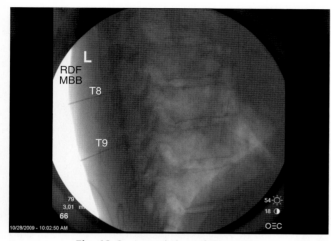

Fig. 13-8   Lateral view of T8 and T9.

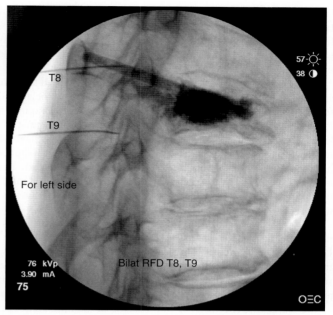

Fig. 13-10   Lateral view of T8 and T9. RFD, radiofrequency denervation.

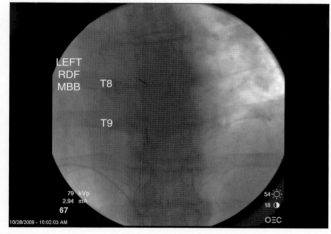

Fig. 13-9   Anteroposterior view of T8 and T9. MBB, medial branch block; RFD, radiofrequency denervation.

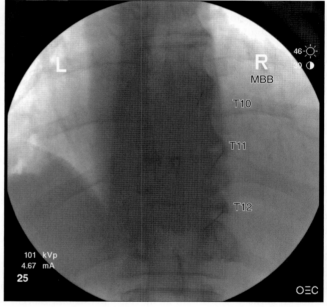

Fig. 13-11   Anteroposterior view of T10, T11, and T12. MBB, medial branch block.

anatomy of the medial branches at this level. The test dose of contrast under live fluoroscopy should show cephalad spread in an elongated ovoid shape covering the area where the target nerve lies (**Figs. 13-8** to **13-11**).

Lumbar

Positioning   Lumbar medial branch blocks can be performed via the posterior approach, but it is not used because of the target obstruction via superior portion of the zygapophyseal joint. Therefore, the oblique approach is usually used. To perform the block with an oblique approach, the patient can lie prone on the fluoroscopy table with a cushion under the hips to decrease lumbar lordosis and have the C-arm of the fluoroscope rotated 10 to 20 degrees from the AP view to the side being blocked. The oblique view can also be obtained with the patient lying semi-prone with a cushion under their abdomen to tilt the target side upward.

Needle Placement   In the lumbar region, the medial branch nerve is located at the level of the transverse process or slightly superior and lateral to the medial border of the superior articulating process. The target for the L1-L4 medial branches is located at the junction of the superior articulating process and transverse process at which the target nerve crosses, midway between the superior border of the transverse process and the location of the mamilloaccessory

notch. To find the target, an oblique view is needed with C-arm fluoroscopy. The goal is to obtain an optimal "Scotty Dog" view, which usually occurs at 10 to 20 degrees. The "nose" represents the transverse process, the "eye" represents the pedicle, and the "ear" corresponds to the superior articulating process. The target point is located behind the "eye" of the "Scotty dog," so the puncture site on the skin is directly in line using a coaxial technique under fluoroscopy. A 1% lidocaine skin wheal is injected subcutaneously. The needle should be advanced directly down the x-ray beam to the target point. The needle tip can be curved to aid in steering the needle to the target point. The needle is advanced until the needle tip contacts bone where the superior articulating process, base of transverse process, and pedicle join each other. When this occurs, the needle tip is "walked" up over the superior aspect of the transverse process just until the tip slides over the top of the transverse process.

In the lateral view, the needle position should be viewed to make sure it is not too far anteriorly and that it is not in the neural foramen. Confirmation of needle position is done with oblique and PA views. In PA view, the tip of the needle should be against the lateral surface of the superior articular process, preferably the most medial end of the transverse process. Contrast 0.1 to 0.3 mL should be injected to confirm the absence of intravascular spread. The needle bevel should be directed caudally to prevent spread of injectate into the neural foramen and allowing the injectate to be deposited on the medial branch.

At the L5 level, is it important to remember the target nerve is not the medial branch of L5. The L5 medial branch is actually the L5 dorsal primary ramus, which is located against the bone along the superomedial aspect of the groove formed by the sacral ala and superior articulating process of S1. The target is along the superior articulating process sacral ala junction just below the upper margin of the sacral ala. The target is found using an oblique view. Less oblique tilt is needed when compared with the L1-L4 levels. Usually 0 to 10 degrees is sufficient for the L5 dorsal primary ramus. Too much oblique causes obstruction of the target point with the "Scotty dog" view because of the iliac crest being in the path of the needle. The skin puncture site should be slightly lateral to the target point but medial to the adjacent iliac crest. Needle advancement should be monitored under fluoroscopic guidance, making sure the needle tip is always below the upper margin of the sacrum with its course being in a ventral and medial direction toward the target point. When the needle contacts the bone forming the superior edge of the sacral ala, the needle is advanced carefully over the bone 2 to 3 mm. PA and oblique views are taken to confirm correct needle position. On the oblique view, the needle tip should be seen resting on the ala of sacrum, at the base of the S1 superior articular process. On the AP view, the needle tip should be against and under the lateral margin of the superior articular process of the sacrum. The needle bevel should be pointed medially to decrease risk of inadvertent spread of injectate into the S1 foramen or to the L5-S1 intervertebral foramen. Contrast should be injected to rule out intravascular spread and to confirm correct placement of the needle (**Figs. 13-12** to **13-16**).

S1 Needle Placement The S1 medial branch is a small nerve located cephalad to the S1 posterior opening in line between the S1 opening and the L5-S1 facet joint. Caudocranial trajectory is needed to contact periosteum along the superolateral margin of the S1 foramen.

Patient Management and Evaluation

When evaluating diagnostic medial branch blocks, the patients should have two comparative blocks with short- and long-acting local anesthetics to rule out false-positive results. Patients should have shorter relief with lidocaine than when using bupivacaine. The pain relief should last at least 2 hours with lidocaine and at least 3 hours or longer than the duration of relief with lidocaine when bupivacaine is used. The patient should not take oral opioid medications before the procedure. Immediately after the procedure, the patient should repeat maneuvers that normally reproduce or aggravate his or her pain. Although it is subject to debate, pain relief should be at least 50% to 80% or greater. In the past, there

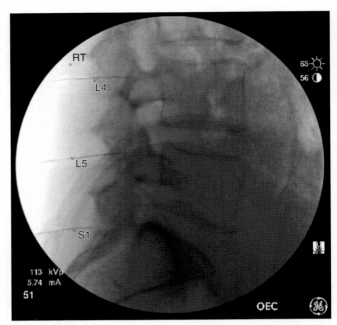

Fig. 13-12 Lateral view of L4, L5, and S1. RT, right.

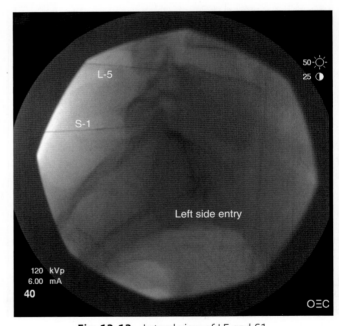

Fig. 13-13 Lateral view of L5 and S1.

has been a lack of consensus on a definition of successful diagnostic block.[57] Schwarzer et al[58] defined positive diagnostic block as 50% or greater reduction in pain. Guidelines by the American Society of Interventional Pain Physicians (ASIPP) use positive diagnostic block response as 80% pain relief with movements that normally cause pain.[11] An observational study by Manchikanti et al[59] examined using 50% or greater versus 80% or greater as a cut-off for positive diagnostic blocks. The authors found that of the patients who received greater than 80% relief from diagnostic medial branch blocks, 89.5% of them continued to have facet joint–mediated pain at 2-year follow-up. In contrast, in the 50% relief arm of the study, only 51% of these patients had continued lumbar-mediated facet pain at 2-year follow-up. They concluded that it is

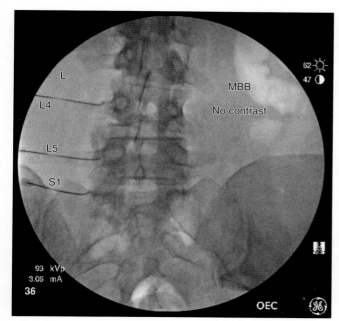

Fig. 13-14 Anteroposterior view of L4, L5, and S1. MBB, medial branch block.

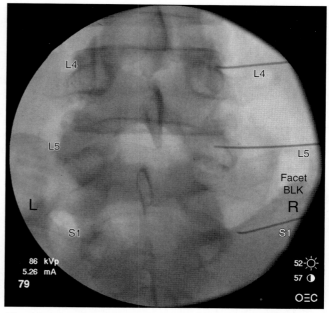

Fig. 13-16 Anteroposterior view of L4, L5, and S1. BLK, block.

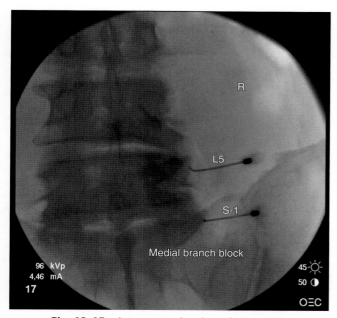

Fig. 13-15 Anteroposterior view of L5 and S1.

optimal to use 80% pain relief and being able to perform previously painful movements as a positive diagnostic response. This is to improve patient outcomes and avoid performing unnecessary procedures.[59]

Before the procedure, the patients' pain score should be recorded. Immediately after the procedure, the pain score should be reassessed when the patient is brought to a sitting or standing position. The patient then can be transported to the recovery room. In an ideal setting, patients should be monitored for at least 2 hours after the procedure to monitor and record the relief of pain. However, if the patient does not experience any postprocedural complications, he or she can be discharged 15 to 30 minutes after the injection. Patients should be accompanied by a responsible person who will drive them home. They should not operate any heavy machinery or drive a vehicle for the rest of the day. Patients should try aggravating maneuvers such as rotation, flexion, or extension and note pain levels before discharge, 30 minutes, 1 hour, 3 hours, and 6 hours after the procedure. Patients should write down when the pain returns to its normal level or when they need to take their home regimen of pain medications because of recurrence of their pain. Patients should report their pain response at 3 to 4 days after the procedure.

For patients having positive controlled diagnostic blocks, they can undergo therapeutic medial branch blocks or radiofrequency ablation. Therapeutic medial branch evidence is level II-1 or II-2. These blocks should provide at least 50% pain relief or greater for a minimum of 8 weeks. Blocks should preferably not be performed at intervals sooner than 2 to 3 months apart.[11]

Outcomes and Evidence

In 2005, it was noted that evidence-based evaluations showed level III for short- and long-term relief with lumbar and cervical medial branch blocks in managing chronic low back or neck pain.[60] A repeat review of the same authors in 2007 showed that the evidence is moderate for short- and long-term pain relief with repeat interventions for cervical, thoracic, and lumbar medial branch nerve blocks with local anesthetics.[50] In a review study by Falco et al[12] in 2009, cervical medial branch blocks were concluded as level II-1 with strong recommendation of 1B or 1C.[12] The ASIPP guidelines show both moderate recommendation for short- and long-term relief of cervical, thoracic, and lumbar medial branch blocks.[11]

The ASIPP guidelines state that for the diagnostic phase, the two medial branch procedures should be at intervals of no sooner than 1 week or preferably 2 weeks. For the therapeutic phase, 2 to 3 months or longer are needed between injections (≥50% relief for at least 3 months). If the therapeutic procedures are planned for different regions, the practitioner should wait at least 1 to 2 weeks to treat the different areas.[11]

The evidence for cervical, thoracic, and lumbar medial branch nerve blocks with local anesthetics (with or without steroids) is moderate for short- and long-term pain relief with repeat interventions.[50] Atluir et al[14] noted that the evidence for thoracic MBB is level 1 or II-1 with strong recommendations of 1A or 1B.

A systematic review by Falco et al[12] noted that the recommendation is a strong 1B or 1C for the use of therapeutic facet joint medial branch blocks in providing both short-term and long-term relief in the treatment of chronic cervical facet joint neck pain. For cervical medial branch blocks, there is level II-1 evidence with strong recommendation of 1B or 1C. For cervical radiofrequency neurotomy, there is level II-1 to level II-2 evidence with strong recommendation of 1B or 1C. There is no evidence available for cervical intraarticular facet joint injections.

Risks and Complications

These include:

1. Bleeding: hemorrhage or hematoma
2. Infection
3. Allergic reaction related to medications or antiseptic skin solution
4. Vasovagal reaction
5. Epidural, subdural, or subarachnoid injection
6. Nerve trauma
7. Postprocedural radicular pain
8. Intraarterial or intravenous injection
9. Radiation exposure
10. Ataxia: risk for upper cervical area, especially third occipital nerve blocks
11. Pneumothorax: possible with low cervical, thoracic, and high lumbar blocks

There are certain risks specific for the cervical region. For patients undergoing third occipital nerve blocks and other upper cervical medial branch blocks, the patients may experience ataxia after the procedure because of the local anesthetics blocking the upper cervical proprioceptors needed for tonic neck reflexes. This temporary sensation usually resolves in 15 to 30 minutes. Patients should be warned before the procedure about this potential side effect. If it does occur, then the patient should be instructed to focus on horizontal objects in the room. The patient should not look downward or sideways because these movements will incur a sense of unsteadiness.

A strict sterile technique should be used to decrease infection. Patients taking coagulopathic medications should have appropriate time off these medications and appropriate laboratory test results checked. Correct needle placement is important to decrease the chance of epidural, subarachnoid spread, or pneumothorax. For thoracic medial branch blocks, needle placement must always be dorsal to target bone to prevent the risk of pneumothorax. A study by Dreyfuss et al[41] showed that needle placement for lumbar medial branch blocks at the middle of the transverse process at its junction with the superior articular process decreased the risk of aberrant spread. For the L5 dorsal ramus, the needle bevel should point medially, and the target point is halfway between the upper end and middle of the ala of the sacrum to reduce aberrant spread. Contrast should be used to rule out intravascular injection. With regards to radiation exposure, new techniques using ultrasound technique and a single-needle technique may decrease or completely eliminate radiation exposure. More studies are needed to confirm the application and feasibility of these techniques.[61,62]

Intravascular injections can cause burning pain and anaphylactic reactions. They can also cause false-negative responses. Contrast injection with fluoroscopy should therefore be used. Dreyfuss et al[41] found 8% intravascular injection when studying lumbar medial branch blocks in 15 subjects and 120 injections. Kaplan et al[63] found that inadvertent venous uptake occurred in 33% of nerve blocks with initial venous uptake carrying 50% false-negative results despite subsequent lack of venous uptake with needle repositioning. Lee et al[64] showed that the overall incidence of intravascular injection in lumbar medial branch blocks was 6% and the prediction of intravascular injection by aspiration test sensitivity was 34%. Spot radiographs demonstrated intravascular uptake in 40% of those documented by real-time ultrasonography. Real-time fluoroscopy with contrast enhancement should be performed during the blocks to increase diagnostic and therapeutic values and to avoid complications because both aspiration and spot radiography frequently missed intravascular uptake.

References

1. Ball J: Enthesopathy of rheumatoid and ankylosing spondylitis. *Ann Rheum Dis* 30:213-222, 1971.
2. de Vlam K, Mielants H, Verstaete KI, et al: The zygapophyseal joint determines morphology of the enthesophyte. *J Rheumatol* 27:1732-1739, 2000.
3. Fujishiro T, Nabeshima Y, Yasui S, et al: Pseudogout attack of the lumbar facet joint: a case report. *Spine* 27:E396-E398, 2002.
4. Campbell AJ, Wells IP: Pigmented villonodular synovitis of a lumbar vertebral facet joint. *J Bone Joint Surg Am* 64:145-146, 1982.
5. Manchikanti L, Pampati V, Fellows B, et al: The Inability of the clinical picture to characterize pain from facet joints. *Pain Physician* 3:158-166, 2000.
6. Mironer YE, Somerville JJ: Protocol for diagnosis and treatment of facet joint. *Pain Digest* 9:188-190, 1999.
7. Sehgal N, Dunbar E, Shah RV, et al: Systematic review of diagnostic utility of facet/zygapophysial joint injections in chronic spinal pain: an update. *Pain Physician* 10:213-228, 2007.
8. Bogduk N: International Spinal Injection Society guidelines for the performance of spinal injection procedures. Part I: zygapophysial joint blocks. *Clin J Pain* 13:285-302, 1997.
9. Revel ME, Listrat VM, Chevalier XJ, et al: Facet joint block for low back pain. Identifying predictors of a good response. *Arch Phys Med Rehabil* 73:824-828, 1992.
10. Revel M, Poiraudeau S, Auleley GR, et al: Capacity of the clinical picture to characterize low back pain relieved by facet joint anesthesia: proposed criteria to identify patients with painful facet joints. *Spine* 23:1972-1976, 1998.
11. Manchikanti L, Boswell MV, Singh V, et al: Comprehensive evidence-based guidelines for interventional techniques in the management of chronic spinal pain. *Pain Physician* 12:699-802, 2009.
12. Falco F JE, Erhart S, Wargo BW, et al: Systematic review of diagnostic utility and therapeutic effectiveness of cervical facet joint interventions. *Pain Physician* 12:323-344, 2009.
13. Manchikanti L, Boswell MV, Singh V, et al: Prevalence of facet joint pain in chronic spinal pain of cervical, thoracic, and lumbar regions. *BMC Musculoskeletal Disorders* 5:15-21, 2004.
14. Atluir S, Datta S, Falco F JE, et al: Systematic review of diagnostic utility and therapeutic effectiveness of thoracic facet joint interventions. *Pain Physician* 11:611-629, 2008.
15. Bogduk N, Holmes S: Controlled zygapophysial joint blocks: the travesty of cost-effectiveness. *Pain Med* 1:24-34, 2000.
16. Barnsley L, Lord S, Bogduk N: Comparative local anaesthetic blocks in the diagnosis of cervical zygapophysial joint pain. *Pain* 55:99-106, 1993.
17. Manchikanti L, Singh V, Pampati V: Are diagnostic lumbar medial blocks valid? Results of a 2-year follow-up. *Pain Physician* 6:147-153, 2003.
18. Lord SM, Barnsley L, Bogduk N: The utility of comparative local anaesthetic blocks versus placebo-controlled blocks for diagnosis of cervical zygapophysial joint pain. *Clin J Pain* 11:208-213, 1995.

19. Hirsch C, Ingelmark BE, Miller M: The anatomical basis for low back pain: Studies on the presence of sensory nerve endings in ligamentous, capsular, and intervertebral disc structures in the human lumbar spine. *Acta Orthop Scand* 33:1-17, 1963.

20. Manchikanti L, Singh V: Review of chronic low back pain of facet joint origin. *Pain Physician* 5:83-101, 2002.

21. Cavanaugh JM, Lu Y, Chen C, et al: Pain generation in lumbar and cervical facet joints. *J Bone Joint Surg Am* 88:63-67, 2006.

22. Cohen SP, Raja SN: Pathogenesis, diagnosis, and treatment of lumbar zygapophysial (facet) joint pain. *Anesthesiology* 106:591-614, 2007.

23. Ashton IK, Ashton BA, Gibson SJ, et al: Morphological basis for back pain: the demonstration of nerve fibers and neuropeptides in the lumbar facet joint capsule but not in ligamentum flavum. *J Orthop Res* 10:72-78, 1992.

24. El-Bohy AA, Cavanaugh JM, Getchell ML, et al: Localization of substance P and neurofilament immunoreactive fibers in the lumbar facet joint capsule and supraspinous ligament of the rabbit. *Brain Res* 460:379-382, 1988.

25. Beaman DN, Graziano GP, Glover RA, et al: Substance P innovation of lumbar spine facet joints. *Spine* 18:1044-1049, 1993.

26. Kallakuri S, Singh A, Chen C, et al: Demonstration of substance P, calcitonin gene-related peptide, and protein gene product 9.5 containing nerve fibers in human cervical facet joint capsules. *Spine* 29:1182-1186, 2004.

27. Panjabi MM, Oxland T, Takata K, et al: Articular facets of the human spine: quantitative three-dimensional anatomy. *Spine* 18:1298-1310, 1993.

28. Ebraheim NA, Xu R, Ahmad M, et al: The quantitative anatomy of the thoracic facet and the posterior projection of its inferior facet. *Spine* 22:1811-1817, 1997.

29. Panjabi MM, Takata K, Geol V, et al: Thoracic human vertebrae: quantitative three-dimensional anatomy. *Spine* 16:888-901, 1991.

30. Masharawi Y, Rothschild B, Dar G, et al: Facet orientation in the thoracolumbar spine: three-dimensional anatomic and biomechanical analysis. *Spine* 29:1755-1763, 2004.

31. Tulsi RS, Hermanis GM: A study of the angle of inclination and facet curvature of superior lumbar zygapophyseal facets. *Spine* 18:1311-1317, 1993.

32. Boden SD, Riew KD, Yamaguchi K, et al: Orientation of the lumbar facet joints: association with degenerative disc disease. *J Bone Joint Surg Am* 78:403-411, 1996.

33. Bogduk N, Marsland A: The cervical zygapophyseal joints as a source of neck pain. *Spine (Phila Pa 1976)* 13(6):610-617, 1988.

34. Bogduk N: The clinical anatomy of the cervical dorsal rami. *Spine* 7:319-330, 1982.

35. Lord S, Barnsley L, Wallis B, et al: Third occipital nerve headache: a prevalence study. *J Neurol Neurosurg Psychiatry* 57:1187-1190, 1994.

36. Zhang J, Tsuzuki N, Hirabayashi S, et al: Surgical anatomy of the nerves and muscles in the posterior cervical spine: a guide for avoiding inadvertent nerve injuries during the posterior approach. *Spine* 28:1379-1384, 2003.

37. Chua WH: *Clinical anatomy of the thoracic dorsal rami*. BMedSci Thesis, University of Newcastle, Australia, 1994.

38. Chua WH, Bogduk N: The surgical anatomy of thoracic facet denervation. *Acta Neurochir (Wien)* 136:140-144, 1995.

39. Selby DK, Paris SV: Anatomy of facet joints and its clinical correlation with low back pain. *Contemp Orthop* 12:1097-1103, 1981.

40. Suseki K, Takahashi Y: Innervation of lumbar facet joints: origins and functions. *Spine* 22:477-485, 1997.

41. Dreyfuss P, Schwarzer AC, Lau P, et al: Specificity of lumbar medial branch and L5 dorsal ramus blocks: a computed tomography study. *Spine* 22:895-902, 1997.

42. Bogduk N: Low back pain. In *Clinical anatomy of lumbar spine and sacrum*, ed 4, New York, 2005, Churchill Livingstone, pp 183-216.

43. Dwyer A, Aprill N, Bogduk N: Cervical zygapophysial joint pain patterns I: a study in normal volunteers. *Spine* 15:453-457, 1990.

44. Aprill C, Dwyer A, Bogduk N: Cervical zygapophyseal joint pain patterns II: a clinical evaluation. *Spine* 15:458-461, 1990.

45. Dreyfuss P, Tibiletti C, Dreyer S: Thoracic zygapophyseal joint pain patterns. *Spine* 19:807-811, 1994.

46. Fukie A, Ohseto K, Shiotan M: Patterns of pain induced by distending the thoracic zygapophyseal joints. *Reg Anesth* 22:332-336, 1997.

47. McCall IW, Park WM, O'Brien JP: Induced pain referral from posterior elements in normal subjects. *Spine* 4:441-446, 1979.

48. Marks R: Distribution of pain provoked from lumbar facet joints and related structures during diagnostic spinal infiltration. *Pain* 39:37-40, 1989.

49. Fukie S, Ohseto K, Shiotani M, et al: Distribution of referred pain from the lumbar zygapophyseal joints and dossal rami. *Clin J Pain* 13:303-307, 1997.

50. Boswell MV, Colson JD, Seghal N, et al: A systematic review of therapeutic facet joint interventions in chronic spinal pain. *Pain Physician* 10:229-253, 2007.

51. Weisel SW, Tsourmas N, Feffer HL, et al: A study of computer assisted tomography: 1. The incidence of positive CAT scans in an asymptomatic group of patients. *Spine* 9:548-555, 1984.

52. Jensen MC, Brant-Zawadzki MN, Obuchowski N, et al: Magnetic resonance imaging of the lumbar spine in people without back pain. *N Engl J Med* 333:69-73, 1994.

53. Stojanovic MP, Sethee J, Mohiuddin M, et al: MRI analysis of the lumbar spine: can it predict response to diagnostic and therapeutic facet procedures? *Clin J Pain* 26:110-115, 2010.

54. Schwarzer AC, Wang SC, O'Driscoll D, et al: The ability of computed tomography to identify a painful zygapophysial joint in patients with chronic low back pain. *Spine* 20:907-912, 1995.

55. Ackerman WE, Ahmad M: Pain relief with intraarticular or medial branch nerve blocks in patients with positive lumbar facet joint SPECT imaging: a 12-week outcome study. *South Med J* 101:931-934, 2008.

56. Houseni M, Chamroonrate W, Zhuang H, et al: Facet joint arthropathy demonstrated on FDG-PET. *Clin Nucl Med* 31:418-419, 2006.

57. Binder DS, Nampiaparampil DE: The provocative lumbar facet joint. *Curr Rev Musculoskeletal Med* 2:15-24, 2009.

58. Schwarzer AC, Aprill CN, Derby R, et al: The false-positive rate of uncontrolled diagnostic blocks of the lumbar zygapophysial joints. *Pain* 58:195-200, 1994.

59. Manchikanti L, Pampati S, Cash KA: Making sense of the accuracy of diagnostic lumbar facet joint nerve blocks: an assessment of the implications of 50% relief, 80% relief, single block, or controlled blocks. *Pain Physician* 13:133-143, 2010.

60. Boswell MV, Colson JD, Spillane WF: Therapeutic facet joint interventions in chronic spinal Pain: a systematic review of effectiveness and complications. *Pain Physician* 8:101-104, 2005.

61. Shin JK, Moon JC, Yoon KB, et al: Ultrasound-guided lumbar medial-branch block: a clinical study with fluoroscopy control. *Reg Anesth Pain Med* 31:451-454, 2006.

62. Stojanovic MP, Zhou Y, Hord D, et al: Single needle approach for multiple medial branch blocks: a new technique. *Clin J Pain* 19:134-137, 2003.

63. Kaplan M, Dreyfuss P, Halbrook B, et al: The ability of lumbar medial branch blocks to anesthetize the zygapophysial joint. A physiologic challenge. *Spine* 23:1847-1852, 1998.

64. Lee CJ, Kim YC, Shin JH, et al: Intravascular injection of lumbar medial branch block: a prospective evaluation of 1433 injections. *Anesth Analg* 106:1274-1278, 2008.

14 Radiofrequency Rhizotomy for Facet Syndrome

Jan Van Zundert, Pascal Vanelderen, Maarten van Eerd, Arno Lataster, Craig Hartrick, Nagy Mekhail, and Maarten van Kleef

CHAPTER OVERVIEW

Chapter Synopsis: Neck pain remains among the most difficult pain conditions to accurately diagnose and therefore to successfully treat. Cervical pain can arise from structures including the disci intervertebrales, the vertebrae themselves, the joints, and the ligaments and muscles that surround them. Although trauma and degeneration can be causes of pain, other neck pain syndromes may require investigation. The quality and temporal characteristics of pain as well as concurrent neurological symptoms can lend clues to its source. Anesthetic injections may be used for a diagnostic block. A classification system for "grades" of neck pain has recently been proposed that may help to standardize neck pain diagnoses. Corticosteroid injection, medial branch blocks, and radiofrequency (RF) nerve ablation may all be considered as interventional therapies after more conservative approaches for chronic neck pain have been exhausted. This chapter considers the procedural details associated with these procedures for lumbar facet pain as well as cervical pain.

Important Points:
- At the cervical level, the facet joint appears to be an important source of pain with degenerative neck symptoms. More than 50% of patients presenting to a pain clinic with neck pain may have facet joint–related pain.
- The most common symptom is unilateral pain without radiation to the arm. The history should exclude risk factors for serious underlying pathology (red flags).
- Conservative treatment options for cervical facet pain, such as physiotherapy, manipulation, mobilization, and pharmacological management, although supported by little evidence, are frequently applied before considering interventional treatments.
- Interventional pain management techniques, including medial branch blocks and RF treatment, may be considered.
- The zygapophyseal (facet) joints account for between 5% and 15% of cases of chronic axial low back pain.
- The most frequent complaint is axial low back pain with referred pain perceived in the flank, hip, and thigh.
- No physical examination findings are pathognomonic for diagnosis.
- The strongest indicator for lumbar facet pain is pain reduction after anesthetic blocks of the rami mediales (medial branches) of the rami dorsales that innervate the facet joints.
- In patients with injection-confirmed facet joint pain, procedural interventions can be undertaken in the context of a multidisciplinary, multimodal treatment regimen that includes pharmacotherapy; physical therapy; regular exercise; and if indicated, psychotherapy.
- The "gold standard" for treating patients with facetogenic pain is RF treatment.

Clinical Pearls: As in any interventional technique, patients need to be carefully selected prior to offering interventional treatment for pain originating from the zygapophyseal (facet) joints. After treatment, outcome assessment and complication evaluation are mandatory.

Cervical
- In the group of patients attending a pain clinic for neck pain, facet joints are probably involved in more than 50% of cases.
- Medial branch block of the ramus dorsalis of the segmental nerve is primarily considered as a diagnostic aid; however, (repetitive) infiltration of local anesthetic was shown to provide therapeutic effect. Infiltrations need to be repeated every 14 to 16 weeks, which makes it burdensome for the patient.
- The evidence of RF treatment of the ramus medialis (medial branch) of the ramus dorsalis for chronic cervical pain originating from the zygapophyseal (facet) joints is derived from observational studies. One RCT in patients with whiplash-associated disorders showed a positive effect for RF treatment compared to sham intervention.

Lumbar
- Lumbar paravertebral tenderness is suggestive of pain originating from the zygapophyseal (facet) joints.
- Confirmation of pain originating from the zygapophyseal (facet) joints is obtained by a positive anesthetic block of the ramus medialis (medial branch) of the ramus dorsalis.

Cervical Facet Pain

Establishing the Diagnosis

Background   Neck pain is defined as pain in the area between the base of the skull and the first thoracic vertebra. Pain extending into adjacent regions is defined as radiating neck pain. Pain may radiate into the head (cervicogenic headache), shoulder, or upper arm (radicular or nonradicular pain).[1] A distinction is made between trauma-related neck pain (whiplash-associated disorders) and degenerative neck problems. Because the causes of neck pain often are unclear, a distinction is made between the cause and source.[2] The following innervated structures in the neck may be sources of pain: vertebrae, discs, uncovertebral (Luschka) joints, ligaments, muscles, and facet (zygapophyseal) joints.

Beside the cervical discus intervertebralis, other structures in the neck, such as facet joints and uncovertebral joints, may also show degenerative signs. A diagnosis is defined as a clinical picture with known etiology and prognosis. A syndrome is a combination of symptoms occurring at a higher frequency in a certain population.

Cervical facet syndrome is defined as a combination of symptoms:

- Axial neck pain (not or rarely radiating past the shoulders)
- Pain with pressure on the dorsal side of the spinal column at the level of the facet joints
- Pain and limitation of extension and rotation
- Absence of neurological symptoms

There is a great deal of research into degenerative signs of the cervical vertebral column. In the discus intervertebralis (1) annular tears, (2) discus intervertebralis prolapse, and (3) endplate damage and internal discus intervertebralis disruption have been identified as potential structural discus intervertebralis pathologies.[3] Other structures in the neck, such as the facet joints and uncovertebral joints, may also show degenerative signs. The hypothesis that discus intervertebralis degeneration and discus intervertebralis narrowing increase facet joint loading and consequently facet osteoarthritis seems plausible but has yet to be proven. Some researchers claim that the discus intervertebralis and the facet joints can be seen as independent pain generators.[4]

Compared with research on lumbar facet pain, research on cervical facet dysfunction is relatively recent. In 1988, Bogduk and Marsland[5] described the positive effect of injection of local anesthetics close to the facet joints in patients with neck pain. Dwyer et al[6] showed that injection of irritating substances into the facet joints results in a specific radiation pattern (**Fig. 14-1**). The same radiation pattern is seen with mechanical and electrical stimulation. However, because it was later demonstrated that stimulation of the discus intervertebralis produces the same radiation pattern as stimulation of the facet joints, this is probably a segmental phenomenon.

Clinical findings of degenerative signs are mainly based on radiological findings. Spondylosis (disorders of the nonsynovial joints) and osteoarthritis (facet osteoarthritis) are frequent in advanced age. Degenerative disorders are usually seen at the low and midcervical levels (C4-C5, C5-C6, C6-C7). A causal relationship with pain symptoms has not been proven.

History   While taking the history, attention should be paid to signs and symptoms potentially indicating a serious underlying pathology ("red flags"). It is important to question the patient about previous trauma and previous or ongoing oncological treatments. Indications for potential spinal metastases are (1) history of malignancy, (2) pain starting after the age of 50 years, (3) continuous pain independent of posture or movement, and (4) pain

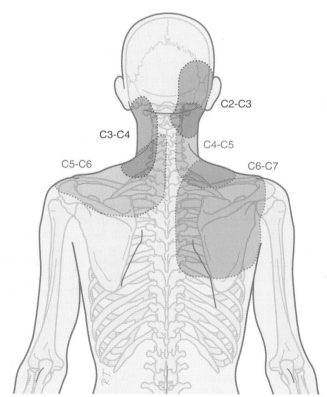

Fig. 14-1   Radiation pattern of cervical facet pain. (Illustrated by Rogier Trompert Medical Art. http://www.medical-art.nl.)

at night. When symptoms such as weight loss, fever, nausea, vomiting, dysphagia, coughing, or frequent infections are reported, an extensive history and further examination are mandatory.

The most common symptom with pain arising from the cervical facet joints is unilateral pain, not radiating past the shoulder. The pain often has a static component because it does not always occur in relation to movement. Rotation and retroflexion are usually reported as painful or limited.

The radiation pattern is not distinctive for facet problems but can indicate the segmental localization. It is important to determine if the pain symptoms cause functional limitations (e.g., dressing, lifting, car driving, reading, sleeping, and in the work situation).

Physical Examination   Neurological tests (reflexes, sensibility, and motor function) are necessary to exclude radiculopathy. To examine the function of the neck, the following tests are important:

> Flexion and extension: passive and active
> Lateroflexion: passive and active
> Rotation: passive and active
> Rotation in maximal flexion: passive and active
> Rotation in extension: passive and active

Rotation in a neutral position determines the rotation movement of the entire cervical spinal column. Rotation in flexion assesses the movement in the higher cervical segments. Rotation in extension assesses the movement in the lower cervical segments.

Local pressure pain over the facet joints can indicate problems arising from the facet joints. Recent research showed that local pressure, defined as pain with pressure of at least 4 kg, is a predictor of success of RF treatment (see Radiofrequency Treament sections).[7] When the neck pain is accompanied by radiation to the shoulder region, shoulder pathology should be excluded.

There is no evidence for the relation between the results of clinical examination and the history with the presence of pain originating from the cervical facet joints.[8] In daily clinical practice, history and physical examination are useful to exclude serious pathology and to obtain a working diagnosis. An indication of the segmental level (high, mid, or low cervical) involved can be obtained.

Diagnostic Blocks
The working diagnosis of facet pain based on history and clinical examination may be confirmed by performing a diagnostic block. Local anesthetic can be injected intraarticularly or adjacent to the ramus medialis (medial branch) of the ramus dorsalis of the segmental nerve.[2,9] Diagnostic medial branch block procedures are performed under fluoroscopy. There is no consensus about the definition of a successful diagnostic block. Some authors claim that 100% pain relief should be achieved.[10] But Cohen et al[7] showed that there is no difference in outcome of the RF treatment of patients reporting 80% and those reporting more than 50% pain reduction after a diagnostic block. In daily clinical practice, we consider a diagnostic block successful if more than 50% pain reduction is reported.

To minimize the number of false-positive results, a number of researchers have suggested that a second block should be carried out using a local anesthetic with different duration of action (e.g., lidocaine and bupivacaine; comparative double blocks). Only if the patient responds concordantly (longer or shorter pain reduction

depending on the duration of action of the local anesthetic) is this indicative of facet joint pain. This is not an etiological but a pharmacological criterion. These researchers suggest that double blocks are the gold standard for the diagnosis of facet pain. A gold standard, however, should be generally accepted and used. The concept of double blocks has theoretical and practical shortcomings. A best evidence synthesis on the assessment of neck pain concluded that diagnostic facet injections have not been validated to identify facet joint pain.[11]

In summary, on the basis of history and physical examination, a working diagnosis of cervical facet pain is defined. One diagnostic block can be recommended for confirming the clinical working diagnosis of facet pain. A block is considered positive when the patient experiences 50% pain reduction.[7]

Differential Diagnosis
Serious causes of neck pain such as tumors, infections, fractures, and systemic diseases are rare. A clinically relevant prolapsed discus intervertebralis and cervical spondylotic myelopathy cause neurological symptoms. Every patient with motor function loss, reflex changes, or sensibility loss must be thoroughly assessed.

Metastases, cervical herniated nucleus pulposus with radiculopathy, discitis, and fractures should be excluded through history and (additional) tests.

Chronic pain diagnoses such as segmental dysfunction, instability, and muscle strain are not sufficiently documented to be included in the differential diagnosis.[2] A summary of the differential diagnosis is represented in **Table 14-1**.

Anatomy
The vertebrae from C2 to S1 articulate with one another at the medial intervertebral joints, or disci intervertebrales between their corpora vertebrae and the lateral intervertebral, zygapophyseal, or facet joints between their processus articulares. The complex of two adjacent vertebrae with their intervertebral joints and ligamentous interconnections is defined as a segment.

The facet joint is located between the processus articularis inferior of a superior vertebra and the processus articularis superior of the adjacent inferior vertebra. It is a synovial joint with joint surfaces, a synovial membrane, and a joint capsule. The bony facets are covered with hyaline cartilage, and the joint capsule is fibrous. The chain of facet joints forms the facet column and permits segmental gliding movements between the vertebrae.

Table 14-1: Differential Diagnosis in Axial Neck Pain without Irradiation	
Tumors	
Infections	Discitis, septic arthritis, osteomyelitis, meningitis, epidural abscess
Trauma	Fractures, whiplash-associated disorders
Rheumatoid arthritis	
Crystal arthropathies	e.g., Gout
Vascular disorders	Aneurysm
Neurological causes*	Neuromas
Degenerative disorders	Spondylosis, osteoarthrosis

*Neurological causes are almost always accompanied with loss of neurological function.

The cervical facet joint capsules are longer and looser than the facet joint capsules in the thoracic and lumbar regions.[12] The more or less flat facet joint surfaces from C2 to C7 form an angle of approximately 45 degrees with the longitudinal axis through the cervical spinal column with a large range of intra- and interindividual variability. Compared with the lumbar facet joints, the cervical facet joints have a high density of mechanoreceptors. McLain took twenty-one cervical facet joint capsules and surrounding tissue from three human subjects by block-excision and processed them in a modified gold chloride technique.[13] In twenty-five micron serial histological sections he identified, according to the classification of Freeman and Wyke, encapsulated Type I, II, and III mechanoreceptors and non-encapsulated Type IV mechanoreceptors. The Type II receptors were found most frequently, mainly localized in the dens, fibrous joint capsule. Fewer Type I receptors were identified in both the capsule and the areolar, loose connective tissue. Only a handful of Type III receptors were found, at the junction between the capsule and the loose connective, sub-synovial tissue. Unencapsulated, nociceptive Type IV free nerve endings were present throughout the capsule, synovium, and areolar tissue.[14]

The facet joints from C3 to C7 are innervated by the ramus medialis (medial branch) of the ramus dorsalis of the segmental nerve (**Fig. 14-2**). Each facet joint is innervated by nerve branches from the upper and lower segments (**Fig. 14-3**).[15]

Imaging

In specific cases, plain radiography of the cervical spinal column (two or three directions) can be indicated to exclude tumor or fracture. Plain radiography does not, however, provide information for establishing the diagnosis of facet problems. This examination can help in estimating the degree of degeneration. The anterior spinal column is inspected for narrowing of the discus intervertebralis and anterior and posterior osteophyte formation. The posterior spinal column is inspected for facet osteoarthritis (facet sclerosis and osteophyte formation). In 1963, Kellgren et al[16] stated

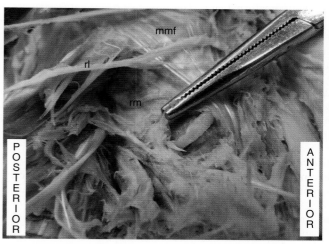

Fig. 14-2   Cervical spinal column, lateral view. Forceps opens arthrotic facet joint C4-C5. mmf, musculus multifidus; rl, ramus lateralis of ramus dorsalis; rm, ramus medialis (medial branch) of ramus dorsalis.

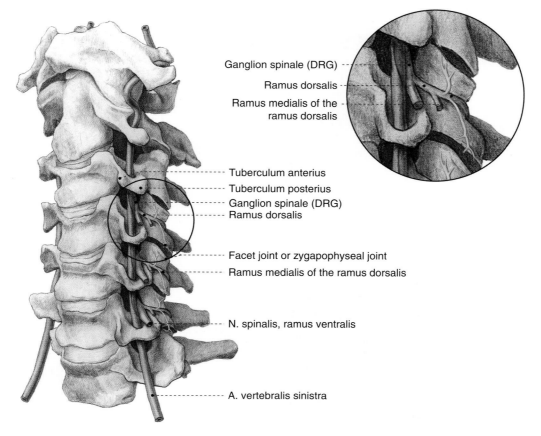

Ganglion spinale (DRG)
Ramus dorsalis
Ramus medialis of the ramus dorsalis

Tuberculum anterius
Tuberculum posterius
Ganglion spinale (DRG)
Ramus dorsalis

Facet joint or zygapophyseal joint
Ramus medialis of the ramus dorsalis

N. spinalis, ramus ventralis

A. vertebralis sinistra

Fig. 14-3   Innervation of the cervical vertebral column and the facet joints. DRG, dorsal root ganglion. (Illustrated by Rogier Trompert Medical Art. http://www.medical-art.nl.)

that when degenerative changes are seen on plain radiography, anatomical degeneration has already reached an advanced stage.

With progressing age, degenerative changes are more frequently seen: 25% at the age of 50 years up to 75% at the age of 70 years.[17] An age-related prevalence study concerning facet joint involvement in chronic neck pain indicates a comparable prevalence among all age groups.[18]

Degenerative changes of the cervical spinal column are present in asymptomatic patients, indicating that degenerative changes do not always cause pain. However, the conclusion that there is no relation between degeneration and pain cannot be drawn. There are studies indicating a relationship between degenerative changes and pain symptoms.[17,19]

In summary, a relationship between radiologic identification of degenerative changes and pain symptoms is not proven. If neurological etiology of the pain symptoms is suspected, magnetic resonance imaging (MRI) or computed tomography (CT) is indicated.

Guidelines
Recently, the following classification for neck pain and associated symptoms has been proposed:[20]

- Grade I neck pain: No symptoms indicating serious pathology and minimal influence on daily activities

- Grade II neck pain: No symptoms indicating serious pathology and influence on daily activities
- Grade III neck pain: No symptoms indicating serious pathology, presence of neurological disorders such as decreased reflexes, muscle weakness, or decreased sensory function
- Grade IV neck pain: Indications of serious underlying pathology such as fracture, myelopathy, or neoplasm

The following interventions are published options for the treatment of cervical joint pain:

- Intraarticular steroid injections
- Local infiltration of the ramus medialis (medial branch) of the ramus dorsalis
- RF treatment of the ramus medialis (medial branch) of the ramus dorsalis

A practice algorithm for the management of facet pain is illustrated in **Fig. 14-4**.

Indications and Contraindications
Chronic neck pain can be caused by the facet joints. Percentages between 25% and 65% are described, depending on the patient group and selection method. In the group of patients attending a pain clinic for neck pain, it is likely to be more than 50%.[21,22]

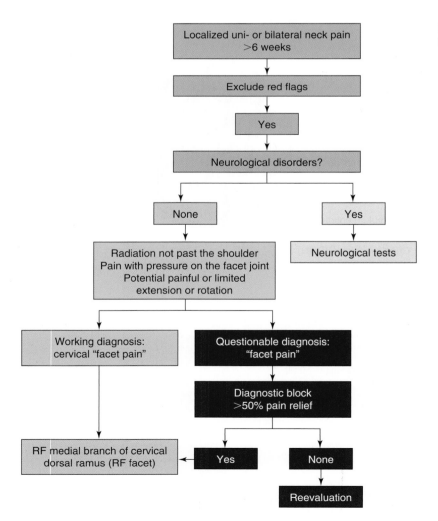

Fig. 14-4 Practice algorithm for the treatment of cervical facet pain. RF, radiofrequency.

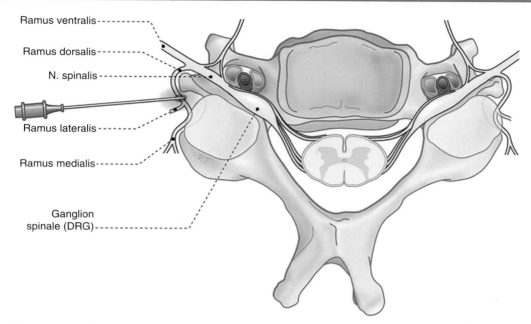

Ramus ventralis
Ramus dorsalis
N. spinalis
Ramus lateralis
Ramus medialis
Ganglion spinale (DRG)

Fig. 14-5 Posterolateral approach of the cervical ramus medialis (medial branch) of the ramus dorsalis. DRG, dorsal root ganglion. (Illustrated by Rogier Trompert Medical Art. http://www.medical-art.nl.)

Conservative treatment options for cervical facet pain such as physiotherapy, manipulation, mobilization, and pharmacological treatment are frequently applied before considering interventional treatments.

Interventional pain management techniques such as medial branch blocks and RF treatment may be considered in any patient with chronic (>3 months) neck pain.

Absolute contraindications for interventional pain management techniques are infection at the injection site and severe coagulation disorders.

Corticosteroid injections are performed after a careful risk-to-benefit analysis in patients with metabolic diseases such as diabetes. Psychological factors such as avoidance behavior and catastrophizing are less commonly related to neck symptoms in contrast to patients with low back problems.[2]

Monitoring of the saturation level and availability of resuscitation equipment is necessary.
Instrumentation: sterile operation gloves, sterile needles (SMK or Racz-Finch), gas-sterilizable RF probes
RF lesion generator
Operation table with possibility to use x-ray
X-ray C-arm
Postoperative recovery facility

RF, radiofrequency.

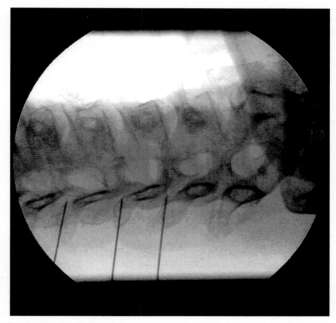

Fig. 14-6 Radiofrequency treatment cervical ramus medialis (medial branch) of the rami dorsales/facet C4, C5, C6, left: three quarters projection.

Technique
Percutaneous Facet Denervation The (postero-)lateral approach in the supine position is described below (**Fig. 14-5**). The advantage of this technique is that it is possible to maintain eye contact with the patient. Sedation is rarely required.

The patient is placed in the supine position with the head slightly extended on a small cushion. The C-arm is placed in an oblique position (±30 degrees). In this position, the beam runs parallel with the exiting nerve root that runs somewhat caudofrontal. Also in this position, the pedicles from the contralateral side are projected on the anterior half of the vertebral body. In the frontal plane (anteroposterior [AP] direction), the C-arm is positioned in a small angle with respect to the transverse plane. In this position, the discus intervertebralis space and neuroforamen are visible (**Fig. 14-6**). The ramus medialis (medial branch) of the ramus dorsalis runs over the base of the processus articularis superior. The injection point is marked on the skin, slightly posterior and caudal to the end point of the needle that is dorsal to the posterior boundary of the facet column. The first needle is introduced in a horizontal plane, slightly cranially so the tip of the needle points in the direction of the end point. It is important to understand that this is not a "tunnel-view" technique. The needle is slowly advanced anteriorly and cranially until bony contact with the facet column occurs. The farther the needle is advanced, the more difficult it becomes to change the direction. Therefore, the position of the needle needs to be checked frequently. If the needle points too much in the direction of the neuroforamen without contacting bone, the direction needs to be corrected to be more posterior. If there is no bone contact in the posterior direction, there is a risk that the needle will enter the spinal canal between the laminae. To prevent this, the needle position can be checked in the AP direction. The final position of the needle in the AP direction is in the concave "waist" of the facet column. After placement of the first needle, the other needles are introduced in the same way. The first needle acts as a guide to direction and depth.

The same technique is used for the facet joints of C3-C4 to C6-C7. For the facet joint of C2-C3, a different end point for the needle is used, just beneath the C2-C3 joint.[23]

After an optimal anatomical localization is reached and controlled using fluoroscopy, the position of the needle tip at the ramus medialis (medial branch) of the dorsal ramus is confirmed using electrical stimulation. The stimulation threshold is determined: an electrical stimulation of 50 Hz must give a reaction (tingling) in the neck at less than 0.5 V. Then stimulation is carried out at 2 Hz. Contractions of the paraspinal muscles can occur. Muscle contractions in the arm indicate a position close to the exiting segmental nerve. The needle should then be placed more posterior. After the correct position has been determined, 0.5 to 1 mL local anesthetic (1% or 2% lidocaine) is given. A RF lesion at 80° C for 60 seconds is carried out.

Patient Management and Evaluation

As outlined under the heading Establishing a Diagnosis, a thorough examination is mandatory. A management plan is discussed with the patient, and only after informed consent, an intervention is planned. Evaluation of the effect of the procedure is standard usually after 4 to 6 weeks.

It can be helpful to use at least a Numerical Rating Scale and a Global Perceived Effect Scale. Other evaluation scales are Pain Medication Quantification; Return to Work; General Functioning scales (SF36); and specifically for the neck, The Neck Disability Index. For scientific purposes, it is advised to use scales out of the six core domains: pain, physical functioning, emotional functioning, global improvement, symptoms and adverse events, and participant disposition.

Outcomes Evidence

The recently published Evidence-Based Practice Guidelines based on clinical diagnoses based the recommendations on the "grading strength of recommendations and quality of evidence in clinical guidelines" described by Guyatt et al[24] and adapted by van Kleef et al[25] in an editorial in *Pain Practice* (**Table 14-2**).

Intraarticular Steroid Injections

No reports on quality studies regarding the effect of intraarticular steroid injections are known until now.[26] There are also no comparative studies between intraarticular steroid injections and RF therapy.

Table 14-2: Summary of Evidence Scores and Implications for Recommendation

Score	Description	Implication
1A+	Effectiveness demonstrated in various RCTs of good quality. The benefits clearly outweigh the risks and burdens.	Positive recommendation
1B+	One RCT or more RCTs with methodological weaknesses demonstrate effectiveness. The benefits clearly outweigh the risks and burdens.	Positive recommendation
2B+	One or more RCTs with methodological weaknesses demonstrate effectiveness. The benefits are closely balanced with the risks and burdens.	Positive recommendation
2B±	Multiple RCTs, with methodological weaknesses, yield contradictory results better or worse than the control treatment. The benefits are closely balanced with the risks and burdens or there is uncertainty in the estimates of benefits, risks, and burdens.	Considered, preferably study related
2C+	Effectiveness is only demonstrated in observational studies. Given that there is no conclusive evidence of the effect, benefits are closely balanced with the risks and burdens.	Considered, preferably study related
0	There is no literature or there are case reports available, but these are insufficient to prove effectiveness or safety. These treatments should only be applied in relation to studies.	Only study related
2C−	Observational studies indicate no or too short-lived effectiveness. Given that there is no positive clinical effect, the risks and burdens outweigh the benefits.	Negative recommendation
2B−	One or more RCTs with methodological weaknesses or large observational studies that do not indicate any superiority to the control treatment. Given that there is no positive clinical effect, the risks and burdens outweigh the benefits.	Negative recommendation
2A−	RCT of a good quality that does not exhibit any clinical effect. Given that there is no positive clinical effect, the risks and burdens outweigh the benefits.	Negative recommendation

RCT, randomized controlled trial.

Local Infiltration of the Ramus Medialis of the Ramus Dorsalis

Medial branch block of the ramus dorsalis is primarily considered as a diagnostic aid; however, (repetitive) infiltration of local anesthetic was shown to provide therapeutic effect.[27,28]

In a randomized controlled trial (RCT) comparing the effect of medial branch blocks with bupivacaine alone versus blocks with the same local anesthetic plus steroid a comparable pain reduction was observed in both groups for mean duration of 14 and 16 weeks, respectively. During the follow-up period of 1 year, the mean numbers of procedures were 3.5 and 3.4, respectively. Patients were selected for participation in this study by controlled blocks providing ≥80% pain relief.[28] These findings suggest that the addition of corticosteroid to local anesthetic does not provide better outcome. Moreover, as described above, the diagnostic procedure used in the RCT is burdensome for the patient, and repeat infiltrations are needed every 14 to 16 weeks. Therefore, this therapy cannot be recommended as an initial option.

Radiofrequency Treatment of the Ramus Medialis of the Ramus Dorsalis

Percutaneous RF treatment of cervical pain has been intensively studied. The data from original articles were summarized in seven systematic reviews.[9,26,29-32] However, only one RCT studied RF treatment of the ramus medialis of the ramus dorsalis in patients with whiplash-associated disorder.[10] The effectiveness of RF treatment for degenerative neck pathology was shown in observational studies.[7,33,34]

A retrospective chart analysis on the effect of repeat RF facet denervations illustrated that the mean duration of effect of the first intervention was 12.5 months. Patients who responded positively to the first intervention received a second up to a seventh intervention. Percentages of success were over 90% after each repeat intervention, and the duration of effect was between 8 and 12 months.[35]

The summary of the evidence for interventional management of cervical facet pain is given in **Table 14-3**.

Risk and Complication Avoidance

Complications are rare. Nevertheless, one should be aware that the arteria vertebralis may be punctured if the needle is pushed too far anterior into the neuroforamen. Verification of the needle point position should be made under AP fluoroscopy to prevent intrathecal injection of the local anesthetic. In an observational study,[36] the incidence of inadvertent intravascular penetration for medial branch blocks at spinal level was reported to be 3.9%, comparable to the incidence at lumbar lever (3.7%). Some patients experienced

short-term vasovagal reactions. The intravascular uptake of local anesthetic and contrast solution was thought to be responsible for false-negative diagnostic blocks. No systemic effects were reported.[36] A report on transient tetraplegia after cervical facet joint injection, done without imaging, illustrates the vulnerability of the cervical arteries.[37]

Monitoring of the saturation level and availability of resuscitation equipment are essential. Infections have been described, but the incidence is unknown and probably very low.

A recent report on septic arthritis of the facet joints included two cases of cervical facet joints. In these cases, the port of entry could not be identified, but in one lumbar case, percutaneous injection was directly linked to this severe complication.[38] Other potential complications of facet joint interventions are related to needle placement and drug administration; they include dural puncture, spinal cord trauma, spinal anesthesia, chemical meningitis, neural trauma, pneumothorax, radiation exposure, facet capsule rupture, hematoma formation, and side effects of corticosteroids.[39]

After RF treatment, postoperative burning pain is regularly reported. This pain disappears after 1 to 3 weeks.[40] Smith et al[41] found contrast enhancement on MRI typical for paraspinal abscess, even without apparent infection, which was attributed to a noninfectious post inflammatory process.

There are no incidence data on side effects and complications after cervical RF facet denervation. At the lumbar level, the incidence of complications was lower than 1%.[42]

Pain Originating from the Lumbar Facet Joints

Establishing a Diagnosis

Background   Pain emanating from the lumbar facet joints is a common cause of low back pain in the adult population. Golthwaite was the first to describe the syndrome in 1911, and Ghormley is generally credited with coining the term "facet syndrome" in 1933. Facet pain is defined as pain that arises from any structure that is part of the facet joints, including the fibrous capsule, synovial membrane, hyaline cartilage, and bone.[43-45] The reported prevalence rate varies widely in different studies from less than 5% to as high as 90%, being heavily dependent on diagnostic criteria and selection methods.[46-53] Based on information from studies that were done on well-selected patient populations, we estimate the prevalence to range between 5% and 15% of the population with axial low back pain.[21,54-56] Because arthritis is a prominent cause of facetogenic pain, the prevalence rate increases with age.[18,57] Although some experts have expressed doubts about the validity of "facet syndrome," studies conducted in patients and volunteers have confirmed its existence.[58-63] In rare cases, facet joint pain can result from a specific traumatic event (i.e., high-energy trauma associated with a combination of hyperflexion, extension, and distraction).[64] More commonly, it is the result of repetitive stress or cumulative low-level trauma. This leads to inflammation, which can cause the facet joint to fill with fluid and swell, which in turn results in stretching of the joint capsule and subsequent pain generation.[65] Inflammatory changes around the facet joint can also irritate the spinal nerve via neuroforaminal narrowing, resulting in sciatica. In addition, Igarashi et al[66] found that inflammatory cytokines released through the ventral joint capsule in patients with facet joint degeneration may be partially responsible for the neuropathic symptoms in individuals with spinal stenosis. Predisposing factors for facet joint pain include spondylolisthesis or lysis, degenerative discus intervertebralis disease, and advanced age.[45] The treatment of facet pain is the subject of great controversy. In 1963, Hirsch et al[59] were the first group to describe the technique

Table 14-3: Evidence for Interventional Management of Cervical Facet Pain

Technique	Score
Intraarticular injections	0
Therapeutic (repetitive) medial branch block (local anesthetic with or without corticosteroids)	2B+
RF treatment of the ramus medialis of the cervical ramus dorsalis (for degenerative facet pain)	2C+
RF treatment of the ramus medialis of the cervical ramus dorsalis (for whiplash-associated disorders)	2B+

RF, radiofrequency.

Table 14-4: Causes of Low Back Pain

Lumbar causes	Intervertebral disc	Annular tears Internal disc disruption Discitis
	Vertebral body	Fractures Malignant tumors Osteomyelitis Endplate damage
	Facet joint	Osteoarthrosis Synovitis Inflammatory arthritides Fractures
	Sacroiliac joint	Synovitis Inflammatory arthritides Fractures Osteoarthrosis Ligamentous injury Enthesopathy
	Musculoligamentous	Strain Infection, abscess
Abdominal causes	Vascular Renal	Aortic aneurysm Pyelonephritis Kidney stones Malignancy
	Intestines	Malignancy

of facet joint injections, and in the mid-1970s, Shealy[67,68] published the first reports of RF treatment of the facet joints under radiographic guidance. Because each facet joint receives dual innervation from adjacent levels, and most individuals have multilevel pathology, several levels usually need to be treated.[69-71]

The possible causes of lumbar pain are listed in **Table 14-4**.

History A number of researchers have attempted to elucidate the clinical entity "facetogenic pain," mostly through provocation of pain in volunteers.[61,72-77] The most frequent complaint is axial low back pain. Although bilateral symptoms are more common than for sacroiliac joint pain, centralization of pain is less predictive of response to analgesic blocks than it is for discogenic pain.[78,79] Sometimes pain may be referred into the groin or thigh.[61] Whereas pain originating from the upper facet joints often extends into the flank, hip, and lateral thigh regions, pain from the lower facet joints typically radiates into the posterior thigh. Pain distal to the knee is rarely associated with facet pathology. Other causes of predominantly axial low back pain that must be considered in the differential diagnosis include discogenic pain, sacroiliac joint pathology, ligamentous injury, and myofascial pain. Within the context of facet pathology, inflammatory arthritides, such as rheumatoid arthritis, ankylosing spondylitis, gout, psoriatic arthritis, reactive arthritis, and other spondyloarthropathies, as well as osteoarthrosis and synovitis, must also be considered.

Physical Examination There are no physical examination findings that are pathognomonic for diagnosis. Because facet pain originates from the mobile elements of the back, examination of motion seems relevant. In a series of cadaveric studies, Ianuzzi et al[80] determined that the largest strain on the lower lumbar facet joints occurred during flexion and lateral bending, with extension also stressing L5/S1. It is therefore possible that pain worsened by flexion and extension is suggestive of pathology originating from the lowest lumbar segment(s). Revel et al[54,77] were the first to correlate symptoms and physical examination signs with the response to placebo-controlled blocks.

The Revel criteria for lumbar facet joint pain are as follows:

- Pain not worsened by coughing
- Pain not worsened by straightening from flexion
- Pain not worsened by extension-rotation
- Pain not worsened by hyperextension
- Pain improved in the supine position

However, previous and subsequent studies have failed to corroborate these findings.[81-83] It is widely acknowledged that lumbar paravertebral tenderness is indicative of facetogenic pain, which is a claim supported by clinical trials.[84] Recently, indicators of facet pain have been described based on a survey of an expert panel. They specified a panel of 12 indicators that creates the framework for a diagnosis of facet pain.[85] These indicators are not in line with previous studies.[77,84,86]

Anatomy

The general joint features already described are also applicable to the lumbar spine.

The processus articularis superior of the facet joint bears slightly concave vertical facets that face medially and posteriorly. The processus articularis inferior has slightly convex vertical facets directed laterally and anteriorly (**Fig. 14-7**). In maximal retroflexion (lordosis), the curved joint surfaces of these "pins and claws" enable flexion and extension of the lumbar spine. Axial rotation and lateroflexion are only possible when the segment comes out of this maximal retroflexion.

Compared with the cervical facet joint, the synovial lumbar facet joint is surrounded by a shorter and thicker joint capsule, still enclosing a variable extending synovium and joint space.

Xu et al[87] correlated axial MRI, CT, and cryomicrotome sections of 66 lumbar facet joints in nine cadavers (three female, six male; ages 21 to 95 years). Although one should be skeptical of interpretations of in vivo tissue continuities using cadaveric specimens, the authors, by intraarticular injection of a contrast-fast green dye medium, in the MRI, but to a lesser extent in the CT images, could recognize extensions of the synovium and joint space along the processus articularis superior and inferior, under and into the ligamentum flavum. On the anterior aspect of the lumbar facet joint, the images showed the joint space extending into the ligamentum flavum or between the ligamentum flavum and the lamina. On the posterior aspect, the images showed a prominence of the fibrous joint capsule where the joint space extended under it along the processus articularis inferior or superior. The results were correlated to cryomicrotome sections of the scanned specimens in planes and levels corresponding to those of the MRI and CT.

The posterior enlargement of the processus articularis superior in the lumbar spine is called the processus mamillaris. The posteroinferior aspect of the thin and long processus transversus of the lumbar vertebra is marked by a small processus accessorius. These two processes are bridged by an aponeurotic fibrous ligament, the mamillo-accessory ligament.

As in all spinal segments, the facet joints from L1 to L5 are innervated by the ramus medialis (medial branch) of the ramus dorsalis of the segmental nerve. Each facet joint is innervated by nerve branches from the upper and lower segment (**Fig. 14-8**).[69-71]

The ramus dorsalis L5 runs along the junction between the ala ossis sacri and the processus articularis ossis sacri. It is much longer than the other lumbar rami dorsales.

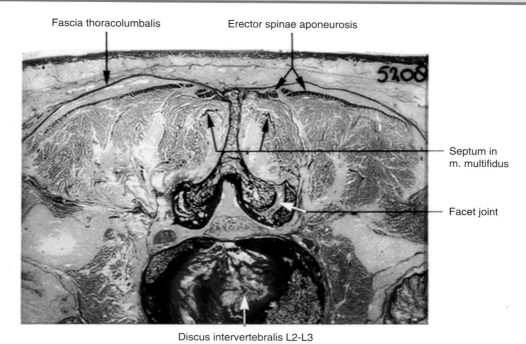

Fascia thoracolumbalis

Erector spinae aponeurosis

Septum in
m. multifidus

Facet joint

Discus intervertebralis L2-L3

Fig. 14-7 Transverse histological section of the lumbar spinal column.

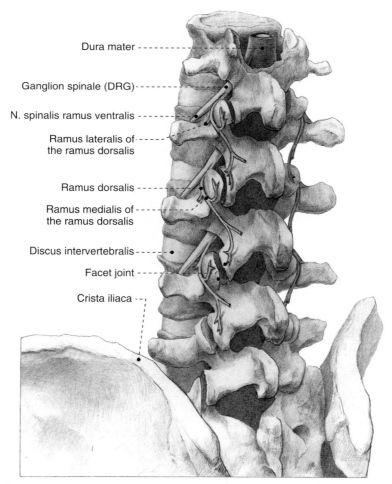

Dura mater

Ganglion spinale (DRG)

N. spinalis ramus ventralis

Ramus lateralis of
the ramus dorsalis

Ramus dorsalis

Ramus medialis of
the ramus dorsalis

Discus intervertebralis

Facet joint

Crista iliaca

Fig. 14-8 Anatomy of the lumbar spinal column. DRG, dorsal root ganglion. (Illustrated by Rogier Trompert Medical Art.
http://www.medical-art.nl.)

For the rami dorsales L1-L4, besides the medial branch, Bogduk et al[88] described a lateral and an intermediate branch. Medial, lateral, and intermediate branches distribute, respectively, to the musculus multifidus, musculus iliocostalis, and musculus longissimus. The ramus dorsalis L5 forms only a medial and intermediate branch, which is not surprising because the musculus iliocostalis does not attach to L5.

Imaging

The prevalence rate of pathological changes in the facet joints on radiological examination depends on the mean age of the subjects, the radiological technique used, and the definition of "abnormality." Degenerative facet joints can be best visualized via CT examination.[89] CT studies conducted in patients with low back pain show a prevalence rate of facet joint degeneration ranging between 40% and 80%.[52,90] MRI scans may be somewhat less sensitive in the detection of facet pathology.[47,89] Interestingly, the number of studies demonstrating a positive correlation between radiological abnormalities and the response to diagnostic blocks is roughly equivalent to the number showing no correlation.[47,51-54,57,70,74,81,90-92] Supplementary radiological examination may also be necessary to rule out so-called "red flags" such as malignancy, compression fracture, or spinal infection.[93]

Guidelines

Conservative Management   The treatment of patients with facet pain should ideally occur in a multidisciplinary fashion and include conservative (pharmacological treatment; cognitive behavioral therapy; manual medicine; exercise therapy and rehabilitation; and if necessary, a more detailed psychological evaluation) as well as interventional pain management techniques. Because there have been no clinical studies evaluating pharmacological or noninterventional treatments for patients with injection-confirmed facet joint pain, one must extrapolate from studies that have been conducted on patients with chronic nonspecific low back complaints. Although nonsteroidal antiinflammatory drugs are often used, scientific evidence supporting their long-term use for low back complaints is scant.[93] Antidepressants appear to be effective, but the treatment effect is small.[94] Manipulation can also be effective,[95,96] although one study showed no difference with "sham" therapy.[97]

Interventional Management   Currently, the gold standard for treating facetogenic pain is RF treatment. The major advantage of temperature-controlled RF treatment compared with voltage-controlled and other "neurolytic" techniques is that it produces controlled and reproducible lesion dimensions.[98] RF facet treatment can also be repeated without a loss of efficacy, which is important because the duration of benefit is limited by the inexorable rate of nerve regeneration.[99] There are currently no randomized studies comparing RF facet treatment with intraarticular injections.[45]

Intraarticular Corticosteroid Injections

The use of intraarticular corticosteroid injections in the facet joints is controversial. Uncontrolled studies have mostly demonstrated transient beneficial effects, but the results of controlled studies have been mostly disappointing. Lilius et al[100] performed the largest randomized study, involving 109 patients. They found no difference between large-volume (8 mL) intraarticular saline injections, intraarticular corticosteroid and local anesthetic, and the same mixture injected around two facet joints. In a randomized, controlled study, Carette et al[101] found only a small difference between the injection of saline (10% good effect) and depot corticosteroid (22% good effect) up to 6 months after treatment. One caveat with placebo-controlled trials that is not commonly recognized is that the intraarticular injection of saline may itself provide therapeutic benefit.[102] Observational studies involving intraarticular local anesthetic and corticosteroid typically show symptom palliation lasting for up to 3 months.[91,103] Based on the literature, one can conclude that intraarticular corticosteroid injections are of very limited value in the treatment of unscreened patients with suspected facetogenic pain. However, subgroup analyses have revealed that patients with positive single-photon emission computed tomography scans may be more likely to respond than patients without an acute inflammatory process.[103,104]

Radiofrequency Treatment

RF treatment is frequently performed for various forms of spinal pain, although the scientific evidence for this intervention remains controversial. The first controlled study was published by Gallagher et al[105] in 1994. The authors selected 41 patients with chronic low back complaints who responded with some pain relief to diagnostic intraarticular injections and randomized them to receive either "sham" or true RF treatment of the rami mediales (medial branches). The two study groups were then subdivided into patients who obtained "good" and "equivocal" relief after the diagnostic block. After 6 months, a significant difference was found only between treatment and control subjects who had experienced good relief from the test blocks. In a well-designed placebo-controlled study, Van Kleef et al[106] demonstrated good results after RF treatment lasting up to 12 months after treatment. Leclaire et al[107] did not establish a therapeutic effect for RF treatment in a placebo-controlled trial, but this study has been criticized because the criterion for a positive "diagnostic" block was 24 hours or more of pain relief after lidocaine infiltration, which is inconsistent with the drug's pharmacokinetics. In addition, 94% of the screened patients with back pain were selected for participation, which is much greater than the presumed prevalence for lumbar facetogenic pain (17% 30%) in this cohort. For these reasons, this study is judged to have major methodological flaws.

Van Wijk et al[108] also found no difference between the treatment and control groups with regard to visual analog scale pain score, medication usage, and function. However, the RF group in this study did report 50% or more reduction in complaints significantly more often (62% vs. 39%) than those who received a sham procedure. However, the evaluation method was subject to discussion.

Finally, in the most recent randomized placebo-controlled trial, which was undertaken in 40 patients who obtained significant pain relief after three diagnostic blocks, a significantly greater improvement in pain symptoms, global perception of improvement, and quality of life was observed after 6 months in subjects allocated to RF treatment.[56] In two randomized studies comparing pulsed and conventional RF treatment for facetogenic pain, both showed conventional RF to be superior.[109,110]

From these seven controlled studies, one can conclude that RF treatment of the facet joints can provide intermediate-term benefit in carefully selected patients. However, in a recent review, the value of this intervention was questioned.[111] In a letter to the editor, the methodology was questioned, and a meta-analysis was performed. When including the six RCTs, RF was significantly better than placebo. Even when only the two trials without shortcomings were included, the difference in favor of RF treatment remained significant.[112]

There is presently no evidence to support the use of operative interventions for injection-confirmed facetogenic pain.[45]

Although several devices have been used and advocated for percutaneous facet joint fusion, none has been evaluated in rigorous trials.

Indications and Contraindications

Patients fulfilling the following criteria are eligible for RF treatment of the ramus medialis (medial branch) of the ramus dorsalis innervating the facet joints:

- Localized unilateral low back pain
- Absence of radicular symptoms
- Eliciting or worsening of the pain by unilateral pressure on the facet joint or the processus transversus
- Pain with extension, lateroflexion, or rotation toward the ipsilateral side
- Unilateral muscle hypertonus at the level of the involved facet joint
- Referred pain in the leg remains limited to the area above the knee
- Pain with extension
- Local unilateral movement shows a limitation of movement or increased stiffness on the side of the facet pain
- Pain lessened by flexion
- Pain reduction after anesthetic blocks carried out under radiographic examination of the ramus medialis (medial branch) of the ramus dorsalis that innervates the facet joints

Technique and Equipment

Diagnostic Blocks Diagnostic blocks are most frequently performed under radiographic guidance but can also be done under ultrasonography.[94,113] Although intraarticular injection and medial branch (facet joint nerve) blocks are often described as "equivalent," this has yet to be demonstrated in a comparative, crossover study design.[45] Neither of these approaches has been shown to be superior.[60] Both medial branch and intraarticular blocks are associated with significant false-positive and false-negative rates. For both techniques, the rate of false-positive results is most often cited as ranging between 15% and 40%.[45] Regarding the false-negative rate, Kaplan et al[114] found that 11% of volunteers retained the ability to perceive capsular distention after appropriately performed medial branch blocks, which was attributed to aberrant innervation.

Other causes of false-negative blocks include inappropriate needle placement, failure to detect vascular uptake, and inability of the patient to discern baseline from procedure-related pain.[115] False-positive results can be ascribed to several phenomena, including placebo response; use of sedation; or the excessive use of superficial local anesthesia, which can obscure myofascial pain.[116,117] In addition, the local anesthetic can spread to surrounding pain-generating structures. More than 70 years ago, Kellegren[118] noted that an intramuscular injection of 0.5 mL of fluid spreads over an area encompassing 6 cm^2 of tissue; this was later confirmed by Cohen and Raja.[45,118] Dreyfuss et al[115] found that either epidural or neuroforaminal spread occurred in 16% of blocks using the traditional target point at the superior junction of the processus transversus and the processus articularis superior. Given the close proximity of the ramus lateralis and intermedius to the ramus medialis (medial branch) of the primary ramus dorsalis, it is not possible to selectively block one without the others. During intraarticular facet blocks, the capsule can rupture after the injection of 1 to 2 mL of fluid with the resultant spread of the local anesthetic to other potential pain-generating structures. Perhaps because of their safety, simplicity, and prognostic value, diagnostic medial branch blocks are done more frequently than intraarticular injections.

Dreyfuss et al[115] researched the ideal needle position for diagnostic medial branch blocks. They compared two different target sites—one with the needle tip positioned on the upper edge of the processus transversus and the other with the needle tip located halfway between the upper edge of the processus transversus and the mamillo-accessory ligament. The authors found that the lower (i.e., latter) target position was associated with a lower incidence of inadvertent injectate spread to the segmental nerves and epidural space when a volume of 0.5 mL was used. It is thus recommended to use the lower target site when performing diagnostic medial branch blocks. After the procedure, the patient is given a pain diary with instructions to discount procedure-related discomfort and engage in normal activities to permit adequate assessment of effectiveness. Failure to properly discriminate between baseline pain and that related to the procedure is a common cause of false-negative blocks. In general, a definitive treatment is carried out if a patient experiences 50% or greater pain reduction lasting for the duration of action of the local anesthetic (e.g., >30 minutes with lidocaine and 3 hours with bupivacaine). Because double, comparative blocks are associated with a significant false-negative rate and have not been shown to be cost-effective, the "double-block" paradigm is not advisable at this time.[119-121]

Radiofrequency Treatment of the Lumbar Facet Joints

There are several ways to perform lumbar facet RF treatment, and comparative studies among different techniques are lacking. This section describes just one technique. RF treatment is a procedure that requires continuous feedback from the patient during the procedure. Therefore, if sedation is used, it should be light enough to enable conversation. The patient is placed in a prone position on an examination table. A cushion is placed under the abdomen to straighten the physiological lumbar lordosis. First, the anatomical structures are identified with an AP examination. Next, the C-arm is rotated axially to align the x-ray beam parallel with the L4-L5 discus intervertebralis to remove parallax of the endplates. The C-arm is then rotated approximately 15 degrees obliquely to the ipsilateral side so the junction between the processus articularis superior and the processus transversus, the traditional target point, is more easily accessible. Several preclinical studies have demonstrated that placing the active tip parallel to the course of the nerve maximizes lesion size.[122,123] Hence, if the practitioner desires to orient the electrode parallel to the targeted nerve in a coaxial view to facilitate placement, the image intensifier can be further angled in the caudad direction. The injection point is then marked on the skin. The traditional target is the cephalad junction between the processus articularis superior and the processus transversus. However, one cadaveric study and literature review determined the optimal needle position to be with the electrode tip lying across the lateral neck of the processus articularis superior.[122] When inserting the electrode, one should first make contact with the processus transversus as close as possible to the processus articularis superior. After contacting bone, the needle is advanced slightly in a cranial direction so the tip slides over the processus transversus (**Fig. 14-9**). In the lateral fluoroscopic view, the electrode tip should now lie at the base of the processus articularis superior in the plane formed by the so-called facet column at the lower aspect of the neuroforamen, approximately 1 mm dorsal to its posterior border (**Fig. 14-10**). When proper needle position is confirmed in multiple views, the impedance is checked, and a sensory stimulus current of 50 Hz is applied. The electrode position is generally deemed adequate if concordant stimulation is obtained at 0.5 V or less. Motor

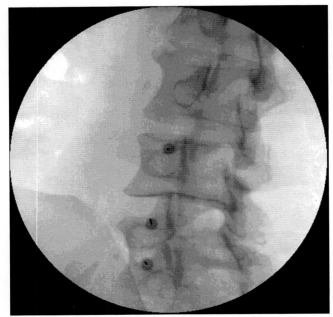

Fig. 14-9 Radiofrequency treatment of L3, L4, and L5 rami dorsales/facet, oblique view.

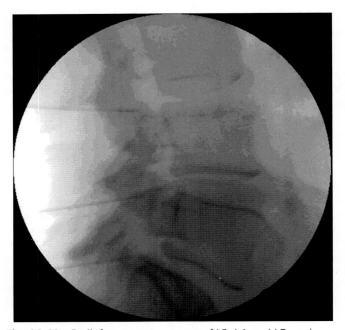

Fig. 14-10 Radiofrequency treatment of L3, L4, and L5 rami dorsales/facet, lateral view.

stimulation at 2 Hz serves to confirm correct needle placement via contraction of the musculus multifidus and to ensure the absence of distal muscle contractions in the leg, which indicates improper placement. Local muscle contractions in the back can generally be observed and palpated by the practitioner, but these are not always detectable. If leg movement is observed or the patient feels contractions in the leg, the needle must be repositioned. When the practitioner is confident the needle is properly positioned, 0.5 mL of local anesthetic is injected. After a brief interval in which the local anesthetic takes effect, a ≥67-degree lesion is applied for at least 1 minute. The nerve location and technique are the same for the

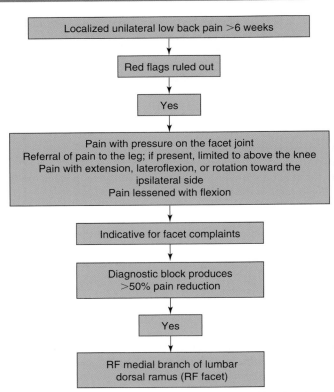

Fig. 14-11 Practice algorithm for the treatment of lumbar facet pain.

Localized unilateral low back pain >6 weeks

Red flags ruled out

Yes

Pain with pressure on the facet joint
Referral of pain to the leg; if present, limited to above the knee
Pain with extension, lateroflexion, or rotation toward the ipsilateral side
Pain lessened with flexion

Indicative for facet complaints

Diagnostic block produces >50% pain reduction

Yes

RF medial branch of lumbar dorsal ramus (RF facet)

Table 14-5: Evidence for Interventional Pain Management of Lumbar Facet Pain

Technique	Assessment
Intraarticular injections	2B±
RF treatment of the ramus medialis (medial branch) of the L1-L4 primary rami dorsales and of the L5 primary ramus dorsalis	1B+

RF, radiofrequency.

ramus medialis (medial branch) of the nerves L1-L4. For L5, it is the ramus dorsalis itself that is amenable to lesioning because it courses along the junction between the ala ossis sacri and the processus articularis ossis sacri. At this level, 2 Hz of stimulation does not always produce prominent contraction of the musculus multifidus, yet motor stimulation should be performed to prevent inadvertent lesioning too close to the segmental nerve.

Patient Management and Evaluation
Patients should be informed that pain might worsen temporarily after RF denervation of the facet joints. Typically, this pain lasts for 2 weeks and is attributed to neuritis of the medial branch nerve. After this period, pain should improve gradually. If pain persists after RF treatment, other causes of low back pain should be examined.

Outcomes Evidence
In the Evidence-Based Practice Guideline on the management of lumbar facet pain, the grade of recommendations defined as described above are listed in **Table 14-5**. The practice algorithm derived from the evidence assessment is illustrated in **Fig. 14-11**.

Risk and Complication Avoidance

Complications of Diagnostic Blocks The most prevalent complication of a diagnostic block results from an overflow of local anesthetic to the segmental nerves. This can cause temporary paresthesias in the legs and loss of motor function.

Complications of Radiofrequency Treatment The complications and side effects of RF treatment have been previously described in a small retrospective study by Kornick et al.[42] Of 116 procedures, the two most commonly occurring complications were transient, localized burning pain and self-limiting back pain lasting longer than 2 weeks, each occurring with a frequency of 2.5% per procedure. In this study, no infections or motor or new sensory deficits were identified. Unlike diagnostic blocks, which in rare instances have been complicated by spinal infection(s), RF treatment has never been associated with infectious complications.[124] This may be because heat lesioning serves a protective function. In rare instances, local burns and motor weakness have been reported.[45,125]

Acknowledgements

This chapter is based on the articles on cervical and lumbar facet joint pain in the series "Evidence-based interventional pain medicine based on clinical diagnoses" previously published in *Pain Practice*. Excerpts from van Eerd M, Patijn J, Lataster A, et al: Cervical facet pain, *Pain Pract* 10(2):113-123, 2010 and van Kleef M, Vanelderen P, Cohen SP, et al: Pain originating from the lumbar facet joints, *Pain Pract* 10(5):459-469, 2010 are used with the permission of the World Institute of Pain and Wiley-Blackwell. The following persons contributed to those articles: Jaap Patijn, Richard Rosenquist, and Steven P. Cohen. The authors thank Nicole Van den Hecke for coordination and suggestions regarding this chapter.

References

1. Guzman J, Hurwitz EL, Carroll LJ, et al: A new conceptual model of neck pain: linking onset, course, and care: the Bone and Joint Decade 2000-2010 Task Force on Neck Pain and Its Associated Disorders. *Spine* 33(suppl):S14-S23, 2008.
2. Bogduk N, McGuirk B: Management of acute and chronic neck pain. In *Pain research and clinical management*, St. Louis, 2006, Elsevier.
3. Adams MA, Roughley PJ: What is intervertebral disc degeneration, and what causes it? *Spine* 31:2151-2161, 2006.
4. Bogduk N, Aprill C: On the nature of neck pain, discography and cervical zygapophysial joint blocks. *Pain* 54:213-217, 1993.
5. Bogduk N, Marsland A: The cervical zygapophysial joints as a source of neck pain. *Spine* 13:610-617, 1988.
6. Dwyer A, Aprill C, Bogduk N: Cervical zygapophyseal joint pain patterns. I: a study in normal volunteers. *Spine* 15:453-457, 1990.
7. Cohen SP, Bajwa ZH, Kraemer JJ, et al: Factors predicting success and failure for cervical facet radiofrequency denervation: a multi-center analysis. *Reg Anesth Pain Med* 32:495-503, 2007.
8. Kirpalani D, Mitra R: Cervical facet joint dysfunction: a review. *Arch Phys Med Rehabil* 89:770-774, 2008.
9. Manchikanti L, Boswell MV, Singh V, et al: Comprehensive evidence-based guidelines for interventional techniques in the management of chronic spinal pain. *Pain Physician* 12:699-802, 2009.
10. Lord SM, Barnsley L, Wallis BJ, et al: Percutaneous radio-frequency neurotomy for chronic cervical zygapophyseal-joint pain. *N Engl J Med* 335:1721-1726, 1996.
11. Nordin M, Carragee EJ, Hogg-Johnson S, et al: Assessment of neck pain and its associated disorders: results of the Bone and Joint Decade 2000-2010 Task Force on Neck Pain and Its Associated Disorders. *J Manipulative Physiol Ther* 32(suppl):S117-S140, 2009.
12. Moore K: *Clinically oriented anatomy*, ed 3, Baltimore, 1992, Williams & Wilkins.
13. De Avila GA, O'Connor BL, Visco DM, Sisk TD: The mechanoreceptor innervation of the human fibular collateral ligament. *J Anat* 162:1-6, 1989.
14. McLain RF: Mechanoreceptor endings in human cervical facet joints. *Iowa Orthop J* 13:149-154, 1993.
15. Groen GJ, Baljet B, Drukker J: Nerves and nerve plexuses of the human vertebral column. *Am J Anat* 188:282-296, 1990.
16. Kellgren J, Jeffrey M, Ball J: *The epidemiology of chronic rheumatism*, Oxford, 1963, Blackwell.
17. Friedenberg ZB, Miller WT: Degenerative disc disease of the cervical spine. *J Bone Joint Surg Am* 45:1171-1178, 1963.
18. Manchikanti L, Manchikanti KN, Cash KA, et al: Age-related prevalence of facet-joint involvement in chronic neck and low back pain. *Pain Physician* 11:67-75, 2008.
19. van der Donk J, Schouten JS, Passchier J, et al: The associations of neck pain with radiological abnormalities of the cervical spine and personality traits in a general population. *J Rheumatol* 18:1884-1889, 1991.
20. Haldeman S, Carroll L, Cassidy JD, et al: The Bone and Joint Decade 2000-2010 Task Force on Neck Pain and Its Associated Disorders: executive summary. *Spine* 33(suppl):S5-S7, 2008.
21. Manchikanti L, Boswell MV, Singh V, et al: Prevalence of facet joint pain in chronic spinal pain of cervical, thoracic, and lumbar regions. *BMC Musculoskelet Disord* 5:15, 2004.
22. Yin W, Bogduk N: The nature of neck pain in a private pain clinic in the United States. *Pain Med* 9:196-203, 2008.
23. Govind J, King W, Bailey B, Bogduk N: Radiofrequency neurotomy for the treatment of third occipital headache. *J Neurol Neurosurg Psychiatry* 74:88-93, 2003.
24. Guyatt G, Gutterman D, Baumann MH, et al: Grading strength of recommendations and quality of evidence in clinical guidelines: report from an American College of Chest Physicians task force. *Chest* 129:174-181, 2006.
25. van Kleef M, Mekhail N, van Zundert J: Evidence-based guidelines for interventional pain medicine according to clinical diagnoses. *Pain Pract* 9:247-251, 2009.
26. Falco FJ, Erhart S, Wargo BW, et al: Systematic review of diagnostic utility and therapeutic effectiveness of cervical facet joint interventions. *Pain Physician* 12:323-344, 2009.
27. Barnsley L, Lord S, Bogduk N: Comparative local anaesthetic blocks in the diagnosis of cervical zygapophysial joint pain. *Pain* 55:99-106, 1993.
28. Manchikanti L, Singh V, Falco FJ, et al: Cervical medial branch blocks for chronic cervical facet joint pain: a randomized, double-blind, controlled trial with one-year follow-up. *Spine* 33:1813-1820, 2008.
29. Geurts JW, van Wijk RM, Stolker RJ, Groen GJ: Efficacy of radiofrequency procedures for the treatment of spinal pain: a systematic review of randomized clinical trials. *Reg Anesth Pain Med* 26:394-400, 2001.
30. Niemisto L, Kalso E, Malmivaara A, et al: Radiofrequency denervation for neck and back pain: a systematic review within the framework of the Cochrane Collaboration back review group. *Spine* 28:1877-1888, 2003.
31. Manchikanti L, Singh V, Vilims BD, et al: Medial branch neurotomy in management of chronic spinal pain: systematic review of the evidence. *Pain Physician* 5:405-418, 2002.
32. Boswell MV, Trescot AM, Datta S, et al: Interventional techniques: evidence-based practice guidelines in the management of chronic spinal pain. *Pain Physician* 10:7-111, 2007.
33. McDonald GJ, Lord SM, Bogduk N: Long-term follow-up of patients treated with cervical radiofrequency neurotomy for chronic neck pain. *Neurosurgery* 45:61-67; discussion 67-68, 1999.
34. Barnsley L: Percutaneous radiofrequency neurotomy for chronic neck pain: outcomes in a series of consecutive patients. *Pain Med* 6:282-286, 2005.

35. Husted DS, Orton D, Schofferman J, Kine G: Effectiveness of repeated radiofrequency neurotomy for cervical facet joint pain. *J Spinal Disord Tech* 21:406-408, 2008.

36. Verrills P, Mitchell B, Vivian D, et al: The incidence of intravascular penetration in medial branch blocks: cervical, thoracic, and lumbar spines. *Spine* 33:E174-E177, 2008.

37. Heckmann JG, Maihofner C, Lanz S, et al: Transient tetraplegia after cervical facet joint injection for chronic neck pain administered without imaging guidance. *Clin Neurol Neurosurg* 108:709-711, 2006.

38. Michel-Batot C, Dintinger H, Blum A, et al: A particular form of septic arthritis: septic arthritis of facet joint. *Joint Bone Spine* 75:78-83, 2008.

39. Boswell MV, Colson JD, Sehgal N, et al: A systematic review of therapeutic facet joint interventions in chronic spinal pain. *Pain Physician* 10:229-253, 2007.

40. Haspeslagh SR, Van Suijlekom HA, Lame IE, et al: Randomised controlled trial of cervical radiofrequency lesions as a treatment for cervicogenic headache [ISRCTN07444684]. *BMC Anesthesiol* 16:1, 2006.

41. Smith M, Ferretti G, Mortazavi S: Radiographic changes induced after cervical facet radiofrequency denervation. *Spine J* 5:668-671, 2005.

42. Kornick C, Kramarich SS, Lamer TJ, Todd Sitzman B: Complications of lumbar facet radiofrequency denervation. *Spine* 29:1352-1354, 2004.

43. Goldthwaite J: The lumbosacral articulation: an explanation of many cases of lumbago, sciatica, and paraplegia. *Boston Med Surg J* 365-372, 1911.

44. Ghormley R: Low back pain with special reference to the articular facts, with presentation of an operative procedure. *JAMA* 1773-1777, 1933.

45. Cohen SP, Raja SN: Pathogenesis, diagnosis, and treatment of lumbar zygapophysial (facet) joint pain. *Anesthesiology* 106:591-614, 2007.

46. Long DM, BenDebba M, Torgerson WS, et al: Persistent back pain and sciatica in the United States: patient characteristics. *J Spinal Disord* 9:40-58, 1996.

47. Murtagh FR: Computed tomography and fluoroscopy guided anesthesia and steroid injection in facet syndrome. *Spine* 13:686-689, 1988.

48. Destouet JM, Gilula LA, Murphy WA, Monsees B: Lumbar facet joint injection: indication, technique, clinical correlation, and preliminary results. *Radiology* 145:321-325, 1982.

49. Lau LS, Littlejohn GO, Miller MH: Clinical evaluation of intra-articular injections for lumbar facet joint pain. *Med J Aust* 143:563-565, 1985.

50. Moran R, O'Connell D, Walsh MG: The diagnostic value of facet joint injections. *Spine* 13:1407-1410, 1988.

51. Raymond J, Dumas JM: Intraarticular facet block: diagnostic test or therapeutic procedure? *Radiology* 151:333-336, 1984.

52. Carrera GF: Lumbar facet joint injection in low back pain and sciatica: description of technique. *Radiology* 137:661-664, 1980.

53. Lewinnek GE, Warfield CA: Facet joint degeneration as a cause of low back pain. *Clin Orthop Relat Res* 216-222, 1986.

54. Revel ME, Listrat VM, Chevalier XJ, et al: Facet joint block for low back pain: identifying predictors of a good response. *Arch Phys Med Rehabil* 73:824-828, 1992.

55. Dreyfuss P, Halbrook B, Pauza K, et al: Efficacy and validity of radiofrequency neurotomy for chronic lumbar zygapophysial joint pain. *Spine* 25:1270-1277, 2000.

56. Nath S, Nath CA, Pettersson K: Percutaneous lumbar zygapophysial (Facet) joint neurotomy using radiofrequency current, in the management of chronic low back pain: a randomized double-blind trial. *Spine* 33:1291-1297; discussion 1298, 2008.

57. Hicks GE, Morone N, Weiner DK: Degenerative lumbar disc and facet disease in older adults: prevalence and clinical correlates. *Spine (Phila Pa 1976)* 34:1301-1306, 2009.

58. Cavanaugh JM, Ozaktay AC, Yamashita HT, King AI: Lumbar facet pain: biomechanics, neuroanatomy and neurophysiology. *J Biomech* 29:1117-1129, 1996.

59. Hirsch C, Ingelmark BE, Miller M: The anatomical basis for low back pain. Studies on the presence of sensory nerve endings in ligamentous, capsular and intervertebral disc structures in the human lumbar spine. *Acta Orthop Scand* 33:1-17, 1963.

60. Marks RC, Houston T, Thulbourne T: Facet joint injection and facet nerve block: a randomised comparison in 86 patients with chronic low back pain. *Pain* 49:325-328, 1992.

61. McCall IW, Park WM, O'Brien JP: Induced pain referral from posterior lumbar elements in normal subjects. *Spine* 4:441-446, 1979.

62. Kuslich SD, Ulstrom CL, Michael CJ: The tissue origin of low back pain and sciatica: a report of pain response to tissue stimulation during operations on the lumbar spine using local anesthesia. *Orthop Clin North Am* 22:181-187, 1991.

63. Mooney V, Robertson J: The facet syndrome. *Clin Orthop Relat Res* 149-156, 1976.

64. Song KJ, Lee KB: Bilateral facet dislocation on L4-L5 without neurologic deficit. *J Spinal Disord Tech* 18:462-464, 2005.

65. Yang KH, King AI: Mechanism of facet load transmission as a hypothesis for low-back pain. *Spine* 9:557-565, 1984.

66. Igarashi A, Kikuchi S, Konno S: Correlation between inflammatory cytokines released from the lumbar facet joint tissue and symptoms in degenerative lumbar spinal disorders. *J Orthop Sci* 12:154-160, 2007.

67. Shealy CN: Facet denervation in the management of back and sciatic pain. *Clin Orthop Relat Res* 157-164, 1976.

68. Shealy CN: Percutaneous radiofrequency denervation of spinal facets. *J Neurosurg* 43:448-451, 1975.

69. Bogduk N, Long DM: The anatomy of the so-called "articular nerves" and their relationship to facet denervation in the treatment of low-back pain. *J Neurosurg* 51:172-177, 1979.

70. Schwarzer AC, Aprill CN, Derby R, et al: The false-positive rate of uncontrolled diagnostic blocks of the lumbar zygapophysial joints. *Pain* 58:195-200, 1994.

71. Schwarzer AC, Wang SC, Bogduk N, et al: Prevalence and clinical features of lumbar zygapophysial joint pain: a study in an Australian population with chronic low back pain. *Ann Rheum Dis* 54:100-106, 1995.

72. Marks R: Distribution of pain provoked from lumbar facet joints and related structures during diagnostic spinal infiltration. *Pain* 39:37-40, 1989.

73. Fukui S, Ohseto K, Shiotani M, et al: Distribution of referred pain from the lumbar zygapophyseal joints and dorsal rami. *Clin J Pain* 13:303-307, 1997.

74. Fairbank JC, Park WM, McCall IW, O'Brien JP: Apophyseal injection of local anesthetic as a diagnostic aid in primary low-back pain syndromes. *Spine* 6:598-605, 1981.

75. Helbig T, Lee CK: The lumbar facet syndrome. *Spine* 13:61-64, 1988.

76. Schwarzer AC, Aprill CN, Derby R, et al: The relative contributions of the disc and zygapophyseal joint in chronic low back pain. *Spine* 19:801-806, 1994.

77. Revel M, Poiraudeau S, Auleley GR, et al: Capacity of the clinical picture to characterize low back pain relieved by facet joint anesthesia. Proposed criteria to identify patients with painful facet joints. *Spine* 23:1972-1976; discussion 1977, 1998.

78. Cohen SP: Sacroiliac joint pain: a comprehensive review of anatomy, diagnosis, and treatment. *Anesth Analg* 101:1440-1453, 2005.

79. Laslett M, McDonald B, Aprill CN, et al: Clinical predictors of screening lumbar zygapophyseal joint blocks: development of clinical prediction rules. *Spine J* 6:370-379, 2006.

80. Ianuzzi A, Little JS, Chiu JB, et al: Human lumbar facet joint capsule strains: I. During physiological motions. *Spine J* 4:141-152, 2004.

81. Jackson RP, Jacobs RR, Montesano PX: 1988 Volvo award in clinical sciences. Facet joint injection in low-back pain. A prospective statistical study. *Spine* 13:966-971, 1988.

82. Schwarzer AC, Aprill CN, Derby R, et al: Clinical features of patients with pain stemming from the lumbar zygapophysial joints. Is the lumbar facet syndrome a clinical entity? *Spine* 19:1132-1137, 1994.

83. Laslett M, Oberg B, Aprill CN, McDonald B: Zygapophysial joint blocks in chronic low back pain: a test of Revel's model as a screening test. *BMC Musculoskelet Disord* 5:43, 2004.

84. Cohen SP, Hurley RW, Christo PJ, et al: Clinical predictors of success and failure for lumbar facet radiofrequency denervation. *Clin J Pain* 23:45-52, 2007.

85. Wilde VE, Ford JJ, McMeeken JM: Indicators of lumbar zygapophyseal joint pain: survey of an expert panel with the Delphi technique. *Phys Ther* 87:1348-1361, 2007.

86. Cohen SP, Argoff CE, Carragee EJ: Management of low back pain. *BMJ* 337:a2718, 2008.

87. Xu GL, Haughton VM, Carrera GF: Lumbar facet joint capsule: appearance at MR imaging and CT. *Radiology* 177:415-420, 1990.

88. Bogduk N, Wilson AS, Tynan W: The human lumbar dorsal rami. *J Anat* 134:383-397, 1982.

89. Weishaupt D, Zanetti M, Boos N, Hodler J: MR imaging and CT in osteoarthritis of the lumbar facet joints. *Skeletal Radiol* 28:215-219, 1999.

90. Carrera GF, Williams AL: Current concepts in evaluation of the lumbar facet joints. *Crit Rev Diagn Imaging* 21:85-104, 1984.

91. Dolan AL, Ryan PJ, Arden NK, et al: The value of SPECT scans in identifying back pain likely to benefit from facet joint injection. *Br J Rheumatol* 35:1269-1273, 1996.

92. Schwarzer AC, Wang SC, O'Driscoll D, et al: The ability of computed tomography to identify a painful zygapophysial joint in patients with chronic low back pain. *Spine* 20:907-912, 1995.

93. Airaksinen O, Brox JI, Cedraschi C, et al: Chapter 4. European guidelines for the management of chronic nonspecific low back pain. *Eur Spine J* 15(suppl 2):S192-S300, 2006.

94. Greher M, Kirchmair L, Enna B, et al: Ultrasound-guided lumbar facet nerve block: accuracy of a new technique confirmed by computed tomography. *Anesthesiology* 101:1195-1200, 2004.

95. Andersson GB, Lucente T, Davis AM, et al: A comparison of osteopathic spinal manipulation with standard care for patients with low back pain. *N Engl J Med* 341:1426-1431, 1999.

96. Giles LG, Muller R: Chronic spinal pain: a randomized clinical trial comparing medication, acupuncture, and spinal manipulation. *Spine* 28:1490-1502; discussion 1502-1493, 2003.

97. Licciardone JC, Stoll ST, Fulda KG, et al: Osteopathic manipulative treatment for chronic low back pain: a randomized controlled trial. *Spine* 28:1355-1362, 2003.

98. Silvers HR: Lumbar percutaneous facet rhizotomy. *Spine (Phila Pa 1976)* 15:36-40, 1990.

99. Schofferman J, Kine G: Effectiveness of repeated radiofrequency neurotomy for lumbar facet pain. *Spine* 29:2471-2473, 2004.

100. Lilius G, Laasonen EM, Myllynen P, et al: [Lumbar facet joint syndrome. Significance of non-organic signs. A randomized placebo-controlled clinical study]. *Rev Chir Orthop Reparatrice Appar Mot* 75:493-500, 1989.

101. Carette S, Marcoux S, Truchon R, et al: A controlled trial of corticosteroid injections into facet joints for chronic low back pain. *N Engl J Med* 325:1002-1007, 1991.

102. Egsmose C, Lund B, Bach Andersen R: Hip joint distension in osteoarthrosis. A triple-blind controlled study comparing the effect of intra-articular indoprofen with placebo. *Scand J Rheumatol* 13:238-242, 1984.

103. Pneumaticos SG, Chatziioannou SN, Hipp JA, et al: Low back pain: prediction of short-term outcome of facet joint injection with bone scintigraphy. *Radiology* 238:693-698, 2006.

104. Holder LE, Machin JL, Asdourian PL, et al: Planar and high-resolution SPECT bone imaging in the diagnosis of facet syndrome. *J Nucl Med* 36:37-44, 1995.

105. Gallagher J, Vadi PLP, Wesley JR: Radiofrequency facet joint denervation in the treatment of low back pain-a prospective controlled double-blind study in assess to efficacy. *Pain Clin* 7:193-198, 1994.

106. van Kleef M, Barendse GA, Kessels F, et al: Randomized trial of radiofrequency lumbar facet denervation for chronic low back pain. *Spine* 24:1937-1942, 1999.

107. Leclaire R, Fortin L, Lambert R, et al: Radiofrequency facet joint denervation in the treatment of low back pain: a placebo-controlled clinical trial to assess efficacy. *Spine* 26:1411-1416; discussion 1417, 2001.

108. van Wijk RM, Geurts JW, Wynne HJ, et al: Radiofrequency denervation of lumbar facet joints in the treatment of chronic low back pain: a randomized, double-blind, sham lesion-controlled trial. *Clin J Pain* 21:335-344, 2005.

109. Tekin I, Mirzai H, Ok G, et al: A comparison of conventional and pulsed radiofrequency denervation in the treatment of chronic facet joint pain. *Clin J Pain* 23:524-529, 2007.

110. Kroll HR, Kim D, Danic MJ, et al: A randomized, double-blind, prospective study comparing the efficacy of continuous versus pulsed radiofrequency in the treatment of lumbar facet syndrome. *J Clin Anesth* 20:534-537, 2008.

111. Chou R, Atlas SJ, Stanos SP, Rosenquist RW: Nonsurgical interventional therapies for low back pain: a review of the evidence for an American Pain Society clinical practice guideline. *Spine (Phila Pa 1976)* 34:1078-1093, 2009.

112. Van Zundert J, Vanelderen P, Kessels AG, et al: Nonsurgical interventional therapies for low back pain: a review of the evidence for an American Pain Society clinical practice guideline. *Spine (Phila Pa 1976)* 34:1078-1093, 2009; *Spine (Phila Pa 1976)* 35:841; author reply 841-842, 2010.

113. Shim JK, Moon JC, Yoon KB, et al: Ultrasound-guided lumbar medial-branch block: a clinical study with fluoroscopy control. *Reg Anesth Pain Med* 31:451-454, 2006.

114. Kaplan M, Dreyfuss P, Halbrook B, Bogduk N: The ability of lumbar medial branch blocks to anesthetize the zygapophysial joint. A physiologic challenge. *Spine (Phila Pa 1976)* 23:1847-1852, 1998.

115. Dreyfuss P, Schwarzer AC, Lau P, Bogduk N: Specificity of lumbar medial branch and L5 dorsal ramus blocks. A computed tomography study. *Spine* 22:895-902, 1997.

116. Ackerman WE, Munir MA, Zhang JM, Ghaleb A: Are diagnostic lumbar facet injections influenced by pain of muscular origin? *Pain Pract* 4:286-291, 2004.

117. Cohen SP, Larkin TM, Chang AS, Stojanovic MP: The causes of false-positive medial branch (facet joint) blocks in soldiers and retirees. *Mil Med* 169:781-786, 2004.

118. Kellegren J: On the distribution of pain arising from deep somatic structures with charts of segmental pain areas. *Clin Sci* 4:35-46, 1939.

119. Lord SM, Barnsley L, Bogduk N: The utility of comparative local anesthetic blocks versus placebo-controlled blocks for the diagnosis of cervical zygapophysial joint pain. *Clin J Pain* 11:208-213, 1995.

120. O'Neill C, Owens DK: Lumbar facet joint pain: time to hit the reset button. *Spine J* 9:619-622, 2009.

121. Bogduk N, Holmes S: Controlled zygapophysial joint blocks: the travesty of cost-effectiveness. *Pain Med* 1:24-34, 2000.

122. Lau P, Mercer S, Govind J, Bogduk N: The surgical anatomy of lumbar medial branch neurotomy (facet denervation). *Pain Med* 5:289-298, 2004.

123. Bogduk N, Macintosh J, Marsland A: Technical limitations to the efficacy of radiofrequency neurotomy for spinal pain. *Neurosurgery* 20:529-535, 1987.

124. Cheng J, Abdi S: Complications of joint, tendon, and muscle injections. *Tech Reg Anesth Pain Manag* 11:141-147, 2007.

125. Ogsbury JS, 3rd, Simon RH, Lehman RA: Facet "denervation" in the treatment of low back syndrome. *Pain* 3:257-263, 1977.

15 Sacroiliac Joint Injections and Lateral Branch Blocks, Including Water-Cooled Neurotomy

Bryan S. Williams

CHAPTER OVERVIEW

Chapter Synopsis: The sacroiliac joint (SIJ) represents a significant but underappreciated source of back pain in the population. SIJ dysfunction may cause pain stemming from any number of conditions, including structural abnormalities, infection, metabolic or inflammatory conditions, or degeneration. Although it may be difficult to differentiate from some other clinical conditions with a similar pain pattern (e.g., discogenic or herniated disc pain), SIJ dysfunction displays a distinctive referral pattern. This chapter describes this pattern and other considerations in the treatment of SIJ pain. The chapter provides a detailed look at the anatomy of the body's largest axial joint and its innervation. The chapter considers forms of SIJ therapy, including intraarticular injection, surgical interventions, and ablation procedures, with a focus on cooled radiofrequency (RF) denervation. Various means of imaging this complex joint are also considered; fluoroscopically or computed tomography–guided imaging with contrast injection of the SIJ appears to be the only reliable method for the diagnosis or exclusion of SIJ pain. As with any injection or ablation therapy, patient selection is a key to success, and more conservative therapies should be exhausted before considering neurotomy. Cooled RF neurotomy for SIJ pain has been used for such a short time that little outcome evidence is available, but early data suggest intermediate-term pain relief for the condition.

Important Points:
- Pain attributable to SIJ dysfunction is an area approximately 3×10 cm just inferior to the posterior superior iliac spine and usually not superior to L5.
- Referral patterns in patients with SIJ dysfunction are usually reported as radiating into the buttock.
- Combination of tests increases the likelihood of a diagnosis of SIJ dysfunction and positive response to SIJ injections.
- Controlled, comparative, image-guided local anesthetic diagnostic blocks are beneficial in the diagnosis of SIJ dysfunction.
- Minimally invasive procedures (intraarticular injections, ablative procedures) are minimally destructive to anatomy and have shown benefit in symptom attenuation.

Clinical Pearls:
- Exclude other etiologies (e.g., lumbar facet joint arthropathy, hip joint arthropathy) as pain generators.
- Ensure that all equipment is available and in proper working order.
- Utilize multiplanar imaging for proper probe placement.
- Deposition of steroidal antiinflammatory medication may reduce the chance of neuritis.

Clinical Pitfalls:
- Inappropriate patient selection
- Lack of knowledge of fluoroscopic anatomy

Establishing a Diagnosis

Goldthwaite and Osgood, in 1905, first described "sacroiliac strain" as a possible source of low back pain[1] and the sacroiliac joint (SIJ) was considered the primary source of low back pain in the early 20th century.[2] In 1936, Pitkin and Pheasant described lower extremity pain as originating in the sacroiliac and lumbosacral joints and their accessory ligaments and coined the term *sacroarthrogenic telalgia*. SIJ fusion became the treatment of choice for radicular pain originating from the low back.[3] It was not until Mixter and Barr that focus was placed on the lumbar spine, the intervertebral disc, and the herniation of nucleus pulposus contents.[4] Today, there is a reemergence implicating the SIJ as a potential source of low back pain with an estimated prevalence among patients with low back pain of 18% to 30%.[5,6]

Pathology of the SIJ has been documented in a variety of conditions; structural abnormalities, joint infections, metabolic and inflammatory disorders, and degeneration have all been implicated.[7] SIJ dysfunction or SIJ syndrome is a condition in which pain localized to the SIJ cannot otherwise be explained by an identifiable pathological process (e.g., joint infection). Clinically distinguishing primary SIJ dysfunction from the other etiologies that overlap in pain referral patterns may be difficult. Much of the confusion regarding the diagnosis of SIJ dysfunction revolves around the inability to differentiate SIJ pain from pain that originates from surrounding structures. For example, discogenic and facet joint pathology have a clinical presentation similar to that of SI joint pathology. Not only are the pain distributions considered similar in many references, but the clinical tests used in diagnosis (e.g., Patrick's, Gaenslen's) are known to stress surrounding structures.[7] The familiar symptom in SIJ dysfunction is the pain or other symptoms ascribed to a rectangular area approximately 3 × 10 cm just inferior to the posterior superior iliac spine (PSIS) identified on a pain drawing; however, no clinical studies have demonstrated this as a consistent finding for diagnosing SIJ dysfunction.[8] Through patient history and diagnostic testing, several referral patterns have been proposed, although these referral patterns may be present in other sources of low back pain.[9]

Furthermore, referral of pain into various locations of the lower extremity does not distinguish SIJ pain from other pain states.[5,10] However, only 4% of patients with SIJ pain mark any pain above the L5 on self-reported pain drawings.[10] The multiple patterns of SIJ pain referral zones may arise for several reasons: SIJ innervation is highly variable and complex; pain may be somatically referred from other primary osseous and ligamentous nociceptors such as the zygapophyseal joint, intervertebral disc, or adjacent structures (e.g., piriformis muscle, sciatic nerve, and L5 nerve root); and the referral pattern may be affected by intrinsic joint pathology and become active nociceptors.[1] Slipman et al[11] examined pain referral patterns in patients with SIJ dysfunction and reported that 94% of patients had pain radiating into the buttock, lower lumbar region (72%), lower extremity (50%), groin area (14%), upper lumbar region (6%), and abdomen (2%). In 28% of patients, the pain radiated distal to the knee, and 14% described foot pain (**Fig. 15-1**).

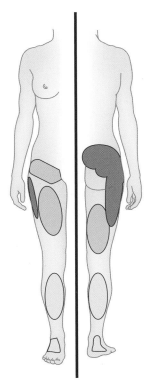

Fig. 15-1 Pain referral pattern from the sacroiliac joint. In descending order, the most common referral patterns extend from the *darkest* (low back and buttock) to the *lightest* regions (foot).

SIJ syndrome may occur acutely from trauma, sudden heavy lifting, prolonged lifting and bending, torsional strain, rising from a stooped position, a fall onto the buttock, or rear-end motor vehicle accident with the ipsilateral foot on the brake.[1] Characteristically associated with SIJ dysfunction include buttock pain caudal to the PSIS; pseudoradiculopathy with pain radiating to the posterolateral aspect of the thigh (at times caudal to the knee); and aggravation of pain in sitting position, rising from a sitting position (exiting an automobile), and relieved by changing positions. The most consistent factor for identifying patients with unilateral SIJ pain is unilateral pain localized predominantly below the L5 spinous process.[5,7,8,10,12]

Physical Examination

In 1994, the International Association for the Study of Pain (IASP) proposed a set of criteria for diagnosing SIJ pain, referring to patients with pain in the area of the SIJ, which should be reproducible by performing specific pain provocation tests or should be completely relieved by infiltration of the symptomatic SIJ with local anesthetics.[13] An assortment of SIJ examination maneuvers has been described to diagnose SIJ dysfunction (**Box 15-1**). Problematic to this is that provocation in this area may incite pain in adjacent structures, confounding the diagnosis of SIJ dysfunction. Additionally, using individual tests (provocative, motion, or palpation) has yielded low sensitivity or specificity for detecting a pathological SIJ.[14-16] Dreyfuss et al,[10] examining the usefulness of medical history and physical examination, concluded that no historical feature, none of the 12 tested SIJ maneuvers, and no ensemble of these 12 maneuvers demonstrated worthwhile diagnostic value. These results are replicated in a prospective cohort study in which provocative maneuvers were not predictive of diagnosis of SIJ dysfunction.[17] Additionally, 20% of asymptomatic patients have been found to possess pain on provocative tests at the SIJ.[18] In contrast, other reports indicate the usefulness of a combination of tests that increases the likelihood of response to SIJ injections.[19-21] In a study examining the diagnostic validity of tests that could be ascribed to the IASP criteria for diagnosing SIJ pain, tests such as pain mapping or pain referral patterns have an ability to correctly identify patients with SIJ pain. However, they fail in discriminating patients without SIJ pain. The compression and thigh thrust test were regarded as positive examination finding in diagnosing SIJ pain.[22] The general consensus appears to be that SIJ pain can be diagnosed with reasonable certainty with controlled comparative local anesthetic diagnostic blocks.[23,24]

Anatomy

The SIJ is the largest axial joint in the body, with an average surface area of 14 to 17.5 cm[2].[25,26] It is a diarthrodial joint, with the anterior third being synovial and the remaining posterior aspect a syndesmosis, composed of interosseous ligament connections (**Fig. 15-2**). An auricular-shaped joint oriented in an oblique medial to lateral direction, morphological variability exists in the adult SIJ with respect to size, shape, and surface contour.[27] The posterior aspect of the joint has a fibrous capsule but may lack synovial continuity with the anterior aspect of the joint. Designed for stability, the SIJ is a triplanar shock absorber, transmitting and dissipating upper trunk loads to the pelvis, force from the lower extremities during ambulation, and facilitates parturition. The SIJ rotates about all three axes, although the predominant motion appears to be x-axis rotation with some z-axis translation.[1] Motion of the SIJ is usually limited to 1 to 3 degrees of rotation and 1.6 mm of translation, with 90 percent of rotation occurring along the x-axis.[1] The SIJ

Box 15-1: Sacroiliac Joint Examination Stress Maneuvers

Patrick (FABERE) test	With the patient supine, the thigh is flexed, and the ankle is placed above the knee of the contralateral leg. The ipsilateral knee is depressed, the contralateral hip is stabilized, and the ankle is maintained in its position above the contralateral knee. A positive test result is indicated by the patient's complaints of pain over the ipsilateral SIJ as the knee is depressed toward the examination table.
Gaenslen's test	With the patient supine, the ipsilateral leg hangs over the examination table and the contralateral leg is flexed, bringing the knee towards the abdomen. Counterpressure is applied to the knee of the hanging leg, toward the floor, and the contralateral leg toward the abdomen. A positive test result is indicated by the patient's complaints of pain over the ipsilateral SIJ as counterpressure is applied.
Fortin's finger test (sacral sulcus tenderness)	The patient is asked to point to the region of pain with one finger. A positive test result is indicated by consistent localization of pain in an area immediately inferomedial to the PSIS within 1 cm.
Shear test	With the patient prone, pressure is applied in a caudal direction. A positive test result is indicated by the patient's complaints of pain over the SIJ as pressure is applied.
Compression test	With the patient in lateral decubitus position, the hips and knees are flexed. Downward force is applied to the uppermost iliac crest. A positive test result is indicated by the patient's complaints of pain over the SIJ as pressure is applied.
Gillet test	With the patient standing, the PSIS is palpated along with the sacral spinous processes. The patient flexes the ipsilateral hip and knee to a minimum of 90 degrees. A positive test result is indicated by the thumb on the PSIS moving cephalad in relation to the thumb on the sacrum.
Yeoman's test	With the patient prone, the hip is extended, and the ipsilateral ilium is rotated. A positive test result is indicated by the patient's complaints of pain over the SIJ as pressure is applied.

PSIS, posterior superior iliac spine; SIJ, sacroiliac joint.

Fig. 15-2 Sacroiliac joint and ligamentous structures.

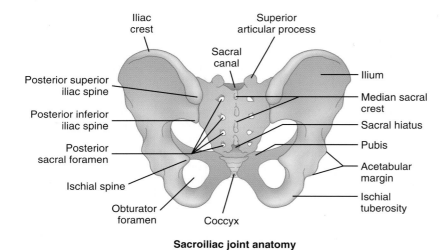

Sacroiliac joint anatomy

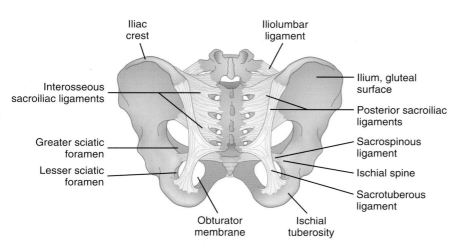

Ligamentous anatomy

motion progressively decreases, and motion at the joint may become markedly restricted secondary to increased cartilage; reduced density of chondrocytes, causing deep fissures in the cartilage; and fibrous connections among the auricular facets.[28] As the capsule becomes increasingly collagenous and fibrous, ankylosis occurs, and by the eighth decade of life, erosions and plaque formation are inevitable and ubiquitous.[29]

Innervation

Variability and lack of precise innervation of the SIJ remains, but it has been suggested that the ventral side of the SIJ is usually supplied by L4 through S2 spinal nerves, the caudal side by the superior gluteal nerve, and the dorsal side by S1 and S2 spinal nerves.[30] Others have implicated the ventral rami of L4 and L5, the superior gluteal nerve, and the dorsal rami of L5, S1, and S2.[31] Some authors have even suggested that the anterior SIJ is devoid of nervous tissue[32] and that the posterior SIJ is supplied by L3 and S4.[33] Additionally implicated are the L5 dorsal ramus and the lateral branches of the S1-S3,[34] and this description is the focus of ablative therapy in the attenuation of SIJ pain.

Basic Science

Intraarticular structures possess nerve fibers, which are sensitive for pain and support the theory that nociceptive signals may originate from the intraarticular structures of the SIJ.[35] Additionally, as previously described, innervation exists for the SIJ, and the intraarticular nociceptive fibers and the lumbosacral innervation are intended for interventions. There is not a "gold standard" for the diagnosis of SIJ dysfunction, but the rationale for the use of SIJ blocks as standard for diagnosing SIJ pain is based on the fact that SIJs are richly innervated and have been shown to be capable of being a source of low back pain and referred pain in the lower extremity.[36]

Therapeutic interventions in the treatment of SIJ pain include manual manipulation, prolotherapy, intraarticular injections, ablative procedures, and surgical interventions. Minimally invasive procedures, including intraarticular injections and ablative procedures, are minimally destructive to anatomy. Serial intraarticular injections of local anesthetics and steroids are thought to reduce the inflammatory response and the resultant joint symptomatology. Multiple studies have evaluated the effectiveness of intraarticular injections and ablative procedures (see Outcomes Evidence). Ablative procedures have included conventional radiofrequency (RF), pulsed RF (PRF) denervation, and cooled RF denervation of the SIJ. Conventional RF[37] and PRF[38] of the lateral branches have been reviewed and discussed by others.

The inherent challenge when treating patients with SIJ pain with RF energy is the inconsistent location of targeted lateral branch nerves.[39,40] The lateral branches supplying afferent information from pain-generating SIJs form a complex arcade of small nerve fibers anastomosing with multiple dorsal rami at each foramen. The location of these branches is unpredictable, varying from patient to patient, side to side, and level to level.[39] Additionally, conventional RF tissue ablation efficacy is limited by the lesion size secondary to impedance created by tissue desiccation, tissue boiling, and carbonization around the electrode tip. Carbonization is probably the most important cause of the increased impedance and leads to an abrupt decrease in lesion current (and delivered power), such that no more energy is delivered around the electrode and no additional tissue heating occurs.[41] Cooled RF energy generates heat in the surrounding tissue, and internal cooling of the electrode moderates temperature near the tip (**Fig. 15-3**). Internal

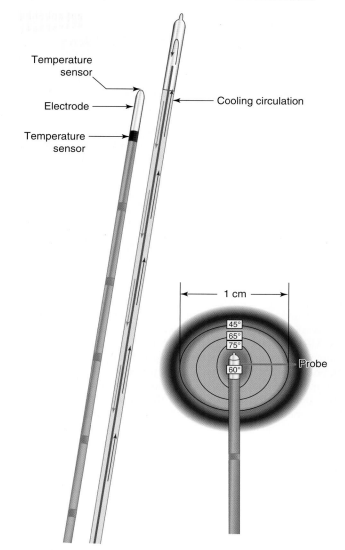

Fig. 15-3 Isotherm probe and temperature moderation.

cooling enhances lesion size by removing the constraint of high-temperature charring in tissue adjacent to the electrode, thus allowing effective ionic heating at a greater distance.[42]

Imaging

No imaging studies consistently provide findings that are helpful to diagnose primary SIJ pain. Computed tomography (CT), magnetic resonance imaging (MRI), and bone scan are done predominantly to exclude other causes of pain rather than to diagnose idiopathic SIJ pain.[9] Because of limitations of the history, physical examination, and imaging modalities, controlled fluoroscopically-guided or CT-guided, contrast-enhanced injections may be the only methods for definitively diagnosing or excluding the SIJ as a source of pain.[9]

The SIJ has several unique anatomical features that make it one of the more challenging joints to image. The joint is difficult to profile well on radiographic views, and therefore the radiographic findings of sacroiliitis are often equivocal.[43] MRI without and with intravenous gadolinium is currently the recommended modality for imaging patients with clinically suspected sacroiliitis and negative or equivocal radiographic findings.[43] MRI does not use

---

Box 15-2: Criteria for Diagnostic and Therapeutic Sacroiliac Joint Injections

- In the diagnostic phase, a patient may receive two procedures at intervals of no sooner than 2 weeks.
- In the therapeutic phase (after the diagnostic phase is completed), the suggested frequency is at least 2 months between injections, provided that >50% relief is obtained for 6 weeks.
- If the procedures are done for different joints, they should be performed at intervals no sooner than 2 weeks. It is suggested that therapeutic frequency remain at least 2 months for each joint. It is further suggested that both joints be treated at the same time, provided the injections can be performed safely.
- In the treatment or therapeutic phase, the interventional procedures should be repeated only as necessary according to the medical necessity criteria.
- Under unusual circumstances with a recurrent injury, procedures may be repeated after stabilization in the treatment phase.

Box 15-3: Selection and Exclusion Criteria for Sacroiliac Joint Neurotomy

Selection Criteria
- Predominantly axial pain below the L5 vertebrae
- Greater than 80% pain relief from two separate intraarticular blocks with no more than 2 cc of injectate per block. It is recommended to use higher concentration anesthetic such as 0.75% bupivacaine or 4% lidocaine for a more effective block.
- Chronic axial pain lasting for >6 months
- Age older than 18 years
- Failure to achieve adequate improvement with comprehensive nonoperative treatments, including but not limited to activity alteration, NSAIDs, physical or manual therapy, and fluoroscopically-guided steroid injections in and around the area of pathology.
- All other possible sources of low back pain have been ruled out, including but not limited to the intervertebral discs, the zygapophyseal joints, the hip joint, symptomatic spondylolisthesis, and other regional soft tissue structures.

Exclusion Criteria
- Pregnancy
- Systematic infection or localized infection at the anticipated introducer entry site
- History of coagulopathy or unexplained bleeding
- Irreversible psychological barriers to recovery
- Active radicular pain or radiculopathy
- Immunosuppression

NSAID, nonsteroidal antiinflammatory drug.

---

ionizing radiation, but CT typically uses 1 to 2 rad compared with 0.5 rad for an anteroposterior (AP) radiograph,[44] and MRI can detect edema and enhancement before bone changes are visible on CT. MRI is also helpful in identifying active disease and following therapy response in patients with moderate and severe radiographic changes;[43] however, CT is superior to MRI for diagnosing chronic bone changes in the superior ligamentous aspect of the SIJ.[45] Imaging for diagnostic and therapeutic SIJ injections and lateral branch blocks (LBBs) requires fluoroscopic guidance, but ultrasound guidance has been used with varying success.[46,47] In SIJ RF neurotomy, radiographic assistance is necessary for placement of lesioning probes.

Guidelines

SIJ injections with local anesthetic and steroid serves as a diagnostic tool and therapeutic intervention. LBBs may serve as diagnostic or prognostic procedures, for lateral branch denervation. As previously stated, controlled fluoroscopically-guided or CT-guided, contrast-enhanced injections may be the only methods for definitively diagnosing or excluding the SIJ as a source of pain. Analgesic response to a diagnostic block serves as a method to diagnose SI joint pain; however, it is imperative that before performing an SIJ injection that proper history, symptom presentation, physical examination, and imaging studies are reviewed to assess the SIJ as a pain generator and other structures as a mimicker of SIJ pain. Single diagnostic blocks carry a false-positive rate of 20%[6] and 22%,[48] so it is imperative to assess every patient for a true positive response and not the other factors contributing to analgesia or as a pain generator. These factors may include the placebo effect, convergence and referred pain, neuroplasticity and central sensitization, expectation bias, unintentional sympathetic blockade, systemic absorption of local anesthetic, and psychosocial issues.[8]

Guidelines for diagnostic and therapeutic treatment of SIJ dysfunction with injections at the SIJ and SIJ RF neurotomy has been proposed (**Boxes 15-2 and 15-3**).[24]

Indications and Contraindications

Selecting appropriate candidates for interventional pain medicine procedures is important, and SIJ RF neurotomy is no exception. Conservative treatment should be used before interventional treatments are initiated. These include nonsteroidal antiinflammatory

---

Equipment

Sacroiliac Joint Injection
- Preparation kit, sterile gloves, surgical cap and mask, 22-gauge 3.5-inch spinal needle, extension tubing
- Fluoroscope
- Medication
  - Lidocaine 1%
  - Contrast media (e.g., iohexol)
  - Bupivacaine 0.5%
  - Depo-methylprednisolone 40–80 mg (or equivalent)

Lateral Branch Block
- Preparation kit, sterile gloves, surgical cap and mask, 22-gauge 3.5-inch spinal needle, extension tubing
- Fluoroscope
- Medication
  - Lidocaine 1%
  - Contrast media (e.g., iohexol)
  - Bupivacaine 0.5% or ropivacaine 0.5%

Cooled Radiofrequency Sacroiliac Joint Neurotomy
- Preparation kit, sterile gloves, surgical cap and mask, sterile surgical drape, 27-gauge 3.5-inch spinal needle, extension tubing
- Fluoroscope
- Grounding pad
- Baylis Pain Management Generator, Pain Management Pump Unit, Pain Management Cooled Radiofrequency Connector Cable, Pain Management SInergy Probe, Pain Management SInergy Introducer, Pain Management Tube Kit, Pain Management Epsilon Ruler
- Medication
  - Lidocaine 1%
  - Bupivacaine 0.5%
  - Contrast media (e.g., iohexol)
  - Depo-methylprednisolone 40–80 mg (or equivalent)

drugs, physical therapy, manual manipulation, and other modalities addressing dysfunction at the joint. Interventional strategies include intraarticular joint injections, lateral branch nerve blocks, and denervative or ablative procedures. The ideal candidates for intraarticular injections include patients with known SIJ dysfunction, failed conservative therapy, or positive physical examination findings on more than two provocative maneuvers that stress the SIJ and ligaments. Contraindications for intraarticular injections include patient refusal, infection at the site of injection, history and physical examination finding inconsistent with sacroiliac etiology, and lack of imaging modality.

Indications for sacral joint RF neurotomy include axial low back or buttock pain lasting longer than 3 to 6 months, tenderness overlying the SIJ, positive physical examination findings on more than two provocative maneuvers that stress the SIJ and ligaments, failure to respond to conservative therapy, pain attenuation upon SIJ corticosteroid injections, or pain relief with LBBs at L4 and L5 primary dorsal rami and at S1-S3. Cohen et al[49] examined outcome predictors for RF denervation of the LBB and reported that no single variable strongly predicted outcome, suggesting that most patients with SIJ pain, irrespective of cause, can potentially benefit from the procedure.

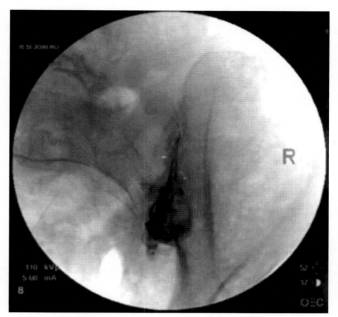

Fig. 15-4   Right sacroiliac joint arthrogram.

Technique

Sacroiliac Joint Injection

Fluoroscopy guidance is recommended and is described. The patient is placed on the fluoroscopy table in the prone position. After sterile preparation and drape have been accomplished, an AP fluoroscopic image of the SIJ is obtained. The fluoroscope is angled caudad, placing the PSIS and iliac crest overlying the joint image. The fluoroscope is obliqued to the contralateral side (20 to 30 degrees), placing the anterior and posterior aspect of the joint in line. A point along the inferior third of the joint is the target for injection. This area is anesthetized, and a 22-gauge spinal needle is advanced under coaxial technique and intermittent fluoroscopy until the joint has been entered; adjustment should be made accordingly. Entrance into the joint experienced as lack of ease to withdrawal the needle and arcing of the needle along the curvilinear joint and is confirmed by delivery of radiopaque contrast showing an arthrogram indicating intraarticular spread of contrast (**Fig. 15-4**). A solution containing local anesthetic and steroid is delivered showing spread of the residual intraarticular contrast. The needle is retracted from the joint, subcutaneous tissue, and skin.

Lateral Branch Block

Fluoroscopy guidance is recommended and is described. The patient is placed on the fluoroscopy table in the prone position. After sterile preparation and drape have been accomplished, an AP fluoroscopic image of the SIJ is obtained. The L5 dorsal rami block is approached by advancing a 22-gauge spinal needle into the groove between the sacral ala and articular process of the sacrum. The S1-S3 LBB are accomplished by advancing a 22-gauge spinal needle lateral to the foramen at the 2:30 and 4:30 positions on the right side and 7:30 and 9:30 positions on the left. After the periosteum is engaged, 0.3 to 0.5 mL of bupivacaine 0.5% is delivered. The needle is retracted from the subcutaneous tissue and skin.

Cooled Radiofrequency Sacroiliac Joint Neurotomy

The patient should be NPO (nothing by mouth). Bowel preparation is optional, and prophylactic antibiotics can be administered based on physician preference. This is a minimally invasive procedure, and monitored anesthesia care is adequate sedation during the procedure.

Identifying Target   The patient is positioned prone, and sterile prep and surgical drape are applied. An AP fluoroscopic image is obtained of the sacrum, including the intervertebral space at L5-S1. The endplate at S1 is aligned, reducing parallax at the first target (L5 dorsal ramus). The target location is the notch between the ala of the sacrum and the superior articular process (SAP) of the sacrum. The target for the S1-S3 levels is the lateral aspect of the sacral foramina.

Needle Placement   For the L5 dorsal ramus, needle placement is not necessary, and the introducer cannula is advanced without prior needle placement. The puncture point on the skin is just lateral and inferior to the target. The introducer is advanced until contact is made with the periosteum (**Fig. 15-5**). In the AP fluoroscopic view, the tip of the needle should be immediately adjacent to the base of the SAP and under its lateral margin. A lateral view is obtained to confirm depth of needle placement. The most ventral extent of the cannula in lateral view should be the zygapophyseal joint (**Fig. 15-6**). The stylet is removed, and bupivacaine 0.5% or lidocaine 2% can be delivered but is optional before lesioning. The SInergy probe is placed through the introducer cannula. The probe is 2 mm shorter than the stylet and will seat in the cannula 2 mm off of the dorsal sacral surface. Displayed on the pain management generator, impedance should not exceed 500 ohm. Impedances greater than 500 ohm may indicate that the probe is seated in tissue not suitable for lesioning or that the probe is not fully seated in the hub of the introducer cannula. The "skin stopper" is advanced along the shaft of the introducer cannula to serve as a depth marker, ensuring that the cannula and probe are not inadvertently advanced.

The lateral branches at S1-S3 are approached by raising a skin wheal over the skin entrance sites and subcutaneous tissue with lidocaine 1% to 2% toward the lateral aspect of S1-S3 dorsal sacral foramina. The 25- and 27-gauge spinal needles are advanced to the lateral aspect of the dorsal sacral foramina. These needles function

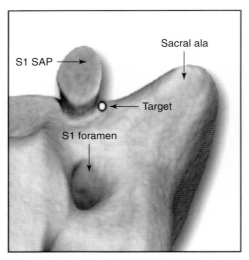
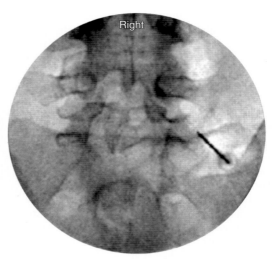

Fig. 15-5 L5 dorsal ramus target and probe insertion. SAP, superior articular process.

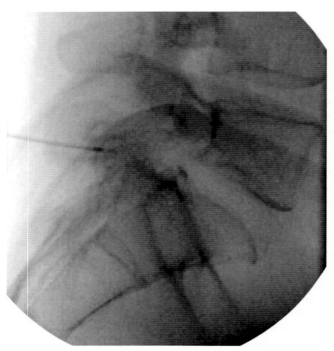

Fig. 15-6 Lateral view of probe placement. Note that the cannula and introducer are initially placed to the zygapophyseal joint.

as reference points for the placement of the introducer and probe in the absence of reliable osseous structures. A lateral fluoroscopic view is obtained to confirm entrance of the dorsal sacral foramina canal (**Fig. 15-7**).

Probe Placement In the AP view, the Epsilon ruler is placed on the skin overlying the sacral foramina. The S1, S2, and S3 levels should have the Epsilon ruler placed with the central spoke aligned with the lateral border of the S1, S2, and S3 foramina, which is marked by the previous needle placement. The ruler is rotated around the central spoke axis such that the upper spoke is marking a location at a 2:30 position (right side) or 9:30 (left side).

The first target for the introducer cannula placement is the 4:00 position for the right side and 8:00 for the left side (**Fig. 15-8**). Using coaxial technique and intermittent fluoroscopy, the cannula is advanced until the stylet has made contact with the dorsal sacral surface. A lateral fluoroscope view is obtained to confirm depth and contact with the dorsal surface and is not transforaminal. The stylet is removed, and bupivacaine 0.5% or lidocaine 2% can be delivered but is optional before lesioning. The SInergy probe is placed through the introducer cannula. The probe is 2 mm shorter than the stylet and will seat in the cannula 2 mm off of the dorsal sacral surface. Displayed on the pain management generator, the impedance should not exceed 500 ohm. The "skin stopper" is advanced along the shaft of the introducer cannula to serve as a depth marker, ensuring that the cannula and probe are not inadvertently advanced into the foramen. The same sequence is used to place SInergy probes at the 2:30 position and the 5:30 position for the right side (9:30 and 6:30 for left) at the S2 level. The S3 level varies in that two lesions are created by placing probes at 2:30 and 4:00 for the right side and 9:30 and 8:00 for the left side (**Fig. 15-9**). Because simultaneous lesions cannot be created with the present pain management generator, the sequence is repeated for each probe placement.

Lesioning The standard lesion parameters are set in the pain management generator. The set temperature is 60° C with a total lesion time of 2:30 minutes. Lesioning is initiated by pressing the output on/off button. Upon pressing the output on/off button, lesioning will begin after priming of the circuit is complete. The pain management generator will shut off when lesioning is complete. After each probe placement, the lesion sequence will be initiated.

Patient Management and Evaluation

Postprocedure instructions are presented in **Box 15-4**. A benchmark for successful treatment of SIJ pain has been reported in the literature as a 50% reduction on visual analog scale (VAS) scores from baseline.[40] Patients should be evaluated within 4 weeks for efficacy and complications. If bilateral neurotomies are indicated, the contralateral side can be lesioned 7 to 10 days after the initial procedure.

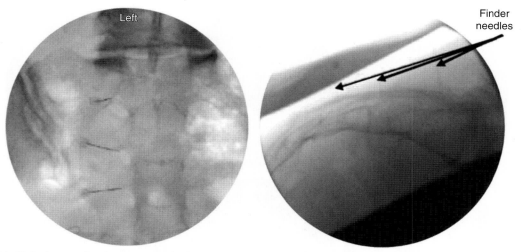

Fig. 15-7 Left S1-S3 finder needle placement at the lateral aspect of the dorsal sacral foramina with entrance of the dorsal sacral canal.

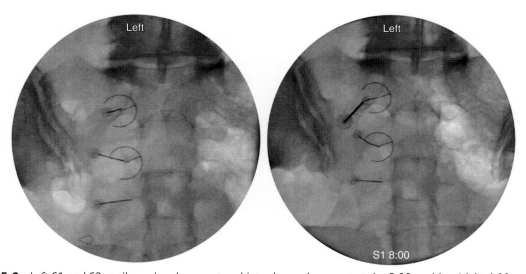

Fig. 15-8 Left S1 and S2 epsilon ruler placement and introducer placement at the 8:00 position (*right 4:00 position*).

Outcomes Evidence

Cooled RF neurotomy for SIJ pain is novel procedure presently without substantial outcome evidence. Although a new technology, Kapural et al[40] in a retrospective study investigated cooled RF of the lateral branches. The primary outcome measures were pain relief (VAS scores), changes in function (pain disability index [PDI]), and global patient satisfaction (GPE). Improvements were observed in VAS pain scores 7.1 ± 1.6 to 4.2 ± 2.5 ($P < .001$) and PDI from 32.7 ± 9.9 to 20.3 ± 12.1 ($P < .001$) at 3 to 4 months after the procedure. Of 26 patients, 18 rated their improvement in pain scores using GPE as improved or much improved, and eight claimed minimal or no improvement. In a randomized placebo-controlled study evaluating lateral branch RF denervation, Cohen et al[50] used the numeric rating scale (NRS) as a primary outcome measure and Oswestry Disability Index (ODI) score, reduction in analgesic medications, and GPE as secondary measures. At 1 month, the treatment group had significantly lower NRS scores than the placebo group (2.4 ± 2.0; range, 0 to 8 vs. 6.3 ± 2.4; range, 2 to 10; $P < .001$). One, 3, and 6 months after the procedure, 11 (79%), nine (64%), and eight (57%) RF-treated patients

experienced pain relief of 50% or greater and significant functional improvement. The authors concluded L4 and L5 primary dorsal rami and S1-S3 lateral branch RF denervation may provide intermediate-term pain relief and functional benefit in selected patients with suspected SIJ pain.

Box 15-4: Postprocedure Instructions

- Do not drive or operate machinery.
- Do not engage in any strenuous activity.
- Do not soak in the bathtub, but a shower is okay.
- Bandages may be removed the following day.
- Resume normal activities as tolerated the day after the procedure.
- Avoid excessive activity, lifting, and other forms of increased physical activity for 1 to 3 days after the procedure.
- If you experience fever, chills, or severe pain accompanied by swelling and redness at the injection site, contact your treating physician.
- If you experience shortness of breath or chest pains, go to the nearest emergency department.

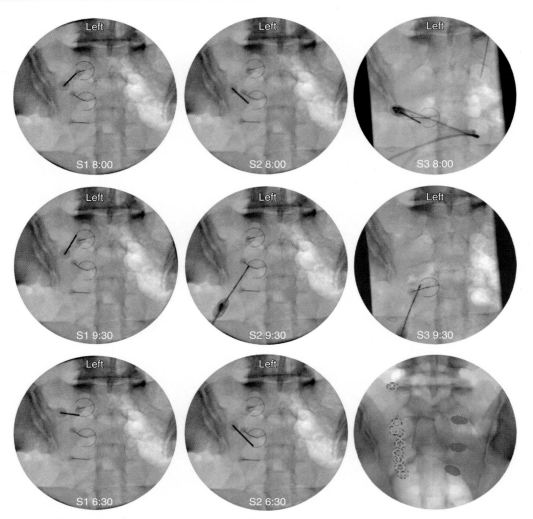

Fig. 15-9 Left L5 and S1-S3 probe placement. Foramina (purple). The lesion targets or lateral branch denervation sites (orange) are the areas of probe placement.

Risk and Complication Avoidance

Fluoroscopic guidance and a firm grasp of anatomy are paramount to performing this procedure safely and effectively. Reported complications from the procedure include temporary worsening of pain attributed to procedure-related pain or temporary neuritis[50,51] and temporary, self-limiting (<14 days) paresthesias.[49,51] Before lesioning, corticosteroid delivery may attenuate the symptoms secondary to neuritis.[52]

The placement of the introducer cannula and subsequent probe should be confirmed using multiplanar fluoroscopy. At the L5 dorsal rami, the cannula should be directed at the dorsal surface of the notch between the sacral ala and the SAP of the sacrum. The most ventral extent of the cannula in lateral view should be the zygapophyseal joint. At the sacral levels (lateral branch), the probe should be placed such that the active tip is at least 7 mm from the edge of the nearest posterior sacral foramina. The practitioner should verify in lateral fluoroscopic view that the probe is dorsal to the sacral surface and not in the sacral foramen.

Conclusion

The SIJ is a reemerging yet underappreciated potential source of axial low back pain. Historically, individual physical examination maneuvers have proven equivocal in diagnosing SIJ dysfunction, but combinations of physical examination maneuvers and the use of image-guided local anesthetic diagnostic blocks increase the likelihood of diagnosis and prognosis of therapeutic procedures such as ablative procedures. Using cooled electrodes has shown promise in the treatment of refractory cases of SIJ pain compared with conventional RF procedures. The cooled electrodes create a larger legion by overcoming impedance created by tissue desiccation, tissue boiling, and carbonization around the electrode tip. Although long-term studies are lacking, the promise of this modality has implications not only for treating patients with SIJ dysfunction but additionally in the treatment of those with pain originating from the zygapophyseal joints.

References

1. Slipman CW, Whyte WS, 2nd, Chow DW, et al: Sacroiliac joint syndrome. *Pain Physician* 4(2):143-152, 2001.
2. Smidt GL, Wei SH, McQuade K, et al: Sacroiliac motion for extreme hip positions. A fresh cadaver study. *Spine (Phila Pa 1976)* 22(18):2073-2082, 1997.
3. Fortin JD, Washington WJ, Falco FJ: Three pathways between the sacroiliac joint and neural structures. *AJNR Am J Neuroradiol* 20(8):1429-1434, 1999.

4. Mixter W, Barr JS: Rupture of the intervertebral disc with involvement of the spinal canal. *N Engl J Med* 211:210-215, 1934.

5. Schwarzer AC, Aprill CN, Bogduk N: The sacroiliac joint in chronic low back pain. *Spine (Phila Pa 1976)*, 20(1):31-37, 1995.

6. Maigne JY, Aivaliklis A, Pfefer F: Results of sacroiliac joint double block and value of sacroiliac pain provocation tests in 54 patients with low back pain. *Spine (Phila Pa 1976)* 21(16):1889-1892, 1996.

7. Fortin JD, Dwyer AP, West S, et al: Sacroiliac joint: pain referral maps upon applying a new injection/arthrography technique. Part I: asymptomatic volunteers. *Spine (Phila Pa 1976)* 19(13):1475-1482, 1994.

8. Cohen SP: Sacroiliac joint pain: a comprehensive review of anatomy, diagnosis, and treatment. *Anesth Analg* 101(5):1440-1453, 2005.

9. Dreyfuss P, Dreyer SJ, Cole A, et al: Sacroiliac joint pain. *J Am Acad Orthop Surg* 12(4):255-265, 2004.

10. Dreyfuss P, Michaelsen M, Pauza K, et al: The value of medical history and physical examination in diagnosing sacroiliac joint pain. *Spine (Phila Pa 1976)* 21(22):2594-2602, 1996.

11. Slipman CW, Jackson HB, Lipetz JS, et al: Sacroiliac joint pain referral zones. *Arch Phys Med Rehabil* 81(3):334-338, 2000.

12. Fortin JD, Aprill CN, Ponthieux B, et al: Sacroiliac joint: pain referral maps upon applying a new injection/arthrography technique. Part II: clinical evaluation. *Spine (Phila Pa 1976)* 19(13):1483-1489, 1994.

13. Merskey H Bogduk N: *Classification of chronic pain: descriptions of chronic pain syndromes and definitions of pain terms*, Seattle, 1994, IASP Press, pp 190-191.

14. Forst SL, Wheeler MT, Fortin JD, et al: The sacroiliac joint: anatomy, physiology and clinical significance. *Pain Physician* 9(1):61-67, 2006.

15. Harrison DE, Harrison DD, Troyanovich SJ: The sacroiliac joint: a review of anatomy and biomechanics with clinical implications. *J Manipulative Physiol Ther* 20(9):607-617, 1997.

16. Dreyfuss P: The sacroiliac joint: a review. *Int Spinal Injection Soc* 2:21-58, 1994.

17. Slipman CW, Sterenfeld EB, Chou LH, et al: The predictive value of provocative sacroiliac joint stress maneuvers in the diagnosis of sacroiliac joint syndrome. *Arch Phys Med Rehabil* 79(3):288-292, 1998.

18. Dreyfuss P, Dryer S, Griffin J, et al: Positive sacroiliac screening tests in asymptomatic adults. *Spine (Phila Pa 1976)* 19(10):1138-1143, 1994.

19. Laslett M, Aprill CN, McDonald B, et al: Diagnosis of sacroiliac joint pain: validity of individual provocation tests and composites of tests. *Man Ther* 10(3):207-218, 2005.

20. Stuber KJ: Specificity, sensitivity, and predictive values of clinical tests of the sacroiliac joint: a systematic review of the literature. *J Can Chiropr Assoc* 51(1):30-41, 2007.

21. Hancock MJ, Maher CG, Latimer J, et al: Systematic review of tests to identify the disc, SIJ or facet joint as the source of low back pain. *Eur Spine J* 16(10):1539-1550, 2007.

22. Szadek KM, van der Wurff P, van Tulder MW, et al: Diagnostic validity of criteria for sacroiliac joint pain: a systematic review. *J Pain* 10(4):354-368, 2009.

23. McKenzie-Brown AM, Shah RV, Sehgal N, et al: A systematic review of sacroiliac joint interventions. *Pain Physician* 8(1):115-125, 2005.

24. Boswell MV, Shah RV, Everett CR, et al: Interventional techniques in the management of chronic spinal pain: evidence-based practice guidelines. *Pain Physician* 8(1):1-47, 2005.

25. Miller JA, Schultz AB, Andersson GB: Load-displacement behavior of sacroiliac joints. *J Orthop Res* 5(1):92-101, 1987.

26. Bernard T, Cassidy JD: The sacroiliac syndrome. Pathophysiology, diagnosis and management. In Frymoyer J, editor: *The adult spine: principles and practice*, New York, 1991, Raven, pp 2107-2130.

27. Bernard T, Cassidy JD: The sacroiliac joint syndrome. Pathophysiology, diagnosis and management. In Frymoyer J, editor: *The adult spine: principles and practice*, New York, 1991, Raven, pp 2343-2363.

28. Kampen WU, Tillmann B: Age-related changes in the articular cartilage of human sacroiliac joint. *Anat Embryol (Berl)* 198(6):505-513, 1998.

29. Bowen V, Cassidy JD: Macroscopic and microscopic anatomy of the sacroiliac joint from embryonic life until the eighth decade. *Spine (Phila Pa 1976)* 6(6):620-628, 1981.

30. Solonen KA: The sacroiliac joint in the light of anatomical, roentgenological and clinical studies. *Acta Orthop Scand Suppl* 27:1-127, 1957.

31. Nakagawa T: [Study on the distribution of nerve filaments over the iliosacral joint and its adjacent region in the Japanese]. *Nippon Seikeigeka Gakkai Zasshi* 40(4):419-430, 1966.

32. Grob KR, Neuhuber WL, Kissling RO: [Innervation of the sacroiliac joint of the human]. *Z Rheumatol* 54(2):117-122, 1995.

33. Murata Y, Takahashi K, Yamagata M, et al: Sensory innervation of the sacroiliac joint in rats. *Spine (Phila Pa 1976)* 25(16):2015-2019, 2000.

34. Fortin JD, Kissling RO, O'Connor BL, et al: Sacroiliac joint innervation and pain. *Am J Orthop (Belle Mead NJ)* 28(12):687-690, 1999.

35. Szadek KM, Hoogland PV, Zuurmond WW, et al: Possible nociceptive structures in the sacroiliac joint cartilage: an immunohistochemical study. *Clin Anat* 23(2):192-198, 2010.

36. Hansen HC, McKenzie-Brown AM, Cohen SP, et al: Sacroiliac joint interventions: a systematic review. *Pain Physician* 10(1):165-184, 2007.

37. Ferrante FM, King LF, Roche EA, et al: Radiofrequency sacroiliac joint denervation for sacroiliac syndrome. *Reg Anesth Pain Med* 26(2):137-142, 2001.

38. Vallejo R, Benyamin RM, Kramer J, et al: Pulsed radiofrequency denervation for the treatment of sacroiliac joint syndrome. *Pain Med* 7(5):429-434, 2006.

39. Yin W, Willard F, Carreiro J, et al: Sensory stimulation-guided sacroiliac joint radiofrequency neurotomy: technique based on neuroanatomy of the dorsal sacral plexus. *Spine (Phila Pa 1976)* 28(20):2419-2425, 2003.

40. Kapural L, Nageeb F, Kapural M, et al: Cooled radiofrequency system for the treatment of chronic pain from sacroiliitis: the first case-series. *Pain Pract* 8(5):348-354, 2008.

41. Lorentzen T: A cooled needle electrode for radiofrequency tissue ablation: thermodynamic aspects of improved performance compared with conventional needle design. *Acad Radiol* 3(7):556-563, 1996.

42. de Baere T, Denys A, Wood BJ, et al: Radiofrequency liver ablation: experimental comparative study of water-cooled versus expandable systems. *AJR Am J Roentgenol* 176(1):187-192, 2001.

43. Tuite MJ: Sacroiliac joint imaging. *Semin Musculoskelet Radiol* 12(1):72-82, 2008.

44. Carrera GF, Foley WD, Kozin F, et al: CT of sacroiliitis. *AJR Am J Roentgenol* 136(1):41-46, 1981.

45. Puhakka KB, Jurik AG, Egund N, et al: Imaging of sacroiliitis in early seronegative spondyloarthropathy. Assessment of abnormalities by MR in comparison with radiography and CT. *Acta Radiol* 44(2):218-229, 2003.

46. Klauser A, De Zordo T, Feuchtner G, et al: Feasibility of ultrasound-guided sacroiliac joint injection considering sonoanatomic landmarks at two different levels in cadavers and patients. *Arthritis Rheum* 59(11):1618-1624, 2008.

47. Hartung W, Ross CJ, Straub R, et al: Ultrasound-guided sacroiliac joint injection in patients with established sacroiliitis: precise IA injection verified by MRI scanning does not predict clinical outcome. *Rheumatology (Oxford)* 49(8):1479-1482, 2009.

48. Manchikanti L, Singh V, Pampati V, et al: Evaluation of the relative contributions of various structures in chronic low back pain. *Pain Physician* 4(4):308-316, 2001.

49. Cohen SP, Strassels SA, Kurihara C, et al: Outcome predictors for sacroiliac joint (lateral branch) radiofrequency denervation. *Reg Anesth Pain Med* 34(3):206-214, 2009.

50. Cohen SP, Hurley RW, Buckenmaier CC, 3rd, et al: Randomized placebo-controlled study evaluating lateral branch radiofrequency denervation for sacroiliac joint pain. *Anesthesiology* 109(2):279-288, 2008.

51. Kapural L, Stojanovic M, Bensitel T, et al: Cooled radiofrequency (RF) of L5 dorsal ramus for RF denervation of the sacroiliac joint: technical report. *Pain Med* 11(1):53-57, 2010.

52. Dobrogowski J, Wrzosek A, Wordliczek J: Radiofrequency denervation with or without addition of pentoxifylline or methylprednisolone for chronic lumbar zygapophysial joint pain. *Pharmacol Rep* 57(4):475-480, 2005.

16 Pulsed Radiofrequency

Khalid Malik and Honorio T. Benzon

CHAPTER OVERVIEW

Chapter Synopsis: Radiofrequency (RF) techniques are used to ablate neural tissue in the treatment of painful conditions by delivering thermal lesions. This chapter focuses on a procedure known as pulsed RF (PRF), which sends pulses of electrical currents to an electrode tip to targeted nerve tissue. The pulsatile nature of the stimulation allows the tip to cool between pulses, keeping the electrode below 42° C, the temperature at which damage to surrounding tissue would occur. The targeted nociceptive tissue is thought to sustain damage from high-density electrical fields generated during the PRF, although the mechanism of destruction is not entirely understood. PRF has been used in a wide variety of both painful and nonpainful conditions. Notably, the technique has been applied at every spinal level of the dorsal root ganglia (DRG) and at many peripheral nerve sites. PRF is most commonly used to treat lumbar or cervical radicular pain. Although data from observational studies indicate that the procedure is quite effective for the treatment of radicular pain, two randomized controlled studies suggest only short-term analgesic benefits.

Important Points:

- During PRF application, an attempt is made to maximize the delivery of RF currents while the thermal tissue injury is minimized by maintaining the tissue temperature below the neurodestructive range.
- The RF currents are applied in a pulsatile manner so the heat can dissipate in between the RF pulses.
- PRF is applied by placing an electrode in the vicinity of the target nociceptive structure; however, because the electrical currents extend radially from the electrode tip, juxtapositioning of the electrode tip parallel to the target nerve is considered unnecessary.
- It is assumed that sustained high-density electrical fields generated during PRF application stress the biomolecules and cause cellular dysfunction and death of the target neural structure.
- Standard PRF protocol constitutes RF currents applied for 20 msec at 2 Hz for a total duration of 120 seconds while the maximum electrode temperature is maintained below 42° C.
- No noticeable side effects or complications have been attributed directly to PRF use.

Clinical Pearl: Due to the relative safety of PRF, its clinical use is widespread, and it has been applied to an array of structures including central nervous system ganglia, peripheral nerves, intervertebral discs, joints, and myofascial trigger points for the treatment of a range of pain syndromes.

Clinical Pitfall: Observational studies on this topic are abundant, and they almost universally support the PRF use. However, only a few controlled trials of PRF use are available, and they report its variable efficacy, which at best is short term.

Introduction and History

Radiofrequency (RF) currents have been used clinically to create predictable and quantifiable thermal lesions since the 1950s and have been used in the treatment of pain since the early 1970s.[1] During conventional RF (CRF) application for the treatment of pain, the RF currents are passed through an electrode that is placed in the vicinity of a nociceptive pathway. Consequently, the electrical energy imparted to the tissues immediately surrounding the active electrode tip creates a thermal lesion, likely interrupting the nociceptive impulses.[2] Because tissue temperatures above 45° C are known to be neurodestructive,[3] tissue temperatures are characteristically raised to well above the neurodestructive range but below the point of gas formation—80° C to 90° C. Although selective destruction of unmyelinated C and A-δ fibers by CRF thermal lesioning has been suggested,[4] further studies showed indiscriminate destruction of all nerve fiber types during thermal CRF lesioning.[5] Because of the possible risk of injury to the motor nerve fibers, local neuritis, loss of sensation, and deafferentation pain, the clinical use of CRF has generally been limited to facet denervation.[6] Observation that low temperature non–tissue-destructive CRF application had results similar to high temperature tissue-destructive CRF generated immense interest. It was theorized that electrical currents rather than temperature determined the outcomes of CRF application.[7] During pulsed RF (PRF), an attempt is made to maximize the delivery of electrical currents to the tissues by using higher voltage RF currents, and the risk of thermal tissue injury is minimized by maintaining the tissue temperatures below the neurodestructive range. These contradictory goals are achieved by applying the RF currents in a pulsatile manner to allow the heat to dissipate in between the RF pulses.[8]

Mechanism of Effect

Sluijter et al[8] in their first description of PRF use described its possible mechanism of action. These authors assumed that by maintaining the electrode temperatures below the thermal destructive range that thermal tissue injury was obviated and the sustained high-density electrical fields that were generated stressed the biomolecules and caused cellular dysfunction and death. However, later investigators observed the slow response time of the temperature-measuring devices used during PRF application and concluded that the generation of brief high-temperature spikes could not be excluded, suggesting a combined role of electrical and thermal tissue injury.[9,10] In laboratory studies, evidence of neuronal activation,[11,12] cellular stress,[13] and damage to cellular substructure[9] have been demonstrated after PRF application. Conversely, other experimental studies showed that the observed PRF effects are predominantly a function of the set temperature and undermined the role of electrical currents.[14,15] Among other postulated mechanisms, neuromodulation as a possible mechanism of PRF effect has also been suggested.[16] The exact mechanism of the clinical effects of PRF is therefore unclear, and no evidence currently exists of nociceptive pathway interruption in response to PRF application.

Technique

PRF is applied via an electrode placed in the vicinity of the target nociceptive structure. However, as the electrical currents extend radially from the electrode tip, unlike the CRF technique, juxtapositioning of the electrode tip parallel to the target nerve is deemed unnecessary. During a typical PRF application, the RF currents are applied for 20 msec, at 2 Hz, for a total duration of 120 seconds; for the majority of the duration of the lesion—480 of 500 msec. Therefore, no RF current is applied. The electrical currents are applied at higher voltage, but the maximum electrode temperature is maintained below 42° C.[8] Variations from this standard PRF protocol have been infrequent with the exception of longer lesion duration, and PRF was been applied for 4, 8, and 20 minutes in clinical studies.

Clinical Uses

The clinical use of PRF is relatively widespread, and it has been used for both painful and some nonpainful conditions.[17] PRF has been applied to the dorsal root ganglia (DRG) at all spinal levels; in the treatment of multiple pain syndromes, including radicular pain, postherpetic neuralgia, herniated intervertebral disc, postamputation stump pain, and inguinal herniorrhaphy pain.[17] It has also been applied to a wide variety of peripheral nerves for the following pain syndromes: medial branch nerve for facet syndrome; suprascapular nerve for shoulder pain; intercostal nerves for postsurgical thoracic pain; lateral femoral cutaneous nerve for meralgia paresthetica; pudendal nerve for pudendal neuralgia; dorsal penile nerves for premature ejaculation; splanchnic nerves for chronic benign pancreatic pain; sciatic nerve for phantom limb pain; obturator and femoral nerves for hip pain; glossopharyngeal nerve for glossopharyngeal neuralgia; occipital nerve for occipital neuralgia; and genitofemoral, ilioinguinal, and iliohypogastric nerves for groin pain and orchialgia.[17] PRF was applied to various central nervous system and autonomic ganglia, including the gasserian ganglion for trigeminal neuralgia; the sphenopalatine ganglion for head, neck, and facial pain; and the lumbar sympathetic chain in the treatment of complex regional pain syndrome.[17] In some reports, the target neural structure for PRF application was unclear, such as sacroiliac joint for sacroiliac joint dysfunction, intradiscally for discogenic pain, myofascial trigger points for myofascial pain, scar neuromas for postsurgical scar pain, spermatic cord for testicular pain, and intraarticularly for arthrogenic pain.[17]

Clinical Efficacy

PRF has been used most frequently for the treatment of lumbar and cervical radicular pains. Seven of the nine studies reporting this PRF use are observational and reported its successful use.[17] Of the two randomized controlled trials (RCT) available on this topic, one is an RCT of 23 patients with chronic cervical radicular pain that compared PRF applied with the DRG in 11 patients to similarly performed sham intervention in 12 patients (Table 16-1).[18] The results of this trial showed statistically significant improvement in pain and patient satisfaction scores at 3 months in the

PRF group. However, in addition to its small size, this trial reported only short-term results at 3 months. The second RCT include 76 patients with lumbar radicular pain and compared PRF with combined PRF and CRF application to the involved DRG.[19] In both study groups, the patients experienced significant pain relief at 2 months, but there was significant loss of analgesic effect by 4 months and return of pain by the eighth month. Although the study results concluded that the PRF of the DRG resulted in short-term benefits and no additional benefit was gained by CRF application, this trial compared PRF with a combined PRF and CRF technique not used clinically and with variable lesion temperatures and durations (i.e., CRF applied until the patient felt radicular pain).

The second most commonly reported PRF application is in the treatment of facet syndrome, (FS) and two RCTs and three observational studies are available on this topic.[17] In one RCT of 60 patients with chronic lumbar FS, the effects of CRF, PRF, and sham treatment were compared.[20] The three study groups were evaluated immediately and at 6 and 12 months after the procedure. The patients in both the CRF and the PRF groups had lower pain and disability scores immediately after the procedure compared with the sham group. However, the pain relief and functional improvement were maintained in the CRF group only at 6 and 12 months. The significance of these lowered pain scores in the postprocedural period in terms of long-term pain relief is unclear. The second RCT included 50 patients with lumbar FS of more than 1 month's duration.[21] Only 26 patients, of whom 13 received CRF and 13 PRF, completed their follow-up evaluations. No significant difference in the pain and disability scores was found at 3 months between the two groups. This trial reported a dropout rate of 48%, and only short-term results at 3 months were reported. The available controlled trials of PRF for the treatment of FS therefore provide inconclusive evidence of its long-term efficacy for this condition. The three available observational studies of PRF application for FS all reported its efficacy.[17]

In an RCT of 40 patients with idiopathic trigeminal neuralgia, the effects of PRF application to gasserian ganglion were compared with CRF.[22] At 3 months, patients in the PRF group reported no significant pain relief or improved satisfaction compared with the CRF group. The results of this study concluded that compared with CRF, PRF was not an effective method of treatment for idiopathic trigeminal neuralgia. One case series reported the efficacy of PRF in the treatment of trigeminal neuralgia.[17]

Successful application of PRF to suprascapular nerve for shoulder pain has been reported in four case reports or case series.[17] A case report and a prospective case series reported successful application of PRF to sphenopalatine ganglion for head, neck, and facial pain.[17] The use of PRF for the remaining clinical conditions described earlier is based on single case report or a case series, almost all of which described the successful use of PRF for that condition.[17]

Thus, although the observational studies almost universally support the use of PRF, the available controlled data are limited in nature and reported variable efficacy of PRF. The efficacy of PRF reported in these RCTs for various clinical conditions was at best short term.

Side Effects and Complications

Although bleeding, infection, and nerve damage from needle placement and burns from incorrect placement of the grounding pad have been reported,[23] no noticeable side effects or complications have been directly attributed to PRF use.

Table 16-1: Controlled Trials of Pulsed Radiofrequency

Date and Author	Methodology, Patients, and Comparison Groups	Follow-up and Outcome Measures	Results and Author Conclusions	Study Analysis
2007: Van Zundert et al[18]	RCT, DB, SCT 23 patients with CRP: 11 had PRF to one level DRG, and 12 had ST	For 3 months, only patients having favorable responses were followed for 6 months; VAS, GPE, SF-36, AU. Success defined as >50% change in GPE and >20 change in VAS	At 3 months, SS success reported in nine of 11 (82%) patients in the PRF group and in four of 12 GPE (33%) and three of 12 VAS (25%) in the ST group. AC: PRF provided SS pain relief compared with ST at 3 months.	This study provide evidence of short-term efficacy of PRF for cervical radicular pain.
2008: Simopoulos et al[19]	RCT 76 patients with LRP: 37 had PRF of DRG, and 39 had combined PRF and CRF (maximally tolerated temperatures)	2 months and monthly thereafter; ≤8 months VAS: success defined as reduction in 2 points in VAS for 8 weeks	Similar decline in VAS scores between the two groups at 2 months. Similar loss of analgesic effect between 2 and 4 months and return of pain to baseline by 8 months. AC: PRF of DRG was safe and resulted in short-term benefit; the additional application of CRF did not offer any additional benefit.	Significant methodological flaws and the use of unconventional RF techniques make the results of this trial irrelevant.
2007: Tekin et al[20]	RCT, DB, SCT 60 patients with LFS: 20 had CRF, 20 had PRF, and 20 had ST	Followed at 6 hours, 6 months, and 1 year after the procedure VAS, ODI	At 6 hours, SS lower VAS and ODI scores for CRF and PRF groups compared with ST. At 6 months and 1 year, the lower scores were maintained only in CRF group. AC: CRF and PRF are both useful interventions in the treatment of chronic facet joint pain.	This trial only provides evidence of the efficacy of PRF at 6 hours after RF facet neurotomy.
2008 Kroll et al[21]	RCT, DB 26 patients with LFS: 13 patients had CRF, and 13 had PRF	For 3 months VAS, ODI	No SS difference between the CRF and PRF groups in relative improvements in either VAS or ODI scores at 3 months. AC: As above	There was no difference in the results of PRF and CRF at 3 months for facetogenic pain.
2007: Erdine et al[22]	RCT, DB 40 patients with TN: 20 had PRF, and 20 had CRF	For 3 months, noncomparative follow-up for 6 months VAS, PSS, AU	At day 1 and 3 months, all of the patients in CRF had SS improvement in VAS and PSS. Only two of 20 patients in the PRF group at day 1 and none at 3 months had SS improved VAS or PSS. AC: Unlike CRF, PRF is not an effective treatment for idiopathic TN.	This trial provided evidence of lack of efficacy of PRF compared with CRF in the treatment of TN.

AC, author's conclusions; AU, analgesic usage; CRP, cervical radicular pain; DB, double blinded; GPE, global perceived effect; LFS, lumbar facet syndrome; LRP, lumbar radicular pain; ODI, Oswestry Disability Index; PRF, pulsed radiofrequency; PSS, patient satisfaction scale; RCT, randomized controlled trial; SCT, sham controlled trial; SF-36, Short Form (36); SS, statistically significant; ST, sham treatment; TN, trigeminal neuralgia; VAS, visual analog scale.

References

1. Hunsperger RW, Wyss O: Production of localized lesions in nervous tissue by coagulation with high frequency current. *Helvetica Physiologica Pharmacologica Acta* 11:283-304, 1953.
2. Shealy CN: Percutaneous radiofrequency denervation of spinal facets: treatment for chronic back pain and sciatica. *J Neurosurg* 43:448-451, 1975.
3. Brodkey J, Miyazaki Y, Ervin FR, et al: Reversible heat lesions, a method of stereotactic localization. *J Neurosurg* 21:49-53, 1964.
4. Letcher FS, Goldring S: The effect of radiofrequency current and heat on peripheral nerve action potential in the cat. *J Neurosurg* 29:42-47, 1968.
5. Smith HP, McWorther JM, Challa VR: Radiofrequency neurolysis in a clinical model. *J Neurosurg* 55:246-253, 1981.
6. Uematsu S, Udvarhelyi GB, Benson DW, et al: Percutaneous radiofrequency rhizotomy. *Surg Neurol* 2:319-325, 1974.
7. Slappendel R, Crul BJ, Braak GJ, et al: The efficacy of radiofrequency lesioning of the cervical spinal dorsal root ganglion in a double-blinded, randomized study: no difference between 40 degrees C and 67 degrees C treatments. *Pain* 73:159-163, 1997.
8. Sluijter ME, Cosman ER, Rittman WB, Van Kleef M: The effects of pulsed radiofrequency fields applied to the dorsal root ganglion—a preliminary report. *Pain Clin* 11:109-117, 1998.
9. Erdine S, Yucel A, Cimen A, et al: Effects of pulsed versus conventional radiofrequency current on rabbit dorsal root ganglion morphology. *Eur J Pain* 9:251-256, 2005.

10. Cosman ER, Cosman ER, Sr: Electric and thermal field effects in tissue around radiofrequency electrodes. *Pain Med* 6:405-424, 2005.

11. Higuchi Y, Nashold BS, Sluijter M, et al: Exposure of dorsal root ganglion in rats to pulsed radiofrequency currents activates dorsal horn lamina I and II neurons. *Neurosurgery* 50:850-855, 2002.

12. Van Zundert J, de Louw AJ, Joosten EA, et al: Pulsed and continuous radiofrequency current adjacent to the cervical dorsal root ganglion of the rat induces late cellular activity in the dorsal horn. *Anesthesiology* 102:125-131, 2005.

13. Hamann W, Abou-Sherif S, Thompson S, Hall S: Pulsed radiofrequency applied to dorsal root ganglia causes a selective increase in ATF3 in small neurons. *Eur J Pain* 10:171-176, 2006.

14. Podhajsky RJ, Sekiguchi Y, Kikuchi S, Myers RR: The histologic effects of pulsed and continues radiofrequency lesions at 42 degrees C to rat dorsal root ganglion and sciatic nerve. *Spine* 30:1008-1013, 2005.

15. Heavner JE, Boswell MV, Racz GB: A comparison of pulsed radiofrequency and continuous radiofrequency on thermocoagulation of egg white in vitro. *Pain Physician* 9:135-137, 2006.

16. Cahana A, Vutskits L, Muller D: Acute differential modulation of synaptic transmission and cell survival during exposure to pulsed and continuous radiofrequency energy. *J Pain* 4:197-202, 2003.

17. Malik K, Benzon HT: Pulsed radiofrequency: a critical review of its efficacy. *Anaesth Intensive Care* 35:863-873, 2007.

18. Van Zundert J, Patijn J, Kessels A, et al: Pulsed radiofrequency adjacent to the cervical dorsal root ganglion in chronic cervical radicular pain: a double blind sham controlled randomized clinical trial. *Pain* 127:173-182, 2007.

19. Simopoulos TT, Kraemer J, Nagda JV, et al: Response to pulsed and continuous radiofrequency lesioning of the dorsal root ganglion and segmental nerves in patients with chronic lumbar radicular pain. *Pain Physician* 11:137-144, 2008.

20. Tekin I, Mirzai H, Ok G, et al: A comparison of conventional and pulsed radiofrequency denervation in the treatment of chronic facet joint pain. *Clin J Pain* 23:524-529, 2007.

21. Kroll HR, Kim D, Danic MJ, et al: A randomized, double-blind, prospective study comparing the efficacy of continuous versus pulsed radiofrequency in the treatment of lumbar facet syndrome. *J Clin Anesth* 20:534-537, 2008.

22. Erdine S, Ozyalcin NS, Cimen A, Celik M, et al: Comparison of pulsed radiofrequency with conventional radiofrequency in the treatment of idiopathic trigeminal neuralgia. *Eur J Pain* 11:309-313, 2007.

23. Cohen SP, Foster A: Pulsed radiofrequency as a treatment for groin pain and orchialgia. *Urology* 61:645, 2003.

17 Discogenic Pain and Discography for Spinal Injections

Stanley Golovac

CHAPTER SYNOPSIS

Chapter Synopsis: Disc pain is primarily axial and it is by nature mechanical: it worsens with activity and is relieved by rest. Aside from those qualities, discogenic pain can be extremely difficult to diagnose and to trace to a particular disc. Discography is a specialized diagnostic tool to determine the source of pain that seems to arise from the intervertebral discs of the spine. This chapter describes the procedure, which entails the injection of contrast dye into the disc nucleus for radiographic evaluation. Similar to palpation during a physical examination, discography directly makes use of the patient's pain experience. In discography, the disc is pressurized to evoke a patient response. This pain report tied to the disc morphology revealed by discography can identify the specific discs that are "pain generators." The most common source of pain revealed by discography is an internal disc disruption. Advanced imaging technologies—computed tomography scans, magnetic resonance imaging, and others—have been used to identify disc damage (including herniation) in advance of disc excision surgery, but none has been able to identify internal disc abnormalities the way discography can. Discography can be used at the lumbar, thoracic, and cervical spinal levels. Subsequent to this provocation discography, a procedure called functional anesthetic discography may be used to test the pain's sensitivity to injected anesthetics at each identified pain generator.

Important Points:
- Discography is the injection of contrast into the disc nucleus for radiographic evaluation.
- Disc stimulation involves pressurizing the disc and recording the response of the patient.
- Provocation discography is the combination of discography and disc stimulation.

Clinical Pearl: The use of discography has to be performed under direct fluoroscopy, and an independent evaluator should assess whether facial grimaces and pain are occurring while the examination is being performed.

Clinical Pitfall: Care needs to be taken to *not* overpressurize any disc or iatrogenic pain and rupture may occur. Serious sequestration of disc material upon a nerve roots or even the spinal cord may occur, leading to a possible permanent injury and paralysis.

History and Background

Discography has become a valuable diagnostic tool since its introduction in the 1940s to diagnose lumbar disc herniation.[1-3] Since discography was introduced, computed tomography (CT) and magnetic resonance imaging (MRI) scanning have also added to our knowledge of the lumbar discs; however, because structural abnormalities such as degenerative disc changes, herniations, and annular tears occur in patients asymptomatic of low back pain,[4,5] discography is the only direct method to asses if a disc is painful or not. Discography has also been shown to reveal abnormalities in symptomatic patients with normal MRI scans.[6,7]

Today, discography is used most often to identify painful internally disrupted discs.[3] Discography is unique in that it is the only diagnostic technique that directly correlates a patient's symptoms with disc morphology.[4] This is analogous to palpation, which is fundamental to physical diagnosis.[5] Tenderness elicited on palpation is analogous to pain provocation on discography.

When evaluating a suspected spinal origin of pain, it is critically important to assess the significance of pathological findings on imaging studies and to determine whether those findings correlate with a patient's symptoms. Discography is distinctive in its ability to make this determination. Discography is used in the lumbar,[6-19] thoracic,[20-25] and cervical[26-35] regions to assess pain that is suspected to be of discogenic origin. Discogenic pain is mechanical in nature (exacerbated with activity and relieved by rest) and is felt primarily in an axial distribution. Performing discography involves the injection of radiographic contrast into the nucleus of the intervertebral disc to visualize disc morphology (**Fig. 17-1**).[4]

The prevalence of discogenic low back pain is 39% in those with low back pain persisting for at least 6 months and who have an unremarkable diagnostic workup and 26% of patients without radicular pain after facet joint pain was eliminated by either performing a diagnostic median branch nerve block or an intraarticular facet joint injection.[36] The advent of new technology such as MRI, CT, and CT myelography has improved anatomical visualization of spine structures. However, these diagnostic modalities have not reliably identified the anatomical location of symptomatic spinal structures. This is evident in the individual who does not have radicular symptoms. Discs that appear normal or abnormal

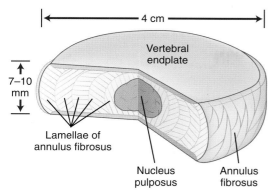

Fig. 17-1 The circumferential area of the surface area of the disc. Both sides come in contact with surface above and below that endplate adhering itself to the vertebral body.

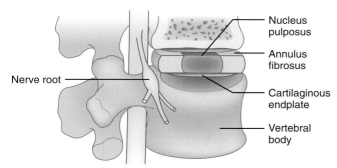

Fig. 17-2 The cross-sectional area denotes how the surface area is viewed and adherent to the vertebral body. The figure demonstrates that relationship of the foramen and the nerve root.

on MRI can either reproduce clinical symptoms during discography or be painless. The lumbar discs are innervated by branches from the lumbar ventral rami, the grey rami communicans, and the sinuvertebral nerve (**Figs. 17-2 and 17-3**). Lumbar discography has been postulated as a diagnostic test to elucidate the specific disc that requires disc excision and fusion with subsequent pain relief. The North American Spine Society (NASS) released its Position Statement on Discography in 1988[37] and again in 1995, summarizing the indications for discography. Both the International Spine Injection Society and NASS agree on the criteria for functional discography. Each organization indicates that a "chemically" sensitive disc is one that a patient feels pain at a low pressure stimulus (basically <15 psi). Between 15 and 50 psi, if a patient experiences pain that is concordant with the pathology of the painful disc, then it is deemed a pressure-sensitive disc. Pressures greater than 51 psi to 90 psi above the opening pressure are noted to be determined. A pressure above 90 psi is stated as being normal. The most common indication for lumbar discography is the need to determine whether one or more lumbar discs are responsible (i.e., the pain generator) for chronic ongoing low back pain. The study by Walsh et al[38] refuted the findings by Holt[19] demonstrating a 0% false-positive rate. Recent literature has demonstrated that compared with present imaging modalities, lumbar discography and lumbar CT discography are superior to MRI in determining abnormal annular pathology.[39-43]

Several studies have demonstrated the limitations of MRI compared with lumbar discography in identifying symptomatic versus asymptomatic discs.[39-42] In 2000, Carragee et al[44] challenged the concept of zero false-positive discography results on the grounds that abnormal psychometrics lead to misleading abnormal results.

Manchikanti et al,[45] in 2001, to the contrary, did not find any impact on discography results in those with or without a somatization disorder. Crock[46] was the first to use the term *internal disc disruption* in 1970 to describe the clinical syndrome of axial low back pain secondary to pathological changes within the disc in the absence of a disc herniation. Radial fissures into the outer innervated annulus can cause pain because of mechanical or chemical irritation. This is the salient pathologic feature of internal disc disruption that cannot be detected on plain radiography, CT, or myelography because these studies are unable to detect internal disc abnormalities.

CT combined with discography allows the detection of annular pathology and determines if it is symptomatic or not. MRI can reveal annular pathology but cannot determine whether or not the disc is the pain generator (**Fig. 17-2**).[38-41] Although the presence of a high intensity zone (HIZ) on T2-weighted MRI sagittal images in the posterior annulus (representative of a radial annular fissure) has a near 90% positive predictive value with concordant discography,[34-36,38,39] this is not absolute, and the absence of an HIZ does not exclude annular pathology or discogenic low back pain.[38-42] HIZ lesions are also found in patients without low back pain symptoms.[47-49] Lumbar discography is not only important in identifying discs that are pain generators but also serves a key role in detecting whether abnormal or normal discs (based on imaging studies) are painful.

Pathophysiology

Two of the most common problems associated with the intervertebral disc are intervertebral disc degeneration and intervertebral disc protrusion or herniation; however, the two processes are not mutually exclusive. Extruded nucleus pulposus spontaneously produces increased amounts of matrix metalloproteinases, nitric oxide, interleukin-6, prostaglandin E2, and other chemical mediators (**Fig. 17-3**). These products may be intimately involved in both the biochemistry of disc degeneration and the pathophysiology of radiculopathy.

Intervertebral disc degeneration is difficult to define and is also difficult to separate from the normal aging process of the intervertebral disc. However, there is a wide variation in the aging and degenerative process of the disc, and some septuagenarians have the intervertebral discs of 30-year-old adults and vice versa. The hallmarks of disc degeneration are loss of fluid and fluid pressure, disruption or breakdown of collagen (including tearing of the annulus fibrosus) and proteoglycans, and sclerosis of the cartilaginous endplate and adjacent subchondral bone. The normal aging and degeneration of the intervertebral disc is closely related to the number of vessels that reach the intervertebral disc, especially the cartilaginous endplate. As the number of vessels decreases and the nutrition provided and waste removed by these vessels decrease, the changes associated with intervertebral disc aging and degeneration increase.[46] The first significant degenerative changes in the intervertebral disc appear around 11 to 12 years of age.

The number of clefts and radial tears increases from 17 to 20 years of age, and the overall number of chondrocytes decreases as cell death, mucoid degeneration, and granular changes begin to appear.[45] The number of clefts and radial fissures continues to increase until late in life (>70 years of age).

Functional Discography

Functional anesthetic discography (FAD)[50] is an additional test that can be carried out after provocation discography. It is based on

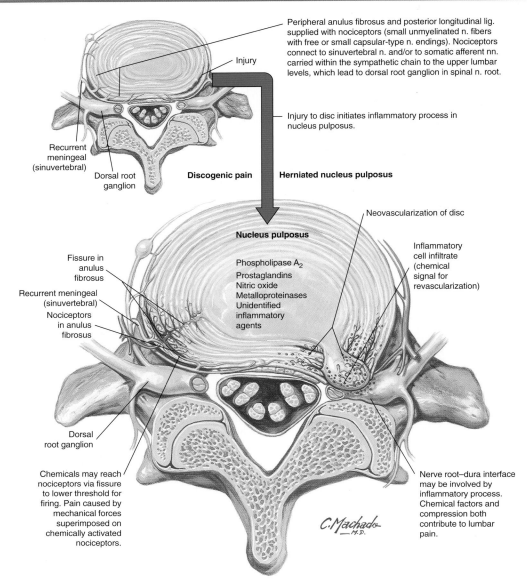

Peripheral anulus fibrosus and posterior longitudinal lig. supplied with nociceptors (small unmyelinated n. fibers with free or small capsular-type n. endings). Nociceptors connect to sinuvertebral n. and/or to somatic afferent nn. carried within the sympathetic chain to the upper lumbar levels, which lead to dorsal root ganglion in spinal n. root.

Injury

Recurrent meningeal (sinuvertebral)

Dorsal root ganglion

Injury to disc initiates inflammatory process in nucleus pulposus.

Discogenic pain

Herniated nucleus pulposus

Neovascularization of disc

Nucleus pulposus

Phospholipase A_2
Prostaglandins
Nitric oxide
Metalloproteinases
Unidentified inflammatory agents

Inflammatory cell infiltrate (chemical signal for revascularization)

Fissure in anulus fibrosus

Recurrent meningeal (sinuvertebral)

Nociceptors in anulus fibrosus

Dorsal root ganglion

Chemicals may reach nociceptors via fissure to lower threshold for firing. Pain caused by mechanical forces superimposed on chemically activated nociceptors.

Nerve root–dura interface may be involved by inflammatory process. Chemical factors and compression both contribute to lumbar pain.

Fig. 17-3 The endoperoxides of the disc, a disc bulge, and annular tear in relation to the nerve root proximity. (Netter illustration from www.netterimages.com © Elsevier Inc. All rights reserved.)

analgesic discography, in which local anesthetic is injected into a painful disc and pain relief is assessed. The theory is similar to diagnostic injections of facet joints or sacroiliac joints. A 17-gauge introducer needle is used for disc access. After the provocation discogram, a balloon-tipped catheter is placed into the center of the disc through the needle (**Fig. 17-4**).[50] The balloon is inflated with contrast, and a stopcock is closed to secure the catheter in the nucleus.

In the recovery area, the patient is instructed to perform specific activities and positions that typically elicit pain, and the visual analog scale (VAS) scores are recorded. In the author's practice, 1 mL of 4% lidocaine is injected into the painful disc through the balloon-tipped catheter after baseline pain scores have been recorded. The same measurements are carried out 8 to 10 minutes later, and the change in VAS is recorded. Provocation discography facilitates diagnosis by eliciting pain, and FAD helps clarify the diagnosis by relieving pain and improving mobility during testing. Each painful disc can be studied sequentially and individually. The

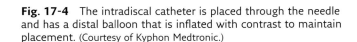

Fig. 17-4 The intradiscal catheter is placed through the needle and has a distal balloon that is inflated with contrast to maintain placement. (Courtesy of Kyphon Medtronic.)

results of the provocation discography are compared with the FAD results to produce a final report. After the FAD is completed, the balloon on each catheter is deflated, and the catheter is removed.

Alamin and coworkers[51] reported that 50% of patients ($n = 32$) had confirmatory findings on FAD after a positive discogram result. The patients with confirmatory FAD underwent fusion and were followed for at least 3 months. The mean preoperative Oswestry Disability Index score was 58.5, and the mean postoperative score was 26.5. The mean preoperative VAS score for back pain was 7.2, and the mean postoperative VAS score was 3.1.

Intradiscal Procedures

Disc biacuplasty is a procedure for treating discogenic pain through neuron ablation by heating intervertebral disc tissue using cooled, bipolar radiofrequency (RF) technology. One study[52] has demonstrated temperature profiles created by disc biacuplasty in human cadavers.

Many practitioners have used various injection formulas to help patients with discogenic pain (**Table 17-1**). From the Saal brothers using intradiscal electrothermal therapy[53] to the use of catheters, medications, and now a "super glue" to help seal off annular tears,

Table 17-1: Intradiscal Procedures

Discogenic Pain	Radicular Pain	Facet Joint Pain
IDET	Dekompressor	Radiofrequency ablation
DiscTRODE	Epidural steroids	Intraarticular injections
Nucleoplasty		Median branch nerve injection
SpineWave		
SpineWand		
Biaculoplasty		

IDET, intradiscal electrothermal therapy.

these techniques enable us to stop pain emitting from the intradiscal areas of the nucleus (**Fig. 17-5**).

DiscTRODE from Radionics did show some promise by using a catheter spiraled in the posterior portion of the disc wall. Allowing heat to be generated helped to seal off the posterior annular tear that may have been provoking the leakage of caustic irritants.

Nucleoplasty from Arthrocare Spine allowed the knowledge and technique to be capitalized on by the use of RF energy to heat up channels within the disc, allowing a coblation and coagulation to occur simultaneously inside the nucleus. By the use of the technique, one could vaporize material and create a negative vacuum in the nucleus, thereby allowing the outer rim to retract back into the disc. Stryker developed the very well-known and proven Dekompressor. This device actually removes intradiscal material and creates a negative vacuum in the disc, allowing the out-bulge defect to retract and lessen the contact on the nerve root (**Fig. 17-6**). The use of a sealant to stop annular stimulation in addition to helping the disc to actually rehydrate is another novel concept. Spinal Restoration in Austin, Texas, is in a third-phase clinical trial analyzing the concept at the present time.

Conclusion

Discography has become an indispensable assessment tool in the evaluation of patients with spinal pain. Current imaging techniques are insufficient to determine if a suspected disc is the source

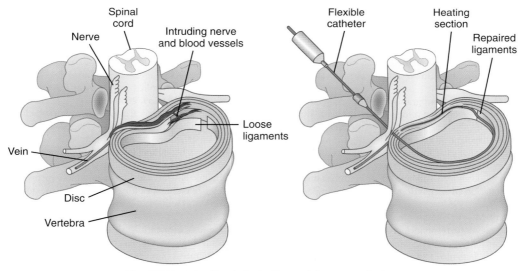

Fig. 17-5 Intradiscal electrothermal therapy catheter.

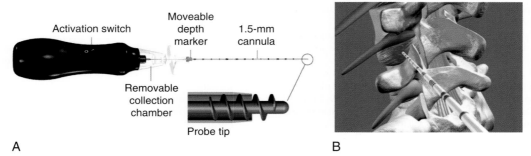

Fig. 17-6 **A,** Dekompressor device. **B,** Dekompressor removing intradiscal material.

of pain. Discography is the only test of the intervertebral disc that is able to stimulate the disc and recreate a patient's pain. This is analogous to palpation, which is fundamental to physical diagnosis. Disc stimulation and pain reproduction can be correlated with analgesia and function if local anesthetic is introduced into the disc. There is both historical and current controversy surrounding the use of discography. This has promoted healthy discussion and advanced the standards for performance of this examination. The use of manometry, FAD, "sham" injection, and strict criteria for identifying positive discs are all intended to limit the likelihood of false-positive results. It is acknowledged that discography has to be interpreted with caution in patients with significant behavioral pathology.

With the continuous evolution of spinal interventions come many new and promising treatments for painful intervertebral discs. These include a host of emerging biological therapies and surgical treatments. All of these require the ability to safely access the intervertebral disc for both diagnosis and treatment. The demand for this procedure is certain to increase. When discography is performed with appropriate clinical indications by skilled, knowledgeable, and experienced proceduralists, it leads to improved clinical outcomes.

References

1. Lindblom K: Technique and results in myelography and disc puncture. *Acta Radiol* 34:321-330, 1950.
2. Aprill C, Bogduk N: High-intensity zone: A diagnostic sign of painful lumbar disc on magnetic resonance imaging. *Br J Radiol* 65:361-369, 1992.
3. Guyer RD, Ohnmeiss DD: Lumbar discography. Position statement from the North American Spine Society Diagnostic and Therapeutic Committee. *Spine* 20:2048-2059, 1995.
4. Lindblom K. Technique and results of diagnostic disc puncture and injection (discography) in the lumbar region. *Acta Orthop Scand* 20:315-326, 1951.
5. Bogduk NC, Aprill C, Derby R: Discography. In White A, Schofferman A, editors: *Spine Care. Diagnosis and conservative treatment*, St. Louis, 1995, Mosby, pp 219-236.
6. Lam KS, Carlin D, Mulholland RC: Lumbar disc high-intensity zone: the value and significance of provocative discography in the determination of the discogenic pain source. *Eur Spine J* 9:36-41, 2000.
7. Schellhas KP, Pollei SR, Gundry CR, Heithoff KB: Lumbar disc high-intensity zone. Correlation of magnetic resonance imaging and discography. *Spine* 21:79-86, 1996.
8. Buirski G, Silberstein M: The symptomatic lumbar disc in patients with low-back pain: magnetic resonance imaging appearance in both symptomatic and control population. *Spine* 18:1808, 1993.
9. Milette PC, Fontaine S, Lepanto L, et al: Differentiating lumbar disc protrusions, disc bulges and discs with normal contour but abnormal signal intensity. Magnetic resonance imaging with discographic correlations. *Spine* 24:44, 1999.
10. Ohnmeiss DD, Vanharanta H, Ekholm J: Relation between pain locations and disc pathology: a study of pain drawings and CT/discography. *Clin J Pain* 15:210, 1999.
11. Walsh TR, Weinstein JN, Spratt KF, et al: Lumbar discography in normal subjects: a controlled, prospective study. *J Bone Joint Surg* 72:1081, 1990.
12. Manchikanti L, Singh V, Pampati V, et al: Provocative discography in low back pain patients with or without somatization disorder: a randomized prospective evaluation. *Pain Physician* 4:227-239, 2001.
13. Horton WC, Daftari TK: Which disc visualized by magnetic resonance imaging is actually a source of pain? A correlation between magnetic resonance imaging and discography. *Spine* 17:S164-S171, 1992.
14. Kornberg M: Discography and magnetic resonance imaging in the diagnosis of lumbar disc disruption. *Spine* 14:1368-1372, 1989.
15. Manchikanti L, Singh V, Pampati V, et al: Evaluation of the relative contributions of various structures in chronic low back pain. *Pain Physician* 4:308-316, 2001.
16. Buenaventura RM, Shah RV, Patel V, et al: Systematic review of discography as a diagnostic test for spinal pain: an update. *Pain Physician* 10:147-164, 2007.
17. Bogduk N: Lumbar disc stimulation (provocation discography). In: Practice Guidelines for Spinal Diagnostic and Treatment Procedures. *ISIS* 20-46, 2004.
18. Derby R, Eek B, Lee SH, et al: Comparison of intradiscal restorative injections and intradiscal electrothermal treatment (IDET) in the treatment of low back pain. *Pain Physician* 7:63-66, 2004.
19. Holt EP, Jr: Fallacy of cervical discography. Report of 50 cases in normal subjects. *JAMA* 188:799-801, 1964.
20. Schellhas KP, Pollei SR, Dorwart RH: Thoracic discography: a safe and reliable technique. *Spine* 19:2103, 1994.
21. Wood KB, Schellhas KP, Garvey TA, Aeppli D: Thoracic discography in healthy individuals: a controlled prospective study of magnetic resonance imaging and discography in asymptomatic symptomatic individuals. *Spine* 24:1548, 1999.
22. Winter RB, Schellhas KP: Painful adult thoracic Scheuermann's disease: diagnosis by discography and treatment by combined arthrodesis. *Am J Orthop* 25:783, 1996.
23. Winter RB, Schellhas KP: Painful adult thoracic Scheuermann's disease: diagnosis by discography and treatment by combined arthrodesis. *Am J Orthop* 25:783-786, 1996.
24. Bogduk N: Thoracic provocation discography. In: Practice Guidelines for Spinal Diagnostic and Treatment Procedures. *ISIS* 287-294, 2004.
25. Singh V: Thoracic discography. *Pain Physician* 7:451-458, 2004.
26. Parfenchuck TA, Janssen ME: A correlation of cervical magnetic resonance imaging and discography/computed tomographic discograms. *Spine* 19:2819, 1994.
27. Schellhas KP, Smith MD, Gundry CR, Pollei SR: Cervical discogenic pain: prospective correlation of magnetic resonance imaging and discography in asymptomatic subjects and pain sufferers. *Spine* 21:300, 1996.
28. Schellhas KP, Garvey TA, Johnson BA, et al: Cervical discography: analysis of provoked responses at C2-C3, C3-C4, and C4-C5. *Am J Neuroradiol* 21:269, 2000.
29. Grubb SA, Kelly C: Cervical discography: clinical implications from 12 years of experience. *Spine* 25:1382, 2000.
30. Fortin JD: Cervical discography with CT and MRI correlations. In Lennard TA, editor: *Pain Procedures in Clinical Practice*, Philadelphia, 2000, Hanley and Belfus, pp 230-240.
31. Bogduk N: Cervical disc stimulation (provocation discography). In: Practice Guidelines for Spinal Diagnostic and Treatment Procedures. *ISIS* 95-111, 2004.
32. Roth DA: Cervical analgesic discography. A new test for the definitive diagnosis of painful-disk syndrome. *JAMA* 235:1713-1714, 1976.
33. Whitecloud TS, III, Seago RA: Cervical discogenic syndrome. Results of operative intervention in patients with positive discography. *Spine* 12:313-317, 1987.
34. Motimaya A, Arici M, George D, Ramsby G: Diagnostic value of cervical discography in the management of cervical discogenic pain. *Conn Med* 64:395-398, 2000.
35. Zeidman SM, Thompson K, Ducker TB: Complications of cervical discography: analysis of 4400 diagnostic disc injections. *Neurosurgery* 37:414-417.1994, 1995.
36. Manchikanti L, Singh V, Pampati V, et al: Evaluation of the relative contributions of various structures in chronic low back pain. *Pain Physician* 4:308-316, 2001.
37. Executive Committee of North American Spine Society: Position Statement on Discography. *Spine* 13:1349, 1988.
38. Walsh TR, Weinstein JN, Spratt K, et al: Lumbar discography in normal subjects. *J Bone Joint Surg Am* 72:1081-1088, 1990.
39. Horton WC, Daftari TK: Which disc visualized by magnetic resonance imaging is actually a source of pain? A correlation between magnetic resonance imaging and discography. *Spine* 17:S164-S171, 1992.

40. Kornberg M: Discography and magnetic resonance imaging in the diagnosis of lumbar disc disruption. *Spine* 14:1368-1372, 1989.

41. April C, Bogduk N: High intensity zone. A diagnostic sign of painful lumbar disc on magnetic resonance imaging. *Br J Radiol* 65:361-369, 1992.

42. Schellhas KP, Pollei SR, Gundry C, Heithoff KB: Lumbar disc high-intensity zone. Correlation of magnetic resonance imaging and discography. *Spine* 21:79-86, 1996.

43. Schwarzer AC, Aprill CN, Derby R, et al: The relative contributions of the disc and zygapophyseal joint in chronic low back pain. *Spine* 19:801-806, 1994.

44. Carragee E, Tanner C, Khurana S, et al: The rates of false-positive lumbar discography in select patients without low back symptoms. *Spine* 25:1373-1380, 2000.

45. Manchikanti L, Singh V, Pampati V, et al: Provocative discography in low back pain patients with or without somatization disorder: a randomized prospective evaluation. *Pain Physician* 4:227-239, 2001.

46. Crock HV: A reappraisal of intervertebral disc lesions. *Med J Augst* 1:983-989, 1970.

47. Smith BM, Hurwitz EL, Solsberg D, et al: Interobserver reliability of detecting lumbar intervertebral disc high-intensity zone on magnetic resonance imaging and association of high-intensity zone with pain and annular disruption. *Spine* 23:2074-2080, 1998.

48. Lam KS, Carlin D, Mulholland RC: Lumbar disc high-intensity zone: the value and significance of provocative discography in the determination of the discogenic pain source. *Euro Spine J* 9:36-41, 2000.

49. Stadnik TW, Lee RR, Coen HL, et al: Annular tears and disk herniation: prevalence and contrast enhancement on MR images in the absence of low back pain or sciatica. *Neuroradiology* 206:49-55, 1998.

50. Functional Anesthetic Discography [Package Insert]. Sunnyvale, California, 2006, Kyphon Inc.

51. Alamin T: International Society for the Study of the Lumbar Spine. Abstracts. Bergen, Norway; June 13-17, 2006, pp 52-53.

52. Karaman H, Tüfek A, Kavak GÖ, et al: 6-month results of transdiscal biacuplasty on patients with discogenic low back pain: preliminary findings. *Int J Med Sci* 8:1-8, 2011.

53. Saal JA, Saal JS: Intradiscal electrothermal therapy for the treatment of chronic discogenic low back pain. *Clin Sports Med* 21(1):167-187, 2002.

18 Minimally Invasive Intradiscal Procedures for the Treatment of Discogenic Lower Back and Leg Pain

Leonardo Kapural and Dawn A. Sparks

CHAPTER OVERVIEW

Chapter Synopsis: Diagnosis and treatment of lumbar discogenic pain remains a challenge. It may account for one third of patients with lower back pain. The mechanism of discogenic pain remains unclear, clinical presentation can vary, and magnetic resonance imaging (MRI) may only suggest the presence of internal disc disruption. Provocative discography can provide unique information about the morphology of the disc and remains the only diagnostic test that can relate the changes observed on imaging tests and the patient's pain. Minimally invasive treatments such as intradiscal biacuplasty or intradiscal electrothermal therapy are likely better alternatives to the currently available surgical options. They are cost-effective and may cause fewer side effects. However, the value of most of these therapies has yet to be established. More basic science and clinical studies are needed to prove the clinical efficacy of such minimally invasive treatments. One thing that is clear, however, is that careful patient selection, based on the present data, significantly improves the success of these procedures.

Percutaneous, minimally invasive intradiscal decompression procedures may be used to relieve pain from a herniated disc; several of these procedures are also considered. As in all interventional therapies for pain, attention to patient selection can vastly improve the odds of success.

Important Points:
- Better selection criteria improve results of annuloplasty and disc decompression procedures for lower back and discogenic leg pain.
- Patients with evidence of one or two levels of disc degeneration on MRI and one or two levels positive on provocative discography are desired candidates for annuloplasty.
- Outcomes of the percutaneous disc decompression procedures were largely positive when used for the treatment of contained lumbar disc herniations. However, more randomized, prospective studies are needed to confirm their effectiveness.

Clinical Pearls:
- Optimal patient positioning, which includes correction of lumbar lordosis using either a soft roll or pillow placed under the mid-abdomen, will facilitate needle placement for any of the intradiscal procedures.
- During provocative discography, excessive amounts of local anesthetic injected deep, closer to the disc and foramina just prior to intradiscal needle placement, may decrease the ability of patient and operator to detect the nerve root impalement.
- During intradiscal biacuplasty, although the temperature is set to 50° C on the radiofrequency generator, tissue temperature reaches about 70° C because of distal ionic heating. During this time, the patient should be awake and communicate with the physician.

Clinical Pitfalls:
- Puncturing an intervertebral disc with a needle may potentially lead to progressive disc disruption. Greater progression of degenerative disc disease has been suggested in post-discography discs, and it seems to be worse in patients who had larger diameter needles inserted in their intervertebral discs.
- Serious but rare complications include discitis, spinal abscesses, and vertebral osteomyelitis. Other neurological complications, such as cauda equina and nerve root damage, may be exclusively caused by misplacement of trocars, probes, or heating elements.

Introduction

Diagnosis and treatment of lumbar discogenic pain remains difficult. It may account for one third of the patients with lower back pain. The mechanism of discogenic pain is still unclear, the clinical presentation can vary, and magnetic resonance imaging (MRI) may only suggest the presence of internal disc disruption. Provocative discography can provide unique information about the morphology of the disc and remains the only diagnostic test that can relate changes observed on imaging tests and the patient's pain.

Minimal invasive treatments such as intradiscal biacuplasty and intradiscal electrothermal therapy (IDET) seem to be more efficacious, less invasive alternatives to currently available surgical options. They are cost-effective and may cause fewer side effects. However, the true therapeutic value of these therapies has yet to be established. More basic science and clinical studies are needed to give an insight on mechanisms of pain relief and to prove the clinical efficacy of such minimally invasive treatments. One thing that is clear, however, is that careful patient selection, based on the present data, significantly improves the successes of these procedures.

A handful of lumbar percutaneous disc decompression procedures are used as minimally invasive approaches to treat back and leg pain caused by contained disc herniation. The clinical outcomes have been generally favorable and complication rates low. However, more research is needed to identify the properly selected patients for a specific disc decompression technique.

Low back pain remains one of the biggest resource-consuming problems in medicine. At least 40% of the U.S. population at one time or another will use medical resources for the treatment of low back pain. Frequent sources of mechanical lower back pains are myofascial, discogenic, and facetogenic, from sacroiliac joint, compression fractures, and lumbar canal stenosis.[1,2]

Low back pain is the one of the most common causes of lost work time in the United States,[1] and discogenic pain is one of the main causes of chronic lower back pain.[3]

It is the aim of this chapter to briefly review new and developing interventional and minimally invasive spinal treatments for discogenic low back (**Figs. 18-1** to **18-3**) and leg pain caused by contained disc herniation. Also, a simple algorithm is offered in **Fig. 18-4** adopted and modified for discogenic back pain[4] and should only be used as a rough intervention guide. This chapter highlights some interesting, novel interventional therapeutic approaches and is not intended to be a complete guide for the treatment of patients with discogenic lower back pain. A comprehensive approach with involvement of multiple specialties and adjunct therapies, such as physical therapy and occupational interventions, are frequently required to produce significant improvement in functional capacity and pain scores of patients with chronic lower back pain.

Discogenic Lower Back Pain

When evaluating patients with the main complaint of long-lasting low back pain, with or without leg pain, it is necessary to investigate the pain generator causing debilitation. More typical features of discogenic source of pain include unrelenting nociceptive low back discomfort or groin or leg pain that worsens with axial loading that improves with recumbency. These signs and reported symptoms alone are usually inadequate to confirm an accurate diagnosis.[1-4] Although MRIs are helpful in visualizing such pathology as disc degeneration, desiccation, high intensity zones, and loss of disc height, these changes frequently correlate poorly with clinical

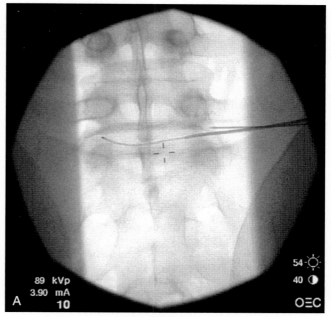

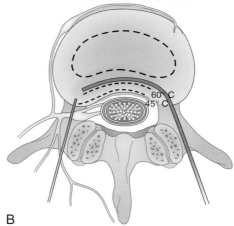

Fig. 18-1 Figs. 18-1 to 18-3 show fluoroscopic views of the final electrode positions during three different intervertebral disc heating procedures used for the treatment of discogenic pain head to head with schematic drawings of the ideal electrode placement. All three fluoroscopic views are anterior-posterior and the schematic drawings are illustrated transverse cuts through the targeted disc.
DiscTRODE (ValleyLab, Boulder, CO) **A,** DiscTRODE electrode properly positioned across the posterior annulus. A second probe visible on the right side is a temperature probe. **B,** Schematic drawing shows proper position of the radiofrequency electrode and temperature probe within the posterior annulus.

findings and the presence of chronic pain, leaving open critical questions of causality.[1-4] Many practitioners use provocative or analgesic diagnostic discography as a way to substantiate their clinical diagnosis of discogenic pain. Provocative or analgesic discography is the only available method to relate anatomical abnormalities seen on MRIs of the lumbar spine with clinically observed lower back pain. However, the predictive value of this test is repeatedly questioned, mainly as a consequence of potentially high false-positive rates.[5-7]

After provisional diagnosis of discogenic pain is introduced, an effective treatment is desired. Several commonly used minimally invasive intradiscal therapies involve careful heating of the

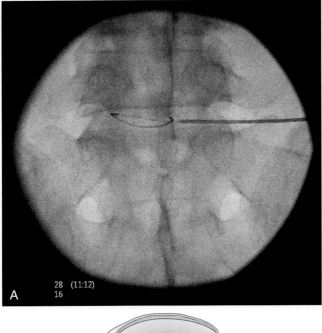

B

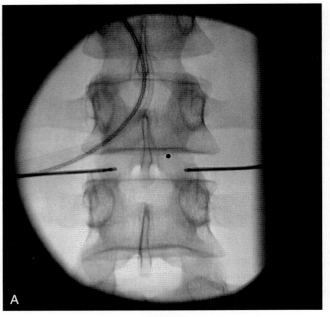

B

Fig. 18-2 Intradiscal electrothermal therapy (IDET) resistive coil is shown within the intervertebral disc. **A,** Anteroposterior fluoroscopic view of the properly positioned IDET coil. **B,** Schematic of the IDET coil proper positioning at interface between the annulus and nucleus. Note a limited temperature spread around the positioned coil.

Fig. 18-3 Bipolar intradiscal biacuplasty probes within the intervertebral disc. **A,** Anteroposterior fluoroscopic view of two biacuplasty probes within the intervertebral disc and away from vertebral endplates. **B,** Schematic transaction through the lumbar spine at the level of the intervertebral disc. Shown are two cooled electrodes for biacuplasty and their approximated positioning within posterior annulus of the lumbar disc. Using such electrodes, appropriate heat distribution is achieved across the posterior annulus without causing injury to posterior neural elements.

annulus fibrosus (so-called annuloplasty procedures) (**Fig. 18-4**). Historically, such therapeutic modalities have been used regardless of the unclear relationship between positive therapeutic effects and absence of the histological changes expected within the annulus of the disc after heat is used.[8-12] Currently, denervation of the annulus by heat destruction of the nociceptors is a plausible mechanism of pain relief. There is no evidence that collagen fibers in the annulus are significantly affected by denaturation and coalescence, possibly suggesting that the collagen alteration is an additional therapeutic mechanism for pain relief.[9-12] The minimally invasive approach, low cost, and relative simplicity of these procedures are the key advantages compared with surgical procedures such as lumbar fusion and disc replacement. IDET (Smith and Nephews, London, UK), DiscTRODE (Valleylab, Boulder, CO), and intradiscal biacuplasty (Baylis Medical, Montreal, Canada) (**Figs. 18-1 to 18-3**) are several annuloplasty methods using heat to treat discogenic pain.

Mechanisms of Pain Relief by Annuloplasty

Dehydration of the intervertebral disc and loss of nuclear material with increasing age are associated with disc degeneration. Consequent delamination and tearing of the lamellar layers are just physical changes that can be associated with biochemical and cellular changes within the disc. Inside the degenerating disc, production of inflammatory cytokines, including tumor necrosis factor-α (TNF-α), nitric oxide, and matrix metalloproteinases are greatly altered.[13,14] Neural elements that are normally limited to the outer third of the annulus penetrate farther into the degenerated disc along the vasculature and fissures.[15-18] Immunohistochemical studies have shown that such nerves in growth is of nociceptive origin (C- and A-δ fibers) and likely responsible for transmitting

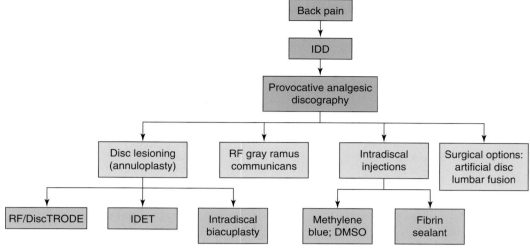

Fig. 18-4 A proposed simplified algorithm for the treatment of discogenic pain. After provocative or analgesic discography, minimally invasive options are those of annuloplasty or intradiscal injections. DMSO, dimethylsulfoxide; IDD, intervertebral disc disease; IDET, intradiscal electrothermal therapy; RF, radiofrequency.

pain responses.[14,17] Elimination of these nociceptors may disrupt the transmission of pain signals.

Thermal annular procedures were developed in an effort to provide minimally invasive delivery of thermal energy to the affected disc via a resistive heating coil (IDET) or an RF catheter (biacuplasty, Kimberly Clark, Atlanta, GA; DiscTRODE) to denervate nociceptive fibers and coagulate collagenous tissues in the annulus. However, scientific evidence to support either mechanism of action is lacking.

During the application of RF, alternating flow of electrical current causes ions in the tissue to move back and forth. This alternating movement by the ions causes molecular vibration within the tissue and results in frictional heating.[19,20] This effect is called ionic heating, and it can lead to thermal injury of the cells when tissue temperature reaches greater than 42° C.[21] The extent of cellular damage usually depends on the amount of temperature and duration of heating.[22] Increase in tissue temperature is a function of current density, or the amount of current per unit area. Current density is greatest at the proximity of the electrode and decreases with increasing distance from the electrode. However, by increasing the power output, current density around the electrode is increased, and thus the lesion size produced by ionic heating is limited by the current density.

One method of increasing lesion size or volume is by cooling the RF electrode internally. This technique was initially developed for tumor and cardiac ablation[23-25] and is currently used in intradiscal biacuplasty procedure.[26-28] Cooled RF probes have hollow lumens that extend to the tip of the electrode. The cooling fluid circulates in a closed loop through the hollow lumens to the tip of the electrode and back to a pump. The coolant acts as a heat sink that removes heat from the tissue adjacent to the electrode. Consequently, larger lesion volumes can be produced by increasing power deposition and the duration at which current is delivered without causing tissue charring around the electrode.[23] A larger lesion volume can be produced by using two internally cooled RF electrodes in a bipolar arrangement at the lower temperature.

Intradiscal Electrothermal Therapy

IDET technology (**Figs. 18-2** and **18-4**) relies on elongated resistive coil of very small diameter to deliver surrounding heat over the limited area of the posterior annulus. Possible mechanisms of pain relief were discussed above. The only difference between the IDET and other disc annuloplasty procedures is that the temperatures attained during the IDET are very high just around the electrode itself, and they dissipate relatively quickly at 2 to 4 mm radius away from the coil. The IDET procedure requires from the proceduralist a relatively long learning curve, and although it seems relatively easy to position resistive coil within the posterior annulus of the disc, multiple attempts may be required or it may be necessary to place another coil from the opposite side of the posterolateral disc to achieve optimal position within the interface between the annulus and nucleus (**Fig. 18-2**). This may contribute to further damage of the intervertebral disc, and sometimes placement of the tip of the coil within the posterior annular fissure may extend too close to the posterior edge of the disc. Indications for IDET include persistent discogenic low back pain despite comprehensive conservative treatments, including physical therapy, a directed home exercise program, and fluoroscopically guided epidural corticosteroid injections. The Saal brothers, inventors of the IDET catheter,[29-31] used initially some additional criteria for the selection of patients, which include those with normal neurological examination results, negative results on straight-leg raise test, absence of any inflammatory arthritic or nonspinal condition that may impersonate lumbar pain, and the absence of prior surgery at the symptomatic intervertebral disc level.[29-31] Provocative discography should replicate the concordant pain at low disc pressurization at up to three intervertebral disc levels. The above selection criteria disparities used in subsequent studies evaluating the effectiveness of IDET are thought to account for divergence seen in clinical results (**Table 18-1**).[29-43]

The IDET results seem to improve if additional patient selection criteria are used.[33,41] Multilevel disc degeneration in patients with discogenic pain was an important predictor of treatment failure compared with a group of patients with one or two degenerated discs as shown on the MRI. Unfortunately, single disc level disease is less frequent, and the majority of the patients present with discogenic pain and multilevel degeneration present on MRI.[41] Overweight patients[44] and patients receiving workers' compensation benefits[40,45] represent additional patient subsets that have a low probability of achieving desired results from IDET.

Table 18-1: Selected Published Articles on Three Annuloplasty Procedures*

Authors	Year	Type of Intervention	Indications of Procedure	Patients (n)	Type of Study	Outcomes	Complications	Conclusions
Assietti et al[42]	2010	IDET	Single-level DDD and positive discogram, >60% disc height	50	Prospective	VAS 68% decrease; ODI from 59.0 ± 7.6% to 20.1 ± 11% at 24 mo	None	Safe and effective
Kapural et al[49,50]	2008	Biacuplasty	Single- or two-level DDD and positive discogram, >50% disc height	15	Prospective pilot	7 of 13 >50% VAS ODI to 17.5 and SF-36-PF from 51 to 67 at 12 mo	None	Safe and effective
Kvarstein et al[46]	2009	DiscTRODE	Chronic LBP, positive discogram	23	Prospective randomized, double blind	No improvement study or sham at 12 mo	None	*Do not recommend use of DiscTRODE*
Pauza et al[35]	2004	IDET	DDD and positive discogram, >80% disc height	64	Randomized sham controlled prospective	56% >2 VAS change; 50% patients >50% relief at 6 mo	None	Safe and effective
Jawahar et al[43]	2008	IDET	DDD and positive discogram, >80% disc height, WC patients	53	Prospective	VAS reduction 63%, ODI 70%	None	Useful in carefully selected WC patients
Kapural et al[41]	2004	IDET	Single- or two-level DDD and positive discogram, >50% disc height vs. multilevel DDD	34	Prospective matched study	1,2-DDD >50% improvement in VAS and PDI	None	IDET procedure effective only in one or two level DDD

*Some variability in patient selection may explain differences in clinical outcomes.
DDD, degenerative disc disease; IDET, intradiscal electrothermal therapy; LBP, low back pain; ODI, Oswestry Disability Index; PDI, pain disability index; SF-36-PF, Short Form 36 Physical Functioning; VAS, visual analog scale; WC, workers' compensation.

Other Annuloplasty and Nucleoplasty Procedures

IDET is not the only minimally invasive annuloplasty procedure (**Fig. 18-4**). The DiscTRODE is a radiofrequency (RF) method in which heat is applied to the posterior annulus. This treatment is generally termed *percutaneous intradiscal RF thermocoagulation.*[46,47] Kvarstein et al[46] used appropriate inclusion criteria, which listed disc height reduction less than 30% and disc protrusion of less than 4 mm, as well as positive one-level pain provocation discography. A disappointing performance resulted because patients reported only modest or no improvements in pain scores and functional capacity.[46,47] Furthermore, the mean reduction of Oswestry Disability Index scores did not reach statistical significance when compared with baseline.[46] This technology proved to be unsuccessful in improving functional capacity and visual analog score (VAS) versus IDET during another study in which strict patient selection criteria were used.[47]

Intradiscal Biacuplasty

Intradiscal biacuplasty is the latest minimally invasive posterior annulus heating technique (**Fig. 18-4**). This technology uses bipolar cooled RF electrodes called transdiscal electrodes (Kimberly Clark, Atlanta, GA). Reviewing the pain scores and functional capacity improvement ratings in patients with discogenic pain, biacuplasty is comparable or better than other minimally invasive annuloplasty

methods.[48-52] Internally cooling electrodes provides for even heating over the wider area of the posterior annulus (**Fig. 18-3, B**).[26-28]

The procedure itself is fluoroscopy guided with the patient lying in the prone position. Electrodes are inserted bilaterally in the posterior annulus of the intervertebral disc as shown in **Fig. 18-3, B**. The generator controls delivery of RF energy by monitoring the temperature measured by a thermocoupler near the tip of the electrode. The temperature increases gradually over a period of 7 to 8 minutes to 50° C with final heating for another 7 minutes. During this time, the patient should be awake and communicating with the physician to decrease the probability of neurological injury.

Currently, clinical biacuplasty data from two case series of eight and 15 patients are available for critical review. Both studies demonstrated significant pain relief after the disc biacuplasty procedure at 3, 6, and 12 months.[50-52] European case series suggested improvement in pain scores greater than 50% at 3 months with general good patient satisfaction. A U.S. pilot study involving 15 patients described reduction in the median VAS pain score from 7 to 3 cm at 6 and 12 months of follow-up, respectively; improvement in Oswestry Disability Index from 23.3 to 16.5 points; and significant increase in the Short Form 36 Physical Functioning scores (**Table 18-1**).[50,52] The sham, prospective randomized study is currently being conducted, and data may be available as soon as mid-2011. Intradiscal biacuplasty may offer several advantages over the earlier techniques. There is negligible disruption to the native tissue architecture, and thus the biomechanics of the spine is likely unchanged, and the relative ease of electrode placement abolishes the need to thread a long-heating catheter (e.g., IDET).

Complications of Annuloplasty Procedures

The incidence of various complications related to annuloplasty could be as high as 10%.[53,54] If the RF electrode or resistive coil is positioned in the close proximity of the neural elements, high temperatures delivered may cause nerve injury possibly manifested as a radicular pain or transient palsy. Transient radiculopathy with the resolution in less than 6 weeks and, rarely, motor deficit with prominent foot drop were previously reported after the IDET procedure.[54]

Catheter breakage,[54] vertebral osteonecrosis,[55] and cauda equina[56] syndrome all have been reported as rare complications of the IDET procedure. The duration of back pain, obesity, smoking, history of leg pain, and diabetes may not be associated with the higher incidence of complications.[53] Compared with nucleoplasty (disc decompressive procedure) alone, the frequency of the complications was not higher in patients who received IDET combined with nucleoplasty procedure.[57]

Discitis is rare complication of any intradiscal procedure.[58-62] Appropriate timing of intravenous antibiotic seems to be effective in preventing discitis after provocative discography and any minimally invasive intradiscal procedure.[58-62] The incidence of disc herniation after annuloplasty could be as high as 0.3%, and it was speculated to be caused by thermally mediated loss of tensile strength of the collagen fibers.[63] At least one case report documented disc herniation with clear increase in the size of disc protrusion after IDET procedure.[53,54]

Mechanisms of Disc Herniation and Pain Relief from Percutaneous Disc Decompression

A herniated disc can cause radicular pain or referred pain in the extremity involved. Whereas radicular pain follows appropriate dermatomal area, referred pain can be elsewhere in the extremity. With an internal disc disruption, nucleus of the disc has altered weight-bearing loads and could cause a change in shape or complete disruption of the annular fibers, which in turn may produce contained disc herniation or extrusion of the disc. Nerve root compression can result from either of those two mechanical events (**Fig. 18-5**).[64]

Occasionally, radicular or referred pain in the extremity can be significant with or without significant mechanical pathology as described above. This is because various inflammatory mediators are present in the intravertebral disc, including phospholipase A_2, prostaglandin E_2, interleukin-1α, interleukin-1β, interleukin-6, TNF-α, and nitric oxide.[65] Exposure of the neural structures to the nuclear material, therefore, may cause chemical painful radiculitis. MRI remains the modality of choice in diagnosing lumbar disc herniations. Intervertebral disc can be well described, as well as the surrounding nerves and bony structures.

Assumption that protruded but contained disc herniation may exert pressure on a nerve root and possibly dorsal root ganglion provided the basis for intradiscal percutaneous disc decompression. Simply, removal of the small amount of the nuclear material from the disc with contained herniation and with absent transannular fissure, or RF within the nucleus, can provide rather precipitous decrease in intradiscal pressure and partial retraction of the herniation away from the nerve. Such a decrease in intradiscal pressure is less likely if the elasticity of the disc is not preserved and

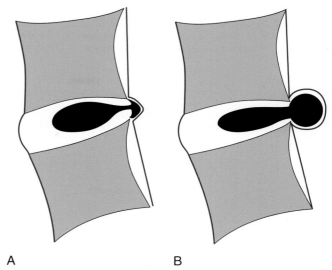

A   B

Fig. 18-5 Two basic types of intervertebral disc herniation: protrusion is characterized by the fact that the greatest distance, in any plane, between the edges of disc material beyond the disc space is less than the distance between the edges of the disc base in the same plane (**A**). Extrusion is present if any one distance between the edges of the disc material beyond the disc space is greater than the distance between the edges of the base in the same plane (**B**).

the outer annulus is damaged containing high-grade (Dallas 5) fissure.

Therefore, the ideal candidate for percutaneous, minimally invasive intradiscal disc decompression is someone with maintained height of the disc (>50%), radicular pain correlating with imaging findings, leg pain more than back pain, and clearly contained disc herniation. Those who are not candidates for such procedures are patients with extruded disc herniation, progressive neurological motor deficits, cauda equina syndrome, and overly calcified disc herniations. Also, the presence of any spinal stenosis needs to be closely evaluated.

The Dekompressor Device

The percutaneous decompression (Dekompressor) technology extracts nuclear disc material by an auger within a cannula that ends inside the nucleus. A significant change in intradiscal pressure follows the reduction of nuclear volume within the closed hydraulic space. It is imperative that the annular wall be intact for this technique to retract the bulging section; therefore provocative discography may occasionally be needed to confirm the affected level and to rule out any annular disruption.[66-68]

To place the Dekompressor introducer and stylet within the disc, a similar oblique angle is used as for the standard discography. The active, rota-rooter probe is advanced via introducer after diluted contrast is injected to delineate the disc nucleus. A transparent collection chamber is attached to the probe, which can be removed and inspected for collected nuclear tissue. Assessment of the tissue volume removed may be difficult because the amount of the tissue in the collection chamber should be added to the amount of the tissue along the probe. Decompression is completed when the physician believes that the sufficient material has been removed from the disc.

Studies published on the efficacy of the Dekompressor device when used for treatment of contained, symptomatic disc

Table 18-2: Selected Clinical Studies on Nucleoplasty and Dekompressor*

Authors	Year	Type of Intervention	Indications of Procedure	Patients (*n*)	Type of Study	Outcomes	Complications	Conclusions
Mirzai et al[72]	2007	Nucleoplasty	Lumbar herniated disc, and radicular pain for at least 3 mo	52	Prospective	VAS from 7.5 to 3.1; ODI 42.2 to 24.8 at 6 mo	None	<6 mm, contained herniations, disc height >50%, annular integrity
Yakovlev et al[73]	2007	Nucleoplasty	Contained herniation; radicular or axial >6 mo; disc height >50%; positive discogram	22	Retrospective	VAS down 3.98; 81.8% improvement in function; analgesics down 72.7% at 1 yr	None	Safe and effective
Singh et al[70]	2002	Nucleoplasty	Contained herniation; radicular >3 mo; disc height >50%; positive discogram	80	Prospective observational	75% decrease in numeric pain score at 12 mo	None	Safe and effective
Lierz et al[66]	2009	Dekompressor	Contained herniation	64	Prospective observational	VAS down 5.2; decreased medication use 80% at 12 mo	None	Safe and effective
Calisaneller et al[74]	2007	Nucleoplasty	Contained herniation	29	Prospective	VAS from 6.95 to 4.53	None	≈50% of the patients had 50% relief
Amoretti et al[67]	2004	Dekompressor	Contained herniation	10	Retrospective	VAS >70% decrease; 80% no analgesics	None	Safe and effective

*Conclusion on clinical effectiveness seems to be largely positive but lacking randomized, sham prospective clinical trials.
ODI, Oswestry Disability Index; VAS, visual analog scale.

herniation are few and observational. In 64 patients, Lierz et al[66] reported an average decrease in pain scores from 7.3 to 2.1 after 12 months with 80% of the patients being able to reduce their pain medications. Amoretti et al[67] reported in 50 patients a more than 70% decrease in pain in 72% of cases, and Alò and colleagues[68] reported an 80% success rate using the same technique. There are still no controlled studies published on Dekompressor efficacy.

Coblation Nucleoplasty

Coblation technology has been used in various arthroscopic procedures and relies on partial ablation of the nuclear tissue followed by coagulation. Similarly, Nucleoplasty Coblation (ArthroCare Corporation, Austin, TX) can ablate and coagulate the nucleus pulposus to decompress the disc and thermally alter disc tissue.[69] It seems that decompression is minimal or nonexistent in degenerated discs and more likely in nondegenerated ones.[70-74] An access to the disc is accomplished through a canula with the obturator stylet using fluoroscopy. It is followed by an RF electrode called the SpineWand. Tissue ablation creates channels through the nucleus to the opposite side. The canula is then slowly withdrawn to the starting position five or six times.[69]

Radicular pain should be greater than axial pain, and patients should have already failed conservative treatments. Less favorable outcomes are seen with large disc protrusions and disc extrusions. A patient with a contained disc protrusion of less than 6 mm whose annular integrity is documented by discography and who has consistent radicular symptoms confirmed by selective nerve root blocks represents the ideal candidate for annuloplasty.[69-75] Improvements in both functional capacity and pain relief were seen with nucleoplasty during observational studies (Table 18-2).[70-74] A recent systematic review, although strongly supporting therapeutic efficacy of this procedure, repeated necessity of randomized, prospective sham study to acquire level 1 evidence for the procedure.[75]

Two other commonly used percutaneous disc decompression methods are somewhat less used over recent years. One is called The Nucleotome (Clarus Medical, Minneapolis, MN) and contains an automated shaver with continuous irrigation to remove nuclear disc material. Although it can remove large amount of disc material, it also uses a bulky probe, which can potentially produce significant annular damage. The same concerns are shared by most practitioners who have had experience using the other commonly used percutaneous lumbar laser discectomy.

Complications of Percutaneous Decompressive Procedures

At least one study found a statistically significant higher prevalence of leg pain and increased weakness in patients who received nucleoplasty compared with those receiving just conservative treatment.

However, the most common side effect was soreness at the site of the catheter insertion.[76] Although side effects with the Dekompressor are rare, so is the volume of the patients reported receiving this procedure (at least when compared with the number of patients in studies on nucleoplasty). The probe break within the disc nucleus has been described where the tip of the probe had to be removed surgically.[77]

Conclusion

Discogenic pain continues to be a debilitating condition that represents a major source of chronic low back pain. At this time, evidence for the overall effectiveness of minimally invasive intradiscal procedures for the treatment of discogenic pain is deficient. However, continued studies provide evidence that the RF annuloplasties can be beneficial to selected subpopulation of patients. DiscTRODE annuloplasty and conventional nuclear RF seem to be ineffective in improving functional capacity in patients with discogenic back pain. IDET and intradiscal biacuplasty types of annuloplasty may produce positive therapeutic effect in highly selected patient groups. More work is ahead of us to clearly determine if certain disc decompression procedures can provide long-term pain relief during randomized, sham-controlled studies.

References

1. Andersson, GBJ: Epidemiological features of chronic low-back pain. *Lancet* 354(9178):581-585, 1999.
2. Kaaria S, Kaila-Kangas L, Kirjonen J, et al: Low back pain, work absenteeism, chronic back disorders, and clinical findings in the low back as predictors of hospitalization due to low back disorders. *Spine* 10:1211-1218, 2005.
3. Schwartzer AC, Aprill CN, Derby R, et al: The prevalence and clinical features of internal disc disruption in patients with chronic low back pain. *Spine* 20:1878-1883, 1995.
4. Kapural L, Goldner JD: Interventional pain management: when/what therapies are best for low back pain. *Current Opin Anesthesiol* 18:569-575, 2005.
5. Carragee EJ, Tanner CM, Khurana S, et al: The rates of false-positive lumbar discography in select patients without low back symptoms. *Spine* 25:1373-1380, 2000.
6. Walsh TR, Weinstein JN, Spratt KF, et al: Lumbar discography in normal subjects. A controlled, prospective study. *J Bone Joint Surg Am* 72:1081-1088, 1990.
7. Derby R, Howard MW, Grant JM, et al: The ability of pressure-controlled discography to predict surgical and nonsurgical outcomes. *Spine* 24:364-371, 1999.
8. Freeman BJ, Walters RM, Moore RJ, et al: Does intradiscal electrothermal therapy denervate and repair experimentally induced posterolateral annular tears in an animal model? *Spine* 28:2602-2608, 2003.
9. Kleinstueck FS, Diederich CJ, Nau WH, et al: Temperature and thermal dose distributions during intradiscal electrothermal therapy in the cadaveric lumbar spine. *Spine* 28:1700-1708, 2003.
10. Shah RV, Lutz GE, Lee J, et al: Intradiskal electrothermal therapy: a preliminary histologic study. *Arch Phys Med Rehabil* 82:1230-1237, 2001.
11. Smith HP, McWhorter JM, Challa VR: Radiofrequency neurolysis in a clinical model. *J Neurosurg* 55:248-253, 1981.
12. Obrzut SL, Hecht P, Hayashi K, et al: The effect of radiofrequency energy on length and temperature properties of the glenohumeral joint capsule. *Arthroscopy* 4:395-400, 1998.
13. Podichetty VK: The aging spine: the role of inflammatory mediators in intervertebral disc degeneration. *Cell Mol Biol (Noisy-le-grand)* 53(5):4-18, 2007.
14. Ashton IK, et al: Neuropeptides in the human intervertebral disc. *J Orthop Res* 12(2):186-192, 1994.
15. Johnson WE, Evans H, Menage J, et al: Immunohistochemical detection of Schwann cells in innervated and vascularized human intervertebral discs. *Spine* 26(23):2550-2557, 2001.
16. Melrose J, Roberts S, Smith S, et al: Increased nerve and blood vessel ingrowth associated with proteoglycan depletion in an ovine anular lesion model of experimental disc degeneration. *Spine* 27(12):1278-1285, 2002.
17. Palmgren T, Grönblad M, Virri J, et al: An immunohistochemical study of nerve structures in the anulus fibrosus of human normal lumbar intervertebral discs. *Spine* 24(20):2075-2079, 1999.
18. Jackson HC, 2nd, Winkelmann RK, Bickel WH: Nerve endings in the human lumbar spinal column and related structures. *J Bone Joint Surg Am* 48(7):1272-1281, 1966.
19. Noe CE, Racz GB: Radiofrequency. In Raj P, editor: *Pain medicine: a comprehensive review*, St. Louis, 1996, Mosby, pp 305-308.
20. Organ LW: Electrophysiologic principles of radiofrequency lesion making. *Appl Neurophysiol* 39(2):69-76, 1976.
21. Dickson JA, Calderwood SK: Temperature range and selective sensitivity of tumors to hyperthermia: a critical review. *Ann NY Acad Sci* 335:180-205, 1980.
22. Curley SA: Radiofrequency ablation of malignant liver tumors. *Ann Surg Oncol* 10(4):338-347, 2003.
23. Lorentzen T: A cooled needle electrode for radiofrequency tissue ablation: thermodynamic aspects of improved performance compared with conventional needle design. *Acad Radiol* 3(7):556-556, 1996.
24. Wittkamp FHM, Hauer RN, Robles de Medina EO: Radiofrequency ablation with a cooled porus electrode catheter [abstract]. *J Am Coll Cardiol* 11(17), 1988.
25. Goldberg SN, Gazelle GS, Solbiati L, et al: Radiofrequency tissue ablation: increased lesion diameter with a perfusion electrode. *Acad Radiol* 3(8):636-644, 1996.
26. Pauza K: Cadaveric intervertebral disc temperature mapping during disc biacuplasty. *Pain Physician* 11(5):669-676, 2008.
27. Kapural L, Mekhail N, Sloan S, et al: Histological and temperature distribution studies in the lumbar degenerated and non-degenerated human cadaver discs using novel transdiscal radiofrequency electrodes. *Pain Med* 9(1):68-75, 2008.
28. Petersohn JD, Conquergood LR, Leung M: Acute histologic effects and thermal distribution profile of disc biacuplasty using a novel water-cooled bipolar Electrode system in an in vivo porcine model. *Pain Med* 9(1):26-32, 2008.
29. Saal JA, Saal JS: Intradiscal electrothermal treatment for chronic discogenic low back pain: prospective outcome study with a minimum 2-year follow-up. *Spine* 27:966-973, 2002.
30. Saal JA, Saal JS: Intradiscal electrothermal treatment for chronic discogenic low back pain: a prospective outcome study with minimum 1-year follow-up. *Spine* 25:2622-2627, 2000.
31. Saal JS, Saal JA: Management of chronic discogenic low back pain with a thermal intradiscal catheter. A preliminary report. *Spine* 25:382-388, 2000.
32. Appleby D, Andersson G, Totta M: Meta-analysis of the efficacy and safety of intradiscal electrothermal therapy (IDET). *Pain Med* 7:308-316, 2006.
33. Bogduk N, Karasek M: Two-year follow-up of a controlled trial of intradiscal electrothermal anuloplasty for chronic low back pain resulting from internal disc disruption. *Spine J* 2:343-350, 2002.
34. Endres SM, Fiedler GA, Larson KL: Effectiveness of intradiscal electrothermal therapy in increasing function and reducing chronic low back pain in selected patients. *WMJ* 101:31-34, 2002.
35. Pauza KJ, Howell S, Dreyfuss P, et al: A randomized, placebo-controlled trial of intradiscal electrothermal therapy for the treatment of discogenic low back pain. *Spine J* 4:27-35, 2004.
36. Wetzel FT, McNally TA, Phillips FM: Intradiscal electrothermal therapy used to manage chronic discogenic low back pain: new directions and interventions. *Spine* 27:2621-2626, 2002.
37. Derby R, Eek B, Chen Y, et al: Intradiscal electrothermal annuloplasty (IDET): a novel approach for treating chronic discogenic back pain. *Neuromodulation* 3:82-88, 2000.

38. Lutz C, Lutz GE, Cooke PM: Treatment of chronic lumbar diskogenic pain with intradiskal electrothermal therapy: a prospective outcome study. *Arch Phys Med Rehabil* 84:23-28, 2003.

39. Lee MS, Cooper G, Lutz GE, et al: Intradiscal electrothermal therapy (IDET) for treatment of chronic lumbar discogenic pain: a minimum 2-year clinical outcome study. *Pain Physician* 6:443-448, 2003.

40. Mekhail N, Kapural L: Intradiscal thermal annuloplasty of discogenic pain: an outcome study. *Pain Pract* 4:84-90, 2004.

41. Kapural L, Korunda Z, Basali AH, et al: Intradiscal thermal annuloplasty for discogenic pain in patients with multilevel degenerative disc disease. *Anesth Analg* 99:472-476, 2004.

42. Assietti R, Morosi M, Block JE: Intradiscal electrothermal therapy for symptomatic internal disc disruption: 24-month results and predictors of clinical success. *J Neurosurg Spine* 12(3):320-326, 2010.

43. Jawahar A, Brandao SM, Howard C, et al: Intradiscal electrothermal therapy (IDET): a viable alternative to surgery for low back pain in workers' compensation patients? *J La State Med Soc* 160(5):280-285, 2008.

44. Cohen SP, Larkin T, Abdi S, et al: Risk factors for failure and complications of intradiscal electrothermal therapy: a pilot study. *Spine* 28:1142-1147, 2003.

45. Webster BS, Verma S, Pransky GS: Outcomes of workers' compensation claimants with low back pain undergoing intradiscal electrothermal therapy. *Spine* 29:435-441, 2004.

46. Kvarstein G, Mawe L, Indahl A, et al: A randomized double-blind controlled trial of intra-annular radiofrequency thermal disc therapy-A 12-month follow-up. *Pain* 145:279-286, 2009.

47. Kapural L, Hayek S, Malak O, et al: Intradiscal thermal annuloplasty versus intradiscal radiofrequency ablation for the treatment of discogenic pain: a prospective matched control trial. *Pain Med* 6:425-431, 2005.

48. Kapural L, Mekhail N: novel transdiscal biacuplasty for the treatment of lumbar discogenic pain: a case report. *Pain Pract* 7(2):130-134, 2007.

49. Kapural L, De la Garza M, Ng A, et al: Novel transdiscal biacuplasty for the treatment of lumbar discogenic pain: a 6 months follow-up. *Pain Med* 9(1):60-67, 2008.

50. Kapural L: Intervertebral disc cooled bipolar radiofrequency (intradiscal biacuplasty) for the treatment of lumbar discogenic pain: a 12 month follow-up of the pilot study. *Pain Med* 9(4):464, 2008.

51. Kapural L, Cata JP, Narouze S: Successful treatment of lumbar discogenic pain using intradiscal biacuplasty in previously discectomized disc. *Pain Pract* 9(2):130-134, 2009.

52. Cooper AR: *Disc biacuplasty for treatment of axial discogenic low back pain: initial case series.* In Glasgow, Scotland, 2007, British Pain Society Annual General Meeting.

53. Cohen SP, Larkin T, Abdi S, et al: Risk factors for failure and complications of intradiscal electrothermal therapy: a pilot study. *Spine* 28:1142-1147, 2003.

54. Kapural L, Cata J: Complications of minimally invasive procedures for discogenic pain. *Tech Reg Anesth Pain Med* 11(3):157-163, 2007.

55. Djurasovic M, Glassman SD, Dimar JR, et al: Vertebral osteonecrosis associated with the use of intradiscal electrothermal therapy: a case report. *Spine* 27(13):E325-E328, 2002.

56. Wetzel FT: Cauda equina syndrome from intradiscal electrothermal therapy. *Neurology* 56:1607, 2001.

57. Cohen SP, Williams S, Kurihara C, et al: Nucleoplasty with or without intradiscal electrothermal therapy (IDET) as a treatment for lumbar herniated disc. *J Spinal Disord Tech* 18(suppl):S119-S124, 2005.

58. Klessig HT, Showsh SA, Sekorski A: The use of intradiscal antibiotics for discography: an in vitro study of gentamicin, cefazolin, and clindamycin. *Spine* 28:1735-1738, 2003.

59. Esimont FJ, Wiesel SW, Brighton CT, et al: Antibiotic penetration into rabbit nucleus pulposus. *Spine* 12:254-256, 1987.

60. Thomas RW, Batten JJ, Want S, et al: A new in-vitro model to investigate antibiotic penetration of the intervertebral disc. *J Bone Joint Surg Br* 77:967-970, 1995.

61. Rhoten RL, Murphy MA, Kalfas IH, et al: Antibiotic penetration into cervical discs. *Spine* 37:418-421, 1995.

62. Boscardin JB, Ringus JC, Feingold DJ, et al: Human intradiscal levels with cefazolin. *Spine* 17(suppl):S145-S148, 1992.

63. Kleinstueck FS, Diederich CJ, Nau WH, et al: Acute biomechanical and histological effects of intradiscal electrothermal therapy on human lumbar discs. *Spine* 26:2198-2207, 2001.

64. Komori H, Shinomiya K, Nakai O, et al: The natural history of herniated nucleus pulposus with radiculopathy. *Spine* 21:225-229, 1996.

65. Takahashi H, Suguro T, Okazima Y, et al: Inflammatory cytokines in the herniated disc of the lumbar spine. *Spine (Phila Pa 1976)* 15:21(2):218-224, 1996.

66. Lierz P, Alò KM, Felleiter P: Percutaneous lumbar discectomy using the Dekompressor system under CT-control. *Pain Pract* 9(3):216-220, 2009.

67. Amoretti N, Huchot F, Flory P, et al: Percutaneous nucleotomy: preliminary communication on a decompression probe (Dekompressor) in percutaneous discectomy. Ten case reports. *Clin Imaging* 29:98-101, 2005.

68. Alò KM, Wright RE, Sutcliffe J, et al: Percutaneous lumbar discectomy: clinical response in an initial cohort of fifty consecutive patients with chronic radicular pain. *Pain Pract* 4:19-29, 2004.

69. Deer T, Kapural L: Imaging for disc decompression procedures. *Tech Reg Anesth Pain Med* 11(2):81-89, 2007.

70. Singh V, Piryani C, Liao K, et al: Percutaneous disc decompression using coblation (Nucleoplasty™). *Pain Physician* 5:250-259, 2002.

71. Sharps LS, Zacharia I: Percutaneous disc decompression using nucleoplasty. *Pain Physician* 5:121-126, 2002.

72. Mirzai H, Tekin I, Yaman O, et al: The results of nucleoplasty in patients with lumbar herniated disc: a prospective clinical study of 52 consecutive patients. *Spine J* 7:88-92, 2007.

73. Yakovlev A, Tamimi MA, Liang H, et al: Outcomes of percutaneous disc decompression utilizing nucleoplasty for the treatment of chronic discogenic pain. *Pain Physician* 10:319-328, 2007.

74. Calisaneller T, Ozdemir O, Karadeli E, et al: Six months post-operative clinical and 24 hour post-operative MRI examinations after nucleoplasty with radiofrequency energy. *Acta Neurochir (Wien)* 149:495-500, 2007.

75. Gerges FJ, Lipsitz SR, Nedeljkovic SS: A systematic review on the effectiveness of the Nucleoplasty™ procedure for discogenic pain. *Pain Physician* 13:117-132, 2010.

76. Bhagia SM, Slipman CW, Nirschl M, et al: Side effects and complications after percutaneous disc decompression using coblation technology. *Am J Phys Med Rehabil* 85:6-11, 2006.

77. Domsky R, Goldberg ME, Hirsh RA, et al: Critical failure of a percutaneous discectomy probe requiring surgical removal during disc decompression. *Reg Anesth Pain Med* 31:177-179, 2006.

19 Vertebral Augmentation

Tristan C. Pico, Basem Hamid, and Allen W. Burton

CHAPTER OVERVIEW

Chapter Synopsis: The spine is susceptible to vertebral compression fractures (VCFs), which can arise from osteoporosis and various types of bone growths and tumors. The downstream consequences of VCF can be significant and go hand in hand with increased mortality, particularly in the aging population. Two minimally invasive procedures to treat VCF are percutaneous vertebroplasty (PV) and percutaneous kyphoplasty (PK). In PV, a substance called polymethylmethacrylate (PMMA), also known as bone cement, is injected into the vertebral body. PK is similar but involves the placement of a balloon, called a tamp, into the vertebral body. The tamp is then inflated and deflated repeatedly to create a space for injection of PMMA. Similar to many axial and mechanical sources of spinal pain, VCF pain abates with rest and can be exacerbated by activity after a fracture. This chapter considers technical aspects and the risks of complications with the injection procedures. As with any spinal injection technique, PV and PK require an intimate understanding of spinal anatomy. Patient selection requires special attention, and the details of the procedure should be specialized to each patient. The data largely support PV and PK as effective measures against pain after VCF.

Important Points:
- PV (bone cement injection into fractured vertebrae) and PK balloon augmentation followed by bone cement injection into fractured vertebrae are safe and effective procedures used in the treatment of patients with painful VCFs.
- Patients with osteoporosis need careful positioning and padding to avoid injury.
- During the PV and PK procedures, careful needle placement is critical with the use of omniplanar fluoroscopic imaging.
- Injection of PMMA must be done slowly and carefully using a viscous opacified cement mixture to avoid extrusion or injection must be halted promptly upon PMMA extrusion.
- Overinjection of PMMA should be avoided, particularly with respect to the posterior cortical wall and spinal canal or neural foramen region.
- Any post-procedure neurological abnormality mandates a careful evaluation, including consideration of prompt computed tomography to define the PMMA injection in three dimensions and guide potential therapeutic options, including surgical decompression.

Clinical Pearls:
- Vertebroplasty and kyphoplasty are effective, relatively simple procedures to treat VCF-related pain.
- These procedures can be safely performed on very frail, medically ill patients with careful attention to positioning, light sedation, copious local anesthetic, and a gentle touch.
- The exact role of "balloon" versus "no balloon" procedures remains to be evaluated by a randomized controlled trial, and currently mainly expert opinion guides this decision making.

Clinical Pitfalls:
- These procedures involve placing a large (at least 13 g) needle deeply into the spine. Care must be taken not to cause harm due to needle misplacement.
- Osteoporotic patients will suffer new fractures in many cases (up to 25% of patients); these patients MUST be on aggressive anti-osteoporotic therapy, or referred for such care.
- In patients with persistent pain after vertebral augmentation, the clinician should consider facetogenic pain as a probable therapeutic target related to spinal kyphosis.
- Patients with neurologic deficit or possible PMMA injection in the spinal canal post procedure need MANDATORY imaging (CT or MRI) and emergent surgical consultation.

Introduction

Vertebral compression fractures (VCFs) can result from a variety of conditions, which include but are not limited to osteoporosis, primary or metastatic spine neoplasms, and some benign bone tumors such as vertebral hemangiomas. Especially with the aging population, osteoporosis remains the most common cause of VCFs.[1] Direct care costs of osteoporotic VCFs have been estimated between $12.2 and $17.9 billion a year. VCFs are associated with significant morbidity and mortality, including impairment of daily activities and psychosocial performance. The kyphotic deformities caused by VCFs are associated with pulmonary dysfunction, constipation, and imbalance. Compared with age-matched control subjects, patients with VCFs have a higher mortality rate, increasing with the numbers of fractures as well as the duration of follow-up.[1-4]

Vertebroplasty and kyphoplasty are minimally invasive techniques used to treat painful VCF. Vertebroplasty is the percutaneous injection of a vertebral body (VB) with bone cement, generally polymethylmethacrylate (PMMA). PMMA has been used in orthopedics since the late 1960s.[5] Percutaneous vertebroplasty (PV) was first reported by a French group in 1987 for the treatment of painful hemangiomas. This case was a "stunner" of a C2 hemangioma, according to the authors. It was painful and got better after cement injection.[6,7] Since then, the indications for PV have expanded to include osteoporotic compression fractures, traumatic compression fractures, and painful vertebral metastasis.[8,9]

Kyphoplasty is a modification of PV. It involves the percutaneous placement of balloons (called "tamps") into the VB with an inflation and deflation sequence to create a cavity before the cement injection. Percutaneous kyphoplasty (PK) may restore some of the VB height and reduce the kyphotic angulation of the compression fracture before PMMA injection.[10]

Ideal candidates for PV or PK have activity-related axial pain corresponding to the level of a recent compression fracture. This pain lessens or abates completely with recumbency, sitting still, or both. A complete neurological examination and recent radiographic imaging are mandatory to rule out spinal cord compromise or retropulsed bony fragments in the canal. Magnetic resonance imaging (MRI) shows an increased T2-weighted signal caused by bone edema at the level with a recent fracture. Bone scan has also been used to target the most recent fracture(s) in patients with multiple fractures because uptake of radiotracer has been associated with a higher rate of excellent pain relief compared with PV without correlation with scintigraphy.[11,12] Spinal cord compression on MRI (in the absence of neurological findings) is a relative contraindication. There may be cases in which the procedure is still indicated in a patient with a "tight canal" such as this, but the margin of error is very small, so if a small amount of PMMA extrudes, neurological deficits may ensue. If a posterior cortical fracture is suspected on MRI, a computed tomography scan will reveal the bony architecture more precisely.

Procedural Overview and Complication Avoidance

Standards for the safe practice of these techniques have been published by the Society of Interventional Radiology (SIR) in 2003 and recently updated by the Cardiovascular and Interventional Radiological Society of Europe; highlights of this document can be found in **Box 19-1**.[13,14]

Box 19-1: Summary of Guidelines for Percutaneous Vertebroplasty and Percutaneous Kyphoplasty According to the Society of Interventional Radiology and Cardiovascular and Interventional Radiological Society of Europe

Indications
- Painful osteoporotic VCF refractory to 3 weeks of analgesic therapy
- Painful vertebrae caused by benign or malignant primary or secondary bone tumors
- Painful VCF with osteonecrosis (Kummell disease)
- Reinforcement of vertebral body before surgical procedure
- Chronic traumatic VCF with nonunion

Absolute Contraindications
- Asymptomatic VCF
- Patient improving on medical therapy
- Active infection
- Prophylaxis in a patient with osteoporosis
- Uncorrectable coagulopathy
- Myelopathy caused by retropulsion of bone or canal compromise
- Allergy to PMMA or opacification agent

Relative Contraindications
- Radicular pain
- VCF >70% height loss
- Severe spinal stenosis or asymptomatic retropulsion
- Tumor extension into canal or epidural space
- Lack of surgical backup

PMMA, polymethylmethacrylate; VCF, vertebral compression fracture.

Before the procedure, the patient should be taken off all anticoagulants, and the coagulation profile should be normal. The platelet count should be at least 50,000 per microliter at the time of the procedure, although no data exist to clearly define a "cut-off" platelet count. In the cancer population, we are asked, "How high do we want the number," and there have been cases reported of hemorrhage requiring open surgery. We have had patients with prolonged "oozing" after the procedure with marginal coagulation status. There may be instances when the risk-to-benefit ratio favors performing these procedures in patients with lower platelet counts. Active infection and sepsis are contraindications. We recommend waiting at least 2 weeks after treatment of an infection to minimize the risk of infection.

Informed consent should include lack of pain relief, osteomyelitis, fracture of the vertebra or pedicle, extravasation of cement into the spinal canal or neural foramen, paralysis or nerve root damage, and venous embolism. Rare but fatal anaphylaxis to PMMA has been reported in four cases. Also, the rare but potential need for open surgery should be discussed with the patient.

Vertebroplasty and kyphoplasty require the clinician to be trained in spinal anatomy, fluoroscopic imaging, and the use of these techniques to perform interventional procedures. The procedure should be performed in a sterile operating room suite that allows fluoroscopic imaging of the thoracolumbar spine. Biplanar or C-arm fluoroscopy of good quality is mandatory for maximal procedural safety. A radiolucent table is mandatory, as is appropriate padding for prone slightly flexed positioning. Other procedural materials needed include local anesthetic solution (the authors use a 50:50 mixture of 1% lidocaine with 0.25% bupivacaine), PMMA material, and barium or other radio-opacification material, although most cements now come opacified by the manufacturer. Eleven- or 13-gauge bone biopsy needles with connection tubing and cement injection syringes are needed. Numerous commercial "kits" are available.

General anesthesia or monitored anesthesia care (MAC) can be used. If MAC is used, the surgeon must use generous amounts of local anesthetic, especially injected onto the periosteum, where much nociception occurs. Some patients experience discomfort with advancement of the trocars across the posterior cortical margin with balloon inflation (in the case of kyphoplasty) and with PMMA injection. The anesthesiologist must be prepared to "deepen" the MAC during these phases of the procedure. Patient selection is important with consideration to the anesthesia choice. Very anxious or nervous patients may have a better experience with a general anesthetic. Careful consideration must be given to padding the pressure points of this fragile group of patients. After uni- or bipedicular VB access has been obtained, some clinicians proceed directly with injection of PMMA, but others prefer to do venography before cement injection. In theory, venography provides anatomical knowledge of large venous channels' proximity to the trocar. This information is used to more carefully inject the PMMA. For example, if a small amount of contrast injection reveals a direct spread into a venous channel, the operator may move the trocar before injection or carefully inject relatively solidified PMMA to embolize the large vein before injecting more PMMA into the VB. The literature reveals variable efficacy of the use of venography.[15,16] Most groups no longer use venography.

PMMA injection into the VB is undertaken after careful imaging confirming location of the trocar or trocars into the anteromedial portion of the VB. The PMMA should be opacified and beginning to harden to the consistency of toothpaste before injection. Injection can be done by small syringes filled with PMMA or one of several commercially available kits. The injection must be done

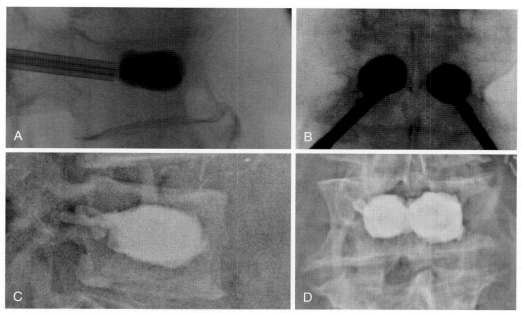

Fig. 19-1 Anteroposterior and later radiographs of correct balloon placement and of postkyphoplasty results. **A,** Lateral fluoroscopic view of inflated kyphon balloon tamps intraoperatively. **B,** Anterior-posterior fluoroscopic view of inflated kyphon balloon tamps intraoperatively. **C,** Post kyphoplasty lateral radiograph. **D,** Post kyphoplasty anterior-posterior radiograph.

under live lateral or biplanar fluoroscopic guidance. If PMMA begins to go into a blood vessel or toward the posterior cortical margin, it must be halted immediately. The authors halt cement injection when it spreads to the posterior third of the VB. To minimize PMMA leakage, several groups recommend the use of high-viscosity cement and relatively small volume injection (**Fig. 19-1**).[17-19]

Outcomes and Potential Complications

Both PK and PV have a very high acceptance and use rate. There is substantial improvement in pain and significant improvement in function after treatment by either of these techniques. Kyphoplasty improves height of the fractured vertebra and improves kyphosis by more than 50% if performed within 3 months from the onset of the fracture (onset of pain). There is some height improvement, although not as marked, along with significant clinical improvement, if the procedure is performed after 3 months.[20]

In multiple studies, PV has been shown to provide substantial pain relief or improved mobility in 75% to 92.4% of patients with osteoporotic VCFs and in 50% to 86% of patients with pathologic VCFs secondary to neoplasm.[1,8,13]

Two studies published in 2009 called the efficacy of PV into question. Although both were randomized controlled trials (RCTs), several problems exist within the methodology of each study. Kallmes et al[21] published the larger of the two studies, in which during a 4-year period, 131 patients with VCF from 11 centers were randomized to either PV or a "sham" procedure, which was a medial branch block. Pain scores decreased in both the control and PV groups with no statistically significant difference at 1 month (3.9 ± 2.9 for the PV group vs 4.6 ± 3.0 for the control group; $P = .19$). The authors did note a trend toward a statistically significant difference in clinically meaningful improvement in pain (64% in the PV group vs. 48% in the control group at 1 month; $P = .06$). Unfortunately, this study has several flaws. Crossover was significant, with 43% of the control group crossing over to PV but only 12% of the PV crossing over to the control procedure. Patients with

back pain and fractures up to 1 year old were included, but chronic back pains with an acute VCF were not specifically excluded. Also, the study had a small sample size, necessitating the liberalization of the inclusion criteria and later decreasing the target enrollment because of difficulty in patient recruitment.[21]

Another study published at the same time was performed by Buchbinder et al.[22] Seventy-eight patients were recruited over a 4-year period at five institutions and randomized to PV or medial branch block. Patients were not allowed to cross over if pain control was inadequate. The PV group had a decrease in pain from 7.4 ± 2.1 preoperatively to 2.6 ± 2.9 at 3 months, and the control group had a decrease from 7.1 ± 2.3 to 1.9 ± 3.3 over the same time period. In addition, no difference was found in disability or quality of life questionnaires between the two groups. The small sample size makes interpretation of the results somewhat difficult, as does the use of a medial branch block for the control group. In addition, the authors do note they also had difficulty recruiting for their study, and approximately 30% of eligible participants declined to participate.[22]

The superiority of one technique over the other remains controversial and is discussed in the following text. As experience grows with these techniques, various groups are pushing the envelope on indications for the procedure, with the possibility of seeing more complications in this patient group. There are some preliminary data and case series on efficacy in patients with radicular pain, traumatic burst fractures, severe VCF or vertebral plana, cervical spine pathology, and intraoperative PMMA augmentation of pedicle screw fixation spinal stabilization.[23-26] In our center, we have pushed "relative" contraindications in cancer patients without increased morbidity even in those with very advanced cancers.[27,28]

Adjacent-Level Fractures

A small increase in adjacent-level fractures was noticed with long-term follow-up. This phenomenon is similar with both PV and PK.[29] Subsequent VCFs may occur at adjacent or remote levels (compared with the treated "vertebroplastied" level). The reported rate of new fractures varies from 7% to 20% over a 1-year follow-up, with sooner refracture occurring at the adjacent levels.[30,31] This suggests a local unfavorable biomechanical situation in some patients who have adjacent-level fracturing and ongoing disease process (usually osteoporosis) in the nonadjacent fracture group. A large database of 106 patients who underwent 212 PV procedures was evaluated over a 3-year follow-up period by Kim et al.[32] They noted 72 new fractures over the 3-year follow-up (7.9%). The 1-year fracture-free rate was 93% by Kaplan-Meier analysis. The mean fracture-free interval was 32 months, with adjacent fractures being predicted by location in the thoracolumbar junction and greater height restoration. A more recent retrospective study by Tseng et al[31] reviewed 852 patients who underwent 1131 PV procedures and a minimum of a 2-year follow-up. Of these patients, 16.6% experienced new VCFs of which 62% were adjacent level fractures. The adjacent-level fractures occurred earlier than the nonadjacent-level fractures (71.9 ± 71.8 days vs. 286.8 ± 232.8 days).[31] There may be certain anatomical configurations in the fracture that predispose to adjacent-level fracture, such as intraosseous clefts.[33] In addition, whereas leakage of cement into the intravertebral disc and lower body mass index appear to predispose patients to adjacent-level fracture, nonadjacent-level fractures are associated with decreased segmental mobility.[34] Also, certain patient populations may be at higher risk for future fractures, including those with osteoporosis, previous vertebral fracture, and organ transplant recipients.[4,31,35] In all series examining this phenomenon, outcomes of pain relief after PV or PK for the adjacent-level fracture are excellent. It should be noted that up to 20% of patients with untreated VCF have a subsequent VCF within 1 year.[36]

Complications

Complications are rare but can be serious. The exact incidence is unknown. Most case series report asymptomatic PMMA extrusion rates of around 10% to 15%.[10,37] SIR divides complications for these techniques into two categories: minor and major. Minor complications are those considered to require no therapy and having no consequence, such as PMMA extrusion into the disc. Major complications are those requiring therapy, including an unplanned increase in the level of care needed or ongoing permanent sequelae (i.e., PMMA into the spinal canal with neurological deficit). SIR noted published complication rates for major complications to be less than 1%, except in those with neoplastic involvement of the vertebrae, in whom the reported level of major complications is less than 5%.[13]

PMMA can flow out of the VB posteriorly into the spinal canal or neural foramina or anteriorly into the paraspinous veins with systemic consequences. There are case reports of nerve root and spinal cord compression from extravertebral PMMA.[38,39] There have been several reports of minimally symptomatic pulmonary emboli, one case of cardiovascular collapse requiring pulmonary embolectomy, one lethal pulmonary embolus, and one case of paradoxical cerebral arterial PMMA emboli.[40-43] The literature suggests that there may be less PMMA leak with PK versus PV.[44]

Infectious complications, although rare, have been reported. There have been several reports of osteomyelitis requiring corpectomy.[45] Meticulous attention to sterile technique is warranted, including preoperative intravenous antibiotic administration. Most have abandoned the older technique of adding tobramycin powder to the PMMA because of uncertainty over both the efficacy and potential impact on the PMMA properties.

Complications have been reported with both procedures (vertebroplasty and kyphoplasty); a review of U.S. Food and Drug Administration safety data revealed 58 reported complications from 1999 through 2003 of approximately 200,000 procedures performed. These were approximately evenly divided among PV and PK, with more cases of pedicle fracture and spinal cord compression in PK than PV.[46] This voluntary reporting system is almost certainly flawed and most likely underreports the overall incidence of complications. As further studies are performed, a more complete risk-to-benefit ratio can be defined.

Vertebroplasty versus Kyphoplasty

Both PV and PK have been shown to be effective to reduce the pain associated with VCFs (**Box 19-2**). These procedures have low complication rates and tend to have islands of supporters (i.e., clinicians who always favor one over the other regardless of clinical circumstances). One study has been published in the past few years addressing PV versus PK. Liu et al[47] enrolled 100 patients with confirmed osteoporotic fractures at the thoracolumbar junction and randomized them to PV or PK. There was no difference in preoperative visual analog scale (VAS) pain score, VB height, or kyphotic wedge angle. Postoperative VAS pain scores (2.6 ± 0.6 for both PK and PV) were significantly different from preoperative pain scores (8.0 ± 0.8 for PK; 7.9 ± 0.7 for PV) but were not statistically different between PV and PK at any time in the postoperative period up to 6 months. Although no difference in pain relief was noted, there was a statistically significant increase in both VB height and reduction of the kyphotic wedge angle in the PK compared with PV. In PK, the VB height increased from 1.13 ± 0.22 cm to 2.04 ± 0.41 cm, and the kyphotic wedge angle decreased from 17.0 degrees ± 7.3 degrees to 9.0 degrees ± 5.7 degrees. This effect was less pronounced in PV, in which the VB height increased from 1.01 ± 0.22 cm to 1.32 ± 0.26 cm and the wedge angle decreased from 15.5 degrees ± 4.2 degrees to 12.2 degrees ± 3.6 degrees.[47] Currently, the authors favor the use of PK in circumstances in which the patient has a collapse of more than 20% of vertebral height and a fracture age of less than 3 months in hopes of restoring vertebral height and maintaining functional anatomy when possible. Deramond et al[48] have stated that PK may be preferable over PV in patients with severe or multiple wedge deformity that has developed in the past 3 weeks.

Advances in Technology

Coblation

Patients with spine tumors have an increased risk of perioperative complications, and in the setting of limited life expectancy, this can lead to an unacceptable quality of life.[49] Using less invasive techniques to treat VCF and other spinal lesions can potentially help

---

Box 19-2: Vertebroplasty versus Kyphoplasty

Vertebroplasty
- Less expensive
- Faster for the operator and patient
- Indicated to treat even older fractures

Kyphoplasty
- More anatomical correction of spinal deformity than vertebroplasty
- Greater height restoration in recent fractures (<3 months old)
- Indicated for patients with extensive kyphosis caused by multiple recent VCFs
- Less PMMA extravasation

PMMA, polymethylmethacrylate; VCF, vertebral compression fracture.

avoid this problem. As described in the introduction, many patients with spinal tumors have VCF. Although PV and PK are highly beneficial in this patient population, additional therapies have been developed that pain physicians can use for treatment of the tumor and to potentially improve the efficacy of PV or PK.

Plasma-mediated radiofrequency ablation (coblation) is currently used in procedures such as tonsillectomy, disc decompression, and tendon and cartilage debridement in which dissolution of the tissue is necessary. A plasma field is created by passing radiofrequency waves through a conducting medium such as saline, creating a precisely focused plasma field composed of ionized particles. This field, formed immediately adjacent to the tip of the device, causes dissolution of soft tissue at the relatively low temperatures of 40° to 70° C.[50] Coblation has the potential to increase safety and efficacy in a number of ways. Such a device allows for cavity creation in the VB with little mechanical disturbance of tissue outside of the plasma field. Minimizing disturbance of the rest of the VB could allow for vertebral augmentation in cases of retropulsion of tumor or cortical wall that would otherwise be a contraindication to PV or PK.[51] Dissolution of the surrounding soft tissue also allows for destruction of spinal primary or metastatic tumors and increases the efficacy of chemotherapy or radiation therapy by cytoreduction. This is accomplished by removing and replacing the coblation device at different positions of the clock, typically at the 12, 2, 4, 6, 8, and 10 o'clock positions, thus forming a void in the VB larger than the device itself (**Fig. 19-2**). In conventional PK for treatment of tumor-related VCF, the tumor is pressed against the healthy bone, forming a rim of tissue between the cement and bone. If the practitioner were to choose to perform PK in addition to coblation, removal of the tumor can allow for better interdigitation of the cement in the VB.[52] In addition, the relatively low temperatures of the plasma field causes less heat transfer to the VB and assists with hemostasis in the VB.[52]

Cortoss Cement

PMMA-based cements have a long history of safety and efficacy in the orthopedic community, and their use in PV was a natural extension of their use in arthroplasty. The usual PMMA formulations were modified to allow their use in PV, but doing so has introduced some problems. Because the cement must be injected through small-bore needles, the liquid monomer component was increased to decrease viscosity. Increasing the liquid monomer component has the unfortunate consequence of lowering the compressive strength of the cured polymer and increases the setting time of the polymer.[53,54] Additionally, PMMA cement is poorly radiopaque, so opacifiers such as barium sulphate, zirconium dioxide, or powdered tantalum are added to the cement mixture.[54] These materials do not undergo polymerization and can act as stress risers within the cured cement.[53] It should be noted, however, that current PMMA-based cements are highly effective despite these drawbacks.

Cortoss is a new cement based on bisphenol-a-glycidyl-dimethacrylate (bis-GMA) resin. Unlike PMMA, it does not require premixing and is supplied as a two-part paste that is mixed upon release from the delivery gun. This allows the filler to be dispensed as needed during the procedure. After it has been mixed, hardening occurs in 5 to 8 minutes and can support weight-bearing loads immediately after setting.[55] Cortoss has a higher compressive strength, bending modulus, and shear strength compared with PMMA[53] and does not appear to develop the interposed fibrous layer between the interface of the composite and extant bone.[56] Last, Cortoss is inherently radiopaque, so no additional opacifying agents are required.[55]

Despite these advantages, Cortoss has been shown to have comparable but not superior efficacy to typical PV PMMA cements. In a study by Middleton et al,[54] 34 patients underwent PV at a total of 42 levels. Cortoss was injected using a unipedicular approach with a mean injectate volume of 2.2 mL. Approximately 82% of patients reported improvement in symptoms after PV, and 79% required less analgesia. There was one incident each of pulmonary embolism (PE), generalized rash, transient radicular leg pain, and retropulsion of cement 1 year later secondary to progression of metastatic disease, with each incident representing 2.9% of the study population; however, 88% of patients had no complications.[54] Previously reported rates of complication of PE are anywhere from 0% to 7% of PMMA vertebroplasties, and for transient radicular pain, there is a reported range of 1% to 8%.[54]

Conclusion

PV and PK are minimally invasive techniques used to treat painful VCFs. There is a growing body of evidence, albeit of limited quality

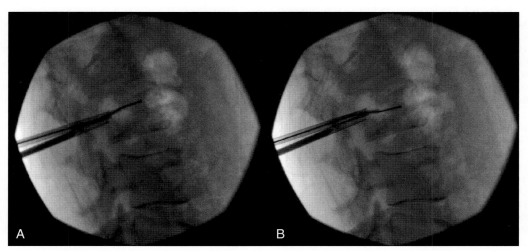

Fig. 19-2 Lateral fluoroscopic images showing creation of void in the vertebral body with a coblation device. **A,** Lateral intraoperative fluoroscopic image of tumor coblation. **B,** Lateral intraoperative fluoroscopic image of tumor coblation in same case showing intra-vertebral body sweeping motion to ablate tumor.

(predominately open case series), indicating that these procedures are efficacious in alleviating the pain associated with VCF. The results of the procedures in these reports are uniformly good. However, there are a growing number of case reports of serious complications.

Recent reviews and editorials have called for a more critical evaluation of these procedures. Watts et al[57] reviewed the literature and concluded that controlled multicenter trials are needed to determine the short- and long-term safety. Garfin et al[20] concluded that there is a 95% improvement in pain and significant improvement in function after these procedures. They emphasized that the procedure is technically demanding with the potential for significant complications. They recommended further efficacy and safety studies. Jarvik and Deyo[58] called for RCTs or some type of control cohort to compare long-term outcomes carefully. Einhorn[59] calls for careful monitoring of outcomes and minimal training standards. Birkmeyer[60] calls for randomized clinical trials, citing insufficient evidence from case series to prove safety, efficacy, and cost-effectiveness. The prospective RCTs described above seem to confuse rather than clarify our understanding of the efficacy of PV. Ideally, a prospective RCT with a larger sample size and appropriate control group can be performed in the future.

It will be difficult to conduct the RCTs needed to compare short- and long-term outcomes of PV or PK versus more conservative therapies. These procedures have gained such widespread popularity that patients would undoubtedly resist being randomized to the conservative treatment group; recent attempts at RCTs for PV have been plagued by low enrollment. Other studies need to be done to compare PV and PK in various disease states in a randomized fashion. Early studies are underway to evaluate biologic materials for spinal injection rather than acrylic (PMMA). Despite the need for more research, PV and PK have shown great promise in the treatment of painful VCFs caused by a variety of different pathologic states. With careful patient selection, adequate training, and attention to details during the procedure, serious complications are rare.

References

1. Stallmeyer MJB, Zoarski G: Patient evaluation and selection. In Mathis JM, Deramond H, Belkoff SM, editors: *Percutaneous vertebroplasty and kyphoplasty*, ed 2, New York, 2006, Springer, pp 60-61.
2. Huang C, Ross PD, Wasnich RD: Vertebral fracture and other predictors of physical impairment and health care utilization. *Arch Intern Med* 156:2469-2475, 1996.
3. Tosteson AN, Hammond CS: Quality-of-life assessment in osteoporosis: health-status and preference-based measures. *Pharmacoeconomics* 20:289-303, 2002.
4. Lindsay R, Silverman SL, Cooper C, et al: Risk of new vertebral fracture in the year following a fracture. *JAMA* 285:320-323, 2001.
5. Charnley J: The reaction of bone to self-curing acrylic cement. A long-term histological study in man. *J Bone Joint Surg Br* 52:340-353, 1970.
6. Galibert P, Deramond H: Percutaneous acrylic vertebroplasty as a treatment of vertebral angioma as well as painful and debilitating diseases. *Chirurgie* 116:326-334; discussion 335, 1990.
7. Galibert P, Deramond H, Rosat P, et al: Preliminary note on the treatment of vertebral angioma by percutaneous acrylic vertebroplasty. *Neurochirurgie* 33:166-168, 1987.
8. Jensen ME, Evans AJ, Mathis JM, et al: Percutaneous polymethylmethacrylate vertebroplasty in the treatment of osteoporotic vertebral body compression fractures: technical aspects. *AJNR Am J Neuroradiol* 18:1897-1904, 1997.
9. Kaemmerlen P, Thiesse P, Jonas P, et al: Percutaneous injection of orthopedic cement in metastatic vertebral lesions. *N Engl J Med* 321:121, 1989.
10. Lieberman IH, Dudeney S, Reinhardt MK, et al: Initial outcome and efficacy of "kyphoplasty" in the treatment of painful osteoporotic vertebral compression fractures. *Spine* 26:1631-1638, 2001.
11. Maynard AS, Jensen ME, Schweickert PA, et al: Value of bone scan imaging in predicting pain relief from percutaneous vertebroplasty in osteoporotic vertebral fractures. *AJNR Am J Neuroradiol* 21:1807-1812, 2000.
12. Karam M, Lavelle WF, Cheney R: The role of bone scintigraphy in treatment planning, and predicting pain relief after kyphoplasty. *Nucl Med Comm* 29:247-253, 2008.
13. McGraw JK, Cardella J, Barr JD, et al: Society of Interventional Radiology quality improvement guidelines for percutaneous vertebroplasty. *J Vasc Interv Radiol* 14:827-831, 2003.
14. Gangi A, Sabharwal T, Irani FG, et al: Quality assurance guidelines for percutaneous vertebroplasty. *Cardiovasc Intervent Radiol* 29:173-178, 2006.
15. Gaughen JR, Jr, Jensen ME, Schweickert PA, et al: Relevance of antecedent venography in percutaneous vertebroplasty for the treatment of osteoporotic compression fractures. *AJNR Am J Neuroradiol* 23:594-600, 2002.
16. Vasconcelos C, Gailloud P, Beauchamp NJ, et al: Is percutaneous vertebroplasty without pretreatment venography safe? Evaluation of 205 consecutives procedures. *AJNR Am J Neuroradiol* 23:913-917, 2002.
17. Fourney DR, Schomer DF, Nader R, et al: Percutaneous vertebroplasty and kyphoplasty for painful vertebral body fractures in cancer patients. *J Neurosurg* 98(suppl 1):21-30, 2003.
18. Laredo JD, Hamze B: Complications of percutaneous vertebroplasty and their prevention. *Semin Ultrasound CT MR* 26:65-80, 2005.
19. Burton AW, Rhines LD, Mendel E: Vertebroplasty and kyphoplasty: a comprehensive review. *Neurosurg Focus* 18:e1, 2005.
20. Garfin SR, Yuan HA, Reiley MA: New technologies in spine: kyphoplasty and vertebroplasty for the treatment of painful osteoporotic compression fractures. *Spine* 26:1511-1515, 2001.
21. Kallmes DF, Comstock BA, Heagerty PJ, et al: A randomized trial of vertebroplasty for osteoporotic spinal fractures. *N Eng J Med* 2009, 361:6.
22. Buchbinder R, Osborne RH, Ebeling PR, et al: A randomized trial of vertebroplasty for painful osteoporotic vertebral fractures. *N Eng J Med* 361:6, 2009.
23. Chung SK, Lee SH, Kim DY, et al: Treatment of lower lumbar radiculopathy caused by osteoporotic compression fracture: the role of vertebroplasty. *J Spinal Disord Tech* 15:461-468, 2002.
24. Nakano M, Hirano N, Matsuura K, et al: Percutaneous transpedicular vertebroplasty with calcium phosphate cement in the treatment of osteoporotic vertebral compression and burst fractures. *J Neurosurg* 97(suppl 3):287-293, 2002.
25. Peh WC, Gilula LA, Peck DD: Percutaneous vertebroplasty for severe osteoporotic vertebral body compression fractures. *Radiology* 223:121-126, 2002.
26. Wetzel SG, Martin JB, Radu EW, et al: Percutaneous vertebroplasty: a minimal-invasive procedure for pain treatment. *Schweiz Rundsch Med Prax* 94:595-598, 2005.
27. Hentschel SJ, Burton AW, Fourney DR, et al: Percutaneous vertebroplasty and kyphoplasty performed at a cancer center: refuting proposed contraindications. *J Neurosurg Spine* 2:436-440, 2005.
28. Burton AW, Reddy SK, Shah HN, et al: Percutaneous vertebroplasty—a technique to treat refractory spinal pain in the setting of advanced metastatic cancer: a case series. *J Pain Symptom Manage* 30:87-95, 2005.
29. Fribourg D, Tang C, Sra P, et al: Incidence of subsequent vertebral fracture after kyphoplasty. *Spine* 29:2270-2276; discussion 2277, 2004.
30. Trout AT, Kallmes DF, Kaufmann TJ: New fractures after vertebroplasty: adjacent fractures occur significantly sooner. *AJNR Am J Neuroradiol* 27:217-223, 2006.

31. Tseng Y, Yang T, Tu, P, et al: Repeated and multiple new vertebral compression fractures after percutaneous transpedicular vertebroplasty. *Spine* 34(18):1917-1922, 2009.

32. Kim SH, Kang HS, Choi JA, et al: Risk factors of new compression fractures in adjacent vertebrae after percutaneous vertebroplasty. *Acta Radiol* 45:440-445, 2004.

33. Trout AT, Kallmes DF, Lane JI, et al: Subsequent vertebral fractures after vertebroplasty: association with intraosseous clefts. *AJNR Am J Neuroradiol* 27:1586-1591, 2006.

34. Ahn Y, Lee J, Le H, et al: Predictive factors for subsequent vertebral fracture after percutaneous vertebroplasty. *J Neurosurg Spine* 9:129-136, 2008.

35. Deen HG, Aranda-Michel J, Reimer R, et al: Balloon kyphoplasty for vertebral compression fractures in solid organ transplant recipients: results of treatment and comparison with primary osteoporotic vertebral compression fractures. *Spine J* 6:494-499, 2006.

36. Silverman SL: The clinical consequences of vertebral compression fracture. *Bone* 13(suppl 2):S27-S31, 1992.

37. McKiernan F, Faciszewski T, Jensen R: Quality of life following vertebroplasty. *J Bone Joint Surg Am* 86-A:2600-2606, 2004.

38. Lee BJ, Lee SR, Yoo TY: Paraplegia as a complication of percutaneous vertebroplasty with polymethylmethacrylate: a case report. *Spine* 27:E419-E422, 2002.

39. Ratliff J, Nguyen T, Heiss J: Root and spinal cord compression from methylmethacrylate vertebroplasty. *Spine* 26:E300-E302, 2001.

40. Jang JS, Lee SH, Jung SK: Pulmonary embolism of polymethylmethacrylate after percutaneous vertebroplasty: a report of three cases. *Spine* 27:E416-E418, 2002.

41. Tozzi P, Abdelmoumene Y, Corno AF, et al: Management of pulmonary embolism during acrylic vertebroplasty. *Ann Thorac Surg* 74:1706-1708, 2002.

42. Chen HL, Wong CS, Ho ST, et al: A lethal pulmonary embolism during percutaneous vertebroplasty. *Anesth Analg* 95:1060-1062, table of contents, 2002.

43. Scroop R, Eskridge J, Britz GW: Paradoxical cerebral arterial embolization of cement during intraoperative vertebroplasty: case report. *AJNR Am J Neuroradiol* 23:868-870, 2002.

44. Phillips FM, Todd Wetzel F, Lieberman I, et al: An in vivo comparison of the potential for extravertebral cement leak after vertebroplasty and kyphoplasty. *Spine* 27:2173-2178; discussion 2178-2179, 2002.

45. Walker DH, Mummaneni P, Rodts GE, Jr: Infected vertebroplasty. Report of two cases and review of the literature. *Neurosurg Focus* 17:E6, 2004.

46. Nussbaum DA, Gailloud P, Murphy K: A review of complications associated with vertebroplasty and kyphoplasty as reported to the Food and Drug Administration medical device related web site. *J Vasc Interv Radiol* 15:1185-1192, 2004.

47. Liu JT, Liao WJ, Tan WC, et al: Balloon kyphoplasty versus vertebroplasty for treatment of osteoporotic vertebral compression fracture: a prospective, comparative, and randomized clinical study. *Osteoporos Int* 21:359-364, 2010.

48. Deramond H, Saliou G, Aveillan M, et al: Respective contributions of vertebroplasty and kyphoplasty to the management of osteoporotic vertebral fractures. *Joint Bone Spine* 73:610-613, 2006.

49. Gerszten PC, Monaco EA, 3rd: Complete percutaneous treatment of vertebral body tumors causing spinal canal compromise using a transpedicular cavitation. *Neurosurg Focus* 27(6):E9, 2009.

50. Woloszko J, Stalder KR, Brown IG: Plasma characteristics of repetitively-pulsed electrical discharges in saline solutions used for surgical procedures. *IEEE Trans Plasma Science* 30:1376-1383, 2002.

51. Shimony JS, Gilula LA, Zeller AJ, et al: Percutaneous vertebroplasty for malignant compression fractures with epidural involvement. *Radiology* 232:846-853, 2004.

52. Georgy BA, Wong W: Plasma-mediated radiofrequency ablation assisted percutaneous cement injection for treating advanced malignant vertebral compression fractures. *AJNR Am J Neuroradiol* 28:700-705, 2007.

53. Gheduzzi S, Webb JJ, Miles AW: Mechanical characteristics of three percutaneous vertebroplasty biomaterials. *J Mater Sci Mater Med* 17:421-426, 2006.

54. Middleton ET, Rajaraman CJ, O'Brien DP, et al: The safety and efficacy of vertebroplasty using Cortoss cement in a newly established vertebroplasty service. *Br J Neurosurg* 22(2): 252-256, 2008.

55. Palussière J, Berge J, Gangi A, et al: Clinical results of an open prospective study of a bis-GMA composite in percutaneous vertebral augmentation. *Eur Spine J* 14(10):982-991, 2005.

56. Erbe EM, Clineff TD, Gualtieri G: Comparison of a new bisphenol-a-glycidal dimethacrylate-based cortical bone void filler with polymethyl methacrylate. *Eur Spine J* 10(suppl 2):S147-S152, 2001.

57. Watts NB, Harris ST, Genant HK: Treatment of painful osteoporotic vertebral fractures with percutaneous vertebroplasty or kyphoplasty. *Osteoporos Int* 12:429-437, 2001.

58. Jarvik JG, Deyo RA: Cementing the evidence: time for a randomized trial of vertebroplasty. *AJNR Am J Neuroradiol* 21:1373-1374, 2000.

59. Einhorn TA: Vertebroplasty: an opportunity to do something really good for patients. *Spine* 25:1051-1052, 2000.

60. Birkmeyer N: Point of view. *Spine* 26:1637-1638, 2001.

20 Ultrasound-Guided Lumbar Spine Injections

Manfred Greher

CHAPTER OVERVIEW

Chapter Synopsis: This chapter focuses on the use of ultrasound imaging for guidance during many different types of injection procedures for back pain. The benefits of using ultrasonography include its economy, portability, and safety. Any spinal injection procedure requires an intimate knowledge of the underlying anatomy, and use of ultrasound guidance requires a similar familiarity with the intricacies of sonographic data. Ultrasound needle guidance has recently supplanted some more traditionally used imaging techniques, including computed tomography and fluoroscopy. Future development of the technique may include the use of three-dimensional sonographic imaging. The techniques guided by ultrasonography described in the chapter include injections for lumbar medial branch or facet nerve block, facet joint injections, lumbar periradicular injections, and intramuscular trigger point injections. Practitioners should take advantage of hands-on learning opportunities, and novices should focus on intramuscular injections to develop expertise in ultrasound-guided injection techniques.

Important Points:
- Ultrasonography is an emerging technique to guide lumbar spine injections.
- Basic sonoanatomic knowledge and needle guidance skills are necessary for good-quality blocks with exact target control.
- Textbooks, Internet resources, cadaver courses, workshops, and hands-on teaching are excellent ways to increase the individual training level.
- For novices, it is best to start with easy blocks such as intramuscular or trigger point injections.
- Whenever vascular uptake could be devastating and cannot be ruled out reliably with ultrasonography, ultrasound-guided techniques should not be performed alone (i.e., selective lumbar nerve root injections).

Clinical Pearls:
- For a medial branch block, reaching the cranial part of the transverse process with the needle tip immediately at the first puncture attempt can be accomplished as follows: With a paramedian short-axis view between two transverse processes and a transducer movement from cranial to caudal, the first bony line encountered is the cranial edge of the transverse process.
- In difficult cases, the practitioner may choose to perform the puncture in a paramedian long-axis view above the transverse processes with an out-of-plane technique and verify the position in the short-axis view afterward.

Clinical Pitfalls:
- The L5 dorsal ramus block has not been described and validated methodologically so far.
- Sacralization or lumbarization can lead to wrong assignment of the segments; the practitioner should always check the radiographs before, if they are available.

Introduction

This chapter summarizes today's knowledge and evidence about ultrasound-guided lumbar spinal injections with a focus on sono-anatomy and clinical practice.

Today low back pain is a big medical and economical challenge not only for the physician and the individual patient but also for the community. Although nonspecific low back pain, in which invasive interventions should be reduced to a minimum if not avoided at all, seems to be the predominant entity, in many cases, specific causes and confined anatomical sources are the reason for pain or have to be ruled out. Traditionally, fluoroscopy or even computed tomography (CT) has been used in these cases as guidance devices, first to increase specificity and second to avoid complications arising from improper needle placement. In the past years, ultrasonography moved into the focus of interest not only in regional anesthesia but also for interventions in

pain medicine. Ultrasound-guided injection techniques are interesting alternatives to fluoroscopy- and CT-guided methods. Today, portable ultrasound machines offer high quality together with a relatively moderate price. Advantages include no exposure to ionizing radiation for both the patient and the physician, availability as a bedside method, and use in remote locations such as developing countries because there is no restriction to specially equipped radiological facilities. As opposed to radiography, there is no contraindication for ultrasonography during pregnancy, which is another great advantage, when treatment of severe low back pain is especially challenging and injections are unavoidable.

Lumbar medial branch or facet nerve blocks, facet joint injections, intramuscular trigger point injections, and lumbar periradicular injections have become technically possible with ultrasound guidance or assistance. A concise presentation and validation of the methods follows.

Basic Principles of Ultrasound-Guided Injections

Ultrasound Machines, Transducers, and Knobology

Today a huge variety of ultrasound machines in different sizes from different companies is available. Portable machines have reached quality levels comparable to larger scale gear. For applications in regional anesthesia and pain therapy, high-resolution technology combined with excellent musculoskeletal imaging properties is of great help to the practitioner. Linear broadband transducers with high frequencies up to 15 MHz are preferred when small structures close to the surface have to be targeted. Curved-array broadband probes with lower frequencies around 5 MHz are used for deeper targets. At least one of each of these two basic types of transducers should be available to physicians routinely performing ultrasound-guided interventions in pain management. **Fig. 20-1** shows a typical linear probe on the left side of the image and a curved-array probe on the right with a schematic shape of the resulting sonographic images. Please note that the side of the mark on the transducer (*arrow*) is corresponding to the mark on the image (*star*). This is important for correct image orientation. Color-flow Doppler ultrasonography helps to identify vessels and is part of the basic machine equipment today. Finally, the operator has to be familiar with basic machine settings such as depth, gain, and focus.

Needles, Techniques, and Sterility

Needle choice depends on both target depth and operator preference. Better visualization is possible with larger diameter needles and shallow insertion angles; however, patient comfort is often associated with the contrary. Good choices are needles with facet tips and diameters between 20 and 25 gauges. Recently, higher reflective ultrasound needles have been developed and are the subject of evaluation at the moment. Image orientation can be short or cross axis (SAX; i.e., transverse plane) or long axis (LAX; i.e., longitudinal plane relative to the target nerve or the spinal column). Needle insertion can be out of plane or in plane relative to the LAX of the transducer's footprint. Whereas out-of-plane techniques offer shorter access but only visualization of the needle tip, in-plane techniques are associated with a longer path to the target but visualization of the entire needle (**Fig. 20-2**). The needle insertion point for the out-of-plane technique is close to the longer side; for the in-plane technique, it is close to the shorter side of the transducer's footprint (**Fig. 20-3**). Sometimes the transducer has to be turned 90 degrees after needle insertion to ensure proper positioning in a second plane. Sterile working conditions are mandatory for invasive procedures, including covering of the probe and use of sterile ultrasound gel. Special covers designed for this purpose are available today; the image shows how to cover a probe with such a shield (**Fig. 20-4**).

Knowledge of Sonoanatomy, Artifacts, and Training

Knowledge of the relevant paravertebral sonoanatomy, including landmark structures, and a basic idea of possible variability is

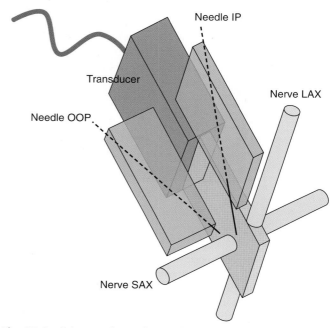

Fig. 20-2 Scheme of transducer relative to the needle and the nerve. IP, in plane; LAX, long-axis view; OOP, out of plane; SAX, short-axis view.

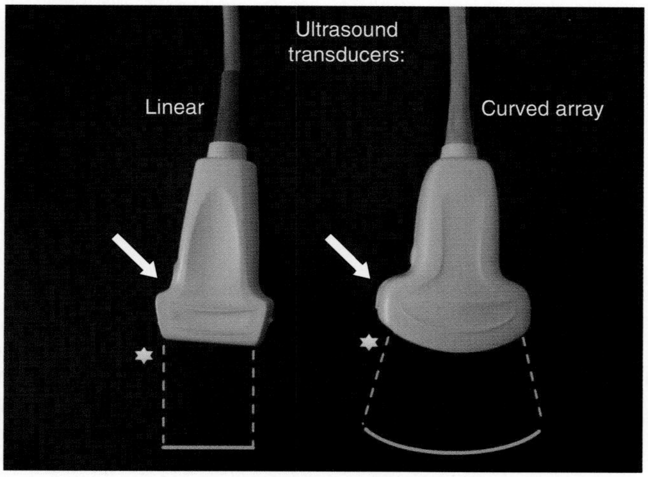

Fig. 20-1 Linear transducer (*left*) and curved array transducer (*right*). The side of the mark on the transducer (*arrow*) is corresponding to the mark on the image (*star*).

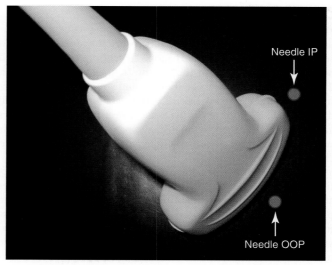

Fig. 20-3 Needle insertion points for out-of-plane (OOP) and in-plane (IP) injections.

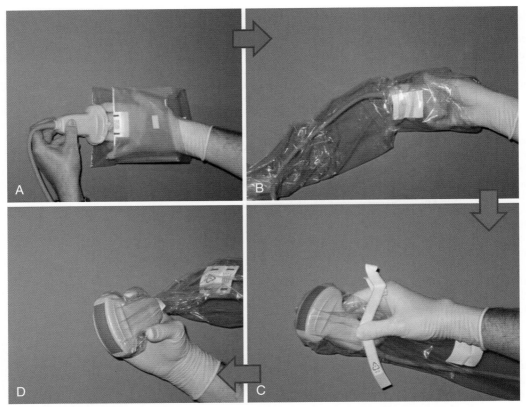

Fig. 20-4 Sterile covering of a probe: **A**, start; **B**, covering; **C**, securing; **D**, ready to use.

paramount for excellent performance. Moreover, the operator has to be familiar with ultrasound artifacts such as shadowing, reverberations, and mirror imaging to not misinterpret examinations. Continuous training in scanning and needle guidance is necessary to maintain high quality. For the beginner, ultrasound phantoms can be helpful. Workshops and hands-on training are most valuable to accelerate the learning process.

Sonography of the Lumbar Spine—Basic Scanning Sequence

With a curved array probe, first a basic scanning sequence of standard planes should be performed to ensure total anatomical and segmental orientation of the region. Depending on the age and body mass index (BMI) of the patient, frequency ranges between 2 and 7 MHz are applied. For slimmer and younger people, higher frequencies are useful because of better detail resolution in small distances. On the contrary, if the target is deeper, lower frequencies are necessary to provide enough tissue penetration, although this means worse image resolution. Normally, 3 to 5 MHz is a good choice.

The basic scanning sequence can be done before skin disinfection and sterile draping with nonsterile gel and no probe cover or after the preparation but then necessarily with sterile gel and a probe cover on. The patient is in prone position with a pillow under the stomach to compensate for lumbar lordosis. The sonographer sits on the patient's left side facing the ultrasound machine next to the head of the patient. The basic scanning sequence consists of five standard planes and starts in the midline above the spinous processes of the lower lumbar spine (**Fig. 20-5**).

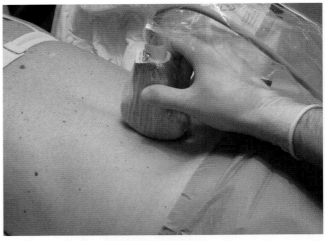

Fig. 20-5 Medial longitudinal scan.

Standard Lumbar Paravertebral Planes and Relevant Sonoanatomy

- **Median LAX (longitudinal view) above the spinous processes** (**Fig. 20-6**): The cranial side is always left on the longitudinal views (note the corresponding marks or stars on the transducer and the image); the spinous processes regularly are lined up very close to the surface with dorsal bony shadowing below and can be counted upwards starting from the continuous bony line on the right side of the image, which is the sacrum.

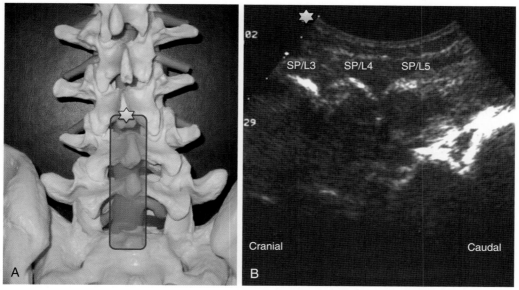

Fig. 20-6 Median long-axis view (longitudinal view) above the spinous processes (SPs). **A,** Spine phantom with, transducer's footprint (*blue area*); **B,** Sonogram. *Star,* cranial.

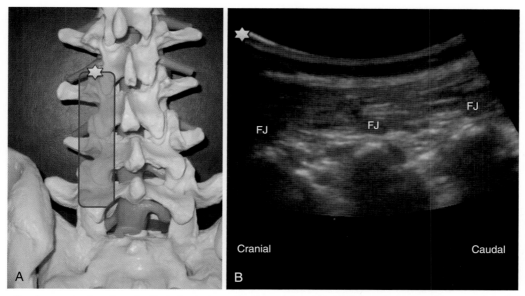

Fig. 20-7 Paramedian long-axis view (longitudinal view) above the facet joints (FJ). **A,** Spine phantom with, transducer's footprint (*blue area*); **B,** Sonogram. *Star,* cranial.

- **Paramedian LAX (longitudinal view) above the facet joints** (Fig. 20-7): Parallel shifting of the transducer to the lateral side without tilting produces an image of the facet joints or superior articular processes with dorsal shadowing; a typical wave line shaped figure can be recognized.
- **Paramedian LAX (longitudinal view) above the transverse processes** (Fig. 20-8): Shifting further lateral results in an image of the transverse processes (TP) alone without other bony landmarks. The scanning plane is longitudinal to the spine and thus the transverse processes are cut in a transverse way. Due to the convention of image orientation, the left part of each transverse process is the cranial end and the right part the caudal end. The transverse processes can be counted upwards from right to left starting from the continuous line of the sacrum like described above. Behind two transverse processes,

the psoas muscle appears, where it is not covered by the shadows of the bone.
- **Paramedian SAX (transverse view) above the transverse processes** (Fig. 20-9): A 90-degree counterclockwise rotation of the transducer above the respective transverse process displays a transverse view with the spinous process, the superior articular process and the transverse process, the erector spinae muscle and the quadratus lumborum muscle. Ventrolateral to the quadratus lumborum, the kidney can be visible in the image.
- **Paramedian SAX (transverse view) between two transverse processes** (Fig. 20-10): Parallel shifting of the transducer to the cranial side displays a transverse view between two transverse processes with the erector spinae muscle most superficial, the facet joint medial, the lateral border of the vertebral body more

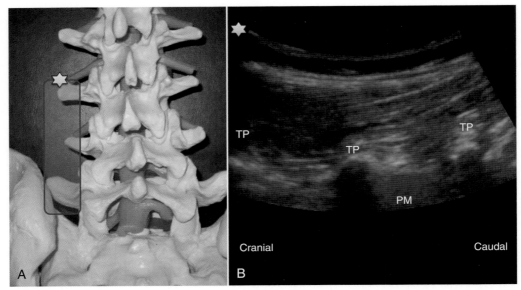

Fig. 20-8 Paramedian long-axis view (longitudinal view) above the transverse processes (TP). PM, psoas muscle. **A,** Spine phantom with transducer's footprint (*blue area*); **B,** Sonogram. *Star,* cranial.

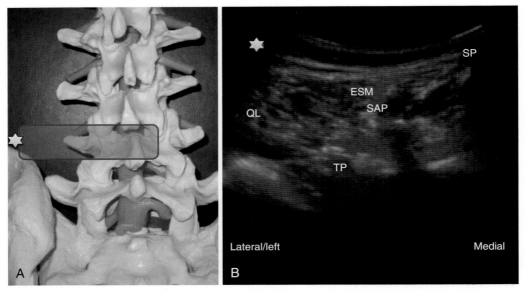

Fig. 20-9 Paramedian short-axis view (transverse view) above the transverse processes (TPs). ESM, erector spinae muscle; SAP, superior articular process; SP, spinous process; TP, transverse process; QL, quadratus lumborum muscle. **A,** Spine phantom with transducer's footprint (*blue area*); **B,** Sonogram. *Star,* lateral.

lateral and deeper, the psoas muscle, and the entry to the neuroforamen (F).

Lumbar Facet Nerve or Medial Branch Block

History and Literature
Lumbar medial branch block (i.e., facet nerve block) with ultrasound guidance instead of fluoroscopy was first described by the author's group in 2004.[1] The new methodology was developed in a model, and the paravertebral SAX and LAX views necessary for proper needle guidance were demonstrated. Lumbar regions of 20 volunteers were scanned to assess the visibility of the sonoanatomical landmarks and to derive estimates of typical distances in a total of 240 views. Finally, the practicability of the new method was

tested in a case series of 28 blocks in clinical patients with suspected facet joint–derived pain. A second study[2] confirmed the accuracy of ultrasound-guided lumbar medial branch blocks in a cadaveric model by means of CT. The target point was defined as the groove at the cephalad margin of the transverse (or costal) process L1-L5 (medial branch T12-L4) adjacent to the superior articular process. Axial transverse CT scans, with and without 1 mL of contrast dye, followed to evaluate needle positions and spread of contrast medium. Forty-five of 50 needle tips were located at the exact target point. The remaining five were within 5 mm of the target. In 47 of 50 cases, the applied contrast dye reached the groove where the nerve is located, corresponding to an overall simulated block success rate of 94% (95% confidence interval, 84% to 98%). Shim and co-workers[3] performed 101 ultrasound-guided lumbar medial

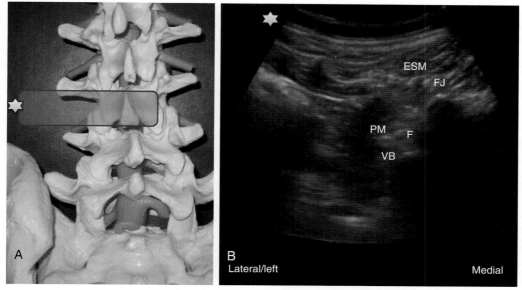

Fig. 20-10   Paramedian short-axis view (transverse view) between two transverse processes. ESM, erector spinae muscle; F, neuroforamen; FJ, facet joint; PM, psoas muscle; VB, vertebral body. **A,** Spine phantom with transducer's footprint (*blue area*); **B,** Sonogram. *Star*, lateral.

branch blocks according to our published technique in 20 patients. Needle position was confirmed with C-arm fluoroscopy. They reported a high success rate of 95% but also two needle positions associated with intravascular spread of contrast dye. A certain limitation of the technique is obesity, as was shown in a recent study by Rauch et al.[4] In 20 patients with BMIs above 30, a success rate of only 62% could be achieved under ultrasound guidance alone.

Facet Joint–Mediated Pain

Facet joint–mediated pain has been identified as a cause of low back pain since 1933. The facet or zygapophyseal joints are often affected by mechanical derangements or degenerative alterations (**Fig. 20-11**). As a consequence, reflex muscular spasm or referred pain can arise. Facet joint–mediated pain commonly appears as lumbosacral pain with or without sciatic pain predominantly proximal to the knee, particularly associated with a twisting or rotary strain of the lumbosacral region. The pain can be uni- or bilateral and is typically enhanced by hyperextension of the spine or locally applied pressure on the facet joints. However, clinical examinations and radiographic imaging as well as scoring systems lack the necessary positive and negative predictive value to diagnose facet joint–mediated pain. A test series of at least two positive highly selective low-volume nerve blocks or intraarticular injections is mandatory to confirm the diagnosis because the false-positive rate of a single successful block is 38%. With a correct diagnosis, radiofrequency treatment can significantly improve patients' symptoms for a long time.

Innervation of the Facet Joint and Target Point for the Block

Each lumbar facet joint is innervated by the two medial branches from the segments above and below. The facet nerve is the medial branch of the dorsal ramus of the spinal nerve. To anesthetize the L3-L4 joint for example, blocks of the L2 and L3 medial branch at the transverse processes of the L3 and the L4 vertebrae are needed. At L5, the entire dorsal ramus instead of a medial branch is present. Each medial branch runs over the junction of the cranial edge of

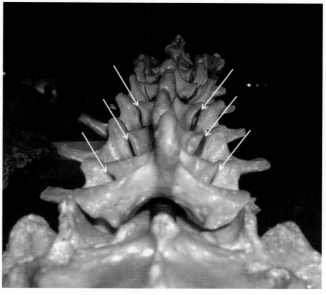

Fig. 20-11   Facet joint (*arrows*).

the transverse and superior articular processes (**Fig. 20-12**). This is the target point for an ultrasound-guided medial branch block (**Figs. 20-13** to **20-16**). It is approached with the transducer in a paramedian SAX and an in-plane needle direction from lateral to medial (**Fig. 20-17**). After bony contact, the transducer has to be rotated 90 degrees clockwise in a paramedian LAX to ensure the tip of the needle on the cranial end of the transverse process in a second plane (**Fig. 20-18**).

Technique

The patient is placed prone with a pillow under the stomach to compensate for lumbar lordosis. The physician sits on the left side of the patient facing the ultrasound machine close to the head of the patient. Disinfection and sterile draping are applied. The transducer is covered, and sterile gel is used. First, a complete basic scanning sequence of the lumbar region as described above is performed to ensure correct localization. If preferred, skin markers can be used. A paramedian SAX plane above the target transverse process is set (**Fig. 20-9**). After performing a skin wheal, the immobile needle with a syringe attached is inserted in plane approximately 45 degrees from lateral to medial (**Figs. 20-14** and **20-17**)

and advanced until bony contact is accomplished. Then the transducer is rotated 90 degrees clockwise into a paramedian LAX (**Fig. 20-18**). Under tiny movements of the needle (to and fro), this second plane is necessary to visualize and verify the position of the needle tip on the cranial end of the transverse process (**Fig. 20-8**). If the tip of the needle is too caudal, it has to be replaced accordingly. Finally, the transducer is rotated back 90 degrees counterclockwise into SAX and the local anesthetic is injected (0.5 to 1 mL) under direct vision. A certain volume spread should be visible at the tip of the needle. Then the procedure is repeated for the next relevant segment.

Facet Joint Injection

History and Literature

A technique for ultrasound-guided periarticular lumbar facet joint injections was published in a German orthopedic journal in 1997 for the first time.[5] Galiano et al[6] showed that intraarticular facet joint injections are feasible under ultrasound guidance alone. In their prospective randomized clinical trial,[7] an ultrasound group was compared with a CT group. In 16 of the 18 patients in the ultrasound group, in which the target was clearly visible, needle placement was successful and comparable to CT-guided interventions. Procedure time was 14.3 minutes in the ultrasound versus 22.3 minutes in the CT group. The aim of another study[8] of this group was to provide a teaching tool to facilitate the acquirement of periradicular and facet joint infiltration techniques in the cervical and lumbar spine. By use of a dedicated image navigation and reconstruction system, sonographic images were generated and fused with the collected CT data set. This allowed instant comparison of both imaging techniques. O'Neill et al[9] used ultrasound-guided stimulating needles for an experimental pain model in volunteers. Two electrode needles were placed on either side of a lumbar facet joint to induce experimental low back pain for 10 minutes with continuous stimulation.

Technique

The target point for an intraarticular facet joint injection is displayed in the corresponding images (**Figs. 20-19** and **20-20**). The

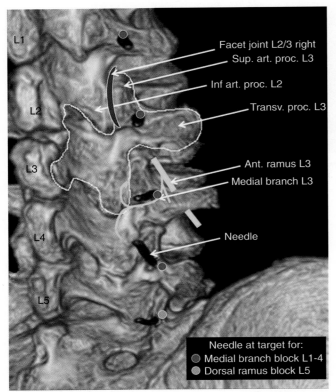

Fig. 20-12 Medial branch anatomy: three-dimensional rendered computed tomography scheme.

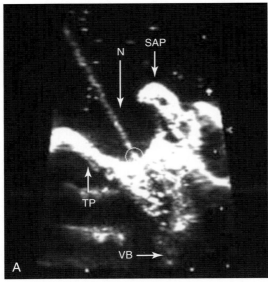

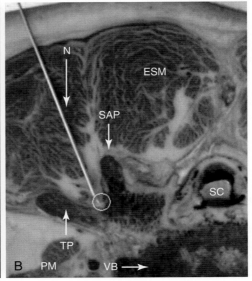

Fig. 20-13 Medial branch block: spine phantom immersed in water (**A**), anatomic slice (**B**). ESM, erector spinae muscle; N, needle; SAP, superior articular process; SC, spinal cord; TP, transverse process; PM, psoas muscle; VB, vertebral body. From Greher M, Scharbert G, Kamolz LP, et al: Ultrasound-guided lumbar facet nerve block: a sonoanatomic study of a new methodologic approach, Anesthesiology 100(5):1242-1248, 2004.

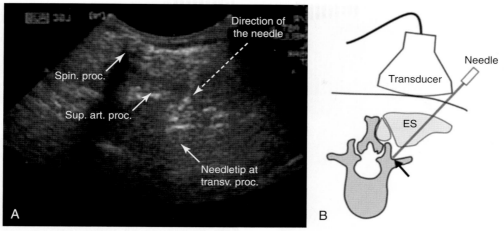

Fig. 20-14 Medial branch block: sonogram in transverse view with needle at target point (**A**), scheme (**B**). ES, erector spinae muscle; Spin. proc., spinous process; Sup. art. proc., superior articular process; transv. proc., transverse process.

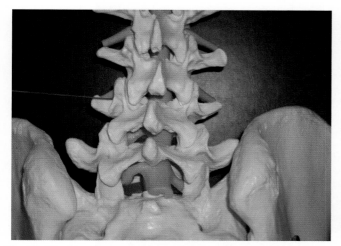

Fig. 20-15 Needle at target point for a medial branch block (anteroposterior view).

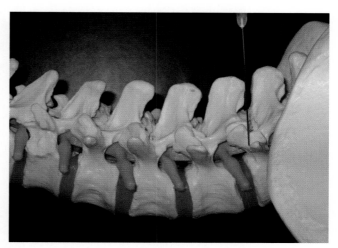

Fig. 20-16 Needle at target point for a medial branch block (lateral).

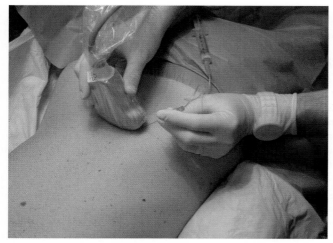

Fig. 20-17 Ultrasound-guided medial branch block: in-plane needle insertion in the short-axis view.

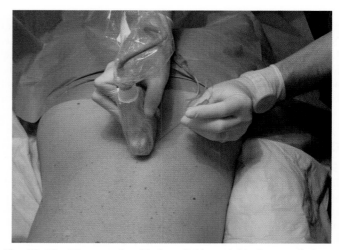

Fig. 20-18 Ultrasound-guided medial branch block: out-of-plane needle control in the long-axis view.

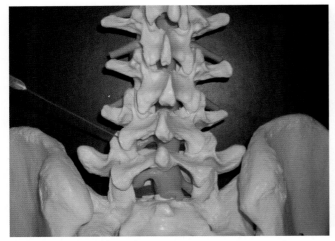

Fig. 20-19 Needle at target point for a facet joint block (anteroposterior view).

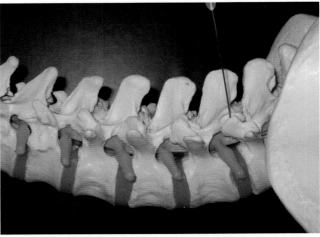

Fig. 20-20 Needle at target point for a facet joint block (lateral).

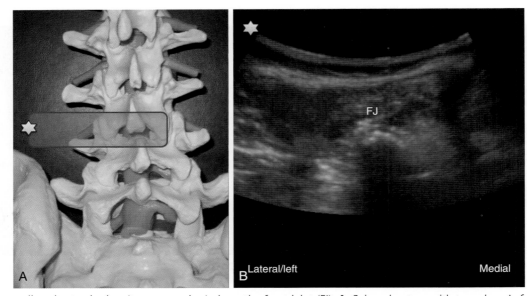

Fig. 20-21 Paramedian short-axis view (transverse view) above the facet joint (FJ). **A,** Spine phantom with transducer's footprint (*blue area*); **B,** Sonogram. *Star,* lateral.

practical performance is similar to that of the medial branch block. Needle insertion is guided in a paramedian SAX view above the facet joint visualizing the double contour of and the entry into the joint (**Fig. 20-21**). Similar to medial branch blocks, the needle is advanced from lateral to medial in plane to the transducer until bony contact is made. Injection of 0.5 mL of volume is enough for one facet joint.

Other Applications

Selective Lumbar Nerve Root or Periradicular Injection
Inadvertent intravascular injections during ultrasound-guided selective lumbar transforaminal nerve root injections cannot be ruled out completely at the moment. Reports of rare but devastating complications such as paraplegia caused by a spinal cord infarction secondary to inadvertent injection of particulate material in a radicular artery[10] under fluoroscopic or CT scan guidance are serious warnings. Because of this, most practitioners recommend

not to perform ultrasound-guided selective nerve root injections at the moment, although they seem to be technically possible.[11]

Intramuscular or Trigger Point Injections
Ultrasound-guided trigger point injections into the muscles of the back can easily be performed and are excellent procedures for the beginner in the field. Thus, the novice gets familiar with the sono-anatomy step by step and can safely learn to guide needles with the in-plane or out-of plane technique into the desired intramuscular target. Observing the spread of local anesthetic during injection into different muscles becomes possible.

Future Developments

Ultrasound-guided injection techniques in low back pain are an evolving field and will definitely gain more importance in the near future, maybe together with the development of sophisticated three-dimensional sonographic imaging techniques. Virtual reality imaging with real-time ultrasound guidance for facet joint injection has recently been described in a pilot study[12] and was successfully used to track both the transducer and the needle in a three-dimensional environment. Further scientific and technological advances are needed to finally bring these fascinating applications into clinical practice.

References

1. Greher M, Scharbert G, Kamolz LP, et al: Ultrasound-guided lumbar facet nerve block: a sonoanatomic study of a new methodologic approach. *Anesthesiology* 100(5):1242-1248, 2004.
2. Greher M, Kirchmair L, Enna B, et al: Ultrasound-guided lumbar facet nerve block: accuracy of a new technique confirmed by computed tomography. *Anesthesiology* 101(5):1195-1200, 2004.
3. Shim JK, Moon JC, Yoon KB, et al: Ultrasound-guided lumbar medial-branch block: a clinical study with fluoroscopy control. *Reg Anesth Pain Med* 31(5):451-454, 2006.
4. Rauch S, Kasuya Y, Turan A, et al: Ultrasound-guided lumbar medial branch block in obese patients: a fluoroscopically confirmed clinical feasibility study. *Reg Anesth Pain Med* 34(4):340-342, 2009.
5. Küllmer K, Rompe JD, Löwe A, et al: [Ultrasound image of the lumbar spine and the lumbosacral transition. Ultrasound anatomy and possibilities for ultrasonically-controlled facet joint infiltration]. *Z Orthop Ihre Grenzgeb* 135(4):310-314, 1997.
6. Galiano K, Obwegeser AA, Bodner G, et al: Ultrasound guidance for facet joint injections in the lumbar spine: a computed tomography-controlled feasibility study. *Anesth Analg* 101(2):579-583, 2005.
7. Galiano K, Obwegeser AA, Walch C, et al: Ultrasound-guided versus computed tomography-controlled facet joint injections in the lumbar spine: a prospective randomized clinical trial. *Reg Anesth Pain Med* 32(4):317-322, 2007.
8. Galiano K, Obwegeser AA, Bale R, et al: Ultrasound-guided and CT-navigation-assisted periradicular and facet joint injections in the lumbar and cervical spine: a new teaching tool to recognize the sono-anatomic pattern. *Reg Anesth Pain Med* 32(3):254-257, 2007.
9. O'Neill S, Graven-Nielsen T, Manniche C, et al: Ultrasound guided, painful electrical stimulation of lumbar facet joint structures: an experimental model of acute low back pain. *Pain* 144(1-2):76-83, 2009.
10. Kennedy DJ, Dreyfuss P, Aprill CN, et al: Paraplegia following image-guided transforaminal lumbar spine epidural steroid injection: two case reports. *Pain Med* 10(8):1389-1394, 2009.
11. Galiano K, Obwegeser AA, Bodner G, et al: Real-time sonographic imaging for periradicular injections in the lumbar spine: a sonographic anatomic study of a new technique. *J Ultrasound Med* 24(1):33-38, 2005.
12. Clarke C, Moore J, Wedlake C, et al: Virtual reality imaging with real-time ultrasound guidance for facet joint injection: a proof of concept. *Anesth Analg* 110(5):1461-1463, 2010.

21 Ultrasound-Guided Cervical Spine Injections

Samer Narouze

CHAPTER OVERVIEW

Chapter Synopsis: In the past few years, there has been a tremendous growth in interest in US-guided cervical injections as ultrasound allows direct, real-time visualization of soft tissue structures (e.g., vessels, nerves). Thus, it is an attractive alternative in cervical spine and neck injections, where there are a multitude of vital soft tissue structures compacted in a small area. This chapter will review various applications of ultrasound in cervical spine injections. Techniques for third occipital nerve block, cervical medial branch nerve block, and cervical facet intraarticular injections are discussed in detail. Advantages as well as limitations of ultrasound relative to fluoroscopy are highlighted. US-guided stellate ganglion block and US-guided atlanto-axial joint injections are discussed in other chapters.

Ultrasonography provides good visualization of bony surfaces, which may make it useful in various superficial spine injections (e.g., medial branch block, facet intraarticular injections, and nerve root blocks).[1] However, it is not as useful in neuraxial blocks because of the bony artifacts and the limited acoustic window.

Important Points:
- Ultrasonography is especially useful in cervical spine injections because there are many soft tissue structures compacted in a small area. The best example is cervical sympathetic (stellate ganglion) block.
- Ultrasonography plays an important role as an adjunct to fluoroscopy in cervical nerve root blocks because it can identify vessels in the vicinity of the nerve root, hence *avoiding* vascular injury and injection, but fluoroscopy can only *detect* intravascular injections after the fact.
- Ultrasonography can be useful in identifying the third occipital nerve as well as the cervical medial branches.
- Ultrasonography can facilitate *atraumatic* cervical facet intraarticular injections.
- By identifying the vertebral artery (both typical and atypical anatomy), ultrasonography can make atlanto-axial injections safer.

Clinical Pearls:
- Most US-guided cervical spine injections centered on differentiating C6 and C7 vertebral level. This can be accomplished by following the course of the vertebral artery as well by the identifying the characteristic C6 transverse process.
- One should always use Doppler US while performing US-guided cervical spine injection to help identify normal and abnormal vessels.
- For novices, it is always recommended to initially use US in conjunction with fluoroscopy, until one acquires the necessary skills and experience.

Clinical Pitfalls:
- US-guided cervical spine injections are advanced US applications that require extra training and experience. Novices should start practicing US musculoskeletal applications first before advancing to spinal applications.
- In cervical nerve root block and atlanto-axial joint injections, it may be wise to use both ultrasound and fluoroscopy, as one modality (ultrasound) helps *avoid* vascular injury and the other modality (fluoroscopy) helps *detect* intravascular injection.

Introduction

Ultrasonography in pain medicine (USPM) is a rapidly growing medical field in interventional pain management. Traditionally, spine interventional procedures for pain management are performed with imaging guidance such as fluoroscopy and computed tomography (CT). In the past few years, there has been a tremendous growth in interest in USPM.

Ultrasonography allows direct real-time visualization of soft tissue structures (e.g., vessels, nerves). Thus, it is an attractive alternative in cervical spine and neck injections, where there is a multitude of vital soft tissue structures compacted in a small area. However, it faces unique challenges in lumbar spine injections because the major shortcoming of ultrasonography is the limited resolution at deep levels.

Ultrasonography provides good visualization of bony surfaces, which may make it useful in various superficial spine injections (e.g., medial branch block, facet intraarticular injections, nerve root blocks).[1] However, it is not as useful in neuraxial blocks because of the bony artifacts and the limited acoustic window.[2]

Ultrasound-Guided Cervical Sympathetic Chain (Stellate Ganglion) Block

Please refer to Chapter 8.

Ultrasound-Guided Cervical Nerve Root Block

Anatomy

The cervical spinal nerve occupies the lower part of the foramen with the epiradicular veins in the upper part. The radicular arteries arising from the vertebral, ascending cervical, and deep cervical arteries lie in close approximation to the spinal nerve.[3]

Huntoon[4] was able to show that the ascending and deep cervical arteries may contribute to the anterior spinal artery (not only the vertebral artery). More than 20% of the foramina dissected had either the ascending or deep cervical artery or a large branch within 2 mm of the needle path for a cervical transforaminal procedure. One third of these vessels were spinal branches that entered the foramen posteriorly, potentially forming a radicular or a segmental feeder vessel to the spinal cord, making it vulnerable to inadvertent injury even during correct needle placement. Variable anastomoses between the vertebral and cervical arteries were found; therefore it is possible to introduce steroid particles into the vertebral circulation via the cervical arteries.[4]

Limitations of the Current Technique

Currently, the guidelines for cervical transforaminal injection technique involve introducing the needle under fluoroscopic guidance into the posterior aspect of the intervertebral foramen just anterior to the superior articular process in the oblique view to minimize the risk of injury to the vertebral artery or the nerve root.[3] Despite strict adherence to these guidelines, adverse outcomes have been reported.[5,6] A potential shortcoming of these current guidelines is the presence of a critical feeder vessel to the anterior spinal artery in the posterior aspect of the intervertebral foramen that could be injured in the pathway of the needle.[4] Ultrasonography may be more adventitious because it allows for visualization of soft tissues, nerves, and vessels, and facilitates real-time visualization of the injectate around the nerve.

Literature Review of Ultrasound-Guided Cervical Nerve Root Block

Galiano et al[7] described the use of ultrasonography in cervical periradicular injections in cadavers. They used CT images for confirmation. However, they were not able to comment on the relevant blood vessels in the vicinity of the vertebral foramen, and this raised some concerns about the safety of performing the procedure with ultrasonography at that time.[8] Now with the introduction of high-resolution ultrasound transducers and gaining more experience, we were able to visualize small critical arteries with ultrasonography.

Narouze et al[9] reported a pilot study of 10 patients who received cervical nerve root injections using ultrasonography as the primary imaging tool with fluoroscopy as the control. In four patients, these authors were able to identify vessels at the anterior aspect of the foramen; two patients had critical vessels at the posterior aspect of the foramen, and in one patient, this artery continued medially into the foramen, forming a segmental feeder artery. In these two cases, such vessels could have been injured easily in the pathway of a correctly placed needle under fluoroscopy.

Sonoanatomy and Ultrasound-Guided Technique for Cervical Selective Nerve Root Block

Ultrasound examination is usually performed using a high-resolution linear array transducer in the lateral decubitus position. The transducer is applied transversely to the lateral aspect of the neck to obtain a short-axis view of the cervical spine (**Fig. 21-1**). The cervical transverse process can be easily identified with the

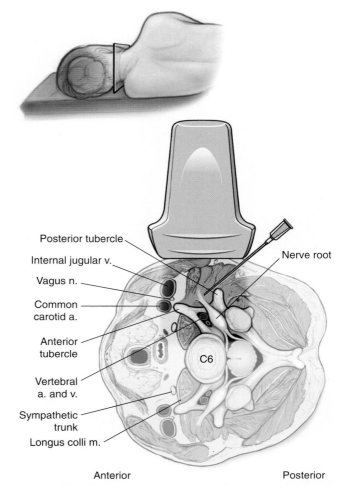

Fig. 21-1 Illustration showing the relevant anatomy at C6 and the orientation of the ultrasound transducer to obtain a short-axis transverse ultrasound view. A, Artery; m, muscle; n, nerve; v, vein. (Reprinted with permission from Cleveland Clinic Foundation, Cleveland, OH.)

anterior and posterior tubercles as hyperechoic structures "two-humped camel" sign, and the hypoechoic round to oval nerve root in between (**Fig. 21-2**).[9] First, the correct cervical level needs to be determined by identifying the transverse process of the seventh and sixth cervical vertebrae (C7 and C6). The seventh cervical transverse process (C7) differs from the above levels because it usually has a rudimentary anterior tubercle and one prominent posterior tubercle.[10] Then by moving the transducer cranially, the transverse process of the sixth cervical spine comes into the image with the characteristic sharp anterior tubercle (**Fig. 21-3**), and then the consecutive cervical spinal level can be easily identified. To confirm the correct spinal level, the vertebral artery can be followed as well. The vertebral artery runs anteriorly at the C7 level before it enters the foramen of the C6 transverse process in about 90% of cases. However, it enters at C5 or higher in the remaining cases (**Fig. 21-4**).[11]

After the appropriate spinal level has been identified, a 22-gauge blunt-tip needle can be introduced just lateral to the lateral end of the transducer and advanced in plane from posterior to anterior under real-time ultrasound guidance to target the corresponding cervical nerve root at the external foraminal opening between the anterior and posterior tubercles of the transverse process, which can be easily identified as the "two-humped camel" sign. One can

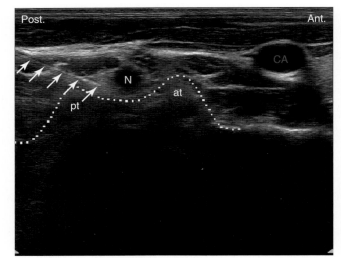

Fig. 21-2 Short-axis transverse ultrasound images showing the anterior tubercle (at) and the posterior tubercle (pt) of the C5 transverse process as the "two-humped camel" sign. The *solid arrows* are pointing to the needle in place at the posterior aspect of the intervertebral foramen. CA, carotid artery; N, nerve root. (Reprinted with permission from Cleveland Clinic Foundation, Cleveland, OH.)

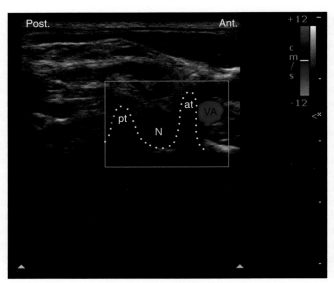

Fig. 21-4 Short-axis transverse ultrasound image showing the sharp anterior tubercle (at) of the C6 transverse process; the vertebral artery (VA) is anterior. N, nerve root; pt, posterior tubercle. (Reprinted with permission from Cleveland Clinic Foundation, Cleveland, OH.)

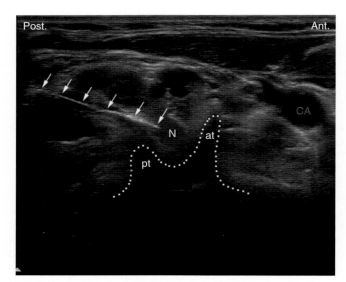

Fig. 21-3 Short-axis transverse ultrasound image showing the sharp anterior tubercle (at) of the C6 transverse process. The *solid arrows* are pointing to the needle in place at the posterior aspect of the intervertebral foramen. CA, carotid artery; N, nerve root; pt, posterior tubercle. (Reprinted with permission from Cleveland Clinic Foundation, Cleveland, OH.)

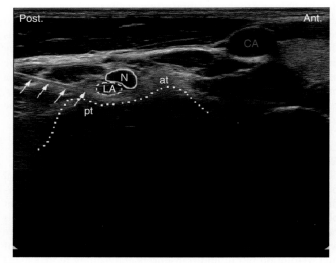

Fig. 21-5 Short-axis transverse ultrasound image showing the spread of the local anesthetic (LA). at, anterior tubercle; CA, carotid artery; N, nerve root; pt, posterior tubercle. (Reprinted with permission from Cleveland Clinic Foundation, Cleveland, OH.)

The author believes that visualization of small vessels (radicular arteries) may be very challenging, especially in obese patients, and requires special training and expertise. Ultrasonography should be used in conjunction with real-time fluoroscopy with contrast injection and digital subtraction (when available) to confirm safe needle placement.[2]

Cervical Medial Branch and Facet Joint Injections

Anatomy
Cervical zygapophyseal (facet) joints are diarthrodial joints formed by the superior articular process of one cervical vertebra articulating with the inferior articular process of the vertebrae above at the

successfully monitor the spread of the injectate around the cervical nerve with real-time ultrasonography; the absence of such spread around the nerve root may suggest unsuspected or inadvertent intravascular injection (**Fig. 21-5**). However, it should be mentioned here that is difficult to monitor the spread of the injectate through the foramen into the epidural space (because of the bony drop-out artifact of the transverse process). This is the reason behind referring to this approach as a "cervical selective nerve root block" rather than cervical transforaminal epidural injection.

level of the junction of the lamina and the pedicle. The angulation of the facet joint increases caudally, being about 45 degrees superior to the transverse plane at the upper cervical level to assuming a more vertical position at the upper thoracic level. The superior articular process also faces more posteromedially at the upper cervical level, and this changes to more posterolateral at the lower cervical level, with C6 being the most common transition level.[12,13]

Each facet joint has a fibrous capsule and is lined by a synovial membrane. The joint also contains varying amounts of adipose and fibrous tissue forming different types of synovial folds contributing to different pathophysiology for joint dysfunction.[14]

The cervical zygapophyseal joints are innervated by articular branches derived from the medial branches of the cervical dorsal rami. The C4-C8 dorsal rami arise from their respective spinal nerves and pass dorsally over the root of their corresponding transverse processes. The medial branches of the cervical dorsal rami curve medially around the corresponding articular pillars and have a constant relationship to the bone at the dorsolateral aspect of the articular pillar as they are bound to the periosteum by an investing fascia and held in place by the tendon of the semispinalis capitis muscle.[15]

The articular branches arise as the nerve approaches the posterior aspect of the articular pillar, one innervating the zygapophyseal joint above and the other innervating the joint below. Consequently, each typical cervical zygapophyseal joint has dual innervation, from the medial branch above and below its location.[15]

The medial branches of the C3 dorsal ramus differ in their anatomy. A deep medial branch passes around the waist of the C3 articular pillar similar to other typical medial branches and supplies the C3-C4 zygapophyseal joint. The superficial medial branch of C3 is large and known as the third occipital nerve (TON). It curves around the lateral and then the posterior aspect of the C2-C3 zygapophyseal joint, giving articular branches to the joint. Articular branches may also arise from a communicating loop that crosses the back of the joint between the TON and the C2 dorsal ramus. Beyond the C2-C3 zygapophyseal joint, the TON becomes cutaneous over the suboccipital region. So pain derived from the C2-C3 zygapophyseal joint can be addressed by blocking the ipsilateral TON as it crosses the lateral aspect of the joint, and pain derived from joints below C2-C3 can be addressed by blocking the cervical medial branches as they pass around the waists of the articular pillars above and below the corresponding joint.[16]

Literature Review of Ultrasound-Guided Third Occipital Nerve and Cervical Medial Branch Block

Eichenberger et al[17] reported ultrasound-guided TON blockade in volunteers. The TON was visualized in all volunteers and showed a median diameter of 2.0 mm. The C2-C3 facet joint was identified correctly by ultrasonography in 27 of 28 cases, and 23 needles were placed correctly into the target zone. They defined the radiologic target point arbitrarily as the intersection of a vertical line passing through the middle of the C2-C3 zygapophyseal joint and an oblique line passing directly over the joint line. They reported accuracy of needle position as confirmed by fluoroscopy in 82% of insertions and a 90% success of nerve blockade.

Although they reported in the above study the feasibility of identifying the medial branch of C3, there have been no other feasibility studies regarding ultrasound-guided lower cervical medial branch block. Nevertheless, the technique was reported before.[18,19]

Literature Review of Ultrasound-Guided Cervical Facet Intraarticular Injections

Galiano et al[20] studied the feasibility of ultrasound-guided cervical facet joint intraarticular injections in cadavers using a lateral approach. They were able to accurately identify the facet joints from C2-C3 to C6-C7 in 36 of 40 attempts. All needle tips were located inside the joint space as verified by CT. Subsequently, they have studied and advocated the use of an ultrasound-guided CT-assisted navigation system as a teaching tool for performing facet injections.[21]

Sonoanatomy and Ultrasound-Guided Technique for Cervical Facet Intraarticular Injections

The author prefers the posterior approach because it is easier to identify the correct cervical level while the patient is in the prone position. Counting can be started from cranial to caudal. (The C1 spine has no or rudimentary spinous process, and the first identified bifid spinous process belongs to C2.) Another advantage of this approach is that the needle is advanced in a caudal to cranial direction, and this matches the caudal angulation of the cervical facet joint, making it easier for the needle to get into the joint space atraumatically. Also, bilateral injections can be performed without the need for position change.[22]

A linear or a curved transducer may be used depending on the size of the patient. A longitudinal scan is obtained initially at the midline (spinous process), and then by scanning laterally, one can easily see the lamina; farther laterally, the facet column appears in the image as the characteristic "saw sign" (**Fig. 21-6**). If in doubt, one can scan even more laterally until the facet joists are no longer in the image and then come back medially toward the facet joints. The inferior articular processes of the level above and the superior articular process of the level below appear as a hyperechoic signals, and the joint space appears as an anechoic gap in between. The needle is then inserted inferior to the caudal end of the transducer and advanced from caudad to cephalad in plane to enter the inferior part of the joint under real-time ultrasonography (see **Fig. 21-6**).

Sonoanatomy and Ultrasound-Guided Technique for Third Occipital Nerve and Cervical Medial Branch Block

Eichenberger et al[17] described the technique in details. The patient is placed in the lateral position, and a high-frequency linear transducer is applied just caudal to the mastoid process exactly perpendicular to the lateral aspect of the neck in a transverse plane to obtain a short-axis view.

Moving the transducer slowly caudally, the lateral mass of the axis and the transverse process of C1 are easily visible. Moving the transducer only 1 to 3 mm more caudally, the vertebral artery appears, and by following this artery caudally, the vertebral artery disappears in the transverse foramen of C2 and the C2-C3 joint appears posteriorly. It presents as a convex density covered by the laminated densities of the overlying neck muscles. The apex of the convexity of the joint was identified and constituted the target point for the needle insertion.

The needle is introduced from immediately below the ultrasound probe and advanced perpendicular to the beam (out of plane) under ultrasound guidance toward the apex of the convexity of the joint until bony resistance was encountered. Then the transducer is rotated to the longitudinal plane because in this view the nerve is best visualized. The TON is identified with the typical sonomorphological appearance of a small peripheral nerve just

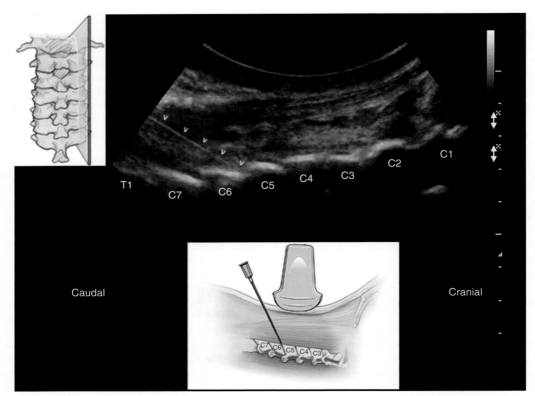

Fig. 21-6 Sagittal (longitudinal) ultrasonographic view showing the hypoechoic articular processes of the facet joints as the "saw sign" and the anechoic facet joint space in between. The needle is introduced caudal to the transducer and advanced in plane into the caudal part of the C5-C6 facet joint (*arrowheads*). *Inset,* Illustration showing the paramedian position of the ultrasound transducer to obtain a longitudinal scan through the facet column. (Reprinted with permission from Cleveland Clinic Foundation, Cleveland, OH.)

lateral to the C2-C3 joint, and the needle is adjusted as needed to lie closer to the nerve (**Fig. 21-7**).

Cervical Medial Branch Block

Lateral Approach

The patient is placed in the lateral position, and a high-frequency linear transducer is applied longitudinally with its upper end just below the mastoid process to obtain a longitudinal view of the cervical spine. After the C2-C3 joint is identified as above, the transducer is slowly moved in a caudal direction to view the lower facet joints until the desired level of the cervical facet joint is reached. The highest points in the bony reflex of the articular pillars represent the facet articulations, and the medial branches can be visualized at the deepest point over the articular pillars between the two articulations in contrast to the TON which runs over the highest point of the articulation.[17]

The needle can be introduced just caudal to the ultrasound transducer and advanced under real-time ultrasonography to the target nerve (in plane). Alternatively, after the correct level has been identified, the transducer is rotated to obtain a short-axis view, and the needle is advanced perpendicular to the beam (out of plane) under ultrasound guidance toward the articular pillar until bony resistance is encountered. Then the transducer can be rotated to the longitudinal plane because the nerve is better visualized in this view, and the needle is adjusted as needed to lie closer to the nerve in the same manner described above for the TON block (see **Fig. 21-7**).[17]

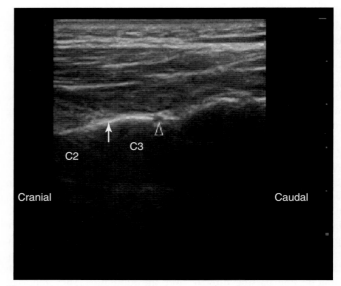

Fig. 21-7 Sagittal (longitudinal) ultrasonographic view at C2-C3 level showing the third occipital nerve (*arrow*) crossing C2-C3 joint and the C3 medial branch (*arrowhead*) as a hypoechoic oval structure at the deepest point (waist) of the articular pillar. (Reprinted with permission from Cleveland Clinic Foundation, Cleveland, OH.)

Ultrasound-Guided Atlanto-Axial Joint Injections

Refer to Chapter 5, Head and Neck Blocks.

References

1. Narouze SN, editor: *Atlas of ultrasound-guided procedures in interventional pain management*, ed 1, New York, 2011, Springer.
2. Narouze S: Ultrasound-guided Interventional procedures in pain management: evidence based medicine. *Reg Anesth Pain Med* 35(suppl):S55-S58, 2010.
3. Rathmell JP, Aprill C, Bogduk N: Cervical transforaminal injection of steroids. *Anesthesiology* 100:1595-1600, 2004.
4. Huntoon MA: Anatomy of the cervical intervertebral foramina: vulnerable arteries and ischemic neurologic injuries after transforaminal epidural injections. *Pain* 117:104-111, 2005.
5. Tiso RL, Cutler T, Catania JA, et al: Adverse central nervous system sequelae after selective transforaminal block: the role of corticosteroids. *Spine J* 4:468-474, 2004.
6. Baker R, Dreyfuss P, Mercer S, et al: Cervical transforaminal injections of corticosteroids into a radicular artery: a possible mechanism for spinal cord injury. *Pain* 103:211-215, 2003.
7. Galiano K, Obwegeser AA, Bodner G, et al: Ultrasound-guided periradicular injections in the middle to lower cervical spine: an imaging study of a new approach. *Reg Anesth Pain Med* 30:391-396, 2005.
8. Narouze SN: Ultrasound-guided cervical periradicular injection: cautious optimism [letter]. *Reg Anesth Pain Med* 31:87, 2006.
9. Narouze S, Vydyanathan A, Kapural L, et al: Ultrasound-guided cervical selective nerve root block: a fluoroscopy-controlled feasibility study. *Reg Anesth Pain Med* 34:343-348, 2009.
10. Martinoli C, Bianchi S, Santacroce E, et al: Brachial plexus sonography: a technique for assessing the root level. *AJR Am J Roentgenol* 179:699-702, 2002.
11. Matula C, Trattnig S, Tschabitscher M, et al: The course of the prevertebral segment of the vertebral artery: anatomy and clinical significance. *Surg Neurol* 48:125-131, 1997.
12. Pal GP, Routal RV, Saggu SK: The orientation of the articular facets of the zygapophyseal joints at the cervical and upper thoracic region. *J Anat* 198:431-441, 2001.
13. Yoganandan N, Knowles SA, Maiman DJ, et al: Anatomic study of the morphology of human cervical facet joint. *Spine* 28:2317-2323, 2003.
14. Inami S, Kaneoka K, Hayashi K, et al: Types of synovial fold in the cervical facet joint. *J Orthop Sci* 5:475-480, 2000.
15. Bogduk N: The clinical anatomy of the cervical dorsal rami. *Spine* 7:319-330, 1982.
16. Lord SM, Barnsley L, Bogduk N: Percutaneous radiofrequency neurotomy in the treatment of cervical zygapophysial joint pain: a caution. *Neurosurgery* 36:732-739, 1995.
17. Eichenberger U, Greher M, Kapral S, et al: Sonographic visualization and ultrasound-guided block of the third occipital nerve: prospective for a new method to diagnose C2-C3 zygapophysial joint pain. *Anesthesiology* 104:303-308, 2006.
18. Gofeld M: Ultrasonography in pain medicine: a critical review. *Pain Pract* 8:226-240, 2008.
19. Siegenthaler A, Narouze S, Eichenberger U: Ultrasound-guided third occipital nerve and cervical medial branch nerve blocks. *Tech Reg Anesth Pain Manage* 13(3):128-132, 2009.
20. Galiano K, Obwegeser AA, Bodner G, et al: Ultrasound-guided facet joint injections in the middle to lower cervical spine: a CT-controlled sonoanatomic study. *Clin J Pain* 22:538-543, 2006.
21. Galiano K, Obwegeser AA, Bale R, et al: Ultrasound-guided and CT-navigation-assisted periradicular and facet joint injections in the lumbar and cervical spine: a new teaching tool to recognize the sonoanatomic pattern. *Reg Anesth Pain Med* 32:254-257, 2007.
22. Narouze S: Ultrasound guided cervical facet intraarticular injections. *Tech Reg Anesth Pain Manage* 13(3):133-136, 2009.

22 Musculoskeletal Injections: Iliopsoas, Quadratus Lumborum, Piriformis, and Trigger Point Injections

Anne Marie McKenzie-Brown, Kiran Chekka, and Honorio T. Benzon

CHAPTER OVERVIEW

Chapter Synopsis: Myofascial pain syndrome arises from the fascia tissue surrounding the muscles that interact with the skeletal support system of the back. The pain results in a trigger point, a localized taut band of muscle tissue that is tender to the touch and may cause radiating pain. The quadratus lumborum and iliopsoas muscles are typically affected by myofascial pain. Their deep location and intimate association with vascular and abdominal organs make injection at these muscles difficult, and identifying trigger points is quite subjective. Trigger points may be classified as active or latent. Similar to many chronic pain states, myofascial pain may begin with a nociceptive process from injury or strain and progress to a central sensitization that can lead to chronic pain. Trigger point injection is only one option for treatment; others include transcutaneous nerve stimulation, acupuncture, and physical therapies. Injected drugs are usually anesthetics or steroids with antiinflammatory effects. Fluoroscopic guidance can improve the success of trigger point injections.

Piriformis syndrome presents its own challenges, starting with proper diagnosis, which often comes by exclusion. This pain syndrome is marked by pain in the entire buttock that can radiate to back and leg areas. In about half of cases, the syndrome arises from trauma (including surgery), although not necessarily with direct or immediate consequences. Injections of the piriformis muscle with local anesthetic and corticosteroids can be used as therapy for pain. Fluoroscopic imaging or ultrasound is recommended for guidance of injections.

Important Points:

- Trigger points in the quadratus lumborum and iliopsoas muscles are a common source of low back pain.
- Quadratus lumborum and iliopsoas muscle injections are more accurately performed under fluoroscopic guidance because of their depth and location in the back.
- When performing these injections, the practitioner should bear in mind that the quadratus lumborum and psoas muscles form the posterior abdominal wall and that there are associated organs and vascular structures anterior to these muscles.
- Good results can be achieved with a thorough history and physical examination and careful patient selection often after other more common diagnoses are eliminated.
- Using dual guidance with fluoroscopy and nerve stimulation allows the practitioner to safely and quickly predictably deposit medications into the belly of the piriformis muscle.
- Practitioners should avoid injecting with any paresthesias or with a dye study that suggests intraneural, intravascular injection or injection into another structure.

Clinical Pearls:

- Patients with quadratus lumborum pain have more pain arising from a supine to a sitting position than going from sitting to standing.
- During the injection, the practitioner should look at the direction of the fibers when injecting the contrast to determine whether the injection has been in the quadratus muscle.
- If the practitioner is unsure whether the injection is deep enough, he or she should stop and inject some contrast before advancing the needle.
- Striated muscle has a characteristics appearance under fluoroscopy.

Myofascial Pain and Trigger Point Injections

Myofascial pain is a common source of discomfort in the lower back. It is a painful condition that results in localized trigger points in the affected muscle. Myofascial pain syndrome was first clearly defined by Simons et al[1] in the 1980s. It is characterized by trigger points in a specific muscle that may or may not respond to snapping palpation with a local twitch response and secondary decreased range of motion caused by the pain.[1] A trigger point is a localized taut band of muscle that is tender to palpation and produces pain that radiates when palpated. Tactile pressure to trigger points result in known, reproducible but nondermatomal referral patterns, also known as zones of reference.[1,2] There is significant variability among practitioners in the identification of trigger points for the diagnosis of myofascial pain syndrome, although there is some evidence that the interrater reliability can be significantly improved with training.[3] There is currently no gold standard test for trigger point identification, leaving a fair amount of subjectivity in the diagnosis. The twitch response is the most specific clinical test of a trigger point.[1] Trigger points are either active or latent.[1] Both active and latent trigger points have tender taut bands within the muscle, but latent trigger points are not associated with spontaneous pain. Latent trigger points may be the result of prior injury that then becomes painful with reinjury. Trigger points may be further subdivided into primary, secondary, and satellite trigger points.[1,2] Primary trigger points become active as a result of trauma, overload or overuse injury, or after leaving a muscle in a prolonged contracted or shortened position.[1] Primary trigger points are in a discrete and separate location, with adjacent secondary trigger points that are often the result of spasm. Satellite trigger points are felt in the area of the referred pain remote from the primary trigger point location. The more irritable the trigger point, the more painful and extensive the referred pain; muscle size does not affect the amount or extent of the referred pain. Producing referred pain requires less pressure applied to an active than to a latent trigger point.[1] Latent trigger points, by definition, are inactivated when key trigger points are inactivated. [1,2] Although in the past their mere existence was questioned, we now know that trigger points can be documented by electromyography (EMG). Hubbard and Berkoff[4] in their 1993 article were the first to report spontaneous needle EMG activity at the trigger point site now described as spontaneous electrical activity (SEA).[4] Endplate noise that has been recorded from specific myofascial trigger points are thought to be attributable to excessive acetylcholine release in the neuromuscular junction.[1] Sympathetic activity appears to play a role in the activity of trigger points, with increased EMG amplitude seen under conditions of psychological stress and reduced firmness after a stellate ganglion block.[5,6]

Myofascial pain is not the same as the pain endured by those with fibromyalgia, which is a more diffuse, centralized musculoskeletal condition with many associated symptoms (e.g., irritable bowel). Predisposing factors are anything that increases or changes the demands on the muscle. These may include repetitive use, deconditioning, poor posture, and occupational or recreational injury related to muscle imbalances.[6] If treated early, the prognosis for myofascial pain is good. Treatment includes physical therapy, including stretching and strengthening or conditioning; trigger point injections; acupuncture; biofeedback; transcutaneous electrical nerve stimulation (TENS); and some medications. It is not entirely clear why trigger points are painful because there is no direct evidence of inflammation or enhanced nociceptors within the trigger point sites. However, after the pain is initiated, sensitization at the level of the dorsal horn may occur, which then progresses to the development of central sensitization and the subsequent development of chronic myofascial pain.[6]

Although local anesthetic is the substance most often used by pain physicians in trigger point injections, there is not much evidence for its superiority over normal saline or dry needling. It does appear that the best response to trigger point injections occurs if a local twitch response is elicited.[7] Part of the problem is that placebo-controlled studies of local anesthetic injections are extremely difficult to accomplish. Many of the studies do not have consistent criteria for trigger points, and some do not distinguish between the tender points of fibromyalgia and the trigger points of myofascial pain. The relief from the local anesthetic consistently outlasts the half-life of the local anesthetic, giving some credence to central sensitization in myofascial pain syndrome. All local anesthetics are somewhat myotoxic, with bupivacaine being the most myotoxic by far, but the muscle quickly regenerates with little long-term ill effect.[8] The mechanism of bupivacaine's effect appears to be on the calcium release related to the channel-ryanodine receptor of skeletal muscle.[8-10] Injected steroid can also be myotoxic and should be used in low doses. Dry needling has been used with varied success but has the disadvantage of postneedling soreness, depending on the sensitivity of the patient before and during the procedure and whether or not acupuncture needles, associated with less soreness, were used.[6] Although not all acupuncture points (e.g., in the ear) are the same as trigger points, there is a striking similarity between acupuncture points and those used for dry needling and for trigger point injections.

The muscles involved in myofascial pain of the lower back can be divided into the posterior (superficial to the transverse process) and anterior (deep to the transverse process) muscles. The posterior muscles include the multifidus (located closest to the spinous process) and the adjacent erector spinae muscles. The latissimus dorsi are attached to the spine by the thoracolumbar fascia, which envelops the multifidus and erector spinae muscles posterior to the quadratus lumborum. The thoracolumbar fascia extends distally and is in contact with the contralateral gluteus maximus and is thus thought an important factor in the transfer of load from the spine to the lower extremities. The quadratus lumborum is replaced distally by the iliolumbar ligament, one of the strongest ligaments in the body and the one responsible for much of the stability of the lumbosacral segment. More anteriorly and inferiorly to the quadratus are the iliopsoas muscles. These descend into the pelvic brim and attach to the lesser trochanter of the femur.[11]

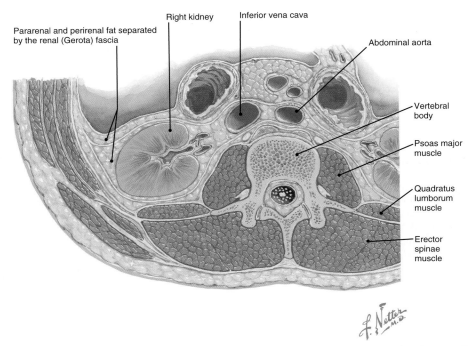

Pararenal and perirenal fat separated by the renal (Gerota) fascia

Right kidney

Inferior vena cava

Abdominal aorta

Vertebral body

Psoas major muscle

Quadratus lumborum muscle

Erector spinae muscle

Fig. 22-1   Lumbar region of back: cross section. (Netter illustration from www.netterimages.com © Elsevier Inc. All rights reserved.)

Pain involving the quadratus lumborum and iliopsoas muscles can be either primary myofascial or secondary in nature, reflecting pathology in the spine or other nearby organs. The quadratus lumborum, psoas major, and iliacus (which comes together to form the iliopsoas) muscles make up the major muscles of the posterior abdominal wall (**Fig. 22-1**).

Quadratus Lumborum Injections

Establishing a Diagnosis

The diagnosis of myofascial pain is a clinical one, largely dependent on the findings of the history and physical examination. The quadratus lumborum muscle allows lateral movement and extension of the mid and lower back. This muscle is a common source of myofascial pain because of its frequent use in normal daily activities such as walking and sitting; it is made worse by poor posture.[2] Pain is felt in the flank, lower back, hip, and sometimes the buttocks but is mostly above the iliac crest and exacerbated by movement of the spine. It may mimic radicular or even sacroiliac joint pain because of its attachment to the iliac crest. Acute myofascial pain of the quadratus lumborum may be precipitated by sudden movements (e.g., lifting in a way that twists the lower back), and even the most mundane of movements such as coughing or deep breathing become painful. Even sleep can be problematic because patients are unable to find a comfortable position in which to sleep because of pain with any lateral movement of the spine. Patients describe pain with arising from the supine position. Because of its proximity to the abdominal organs, disease of these organs, particularly kidney disease, may present as low back pain and must be excluded. Pronounced asymmetry of the dominant quadratus lumborum in elite cricket players (fast bowlers) and resultant pars fractures involving the nondominant side have been reported in the literature in several case reports.[12] Pain from the quadratus lumborum may be confused with pain that comes from injury to the iliolumbar ligament.[13] The iliolumbar ligament connects the transverse process of L5 to the iliac crest. This very strong, thick ligament

stabilizes the L5 body to the ilium and prevents axial rotation and translational movement on the sacrum. Pain from the quadratus lumborum may be distinguished from pain caused by iliolumbar ligament injury because of the absence of pain around the area of the flank with iliolumbar pain. The quadratus lumborum lies deep to the erector spinae muscles and the thoracolumbar fascia, so it may be difficult to distinguish these muscles from the erector spinae just on the basis of palpation.[14]

Physical examination involves observation and palpation for trigger points. When the patient is standing, the practitioner should look from behind for obvious signs of spasm causing a functional scoliosis or tilt and should look for elevation of the posterior superior iliac spine. The practitioner should observe for an antalgic gait and palpate for tender trigger points just below the twelfth rib and around the area of the iliac crest; this may be increased with back rotation. Part of the physical examination includes looking for a functional leg length discrepancy caused by spasm of the quadratus lumborum. The shortened leg is associated with the side of quadratus spasm and subsequent contraction resulting in upward motion of the pelvis.[15] Provocative maneuvers include palpation of trigger points while twisting the back.

Anatomy

The quadratus lumborum is shaped like a quadrangle and has as its origin the aponeurosis of the iliolumbar ligament and part of the iliac crest. It is posterior to the psoas muscle and lateral to the thoracolumbar fascia. It inserts at the twelfth rib and the transverse processes of L1 to L4. It serves as an anchor between the twelfth rib and the pelvis, and the majority of the fibers attach to the twelfth rib.[16] This creates a stable base for the diaphragm, allowing for its function as a basic muscle of respiration.[13] The quadratus lumborum pulls down on the diaphragm and laterally flexes the lumbar spine (unilateral) and aids in back extension (bilateral). Its innervation is from the ventral rami of T12 to L4.

Phillips et al[13] in their cadaver study of the anatomy of the quadratus lumborum showed that although there is considerable variation in the presence and location of the muscle fascicles, the muscle exists in three broad layers, and about half of the quadratus lumborum fascicles acts on the twelfth rib and the rest exert their actions on the lumbar vertebra. The compressive forces exerted by the quadratus lumborum is insignificant compared with that exerted by the erector spinae and multifidus, and thus there is little evidence for a major stabilizing role of the quadratus lumborum on the lumbar spine.[13]

Basic Science
There is no basic science information on quadratus trigger point injections.

Imaging
No special imaging is needed to make the diagnosis. This is a clinical diagnosis except to rule out other causes or bleeding or infectious reasons for the pain.

Guidelines
There are no printed guidelines for injections in the quadratus lumborum muscle.

Indications and Contraindications
The indication is myofascial low back pain with or without radiation to the hip with reproducible trigger points. It is contraindicated in situations in which muscular injections are contraindicated (e.g., coagulopathy or bleeding diathesis, localized infection at the site, or systemic infection).

Equipment
- Materials for sterile prep and drape
- 25-gauge 2- or 3.5-inch spinal needles, depending on the size of the patient
- Local anesthetic with or without a small amount of steroid diluted in the local anesthetic solution
- Fluoroscopy machine or ultrasound machine if the patient is not overweight

Technique
Palpation of Trigger Points   Although in thin patients the quadratus may be theoretically palpated lateral to the erector spinae muscles and injected there, it is more accurate to perform these injections under fluoroscopic guidance. It is certainly reasonable to give a trial of trigger point injections based on palpation before performing the procedure under fluoroscopic guidance.

Quadratus Lumborum Trigger Point Injections Under Fluoroscopic Guidance   Sterile prep and drape of the area to be injected are done. The lateral border of the L4 transverse process is visualized under fluoroscopy. Needle entry is at the lateral inferior edge of the transverse process; the lateral aspect of the transverse process is touched with the needle tip. The needle is advanced approximately 1 cm or less, aiming to go just past the lateral edge of the transverse process. In the lateral view, the needle should not be anterior to the facetal line; bear in mind that the quadratus is just posterior to the posterior abdominal wall and anteriorly is the colon, psoas muscle, and kidneys. The kidney extends to approximately L3, so these injections are performed at L4. One mL of nonionic contrast solution is injected, and the striated appearance of contrast spread is visualized in the muscle along the quadratus lumborum muscle fibers. When it is clear that the needle is in the correct position and again after negative aspiration, local anesthetic

is injected with or without steroid. The authors use a nonparticulate steroid, 5 mg of dexamethasone, but a low dose of particulate steroid (e.g., 20 mg of methylprednisolone diluted in the local anesthetic solution) may also be used. Good pain relief can be obtained with 5 to 7 mL of injectate; this may be done in a fanlike technique as long as intramuscular injection is confirmed. There should be no paresthesias, blood, or cerebrospinal fluid (CSF) with needle insertion.

The authors have not performed these injections under ultrasound guidance; however, an anatomical study[17] has been done involving the use of ultrasound guidance to identify the psoas and quadratus lumborum and erector spinae muscles. The study showed that these muscles are readily identified under ultrasonography, but this technique is not easily translated to overweight (body mass index, 25 to 29.9 kg/m^2) or more obese patients. These authors identified the lumbar spinal levels by counting the images of the transverse processes starting at the level of the sacrum and proceeding in a cephalad direction. When using ultrasonography, the landmarks are first identified using the longitudinal view, where the probe is placed approximately 3 cm parallel to the spinous processes, then when at the desired level, rotating the probe to the short-axis or transverse view.[17]

Patient Management and Evaluation
For the best outcome, these injections are done in conjunction with physical therapy. Because other interventions may be responsive to steroid injections, injection of steroid should be kept to a minimum. As with other trigger point injections, the duration of action of the trigger point injections generally outlasts the duration of the local anesthetic, and in the authors' experience, it varies with the time from symptom onset to injection.

Outcomes Evidence
There is sparse literature on outcomes from quadratus lumborum injections; they are virtually all anecdotal.

Risk and Complication Avoidance
The quadratus has its origin at the iliac crest and iliolumbar ligament and inserts around the twelfth rib and the transverse processes of the lumbar vertebrae. It is posterior to the kidney, so injection, particularly in thin patients, should be done with this in mind.

Iliopsoas Muscle Injections

Establishing the Diagnosis
The major role of the iliopsoas, supported by EMG evidence, is the main hip flexor of the body.[18] Pain coming from the iliopsoas, when ipsilateral, is close to the midline but described as being vertical along the spinal column, sometimes radiating to the groin. Occupations that require patients to sit for many hours (e.g., driving for long hours daily), particularly with their knees above their hips, leave the iliopsoas in prolonged contraction and subsequent possibility of pain.[1] The psoas muscle is continuously active with prolonged sitting or standing, but the iliacus muscle is relatively inactive during standing.[1] Patients often describe pain in the lower back when changing positions from sitting to standing, particularly arising from a deep seated chair. Coughing and deep breathing do not cause pain as they do with myofascial pain of the quadratus lumborum. Patients often elect to sleep in the fetal position at night, but they awaken from the fetal position and extend the back to get out of bed, thereby stretching the iliopsoas muscle. Iliopsoas pain may radiate to the hip and anterior thigh. Pain involving the

iliopsoas bursa can be an important source of unilateral hip and groin pain. Iliopsoas muscle tendinitis is seen with activities that require repetitive hip flexion and may result in a snapping hip. Iliopsoas bursitis is seen with overuse injuries in gymnasts and uphill runners and cyclists, presenting with anterior hip and groin pain.[19] Lumbar spinal stenosis most often affects L4-L5 then L3-L4 levels. Iliopsoas weakness, which may present as difficulty climbing stairs, has been described as an early sign of lumbar spinal stenosis because of its innervations by the muscles of the lumbar plexus.[20]

As with quadratus lumborum, myofascial pain involving the psoas muscle is a clinical diagnosis based on history and physical examination. Pathological processes involving the psoas muscle can be ruled out radiographically (e.g., hematoma and abscess). The physical examination starts with observation of the patient, including observation of the gait to look for an antalgic gait. It is difficult to palpate the iliopsoas muscle from the back, so provocative maneuvers will help with the diagnosis. The *Thomas test*, or inability to straighten the knee with the contralateral leg flexed while the patient is supine, has a positive result with a tight, contracted iliopsoas muscle. Pain is more often felt when rising from a seated position. Active straight-leg raise or resisted knee flexion causes pain. Prone hip extension that results in psoas stretch may also be painful. With iliopsoas bursitis, pain is felt with palpation at the insertion site in the femoral triangle at the lesser trochanter with the knee bent in the position used for the FABER (flexion abduction external rotation) test. Iliopsoas function is tested by passive testing of hip flexion strength; pain elicited by this maneuver may emanate from the iliopsoas.[21]

The iliopsoas muscle can cause hip pain because of snapping hip syndrome. One cause of this syndrome is the iliopsoas tendon's slipping over the lesser trochanter at the level of the osseous ridge. Pain is often felt in the groin and anterior thigh, and clicking is heard when the hip is extended, adducted, and laterally rotated. Otherwise, pain from the iliopsoas muscle is felt lateral to the lumbar spine and in the anterior thigh.

Anatomy

The iliopsoas is a combination of the psoas major, psoas minor, and iliacus muscles. The psoas major has its origin along the anterolateral vertebral column at the levels of T12-L4 and passes under the inguinal ligament to attach, along with the iliacus, as the iliopsoas muscle on the lesser trochanter of the femur. There is a large iliac bursa, which sometimes communicates with the hip joint.[14] The psoas minor is only variably present in a segment of the population and has its origin along the transverse processes of L1-L5; it is anterior to the psoas major. The iliacus muscle originates in the iliac fossa of the pelvis and occupies the anterior portion of the pelvic brim. The psoas major combines with the iliacus muscle at approximately the level of the inguinal ligament and inserts on the lesser trochanter of the femur to become the functional unit called the iliopsoas muscle. The iliopsoas muscle is the most powerful thigh flexor in the body, which is its main function. It lies deep or anterior and medial to the quadratus lumborum. The iliopsoas muscle is covered by the iliacus fascia. It is only directly palpable at the level of the femoral triangle.

The psoas major (ventral rami of L1-L3) and the iliacus (L2 and L3) share similar sources of innervations. The lumbar plexus is embedded in the psoas major. The iliacus muscle lies along the side of the psoas major and attaches to the tendon of the psoas major distally. The iliacus muscle is innervated by the femoral nerve (L2-L4) and the psoas major by the lumbar plexus (L1-L4). The psoas muscle is more associated with the leg and the quadratus with the hip.

The psoas muscles are arranged in a very homogenous fashion such that the bundles from each of the individual segments are of the same length. Compared with its function as the major hip flexor, its significance with respect to the lumbar spine is limited except to use the lumbar spine as a base for its action on the hip.[16,22] It is unique as a primary muscle of the leg in that its origins are from the lumbar spine.[22] It has very little influence in lumbar flexion or extension; however, the psoas muscle does exert significant stress on the lumbar spine in the form of tremendous axial compressive and shear forces on the lower lumbar spine, particularly at the L5-S1 disc space. It also serves to increase the lumbar lordosis of the spine. This is maximized in activities that contract the psoas (e.g., sit-ups).[22] EMG activity is controversial as to whether the iliopsoas plays some role in lateral rotation of the femur.[14,19] The psoas major is innervated by the anterior (ventral) rami of L1-L3. The nerves of the lumbar plexus pass through the psoas major on route to the lower extremity.

Basic Science

Imaging

No special imaging is needed to make the diagnosis; this is a clinical diagnosis.

Guidelines

There are no published guidelines regarding iliopsoas injections.

Indications and Contraindications

The indication is myofascial low back pain with or without radiation to the hip with reproducible trigger points. It is contraindicated in situations in which muscular injections are contraindicated (e.g., coagulopathy or bleeding diathesis, localized infection at the site, or systemic infection).

Equipment

- Materials for sterile prep and drape
- 3.5-inch spinal needle
- Local anesthetic with or without a small amount of steroid diluted in the local anesthetic solution
- Fluoroscopy machine

Technique

Palpation of Trigger Points It is only possible to palpate the psoas muscle at its insertion site in the groin. There are reports of injections at that site with local anesthetic and steroid with good relief of groin pain. However, for low back pain, it is not possible to inject trigger points based on palpation of the psoas in the lower back.

Fluoroscopic Guidance Sterile prep and drape are done. The L4 transverse process is visualized under fluoroscopy. Needle entrance is at the inferior edge of the transverse process, approximately 1 to 1.5 cm medial to the insertion site for the quadratus injection. The needed is advanced approximately 1 to 1.5 cm. One mL of nonionic contrast solution is injected to get good muscle spread along the psoas muscle (distinct pattern) without vascular spread. A lateral confirmatory view is obtained. Local anesthetic with or without steroid is injected. There should be no paresthesias, blood, or CSF with needle insertion. It is important to be mindful of the vascular structures (aorta and inferior vena cava) anterior and medial to the psoas muscle (**Figs. 22-2 and 22-3**).

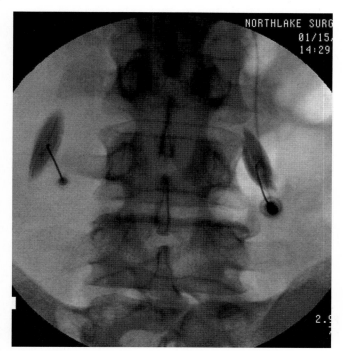

Fig. 22-2 Anteroposterior view of bilateral psoas muscle injections. Note the striated appearance of the contrast.

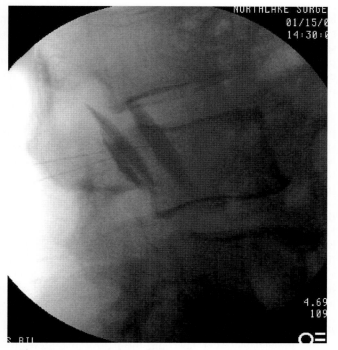

Fig. 22-3 Lateral view of bilateral psoas muscle injections.

Ultrasound Guidance The same comments apply for psoas trigger point injections under ultrasound guidance. Visualization of the muscle in overweight patients is very difficult.

Patient Management and Evaluation

For the best outcome, these injections are done in conjunction with physical therapy. Because some other interventions may be

responsive to steroid injections, injection of steroid should be kept to a minimum.

Outcomes Evidence

There is no outcomes evidence published.

Risk and Complication Avoidance

The iliopsoas muscle is lateral to the vertebral foramen and posterior to the lumbar sympathetic chain and the great vessels of the abdomen, so caution with needle depth is important. The needle is directed perpendicularly, avoiding the foramen medially.

Evaluation and Treatment of Pain from the Piriformis Muscle

Establishing a Diagnosis

Piriformis syndrome is a diagnosis that is often difficult to determine and can lead to misdiagnosis. Because the symptomatology is so variable and so similar to many more common pain pathologies, piriformis syndrome is often a diagnosis of exclusion. The differential diagnosis includes lumbosacral facet syndrome, sacroiliac joint arthropathy, hip arthritic conditions (including greater trochanteric bursitis), and even organic causes such as pelvic masses.

The most common complaint with piriformis syndrome is gluteal (buttock) pain. Nearly the entire buttock (spanning from the sacral margin to the greater trochanter) can be painful and tender. This pain is usually made worse with prolonged sitting (classic complaint of pain during a long car ride) and with sit-to-stand transfers.[23] It is rare to have associated axial back pain, although occasionally there can be associated paraspinal lumbar pain.[23] Furthermore, the gluteal pain may radiate into the entire posterior thigh proximal to the knee as a function of posterior cutaneous nerve of the thigh irritation.[24] If there is associated irritation of the entire sciatic nerve, symptoms can even extend all the way into the toes, although it is not common to develop true focal neurological deficits. Interestingly, because of the anatomical closeness of the piriformis muscle with the pelvic and abdominal walls, symptoms can occur with bowel movements and sexual activity.[23]

Historically, in about 50% of patients, there is an antecedent trauma. The traumatic event is not always direct trauma to the area, and there may be a lag of several months from the inciting trauma to the presentation of classic symptoms. The etiology of piriformis syndrome can even be total hip arthroplasty or spinal surgery.[25] Other causes are quite variable and include true leg length discrepancy (and associated gait abnormality and pelvic tilt), idiopathic piriformis hypertrophy, and altered piriformis anatomy.[26,27]

On examination, piriformis tenderness can be elicited with deep palpation, and a spindle-shaped mass may be felt in the buttock.[23] Although not specific for piriformis syndrome alone, symptoms are exacerbated by hip flexion, adduction, and internal rotation. Straight-leg raise results may or may not be positive based on whether or not the sciatic nerve is significantly affected. Sensory, motor, and reflex testing are almost always normal.[23] Three tests that have more specificity for piriformis syndrome are the Pace sign, Lasègue sign, and Freiberg sign:

- Pace sign: pain and weakness with seated abduction of the hip against resistance[28]
- Lasègue sign: pain with unresisted flexion, abduction, and internal rotation of the hip[29]
- Freiberg sign: pain with forced (i.e., against resistance) internal rotation of the hip with the thigh fully extended[30]

Anatomy

The proximal insertions of the piriformis muscle include the S2-S4 sacral vertebra, the sacroiliac joint capsule, and the posterior iliac spine.[26] From these insertions, the muscle spans laterally through the greater sciatic foramen and attaches distally to the medical surface of the greater trochanter. Innervation to the piriformis muscle is provided by the L5, S1, and S2 spinal nerves. The sciatic nerve (either in divided or undivided form) passes directly through the muscle, under the muscle (most commonly), or above the muscle in very close proximity. The gluteal nerves and vessels and the posterior cutaneous nerve to the thigh also traverse below the muscle.[23]

Basic Science

Similar to most skeletal muscles, direct trauma to the buttock can result in muscle spasm and release of proinflammatory mediators. Proinflammatory prostaglandins, histamine, bradykinin, and serotonin are released into the inflamed muscle belly (further propagating local inflammatory processes). Furthermore, because the sciatic nerve is so close to the piriformis, these same mediators can cause a chemical irritation of the sciatic nerve.[31] An inflamed and spastic piriformis muscle can also cause mechanical compression of the sciatic nerve.[26]

Imaging

Although magnetic resonance imaging (MRI) and computed tomography (CT) may show an enlarged piriformis muscle,[32] piriformis syndrome still is truly a clinical diagnosis made with thorough history and physical examination. Depending on the cut of the MRI and the fluctuations in muscle swelling and reactivity, the imaging study results may be negative despite significant disease of the tissue.

Guidelines

There are no printed guidelines for injections in the piriformis muscle.

Indications and Contraindications

The indication for a piriformis injection is gluteal pain (and associated symptoms) with historical and examination findings suggestive of piriformis muscle irritation. Piriformis injection is contraindicated with local site or systemic infections and any bleeding diathesis or coagulopathy. Because this structure is deep (and noncompressible) and in such close proximity to a major neural structure (the sciatic nerve), it is recommended to use all precautions that are used for a deep nerve block. Also, because fluoroscopic guidance is needed, piriformis injection is contraindicated in pregnant women.

Equipment

- Materials for sterile prep and drape
- 25-gauge 5- or 7-inch insulated nerve block needles, depending on the size of the patient
- Local anesthetic with or without a small amount of steroid diluted in the local anesthetic solution
- Fluoroscopy machine
- Nerve stimulator
- Radiographic contrast medium

Technique

In the technique described by Benzon et al,[31] the patient is placed prone on a fluoroscopy table, and the inferior margin of the

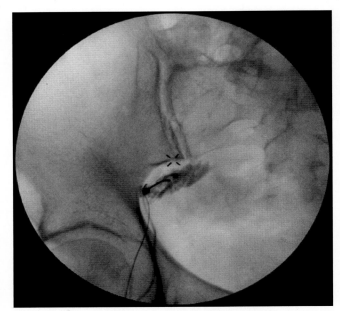

Fig. 22-4 The piriformis muscle is outlined after contrast injection.

sacroiliac joint is imaged and marked. Then an insulated block needle is inserted 1 to 2 cm caudad and 1 to 2 cm lateral to the inferior margin of the sacroiliac joint. The insulated needle should be advanced with the nerve stimulator on until a sciatic nerve–evoked motor response is achieved (dorsiflexion, plantarflexion, eversion, inversion). The needle is slightly withdrawn until the sciatic stimulation disappears. Steroid (40 mg of either methylprednisolone or triamcinolone) plus 5 mL of saline is injected perisciatically. The needle is pulled back 1 cm (into the belly of the piriformis muscle), and the contrast is injected (**Fig. 22-4**). The contrast should outline the piriformis muscle belly, which will either appear as one single muscle unit or two muscle bellies if the piriformis is split by the sciatic nerve. After the characteristic dye spread is achieved, local anesthetic solution and steroid are administered. Typically, good pain relief can be attained with an injection of 5 mL of 0.5% bupivacaine plus 40 mg of methylprednisolone (or triamcinolone).

A similar technique has been described using CT guidance, but the lack of readily available CT suites and the added radiation hazard limit this technique.[33] Further, similar blind techniques have been described as well as a perisciatic stimulator approach without fluoroscopic guidance.[34] Similarly, the piriformis muscle can be visualized with ultrasound although this requires a higher level of expertise with the ultrasound machine, especially in the obese patient.

Patient Management and Evaluation

Rarely, immediately after injection, the patient may develop a sciatic nerve block. This is reason for using saline, not local anesthetic, as the diluent for the perisciatic injection. Sciatic nerve block may still occur from leakage of the local anesthetic from the piriformis muscle or if the needle is not withdrawn far enough into the belly of the muscle. When sciatic nerve block occurs, the patient should be discharged with crutches (or a wheelchair) into the custody of an adult companion. In the long term, injections combined with physical therapy work best. Therapy should focus on correcting any sort of gait abnormality and pelvic tilt or obliquity as well as general core strengthening.

Outcomes Evidence

Using the technique described, Benzon and colleagues[31] were able to achieve some short- or long-term relief of symptoms in 16 of 19 patients. It should be noted that most of these patients had fairly severe and chronic pain with multiple pain generators (not isolated piriformis syndrome).

Risk and Complication Avoidance

Careful attention should be paid to a live fluoroscopic contrast injection to avoid injection into blood vessels. Furthermore, all precautions when performing a standard sciatic nerve block should be used (i.e., injection should be halted with painful paresthesia).

References

1. Simons DG, Travell J, Simons LLS: *Travell and Simons' myofascial pain and dysfunction: the trigger point manual*, ed 2, Philadelphia, 1999, Lippincott Williams & Wilkins.
2. Han SC, Harrison P: Myofascial pain syndrome and trigger-point management. *Reg Anesth* 22:89-101, 1997.
3. Testa M, Barbero M, Gherlone E: Trigger points: update of the clinical aspects. *Eur Med Phys* 39:37-43, 2003.
4. Hubbard DR, Berkoff GM: Myofascial trigger points show spontaneous needle EMG activity. *Spine* 18:1803-1807, 1993.
5. Rivner MH: The neurophysiology of myofascial pain syndrome. *Curr Pain Headache Rep* 5:432-440, 2001.
6. Huguenin LK: Myofascial trigger points: the current evidence. *Physical Ther Sports* 5:2-12, 2004.
7. Cummings TM, White AR: Needling therapies in the management of myofascial trigger point pain: a systematic review. *Arch Phys Med Rehabil* 82:986-992, 2001.
8. Foster AH, Carlson BM: Myotoxicity of local anesthetics and regeneration of the damaged muscle fibres. *Anesth Analg* 58:727-736, 1980.
9. Wald JJ: The effects of toxins on muscle. *Neurol Clin* 18:695-717, 2000.
10. Hong CZ: Myofascial trigger points: pathophysiology and correlation with acupuncture points. *Acupunct Med* 18:41-47, 2000.
11. Salmons S: Muscle. In *Gray's anatomy*, ed 38, St. Louis, 1995, Churchill Livingstone, pp 737-900.
12. Ranson C, Burnett A, O'Sullivan P, et al: The lumbar paraspinal muscle morphometry of fast bowlers in cricket. *Clin J Sport Med* 18:31-37, 2008.
13. Phillips S, Mercer S, Bodguk N: Anatomy and biomechanics of quadratus lumborum. *Proc Inst Mech Eng H* 222(2):151-159, 2008.
14. Porterfield JA, DeRosa C: Lumbopelvic musculature: structural and functional considerations. In *Mechanical low back pain: perspectives in functional anatomy*, ed 2, Philadelphia, 1998, WB Saunders, pp 53-119.
15. Knutson GA: Anatomic and functional leg-length inequality: a review and recommendation for clinical decision-making. Part II, the functional or unloaded leg-length asymmetry. *Chiropr Osteopat* 13:1-6, 2005.
16. Bogduk N: The lumbar muscles and their fascia. In Twomey LT, Taylor JR, editors: *Physical therapy of the low back*, ed 3, Philadelphia, 2000, Churchill Livingston, pp 105-139.
17. Kirchmair L, Entner T, Wissel J, et al: A study of the paravertebral anatomy for ultrasound-guided posterior lumbar plexus block. *Anesth Analg* 93:477-481, 2001.
18. Basmajian JV: Electromyography of the iliopsoas. *Anat Rec* 132(2):127-132, 1958.
19. Hip and thigh. In Percina MM, Bojanic I, editors: *Overuse injuries of the musculoskeletal system*, ed 2, Boca Raton, FL, 2004, CRC Press, pp 153-188.
20. LaBan MM: Iliopsoas weakness: a clinical sign of lumbar spinal stenosis. *Am J Phys Med Rehabil* 83:224-225, 2004.
21. Magee DJ: Hip. In *Orthopedic physical assessment*, ed 5, St. Louis, 2008, Saunders Elsevier.
22. Bogduk N, Pearcy M, Hadfield G: Anatomy and biomechanics of psoas major. *Clin Biomech* 7:109-119, 1992.
23. Parziale JR, Hudgins TH, Fishman LM: The piriformis syndrome. *Am J Orthop* 25:819-823, 1996.
24. Barton PM: Piriformis syndrome: a rational approach to management. *Pain* 47:345-352, 1991.
25. Cameron HU, Noftal F: The piriformis syndrome. *Can J Surg* 31:210, 1988.
26. Hallin RP: Sciatic pain and the piriformis muscle. *Postgrad Med* 74:69-72, 1983.
27. Chen WS: Bipartite piriformis muscle: an unusual cause of sciatic nerve entrapment. *Pain* 58:269-272, 1994.
28. Cameron HU, Noftal F: The piriformis syndrome. *Can J Surg* 31:210, 1988.
29. Robinson D: Piriformis syndrome in relation to sciatic pain. *Am J Surg* 73:355-358, 1947.
30. Freiberg AH: Sciatic pain and its relief by operations on muscle and fascia. *Arch Surg* 34:337-350, 1937.
31. Benzon HT, Katz JA, Benzon HA, Iqbal MS: Piriformis syndrome: anatomic considerations, a new injection technique, and a review of the literature. *Anesthesiology* 98:1442-1448, 2003.
32. Jankiewicz JT, Hennrikus WL, Houkom JA: The appearance of the piriformis muscle in computed tomography and magnetic resonance imaging: a case report and review of the literature. *Clin Orthop* 262:205-209, 1991.
33. Porta M: A comparative trial of botulinum toxin type A and methylprednisolone for the treatment of myofascial pain syndrome and pain from chronic muscle spasm. *Pain* 85:101-105, 2000.
34. Hanania M, Kitain E: Perisciatic injection of steroid for the treatment of sciatica due to piriformis syndrome. *Reg Anesth Pain Med* 23:223-228, 1998.

23 Ultrasound-Guided and Fluoroscopically Guided Joint Injections

Steve J. Wisniewski and Mark-Friedrich B. Hurdle

CHAPTER OVERVIEW

Chapter Synopsis: Injections for the control of painful conditions are not limited to the spine and peripheral nerves; peripheral joints also represent a significant target. This chapter describes the use of joint injections for both diagnostic and therapeutic purposes. Injection of anesthetic into a joint can help identify it as a source of debilitating pain, and injection of steroids can reduce the inflammatory conditions that may underlie the pain. Many clinicians are shifting from a traditional approach of palpatory, or "blind," injection techniques to guidance with various imaging techniques. The potential causes of pain can arise from a dizzying array of conditions that vary depending on the specific joint. The hip joints are subject to degenerative and inflammatory arthritis as well as mechanical stresses, and pain may manifest in many low-body sites. The deep and hidden nature of the hip joint makes it a good candidate for image assistance from fluoroscopy or ultrasonography. The glenohumeral or shoulder joint is similarly subject to arthritic and mechanical disruption that may be an elusive source of unidentified pain. The knee joint is also subject to arthritic conditions as well as bursitis, ligamentous trauma, and patellofemoral pain syndrome. Imaging guidance has also been used for injections of the elbow, wrist, ankle, and small joints of the hands.

Important Points:
- Joint injections are common procedures that have been successfully performed for decades.
- Although not all joint injections need to be performed with imaging guidance, ultrasonography and fluoroscopy are able to accurately guide successful injections when clinically indicated.

Clinical Pearls:
- Ultrasound or fluoroscopic guidance is indicated for certain joint injections when there is increased needle depth required (e.g., hip joint) or when important surrounding neurovascular structures are present.
- These imaging modalities are also helpful to ensure accurate needle placement when joints are being injected for diagnostic purposes.

Clinical Pitfalls:
- A thorough understanding of the advantages and disadvantages of ultrasonography and fluoroscopy is needed for successful use of the imaging modality.
- One must have a good knowledge of the surrounding anatomy involved in joint injections to ensure safe and accurate procedures.

Introduction

Peripheral intraarticular injections have been successfully used for several decades in several locations.[1] Injections may be performed into joints for diagnostic or therapeutic purposes (or both). Diagnostically, local anesthetic injection into a target area can facilitate identification of pain-generating structures and facilitate proper treatment.[2-7] Therapeutically, appropriately placed corticosteroid injections can reduce pain and inflammation and promote functional gains. For both diagnostic and therapeutic intents, precise placement of injectate may be necessary to optimize outcome.[8,9] Although peripheral joint injections have been traditionally performed primarily using palpatory landmarks (i.e., "blind"), the possibility of incorrect needle and injectate placement has led many clinicians to consider the use of image guidance for peripheral joint injections. Whereas an inappropriately placed injection will compromise the diagnostic utility of the procedure, incorrect placement of a therapeutic injectate such as corticosteroid or viscosupplementation may compromise outcome.

Numerous methods of image guidance can be used for peripheral joint injections, including fluoroscopy and ultrasound guidance. Fluoroscopy has been widely used for peripheral joint injections to ensure accurate needle placement. Fluoroscopy assists with intraarticular needle placement using direct visualization and confirmation of correct needle placement with a small injection of contrast.

More recently, ultrasonography has been used to ensure accurate and safe needle placement for a variety of interventional procedures, including joint injections.[10-24] Advantages of ultrasonography include no additional exposure to ionizing radiation, no use of contrast (thus lower cost and less risk of allergic reaction), and the ability to directly visualize surrounding soft tissue and neurovascular structures.

Hip Joint Injections

Establishing a Diagnosis

Pain coming from the hip joint can be caused by a variety of pathologic conditions, including degenerative and inflammatory arthritis, labral tears, avascular necrosis, and femoroacetabular impingement.[25] The pain is often felt in the groin, although pain in the buttocks, lateral hip, and thigh can also be referred from the hip joint. Even after performing a careful history, physical examination, and imaging studies, it can, at times, be challenging trying to differentiate between pain emanating from an intraarticular hip source versus pain referred from surrounding soft tissue structures or being referred pain from the spine. In this clinical situation, an intraarticular hip joint injection with anesthetic may provide useful information to ensure an accurate diagnosis.[2,7] Therapeutically, corticosteroid injections into the hip joint can reduce pain and inflammation.

Anatomy

The hip joint is a ball-and-socket joint that is located deep in the body. Because of this location, the hip joint cannot reliably be palpated. The capsule of the hip joint extends a considerable distance down the femoral neck, thus resulting in a relatively large target area for intraarticular injections. When performing hip joint injections, the location of the neurovascular bundle (femoral nerve, artery, vein), must be identified. These structures often overlie the medial aspect of the femoral head.

Imaging

Because of the deep location of the hip joint along with the femoral neurovascular bundle in close proximity to the target injection site, image guidance is recommended for this injection. Although previous studies have described hip joint injections using palpatory landmarks, the results were suboptimal and may have increased complications.[26,27] Using fluoroscopy, a straight anteroposterior (AP) view of the hip allows accurate visualization of the target area. Alternatively, ultrasonography may be used to visualize the femoral head and neck along with the overlying hip joint capsule in a sagittal oblique plane.[28-30] The proper ultrasound probe needs to be selected for the hip joint, depending on the patient's body habitus. Higher frequency linear ultrasound probes provide better spatial resolution but have less penetration to see deeper structures. Lower frequency curvilinear probes allow better depth penetration and a wider field of view but less spatial resolution.

Indications

Anesthetic injections into the hip joint may be helpful diagnostically to confirm the source of the patient's symptoms.[2,7] Lack of improvement suggests other causes for the patient's pain, such as surrounding soft tissue structures or referred pain from spine pathology. Therapeutically, corticosteroid injections may help with intraarticular pain and inflammation in the appropriate clinical situation.

Contraindications

- Systemic infection
- Skin infection over the injection site
- Pregnancy
- Allergy to medication or contrast dye
- Elevated international normalized ratio (INR), thrombocytopenia, use of anticoagulants or some platelet inhibitors

Equipment

- Needle to draw medications (18 or 19 gauge)
- Syringes (5 or 10 mL) for local anesthetic, injectate, contrast
- Needles for local anesthetic (25 or 27 gauge)
- Sterile towels or drapes
- Spinal needle for injection (usually 22 gauge, 9 cm; longer based on body habitus)
- Skin preparation solution (e.g., povidone–iodine, chlorhexidine)
- Local anesthetic agent (e.g., lidocaine, bupivacaine)
- Corticosteroid if therapeutic injection (e.g., methylprednisolone acetate injectable suspension, triamcinolone, betamethasone)
- Sterile tubing (for aspiration or fluoroscopy)
- Contrast agent (fluoroscopy)
- Surgical marker
- Sterile ultrasound probe cover, sterile ultrasound gel (for ultrasonography)

Technique

Fluoroscopically Guided Hip Joint Injection Fluoroscopically guided hip joint injections can be performed by a variety of approaches, including a direct vertical approach parallel to the fluoroscopic beam and an oblique approach from inferior/lateral to superior/medial. The vertical approach is described here. The patient is placed supine on the fluoroscopy table. A direct AP image over the hip joint to be injected is obtained (**Fig. 23-1**). After clear visualization of the femoral head and neck, a radiopaque object is then used to identify the proper location of needle insertion on the skin. The target site will be the lateral aspect of the femoral head–neck junction to avoid the neurovascular bundle that is usually located medially. Using a surgical marker, this location is then marked on the skin. The femoral artery should be palpated to identify the location of the neurovascular bundle. This location can also be marked on the skin with a surgical marker. The procedure field over the anterior hip should then be sterilely prepped and draped. Using a 25- or 27-gauge needle, the skin and subcutaneous tissue is then anesthetized using 1% lidocaine. Next, a 22-gauge

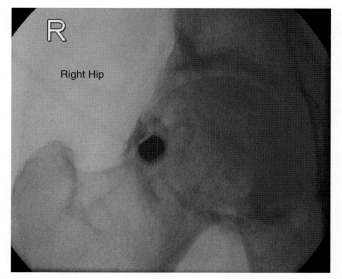

Fig. 23-1 Anteroposterior view of the right hip joint. The needle is placed at the lateral aspect of the femoral head-neck area to avoid the neurovascular bundle.

needle is advanced through the overlying soft tissues using intermittent fluoroscopy to ensure proper needle trajectory. Os should be contacted at the femoral head–neck junction. The needle is then slightly withdrawn 1 to 2 mm. After removal of the stylet from the spinal needle, sterile tubing with a syringe containing contrast is attached. A small amount of contrast is slowly injected under fluoroscopy to ensure intraarticular placement. The contrast should flow smoothly into the hip joint without significant resistance. If resistance is encountered, the needle should be adjusted slightly followed by repeat injection of contrast. Contrast should flow freely and away from the needle tip. A hip arthrogram should be obtained, confirming intraarticular needle placement. The syringe is then changed, and the injectate (anesthetic, corticosteroid, or both) is then slowly injected. After placement of the injectate into the hip joint, the needle is then removed, and the overlying area is cleaned.

Ultrasound-Guided Hip Joint Injection

The choice of ultrasound transducer depends on the patient's body habitus. High-frequency linear array transducers can be used on many patients, although the authors normally prefer to use a curvilinear, lower frequency probe to ensure adequate depth of penetration and to provide a wider field of view.

Numerous previous reports have described intraarticular hip joint injections under ultrasound guidance.[10,14,19-21,23,24] We follow the method previously described by one of the authors, which is described here.[21] The patient is placed in the supine position with the hip in a neutral position. The anterior-superior iliac spine is palpated, and the transducer is oriented in a sagittal plane with the superior end of the transducer located just medial to this structure. The transducer is then kept in the sagittal orientation and moved medially until the hyperechoic (i.e., bright), round femoral head is visualized. The transducer is then rotated into the transverse plane and moved medially to identify the femoral neurovascular bundle. This is easily visualized using color or power Doppler, which is usually now standard on most ultrasound machines. The transducer is then slid back laterally to the femoral head. The transducer is slowly rotated in the orientation of the femoral neck. During this rotation, the superior aspect of the ultrasound probe should keep the femoral head visualized while the inferior aspect of the probe will then bring the femoral neck into view (**Fig. 23-2**).

In this long-axis femoral head–neck view, the ultrasound settings (e.g., depth, gain) can then be further adjusted to provide the optimal image of the femoral head–neck junction and overlying hip joint capsule. While this sagittal oblique orientation is maintained, the examiner slowly slides the transducer medially and laterally to judge the width of the femur neck. The transducer should be positioned at the most lateral aspect possible while all structures are kept clearly in view, thus keeping the neurovascular bundle a greater distance away from the target needle trajectory. With the ultrasound transducer held steady, a surgical marker can then be used to outline the position of the inferior aspect of the ultrasound probe.

The procedure field over the anterior hip should then be sterilely prepped and draped. With a sterile ultrasound transducer cover and sterile ultrasound gel, the transducer is placed back onto the skin as previously marked, and an optimal image is obtained again. Local anesthesia is provided at the puncture site with 1% lidocaine under live ultrasound guidance. A 25-gauge needle is often used for this part of the procedure to anesthetize the skin and deeper subcutaneous layers. Next, a free-hand technique is used with the injectate syringe attached to a 22-gauge 9-cm (or longer based on the clinical situation) spinal needle. The needle is slowly advanced through the overlying soft tissues while the target femoral head–neck junction and needle tip are visualized at all times. The hip joint capsule can be visualized, and a "pop" is often felt as the needle advances through the capsule and into the hip joint. With the needle tip clearly in view, the injectate is then slowly injected while the hip capsule is visualized rising away from the femoral head and neck (**Fig. 23-3**). If corticosteroid is injected, it appears as hyperechoic (bright) under ultrasonography. If only local anesthetic is injected, it appears anechoic (dark) under ultrasonography. After the injection is completed, the needle is removed, and the area is cleaned.

Risk and Complication Avoidance

Complications are rare with hip joint injections if proper patients are selected (i.e., no active infections, no coagulation problems), sterile technique is followed, and proper injection technique is performed. As with other injections, potential complications

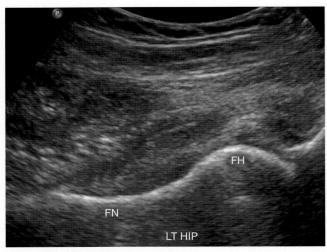

Fig. 23-2 Ultrasound image of the left hip joint with the transducer oriented in a longitudinal view. The top of the image is superficial, and the bottom is deep. FH, femoral head; FN, femoral neck.

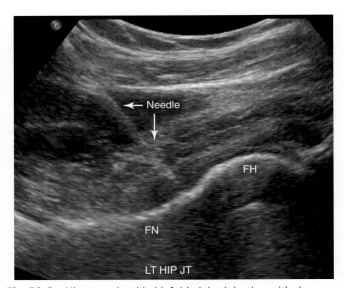

Fig. 23-3 Ultrasound-guided left hip joint injection with the needle tip accurately placed into the joint. *Arrows* point to the needle shaft. The top of the image is superficial, and the bottom is deep. FH, femoral head; FN, femoral neck.

include bleeding or bruising, infection, allergic reaction to medications, and temporarily increased pain. Injury to the neurovascular bundle (femoral nerve, artery, or vein injury) is a potential complication as well but should be minimized with proper preprocedure planning and proper technique.

Glenohumeral Joint Injections

Establishing a Diagnosis

Pain coming from the glenohumeral joint can be caused by a variety of pathological conditions, including degenerative arthritis, inflammatory arthritis, and labral tears. Multiple structures about the shoulder and cervical spine can cause pain. Even after a careful history, physical examination, and imaging studies, it may be difficult to determine the source of pain. In this clinical situation, accurate, selective injections may provide useful information to ensure an accurate diagnosis. Therapeutically, corticosteroid injections into the glenohumeral joint can reduce pain and inflammation.

Anatomy

The glenohumeral joint is a ball-and-socket joint. The humeral head is normally centered in the glenoid, but the labrum of the shoulder helps to deepen the socket of the glenohumeral joint and provide more support. Important neurovascular structures to be aware of during shoulder injections include the brachial plexus (including the axillary nerve) and the axillary artery, which are located medial and inferior to the glenohumeral joint. Posteriorly, the suprascapular nerve and artery are located medial to the glenohumeral joint in the spinoglenoid notch.

Imaging

Glenohumeral joint injections are often performed using only palpatory landmarks without image guidance. Previous studies, however, have shown poor accuracy with non-guided glenohumeral joint injections.[8,31] In the authors' experience, the glenohumeral joint is often located deeper than one would expect. This, in combination with the relatively small target size of the joint space, likely accounts for the reported poor accuracy of this injection performed without imaging guidance. To ensure accurate needle and injectate placement, either fluoroscopy or ultrasound guidance can be used successfully. Using fluoroscopy, a straight AP view of the glenohumeral joint allows accurate visualization of the target area. This injection is most commonly performed from an anterior approach. Alternatively, ultrasonography may be used to accurately perform a glenohumeral joint injection, usually with a posterior approach.[17,32]

Indications

Anesthetic injections into the glenohumeral joint may be helpful diagnostically to confirm the source of the patient's symptoms. Lack of transient pain relief suggests other causes for the patient's pain, such as surrounding shoulder structures or referred pain from cervical spine pathology. Therapeutically, corticosteroid injections may help with intraarticular pain and inflammation when clinically appropriate.

Contraindications

- Systemic infection
- Skin infection over the injection site
- Pregnancy
- Allergy to medication or contrast dye

- Elevated INR, thrombocytopenia, use of anticoagulants or platelet inhibitors

Equipment

- Needle to draw up medications (18 or 19 gauge)
- Syringes (5 or 10 mL) for anesthetic, injectate, contrast
- Needles for local anesthetic (25 or 27 gauge)
- Sterile towels or drapes for injection site
- Needle for injection (usually a 25-gauge, 5-cm needle or 22-gauge, 6.5-cm or 9-cm spinal needle)
- Skin preparation solution (e.g., povidone–iodine, chlorhexidine)
- Local anesthetic agent (e.g., lidocaine, bupivacaine)
- Corticosteroid if therapeutic injection (e.g., methylprednisolone acetate injectable suspension, triamcinolone, betamethasone)
- Sterile tubing (for aspiration or fluoroscopy)
- Contrast agent (fluoroscopy)
- Sterile ultrasound probe cover, sterile ultrasound gel (for ultrasonography)
- Surgical marker

Technique

Fluoroscopically Guided Glenohumeral Joint Injection

Fluoroscopically guided glenohumeral joint injections can be performed with an anterior or a posterior approach. The anterior approach is described here. The patient is placed supine on the fluoroscopy table with the hand supinated. A direct AP image over the glenohumeral joint is obtained. After clear visualization of the joint space between the humerus and glenoid, a radiopaque object is then used to identify the proper location of needle insertion on the skin. The target for the injection is approximately one third of the way up from the inferior aspect of the joint, aiming closer to the humeral head than the glenoid.[33] Using a surgical marker, this location is then marked on the skin. The procedure field over the anterior glenohumeral joint should then be sterilely prepped and draped. Using a 25- or 27-gauge needle, the skin and subcutaneous tissue is then anesthetized using 1% lidocaine. Next, a 22-gauge, 6.5-cm or 9-cm needle is advanced through the overlying soft tissues using intermittent fluoroscopy to ensure proper needle trajectory. Bone is contacted on the medial side of the anterior humeral head. The needle is then slightly withdrawn and redirected medially into the glenohumeral joint (**Fig. 23-4**). After removal of the stylet from the spinal needle, sterile tubing with a syringe containing contrast is attached. A small amount of contrast is slowly injected under fluoroscopy to ensure intraarticular placement. The contrast should flow smoothly into the glenohumeral joint without significant resistance. If resistance is encountered, the needle should be slightly adjusted or the bevel turned followed by repeat injection of contrast. A glenohumeral joint arthrogram should then be obtained, confirming intraarticular needle placement (**Fig. 23-5**). The syringe is then changed, and the injectate (anesthetic, corticosteroid, or both) is then slowly injected. After placement of the injectate into the glenohumeral joint, the needle is then removed, and the overlying area is cleaned.

Ultrasound-Guided Glenohumeral Joint Injection

The choice of ultrasound transducer will depend on the patient's body habitus. High-frequency linear array transducers can be used on most patients, although the authors often use a curvilinear, lower frequency probe to ensure adequate depth of penetration and provide a wider field of view.

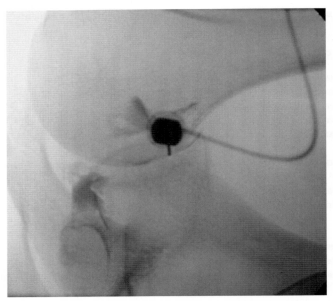

Fig. 23-4 Anteroposterior view of the left glenohumeral joint. Note the needle in the glenohumeral joint just medial to the humeral head.

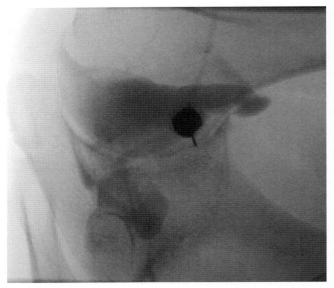

Fig. 23-5 Anteroposterior view of the left glenohumeral joint after significant contrast injection.

Similar to fluoroscopy, there are varying ways to access the glenohumeral joint using ultrasound guidance. The authors prefer a posterior approach that has been previously described.[17,32] The patient is placed in the lateral decubitus position with the target shoulder facing upward. The shoulder can be adducted across the body. The spine of the scapula is palpated, and then the transducer is placed just inferior to this in the posterior/lateral aspect of the shoulder. The hyperechoic (i.e., bright) humeral head is then identified. This can be confirmed with passive shoulder internal or external rotation. The transducer is slid either medial or lateral to identify the posterior labrum, spinoglenoid notch, and posterior humeral head. The target for the injection is between the medial aspect of the humeral head and the triangular-shaped posterior

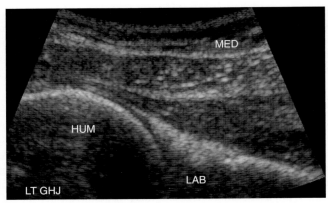

Fig. 23-6 Ultrasound image of the posterior left glenohumeral joint. The top of the image is superficial, and the bottom is deep. HUM, humeral head; LAB, posterior labrum; LT, left; GHJ, glenohumeral joint; MED, medial.

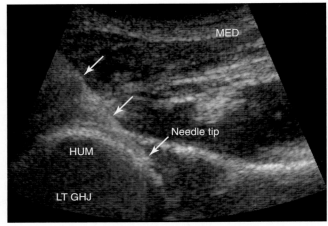

Fig. 23-7 Ultrasound-guided left glenohumeral joint injection with the needle in place. *Arrows* indicate the needle shaft and tip. The top of the image is superficial, and the bottom is deep. HUM, humeral head; LT, left; GHJ, glenohumeral joint; MED, medial.

labrum (**Fig. 23-6**). The target area should be located close to the side of the transducer where the needle will enter the skin. With the ultrasound transducer held steady, a surgical marker can then be used to outline the position of the lateral aspect of the ultrasound probe.

The skin over the posterior shoulder should then be sterilely prepped and draped. With a sterile ultrasound transducer cover and sterile ultrasound gel, the transducer is placed back onto the skin as previously marked, and an optimal image of the glenohumeral joint is again obtained. Local anesthesia is then provided at the insertion site with 1% lidocaine under live ultrasound guidance. A 25-gauge, 5-cm needle is often used for this part of the procedure to anesthetize the skin and deeper subcutaneous layers. Next, a free-hand technique is used with the injectate syringe attached to a 22-gauge, 6.5-cm or 9-cm spinal needle. The needle is slowly advanced through the overlying soft tissues while the targeted posterior glenohumeral joint and needle tip are visualized at all times. The needle tip is advanced into the joint capsule until it is visualized between the humeral head and the posterior labrum (**Fig. 23-7**). The medication is then slowly injected. If corticosteroid is injected, it appears as hyperechoic (bright) under ultrasonography. If only local anesthetic is injected, it appears anechoic (dark) under ultrasonography. After the injection is completed, the needle is removed, and the area is cleaned.

Risk and Complication Avoidance

Complications are rare with glenohumeral joint injections if proper patients are selected (i.e., no active infections, no coagulation problems), sterile technique is followed, and proper injection technique is performed. As with other injections, potential complications include bleeding or bruising, infection, allergic reaction to medications, and temporarily increased pain. Injury to a neurovascular structure is a potential complication as well but should be minimized with proper pre-procedure planning and proper technique.

Knee Joint Injections

Establishing a Diagnosis

Knee pain can be caused by multiple conditions, including bursitis, ligamentous trauma, patellofemoral pain syndrome, inflammatory arthritis, and osteoarthritis. Pain is typically felt directly within the knee, although pain can be referred into both the thigh and lower leg. A detailed history, physical examination, and imaging studies can help localize the pain generator. However, at times, diagnostic intraarticular knee injections can assist in making the correct diagnosis.[34] Therapeutically, corticosteroid and viscosupplementation injections have been shown to reduce pain associated with knee osteoarthritis.[35,36]

Anatomy

The knee is a hinge joint that is relatively superficial. The joint can normally be easily palpated during the physical examination. The capsule of the knee extends proximally to the suprapatellar synovial bursa, laterally into the lateral recesses, posteriorly to the proximal femoral condyles, and distally to the femoral tibial joint space.

Imaging

The superficial structures of the knee joint are readily visualized via ultrasonography. Using ultrasonography, the knee joint capsule (suprapatellar recess) can be visualized deep to the quadriceps tendon between the quadriceps fat pad and the prefemoral fat pad just proximal to the patella. Effusions can often be appreciated at this location. Effusions may also be visualized medially or laterally to the patella under the patellar retinacula. When visualized, these hypoechoic or anechoic (i.e., dark) effusions are usually accessible to aspiration and injection. When no effusion is visible, the medial patellar portal may be used with visualization of the distal patella, Hoffa's fat pad, and the medial femur. In patients with a lower body mass index, a linear probe can be used to visualize the capsule lateral to the patella. In patients with larger knees, a curvilinear probe may be needed to visualize the joint capsule proximal to the patella and deep to the quadriceps tendon. Patients with posterior knee pain may have a Baker's cyst, which is commonly visualized between the gastrocnemius and semimembranosus tendon.[37]

Indications

Multiple pain generators are in close proximity to the knee capsule, including the collateral ligaments and numerous tendons, muscles, and bursae. At times, even after a careful history and physical examination, it may be difficult to discern if the primary pain generator is located within the joint capsule. A guided intraarticular knee injection may help confirm the diagnosis. Injections may also be therapeutic in the treatment of inflammatory arthritis or osteoarthritis.

Contraindications

- Systemic infection
- Skin infection over the injection site
- Pregnancy
- Allergy to medication or contrast dye
- Elevated INR, thrombocytopenia, use of anticoagulants or platelet inhibitors

Equipment

- Syringes (5 or 10 mL) for local anesthetic, injectate, contrast
- Needle to draw up medications (18 or 19 gauge)
- Needle for local anesthetic (25 or 27 gauge)
- Sterile towel or drapes
- Skin prep solution (e.g., povidone–iodine, chlorhexidine)
- Corticosteroid (e.g., methylprednisolone acetate injectable suspension, triamcinolone, betamethasone)
- Sterile tubing (for aspiration or fluoroscopy)
- Contrast agent (Omnipaque 300)
- Sterile ultrasound probe cover, sterile ultrasound gel (for ultrasonography)
- Surgical marker

Technique

Fluoroscopically Guided Knee Joint Injection   There are a variety of approaches to fluoroscopically guided knee injections. These include the lateral or medial patellofemoral joint approach as well as the anterior approach.[38] The lateral patellofemoral joint approach is described here. The patient is placed on the fluoroscopy table in the supine position. The knee to be injected is flexed 20 to 30 degrees with a pillow or towel placed under the joint for comfort. The patella is palpated, and the groove between the patella and femur is marked with a surgical marker. The anterior knee is then sterilely prepped and draped. A 25- or 27-gauge needle is used to anesthetize the skin and subcutaneous tissue. With one hand manually displacing the patella medially, a 19- or 22-gauge needle is advanced under the patella into the patellofemoral joint. After the stylet is removed, sterile tubing and a syringe containing 1 to 2 cc of local anesthetic is attached. There should be minimal resistance when this small volume is injected as a test dose. Next, 1 to 2 cc of contrast agent (either Omnipaque or gadolinium) is injected. If the contrast does not spread easily in the typical capsular pattern or if significant resistance is encountered, the needle should be repositioned. The beginning of a knee arthrogram should be obtained. The injectate is then slowly injected. After the injection is completed, the needle is removed, and the area is cleaned.

Ultrasound-Guided Knee Joint Injection   Patients with a larger body habitus with poorly defined bony anatomical landmarks or advanced osteoarthritis with minimal joint space may benefit from ultrasound-guided knee injections. Typically, a linear probe can be used for visualization of the patellofemoral joint and lateral recesses; a curvilinear probe may be needed to image the suprapatellar synovial bursa.

Two reports have described techniques for ultrasound-guided intraarticular knee injections.[14,39] The authors typically use the methods described by Qvistgaard and colleagues[14] with some modifications. The patient is placed in the supine position. The symptomatic knee is flexed to 30 to 70 degrees, depending on where the fluid is best visualized in the suprapatellar recess. After the patella is palpated, a linear probe is placed over the quadriceps tendon in

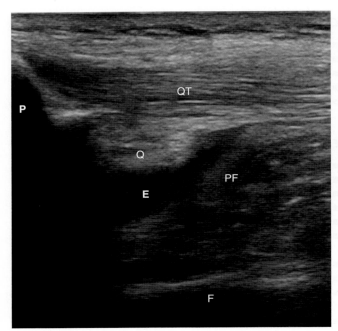

Fig. 23-8 Long-axis ultrasound view of the proximal anterior knee with a subclinical effusion (E). The top of the image is superficial, and the bottom is deep. Left is distal, right is proximal. F, femur; P, patella; PF, prefemoral fat pad; Q, quadriceps fat pad; QT, quadriceps tendon.

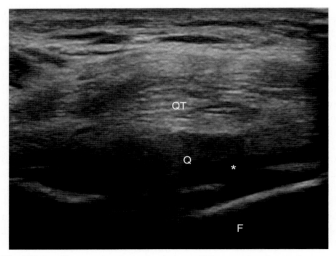

Fig. 23-9 Short-axis ultrasound view of the proximal anterior knee with a subclinical effusion (*) in the suprapatellar pouch. The top of the image is superficial, and the bottom is deep. F, femur; Q, quadriceps fat pad; QT, quadriceps tendon.

the longitudinal axis with the proximal aspect of the patella visible distally. The quadriceps tendon, quadriceps fat pad, and prefemoral fat pad and femur can usually be well visualized. The hypoechoic suprapatellar synovial bursa or collapsed joint recess lies between the quadriceps fat pad and prefemoral fat pad (Fig. 23-8). The probe is then rotated 90 degrees to a short-axis view of the quadriceps tendon (Fig. 23-9). The skin lateral to the transducer is then palpated to estimate the needle trajectory with the goal of avoiding the quadriceps tendon. The skin is then marked with a surgical marker and prepped in the usual sterile fashion.

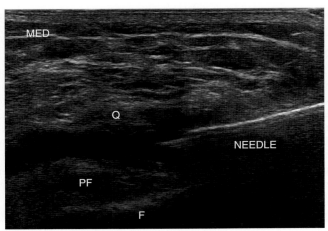

Fig. 23-10 Short-axis ultrasound view of the proximal anterior knee with long-axis view of a 22-gauge needle placed into the suprapatellar pouch from lateral to medial. The top of the image is superficial, and the bottom is deep. F, femur; MED, medial; PF, prefemoral fat pad; Q, quadriceps fat pad.

Using a 25- or 27-gauge needle, 1% lidocaine is injected to anesthetize the superficial tissue and skin. This can be done under direct ultrasound guidance to help visualize the correct path for the larger needle. Next, using a free-hand technique, a 22- or 25-gauge needle is slowly advanced through soft tissue until the needle tip is positioned between the quadriceps fat pad and prefemoral fat pad (Fig. 23-10). If no obvious effusion is visible for aspiration, local anesthetic can be injected to ensure proper needle tip placement. The injectate should flow with minimal resistance. A small effusion should become apparent in the proper tissue plane between the quadriceps tendon and prefemoral fat pad. After proper needle placement is confirmed, either corticosteroid or viscosupplementation can be injected. Corticosteroid particles are usually visible under ultrasonography. After the injection, the needle is then removed, and the site is cleaned.

Risk and Complication Avoidance

The neurovascular structures of the knee are located posterior to the knee capsule. Complications of knee injections are rare if proper precautions are observed and sterile technique is observed. Potential complications include bleeding, infections, allergic reactions, and worsening of symptoms.

Other Peripheral Joint Injections

Practitioners have used ultrasonography to guide multiple other peripheral joint procedures, including the elbow, wrist, ankle, and small joints of the hands (carpometacarpal, metatarsophalangeal, proximal interphalangeal joints). Rheumatologists have found ultrasound guidance helpful when fluid aspiration is needed for diagnostic purposes.[40] In a study to evaluate clinical outcomes, Sibbitt and colleagues[41] found that ultrasound-guided injections of both large and small peripheral joints provided increased pain relief 2 weeks after the procedure. Compared with palpation-guided injections, the response rate increased by 62%.

In conclusion, peripheral joint injections have been completed for both diagnostic and therapeutic purposes for at least 6 decades. Initially, these procedures were completed using only palpatory landmarks for guidance. More recently, fluoroscopy and ultrasonography have been used with increased accuracy.[10-12,20,22,38] To date, limited studies have directly correlated peripheral injection accuracy with efficacy.[41] More studies are needed to firmly establish this relationship. The authors of this chapter believe that when clinically indicated, fluoroscopy and ultrasonography allow physicians to perform safe, accurate peripheral joint injections, which may reduce the risk of complications and improve clinical outcomes.

References

1. Hollander JL, Brown EM, Jr, Jessar RA, Brown CY: Hydrocortisone and cortisone injected into arthritic joints; comparative effects of and use of hydrocortisone as a local antiarthritic agent. *J Am Med Assoc* 147(17):1629-1635, 1951.
2. Braunstein EM, Cardinal E, Buckwalter KA, Capello W: Bupivacaine arthrography of the post-arthroplasty hip. *Skeletal Radiol* 24(7):519-521, 1995.
3. Mitchell MJ, Bielecki D, Bergman AG, et al: Localization of specific joint causing hindfoot pain: value of injecting local anesthetics into individual joints during arthrography. *AJR Am J Roentgenol* 164(6):1473-1476, 1995.
4. Khoury NJ, el-Khoury GY, Saltzman CL, Brandser EA: Intraarticular foot and ankle injections to identify source of pain before arthrodesis. *AJR Am J Roentgenol* 167(3):669-673, 1996.
5. Crawford RW, Ellis AM, Gie GA, Ling RS: Intra-articular local anaesthesia for pain after hip arthroplasty. *J Bone Joint Surg Br* 79(5):796-800, 1997.
6. Lucas PE, Hurwitz SR, Kaplan PA, et al: Fluoroscopically guided injections into the foot and ankle: localization of the source of pain as a guide to treatment—prospective study. *Radiology* 204(2):411-415, 1997.
7. Crawford RW, Gie GA, Ling RS, Murray DW: Diagnostic value of intra-articular anaesthetic in primary osteoarthritis of the hip. *J Bone Joint Surg Br* 80(2):279-281, 1998.
8. Jones A, Regan M, Ledingham J, et al: Importance of placement of intra-articular steroid injections. *BMJ* 307(6915):1329-1330, 1993.
9. Partington PF, Broome GH: Diagnostic injection around the shoulder: hit and miss? A cadaveric study of injection accuracy. *J Shoulder Elbow Surg* 7(2):147-150, 1998.
10. Carson BW, Wong A: Ultrasonographic guidance for injections of local steroids in the native hip. *J Ultrasound Med* 18(2):159-160, 1999.
11. Koski JM: Ultrasound guided injections in rheumatology. *J Rheumatol* 27(9): 2131-2138, 2000.
12. Grassi W, Farina A, Filippucci E, Cervini C: Sonographically guided procedures in rheumatology. *Semin Arthritis Rheum* 30(5):347-353, 2001.
13. Koski JM, Hermunen H: Intra-articular glucocorticoid treatment of the rheumatoid wrist. An ultrasonographic study. *Scand J Rheumatol* 30(5):268-270, 2001.
14. Qvistgaard E, Kristoffersen H, Terslev L, et al: Guidance by ultrasound of intra-articular injections in the knee and hip joints. *Osteoarthritis Cartilage* 9(6):512-517, 2001.
15. Sofka CM, Collins AJ, Adler RS: Use of ultrasonographic guidance in interventional musculoskeletal procedures: a review from a single institution. *J Ultrasound Med* 20(1):21-26, 2001.
16. Sofka CM, Adler RS: Ultrasound-guided interventions in the foot and ankle. *Semin Musculoskelet Radiol* 6(2):163-168, 2002.
17. Adler RS, Sofka CM: Percutaneous ultrasound-guided injections in the musculoskeletal system. *Ultrasound Q* 19(1):3-12, 2003.
18. Migliore A, Martin LS, Alimonti A, et al: Efficacy and safety of viscosupplementation by ultrasound-guided intra-articular injection in osteoarthritis of the hip. *Osteoarthritis Cartilage* 11(4):305-306, 2003.
19. Migliore A, Tormenta S, Martin LS, et al: Open pilot study of ultrasound-guided intra-articular injection of hylan G-F 20 (Synvisc)

20. in the treatment of symptomatic hip osteoarthritis. *Clin Rheumatol* 24(3):285-289, 2005.
20. Sofka CM, Saboeiro G, Adler RS, et al: Ultrasound-guided adult hip injections. *J Vasc Interv Radiol* 16(8):1121-1123, 2005.
21. Smith J, Hurdle MF: Office-based ultrasound-guided intra-articular hip injection: technique for physiatric practice. *Arch Phys Med Rehabil* 87(2):296-298, 2006.
22. Smith J, Hurdle MF, Locketz AJ, Wisniewski SJ: Ultrasound-guided piriformis injection: technique description and verification. *Arch Phys Med Rehabil* 87(12):1664-1667, 2006.
23. Sofka CM, Adler RS, Danon MA: Sonography of the acetabular labrum: visualization of labral injuries during intra-articular injections. *J Ultrasound Med* 25(10):1321-1326, 2006.
24. Smith J, Hurdle, MF, Weingarten TN: Accuracy of sonographically guided intra-articular injections in the native adult hip. *J Ultrasound Med* 28(3):329-335, 2009.
25. DeAngelis NA, Busconi BD: Assessment and differential diagnosis of the painful hip. *Clin Orthop Relat Res* (406):11-18, 2003.
26. Leopold SS, Battista V, Oliverio JA: Safety and efficacy of intraarticular hip injection using anatomic landmarks. *Clin Orthop Relat Res* 391:192-197, 2001.
27. Ziv YB, Kardosh R, Debi R, et al: An in expensive and accurate method for hip injections without the use of imaging. *J Clin Rheumatol* 15(3):103-105, 2009.
28. Koski JM, Anttila PJ, Isomäki HA: Ultrasonography of the adult hip joint. *Scand J Rheumatol* 18(2):113-117, 1989.
29. Moss SG, Schweitzer ME, Jacobson JA, et al: Hip joint fluid: detection and distribution at MR imaging and US with cadaveric correlation. *Radiology* 208(1):43-48, 1998.
30. Iagnocco A, Filippucci E, Meenagh G, et al: Ultrasound imaging for the rheumatologist III. Ultrasonography of the hip. *Clin Exp Rheumatol* 24(3):229-232, 2006.
31. Sethi PM, Kingston S, Elattrache N: Accuracy of anterior intra-articular injection of the glenohumeral joint. *Arthroscopy* 21(1):77-80, 2005.
32. Cicak N, Matasovi T, Bajraktarevi T: Ultrasonographic guidance of needle placement for shoulder arthrography. *J Ultrasound Med* 11(4):135-137, 1992.
33. Peterson JJ, Fenton DS, Czervionke LF: *Image-guided musculoskeletal intervention*, Philadelphia, 2008, Saunders Elsevier.
34. Malfair D: Therapeutic and diagnostic joint injections. *Radiol Clin North Am* 46(3):439-453, v, 2008.
35. Adams ME, Atkinson MH, Lussier AJ, et al: The role of viscosupplementation with hylan G-F 20 (Synvisc) in the treatment of osteoarthritis of the knee: a Canadian multicenter trial comparing hylan G-F 20 alone, hylan G-F 20 with non-steroidal anti-inflammatory drugs (NSAIDs) and NSAIDs alone. *Osteoarthritis Cartilage* 3(4):213-225, 1995.
36. Ravaud P, Moulinier L, Giraudeau B, et al: Effects of joint lavage and steroid injection in patients with osteoarthritis of the knee: results of a multicenter, randomized, controlled trial. *Arthritis Rheum* 42(3):475-482, 1999.
37. Ward EE, Jacobson JA, Fessell DP, et al: Sonographic detection of Baker's cysts: comparison with MR imaging. *AJR Am J Roentgenol* 176(2):373-380, 2001.
38. Freiberger RH, Pavlov H: Knee arthrography. *Radiology* 166(2):489-492, 1988.
39. Im SH, Lee SC, Park YB, et al: Feasibility of sonography for intra-articular injections in the knee through a medial patellar portal. *J Ultrasound Med* 28(11):1465-1470, 2009.
40. Balint PV, Kane D, Hunter J, et al: Ultrasound guided versus conventional joint and soft tissue fluid aspiration in rheumatology practice: a pilot study. *J Rheumatol* 29(10):2209-2213, 2002.
41. Sibbitt WL, Peisajovich A, Michael AA, et al: Does sonographic needle guidance affect the clinical outcome of intraarticular injections? *J Rheumatol* 36(9):1892-1902, 2009.

Index

A

A-alpha fiber damage, 90
Abdominal aortic dissection, CPB complication, 93
Abdominal ganglia, 91f
Abdominal pain, placebo (impact), 43
A-beta fiber damage, 90
Ablative neurosurgical techniques, usage, 52
Achilles tendon, identification, 73
Activity-related axial pain, PV/PK candidates (selection), 194
Acupuncture, 211
Acute herpes zoster, 77
Adductor brevis, posterior branch, 68-69
Adductor canal, proximal patella (median distance), 72
Adductor longus, anterior branch, 68-69
A-delta fiber damage, 90
Adjacent-level fractures, 195-196
    increase, PV/PK (impact), 195-196
Advanced cardiac life support (ACLS), importance, 18
A fibers, 39
    subtypes, 39
Alcock's canal, imaging technique, 112
Alcohol, neurolytic action, 89-90
American Pain Society Clinical Practice Guideline for Low Back Pain, 123-124
American Society of Interventional Pain Physicians (ASIPP) guidelines, 144-145
Amide local anesthetics, pharmacology, 17t
Analgesia, three-in-one block, 43
Anatomical survey, 42
Anesthetic discography, description, 9
Ankle block, 72-73
    landmark approach, 73
    subsustentacular approach, 73
    ultrasound approach, 73
Ankles
    innervation, 72
    lateral aspect, ultrasound image, 73f
    medial aspect, saphenous nerve (blockade), 73
Annuloplasty
    complications, incidence, 189
    procedures, 188
        complications, 189
        documentation, 188t
    usage, 186-187
Antecrural celiac plexus neurolysis, performing, 92f
Anterior neck, short-axis sonogram, 80f
Anterior obturator branch, demonstration, 68f
Anterior superior iliac spine (ASIS), visualization, 96
Anterior tubercle, C5 transverse process (short-axis transverse ultrasound images), 212f

Anterior tubercle, C6 transverse process (short-axis transverse ultrasound images), 212f
Artery, femoral nerve (relationship), 66f
Articular branches, 213
Artifacts, knowledge, 201-202
Ascending cervical artery, impact, 211
Aseptic meningitis, 94
Asthma, history, 23
Astrocyte activation, marker, 21f
Atlanto-axial joint (AAJ) anatomy, 54, 54f
Atlanto-axial joint (AAJ) injections, 54-57
    complications, 56-57
    diagnostic indication, 54
    efficacy, 56
    indications, 54
    needle target, sonogram, 57f
    prognostic injection, 54
    technique, 54-55
    therapeutic indication, 54
Atlanto-axial joint (AAJ) pain, prevalence, 56
Atlanto-occipital joint (AOJ) anatomy, 54, 54f
Atlanto-occipital joint (AOJ) injections, 54-57
    anteroposterior view, 56f
    complications, 54, 56-57
    efficacy, 56
    lateral view, 56f
    sonogram, 56f
    technique, 56
Atlas, inferior articular process (inferior margin), 54-55
At-risk patients, contrast media (requirement), 24
Atypical facial pain, 77
Automated percutaneous lumbar discectomy (APLD), 9
Axial neck pain, 149
    differential diagnosis, irradiation (absence), 150t
Axial pain, complaints, 9
Axilla, probe placement, 41
Axillary brachial plexus, ultrasound image, 61f

B

Backache, CPB complication, 93
Back lumbar region, cross section, 218f
Back pain
    injection
        target identification, 140-141
        techniques, 140-144
    patient management, 134
Balloon placement, anteroposterior/lateral radiographs, 195f
Bathed length principle, 39
Bell palsy, 77
Benzyl alcohol, usage, 19-20
Beta-blocking agents, usage, 24
Betamethasone, micrograph, 19f
B fibers, 39
Biceps femoris, tendon (identification), 44
Bilateral block, incidence (reduction), 64-65

Bilateral psoas muscle injections
    anteroposterior view, 221f
    lateral view, 221f
Biofeedback, 211
Bipolar intradiscal biacuplasty probes, usage, 186f
Bleeding, occurrence, 94
Blind fascia iliaca block, 67-68
Blood vessels, smooth muscle, 83f
Body mass index (BMI)
    measurement, 69
    ultrasound frequency ranges, 202
Body parts, total radiation, 31t
Bony surfaces
    identification, fluoroscopy (usage), 79
    visualization, ultrasonography (usage), 210
Border nerves, 106-110
Brachial plexus
    accessibility, 58
    anatomy, 58-59, 59f
    depth/accessibility, 58
    illustration, 59f
    indications/contraindications, 59
    in-plane lateral/medial ultrasound-guided needle approach, 60
    nerve stimulator, 59
    trunks, interscalene blockade, 60
    ultrasound, 59-60
Brachial plexus blockade
    accomplishment, 59
    axillary technique, 61-62
    equipment, 59-60
    infraclavicular technique, 60-61
    in-plane lateral to medial ultrasound-guided needle approach, usage, 60
    Raj approach, 60-61
    supraclavicular technique, 60
    techniques, 60-62
Brevis muscles, anterior branch, 68-69
Broad-based disc bulging, 123f

C

C1-C2 joint (atlanto-axial joint), attention, 131-132
C2, lateral view, 142f
C2-C3 facet joint
    attention, 131-132
    difference, 138
C2-C3 level, sagittal (longitudinal) ultrasonographic view, 214f
C3, lateral view, 141f-142f
C3, left lateral view, 142f
C3-C4 zygapophyseal joint, C3 articular pillar supply, 213
C3 dorsal ramus, medial branches (difference), 213
C4, anteroposterior view, 142f
C4, lateral view, 141f-142f
C4, left lateral view, 142f
C5, anteroposterior view, 142f
C5, lateral view, 141f

Page numbers followed by *f*, *t*, and *b* indicate figures, tables, and boxes, respectively.

C5, left lateral view, 142f
C6, anteroposterior view, 142f
C6, short-axis sonogram, 80f
C6 anatomy, 211f
C6-C7 zygapophyseal joint, needle
    advancement, 141
C7, short-axis sonogram, 80f
    curved transducer, usage, 81f
C7, transverse process, 141
C7-T1 facet (blocking), C8 medial branch
    block (usage), 141
C8 medial branch, course, 138
C8 medial branch block, requirement, 141
Calcitonin gene-related peptide, presence, 137
C-arm, caudo-cranial angulation
    (requirement), 133-134
Carotid sinus reflex (cessation), procaine
    (usage), 6
Catheter breakage, 189
Cauda equina syndrome, 189
Causalgia, 77
Celiac plexus
    anatomy, 90
    anterocrural nerve approach, 90
    approaches, 90
    cross-sectional view, 92f
    neurolysis, 90-93
        indication, 90
        procedure, 90-91
    posterior view, 92f
    retrocrural nerve approach, 90
    splanchnic nerve approach, 90, 92f
Celiac plexus block (CPB)
    abdominal aortic dissection, 93
    backache, 93
    complications, 91-93
    cross-sectional view, 92f
    diarrhea, 93
    efficacy, 93
    paraplegia, 93
    pneumothorax, 93
Central nervous system (CNS), dysfunction, 39
Central pain, 39
Cerebrospinal fluid (CSF)
    aspiration, 51
    leaks, evidence, 5
    volume, replacement, 5-6
Cervical disc stimulation
    false-positive response, 8-9
    risks/complications, 9
Cervical dorsal rami medial branches, third
    occipital nerve (comparison), 141
Cervical epidural, gadolinium-based contrast
    (usage), 23f
Cervical facet pain, 149-155
    anatomical localization, 154
    background, 149
    equipment, 153b
    evidence scores/implications, summary,
        154t
    history, 149-150
    indications/contraindications, 152-153
    interventional management, evidence, 155t
    intraarticular steroid injections, 154
    outcomes evidence, 154
    patient management/evaluation, 154
    radiation pain, 149f
    risk/complication avoidance, 155
    technique, 153-154
    treatment, practice algorithm, 152f
Cervical facets, 130, 132-133
    anatomy, 150-151
    corticosteroid injections, 153

Cervical facets (Continued)
    degenerative signs, clinical findings, 149
    diagnosis, establishment, 149-150
    diagnostic blocks, 150
    differential diagnosis, 150
    false-positive results, minimization,
        150
    imaging, 151-152
    intraarticular injection
        lateral approach, 133f
        sonoanatomy/ultrasound-guided
            technique, 213
    joints, location, 131
    physical examination, 150
Cervical facet syndrome, definition, 149
Cervical innervation, 138
Cervical joint pain, treatment, 152
Cervical medial branch
    anatomy, 212-213
    injections, 212-214
Cervical medial branch blocks (cervical
    MBBs), 140-141, 214
    lateral approach, 214
    literature review, 213
    needle placement, 140-141
    outcomes evidence, 145-146
    positioning, 140
    risks/complications, 146
    sonoanatomy, 213-214
    target zones, 140f
    ultrasound-guided technique, 213-214
Cervical medial branch neurotomy (cervical
    MBB)
    descriptions, 7
    premise, 7
Cervical periradicular injections,
    ultrasonography (usage), 211
Cervical posterior rami, medial branches,
    138
Cervical radicular pain
    clinical practice algorithm, 124f
    guidelines (World Institute of Pain
        publication), 124
    PRF, application, 175
Cervical ramus medialis
    medial branch, radiofrequency treatment,
        153f
    posterolateral approach, 153f
Cervical spinal column, lateral view, 151f
Cervical spinal nerve
    anatomy, 211
    location, 211
Cervical sympathetic block, 76-81
    anatomy, 76-77
    anterior neck, short-axis sonogram, 80f
    antiseptic skin preparation, 78
    C6, anterior approach, 78
    C6, short-axis sonogram, 80f
    C7, anterior approach, 78
    C7, short-axis sonogram, 80f-81f
    complications, 81-82
        list, 81-82
    fluoroscopy, usage, 78
    injectate, caudal spread (anteroposterior
        view), 81f
    T1, long-axis sonogram, 81f
    T2 anterior approach, 81
    technique, 78
        limitations/evolution, 78-79
    ultrasound-guided cervical sympathetic
        block, 79-80
    ultrasound-guided injection, technique,
        80-81

Cervical sympathetic chain
    anatomical representations, 77f
    components, 76
Cervical transforaminal equipment/technique,
    125
Cervical vertebral column
    degenerative signs, 149
    innervation, 151f
Cervical zygapophyseal joints, innervation,
    213
C-fiber afferents, 90
C fibers, 39
Chemical neurolysis, 89-90
    usage, 89
Chest wall, cross section, 105f
Chondromalaciafacetae, 136
Chronic pain management
    American Society of Anesthesiologists Task
        Force on Chronic Pain Management
        guidelines, 132
    American Society of Regional Anesthesia
        and Pain Medicine guidelines,
        132
    imaging, 134
Clonidine
    effects, 22f
    sciatica treatment, 20
    usage, 20
Cluster headache, parasympathetic outflow
    (activation), 46-47
Coagulation profile, level, 194
Coblation, 196-197
    nucleoplasty, 190
    plasma-mediated radiofrequency ablation,
        usage, 197
Cocaine
    injections, effects, 3
    intrathecal injections, attempt, 4
    usage, 3
Color-flow Doppler ultrasonography, usage,
    201
Complex regional pain syndrome (CRPS), 42
    types, 77
Computed tomography (CT), 29-30
    absorbed dose, 30
    CT-guided image, usage, 30
    discovery, 29
    organ doses, 30
    radiation doses, variation, 30
    safety concerns, 30
    scanners
        expense/sophistication, 29
        installation, 29
    scans, number (estimation), 30f
    usage, 28
Contrast agents, 21-24
    adverse events, 23-24
        anxiety, impact, 23-24
        incidence, 22-23
    injection, 55
    pharmacology, 21-22
    premedication, 24
Contrast-induced nephrotoxicity (CIN), 24
Contrast media
    adverse reactions, severity/manifestations
        (classification), 24t
    osmolality, impact, 21-22
    radiopaque characteristics, 21
    reactions, delay, 24
    requirement, 24
Contrast opacities, 22f
Contrast reaction, prediction, 23
Controlled diagnostic blocks, usage, 137

Conventional radiofrequency (CRF), 174
  application, 174
Cooled bipolar radiofrequency technology,
  usage, 181
Cooled radiofrequency SIJ neurotomy, 168b
  technique, 169-170
Cord damage, risk (increase), 40
Corticosteroids, 18-20
  complications, 19-20
  introduction/application, 18
  particulate steroid complications, 19
Cortisone (Compound E), discovery, 4
Cortoss
  bis-phenol-a-glycidyldimethacrylate
    (bis-GMA) resin, basis, 197
  cement, 197
Current perception thresholds (CPTs), usage,
  44
Curved array transducer, 201f
Cytokine, release, 22f

D

Decremental conduction, 40
Deep cervical artery, impact, 211
Deep peroneal nerve, block, 73
  success rate, 73
Dekompressor, 9
  clinical studies, 190t
  device, 181f, 189-190
    efficacy, studies, 189-190
  introducer/stylet, placement, 189
  technology, nuclear disc material extraction,
    189
Descending genicular artery, color-flow
  Doppler (usage), 71f
Diagnostic blocks, positive response (ASIPP
  usage), 144-145
Diagnostic differential nerve blocks (DDNBs)
  anatomical approach, 42-43
    description, 42-43
    interpretation, 43
    limitations, 43
  classic approach, 40
    description, 40
    interpretation, 40
    limitations, 40
  epidural approach, 41-42
    description, 41
    interpretation, 42
    limitations, 42
  modified approach, 38, 41
    description, 41
    interpretation, 41
    limitations, 41
  neural anatomy, variations, 43-44
  neurophysiological data, 43
  opioid approach, 38, 42
    description, 42
    interpretation, 42
    limitations, 42
  sodium channel packing, 40
Diagnostic differential neural blocks (DDNBs),
  37-38
  anatomical approach, 38
  approach, variation, 38
  basis, 39
  decremental conduction, 40
  discussion, 43-44
  epidural approach, 38
  frequency-dependent block, 40
  historical perspective, 38

Diagnostic differential neural blocks (DDNBs)
    (Continued)
  lipophilic local anesthetic, usage, 39
  local anesthetic, concentrations (impact),
    43
  usage, evidence, 43
Diagnostic SIJ injections, criteria, 168b
Diagnostic ultrasonography (sonography), 29
Diaphragmatic crura, 92f
Diarrhea, CPB complication, 93
Differential block strategy, epidural space
  (usage), 7
Differential nerve blockade, concept, 38
Differential neural blockade, 37-38
  mechanisms, proposal, 39-40
Differential spinal block, theory (challenge), 7
Differential spinal blockade, 6-7
Digital imaging and communication in
  medicine (DICOM), 32
Diplopia, development, 49
Disc
  cross-sectional area, 179f
  endoperoxides, 180f
  herniation
    mechanisms, 189-190
    pressure, exertion, 189
  stimulation (provocation discography),
    8-9
  surface area, circumferential area, 179f
  thermal annular procedures, development,
    187
Discitis, 82
  complication, rarity, 189
Discogenic low back pain, prevalence, 178-179
Discogenic lower back pain, 185-186
  pain relief mechanism, annuloplasty
    (usage), 186-187
  radiofrequency, application, 187
Discogenic pain
  pathologic condition, 122
  provisional diagnosis, 185-186
  treatment, algorithm, 187f
Discography
  diagnostic tool, popularity, 178
  history/background, 178-179
  pain elicitation, 180
DiscTRODE, usage, 181
Disease-modifying anti-rheumatic drugs
  (DMARDs), usage, 20
Dissected knee, medial view, 72f
Distal adductor canal, saphenous nerve, 71f
Distal sciatic nerve block, impact, 70
Dorsalis pedis artery, identification, 73
Dorsal root ganglia (DRG), PRF (usage), 175
Dorsal sacral foramina, lateral aspect (left
  S1-S3 finder needle placement), 171f
Dry needling, usage, 211
Dural punctures, headaches (association), 5
Dysesthesias, ethyl alcohol (association), 90

E

Early postherpetic neuralgia, 77
Emphysema, 82
Epidural anesthesia, cocaine injection
  (impact), 3
Epidural blood patch, 5-6
Epidural injections
  experiments, 5
  improvement, fluoroscopy (usage), 5
  modifications, 5
  transition, 5

Epidural space
  access, caudal approach (usage), 4
  transforaminal approach, 5
Epidural steroids
  formulation, chemical entities, 20t
  injection, commonness, 5
Epistaxis, frequency, 49
Erector pili muscles, 83f
Erector spinae aponeurosis (ESA), 157f
Esophageal penetration, 82
Etanercept, immune modulation properties, 20
External iliac artery, long-axis view, 109f
Extremity, radicular/referred pain (impact),
  189
Eye, dryness, 49

F

Facet arthropathy, 130
Facet capsule nerve endings, substances, 137
Facet interventions, indication, 132
Facet intraarticular joint injections
  patient management/evaluation, 134
  prevalence, 129-130
Facet joint block, target point (needle
  position)
  anteroposterior view, 208f
  lateral view, 208f
Facet joint injections, 206-208, 212-214
  history/literature, 206
  possibility, 200
  technique, 206-208
Facet joint–mediated pain, 205
Facet joint–mediated pain (diagnosis),
  placebo-controlled/controlled local
  anesthetic diagnostic blocks (usage),
  136
Facet joints, 137-138
  anatomy, 131-132, 137-138, 212-213
  architecture/orientation, 131
  C3-C7 innervation, 151
  cervical innervation, 138
  fibrous capsule, 213
  hypertrophy, 123f
  hypoechoic articular processes, sagittal
    (longitudinal) ultrasonographic view,
    214f
  imaging, 134
  inflammatory changes, 155-156
  injection, risk/complication avoidance,
    134
  innervation, 131, 138-139, 151f
    blocks, usage, 205
    nerve endings, impact, 137
  local pressure pain, 150
  location, 150
  lumbar innervation, 138-139
  orientation, 138
  paramedian long-axis (longitudinal view),
    203
  paramedian long-axis view (longitudinal
    view), 203f
  paramedian short-axis view (transverse
    view), 208f
  pathological changes, prevalence rate,
    158
  photograph, 205f
  septic arthritis, 155
  term, origination, 137
  thoracic innervation, 138
  zygapophyseal joints, targeting (injections/
    procedures), 7

Facet nerve blocks
    possibility, 200
    ultrasound guidance, 204-205
Facetogenic pain, determination, 130
Facet syndrome (FS)
    PRF application, 175
    validity, 155-156
Fascia iliaca
    block, technique, 68
    local anesthetic, ultrasound-guided
        deposition, 67-68
Fascia lata, needle travel, 67
Fascia split, layers, 108f
Feet, innervation, 72
Femoral iliac artery, long-axis view, 109f
Femoral nerve (FN), 66
    artery, relationship (ultrasound image), 66f
    formation, 66
    target structure, confirmation, 67
    ultrasound-guided block, 66
    ultrasound-guided technique, anatomical
        landmarks, 68
    variable innervation, 68-69
Femoral three-in-one block, 68-69
Fibers
    blockage, 6t
    diameter, 39
Fluoroscopic-guided glenohumeral joint
        injection, 227
Fluoroscopic-guided hip joint injection,
        225-226
Fluoroscopic-guided knee joint injection, 229
Fluoroscopy, 31-32
    beginnings, 31
    disadvantages, 32
    image storage, 32
    radiation safety, 32
    safety concerns, 32
    usefulness, increase, 32
Foramen ovale
    approach, 54f
    needle tip, oblique submental view, 51f
Frequency-dependent block, 40
Functional anesthetic discography (FAD), 9,
        179-180
    confirmatory findings, 180
Functional discography, 179-180

G

Gadodiamide (Omniscan), GBCM categories,
        25
Gadolinium, 24-26
    adverse reactions, 25-26
Gadolinium-based contrast media (GBCM),
        24-25
    acute reactions, frequency, 25
    confirmatory test, 24-25
    GBCM-related adverse events, 25-26
    tolerance/safety, 25
Gadopentate dimeglumine (Magnevist),
        GBCM category, 25
Gamma knife therapy, 50
Ganglion impar, posterior/lateral views, 98f
Ganglion impar neurolysis, 96-99
    anatomy, 96
    complications, 50
    efficacy, 50
    fluoroscopy, usage, 96
    indications, 96
    performing, 99f
    procedure, 96

Gasserian ganglion
    anatomy, 50-52
    neuroablative procedures, complications,
        52t
    percutaneous radiofrequency
        thermocoagulation, 50
    pulsed radiofrequency
        ablation, 50
        application, 175
    radiofrequency thermocoagulation
        efficacy, 52
        technique, 51-52
Gasserian ganglion block, 50-52
    complications, 52
    technique, 50-51
Genital branch, visualization difficulty,
        109-110
Genitofemoral (GF) nerve (border nerves),
        106-110
    anatomical studies, 107
    anatomy, 107
    block, description, 109
    genital branch, ultrasound-guided
        blockade, 109
    origination, 107
    pathway, schematic diagram, 107f
    sonoanatomy, 107
    technique, 108-109
Genitofemoral (GF) neuralgia, 111
Glenohumeral joint injections, 227-229
    contraindications, 227
    diagnosis, establishment, 227
    equipment, 227
    indications, 227
    risk/complication avoidance, 228-229
    technique, 227-228
Glenohumeral joints
    anatomy, 227
    diagnosis, establishment, 227
    imaging, 227
Glia
    activation, occurrence, 21f
    fibrillary acidic protein, 21f
    structure, 20
Global Perceived Effect Scale, 154
Glomerular filtration rate (GFR), level,
        25
Glucocorticoids, production, 19
Gluteus maximus muscle
    identification, 69-70
    local anesthetic, 44
    subgluteal approach, 69
Greater sciatic notch, piriformis muscle
        (interaction), 114
Greater trochanter, lateral border
        (identification), 43-44
Groin
    crease, ultrasound image, 68f
    local anesthetic solution injection,
        ultrasound scan, 67f

H

Head
    blocks, importance, 46
    preganglionic fibers, impact, 77
Helicoil GE (ultra-fast tomography scanner),
        30f
Hematoma formation, occurrence, 49
Herpes zoster, diagnosis, 6
High-frequency linear ultrasound probe scan,
        usage, 42

High-osmolality contrast media (HOCM),
        21
    protection, 24
    usage, 22-23
High-voltage intradiscal PRF, 9
High-volume epidural injections, trials, 5
High-volume local anesthetic injections, usage,
        66
Hip joint injections, 224-226
    complications
        avoidance, 226
        rarity, 226
    contraindications, 225
    equipment, 225
    procedure field, preparation/draping, 226
    risk, avoidance, 226
    technique, 225-226
Hip joints
    anatomy, 225
    diagnosis, establishment, 224-225
    imaging, 225
    location, 225
    pain, diagnosis (establishment), 224-225
Horner syndrome, 82

I

Idiopathic trigeminal neuralgia, PRF impact
        (randomized controlled trial), 175
Iliacus fascia block, 67-68
Iliacus innervation, 220
Iliohypogastric (IH) nerve (border nerves),
        106-110
    anatomical studies, 107
    anatomy, 107
    pathway, schematic diagram, 107f
    presence, 108f
    sonoanatomy, 107
    technique, 108-109
    transversus abdominis muscle, interaction,
        107
    ultrasonography, usage, 108-109
    ultrasound-guided injection technique,
        109-110
    ultrasound scanning, area
        (recommendation), 107
Ilioinguinal (IL) nerve (border nerves),
        106-110
    anatomical studies, 107
    anatomy, 107
    pathway, schematic diagram, 107f
    presence, 108f
    sonoanatomy, 107
    technique, 108-109
    ultrasonography, usage, 108-109
    ultrasound-guided injection technique,
        109-110
    ultrasound scanning, area
        (recommendation), 107
Iliopsoas
    anatomy, 220
    equipment, 220
    imaging, 220
    injections, guidelines (absence), 220
    role, 219-220
Iliopsoas muscle injections, 219-220
    diagnosis, establishment, 219-220
Image storage, 32
Imaging equipment, advantages/disadvantages,
        102t
Inferior thyroid vessel, retropharyngeal
        hematoma source, 79-80

Inflammatory arthritides, 136
Infraclavicular block, 59
Infraclavicular brachial plexus, ultrasound image, 61f
Inguinal area, nerves, 111f
Inguinal hernia repair pain, 6
Injectate, caudal spread (anteroposterior view), 81f
In-plane (IP) injections, needle insertion points, 201f
Intentional dural puncture, documentation, 3
Intercostal muscles, ultrasonographic image, 106f
Intercostal nerve (ICN), 104-106
    anatomy, 105
    block, performing, 105
    branches, 105f
    fluoroscopic technique, performing, 105
    in-plane/out-of-plane technique, recommendation, 106
    skin/musculature supply, 104
    sonoanatomy, 105
    techniques, 105-106
    ultrasound-guided injection technique, 106
    ultrasound scanning, 105
    ventral rami, 105
Intercostal pleura, ultrasonographic image, 106f
Interlaminar cervical epidural, 126f
Interleukin-1β (IL-1β), 20
Interleukin-6 (IL-6), 20
Internal disc disruption, 8, 179
Interneural injection, commonness, 44
Interscalene brachial plexus, ultrasound image, 61f
Interscalene groove, 59
Interspinous vessels, cocaine injection, 3
Interventional pain management
    contraindications, 153
    procedures, image guidance, 28
    techniques, 153
Intervertebral disc
    bipolar intradiscal biacuplasty probes, usage, 186f
    degeneration, 179
    dehydration, 186-187
    heating procedures, electrode positions (fluoroscopic views), 185f
    nuclear material, loss, 186-187
    problems, 179
    protrusion/herniation, 179
Intervertebral disc herniation
    basic science, 122
    radiculopathy, association, 122
    types, 189f
Intraarticular anesthetic injection, outcomes evidence, 134
Intraarticular corticosteroid injections, 158
Intraarticular facet joint corticosteroid injections, description, 7
Intraarticular hip joint injections, 226
Intraarticular steroid injections, 154
Intractable orofacial pain syndromes, 31
Intractable pain, treatment (interventional procedures), 89
Intradiscal biaculoplasty, 9, 188-189
    clinical data, 188-189
    fluoroscopy guidance, 188
    invasiveness, 185
Intradiscal catheter, placement, 180f
Intradiscal electrothermal annuloplasty, 9

Intradiscal electrothermal therapy (IDET), 187
    catheter, 181f
    invasiveness, 185
    procedure, requirement, 187
    resistive coil, 186f
    results, improvement, 187
    technology, reliance, 187
Intradiscal material removal, Dekompressor (usage), 181f
Intradiscal procedures, 181
Intradiscal radiofrequency, 9
Intradiscal treatments, 9
Intramuscular trigger point injections, 208
    possibility, 200
Intrathecal injections
    attempt, 4
    experiments, 5
Intrathecal space, medication (injection), 21
Intravascular injections, 82
    effects, 146
    occurrence, 49
    seizures/cardiac arrest/toxic reactions, 65
Intravenous (IV) access, securing, 69
Iodinated contrast medium, usage, 22-23
Iodine, contrast agent, 21
Iodine-based contrast, CIN problems, 24
Iodine-based contrast media, types, 21-22
Iodine-based intrathecal contrast, 25t
Iohexol (Omnipaque), usage, 22
Iopamidol (Isovue-M), usage, 22
Ischial tuberosity, identification, 43-44
Isotherm probe, temperature moderation, 165f

K

Knee, dissection (medial view), 72f
Knee joint injections, 229-230
    contraindications, 229
    equipment, 229
    indications, 229
    risk/complication avoidance, 230
    technique, 229-230
Knee joints
    anatomy, 229
    diagnosis, establishment, 229
    imaging, 229
Knobology, 201
Kyphoplasty
    clinician training, requirement, 194
    general anesthesia, usage, 194
    invasiveness, minimum, 193-194
    monitored anesthesia care (MAC), usage, 194
    vertebroplasty, contrast, 196, 196b

L

L1-L4 rami, medial branches, 139
L2-L3 left disc extrusion, T2-weighted axial MRI, 122f
L3-L4, cross sectional preparation, 66f
L3 rami dorsales/facet, radiofrequency treatment
    lateral view, 160f
    oblique view, 160f
L4, anteroposterior view, 145f
L4, lateral view, 144f
L4 rami dorsales/facet, radiofrequency treatment
    lateral view, 160f
    oblique view, 160f

L5, anteroposterior view, 145f
L5, lateral view, 144f
L5 dorsal ramus
    needle placement, 169
    probe placement, lateral view, 170f
    target/probe insertion, 170f
L5 medial branch, course, 139
L5 rami dorsales/facet, radiofrequency treatment
    lateral view, 160f
    oblique view, 160f
L5 target nerve, 144
Lateral atlantoaxial joint injection, 54
    anteroposterior view, 55f
    joint space, contrast (containment), 55f
    median, contrast spread, 55f
    needle, location, 55f
Lateral branch block, 168
    technique, 169
Lateral branches, RF/PRF, 167
Lateral femoral cutaneous nerve (LFCN), 110-111
    anatomy, 110-111
    appearance, 111
    branches, 110
    identification problems, 111
    pathway, 110f
    peripheral nerve, 110-111
    sensory innervation, 110
    sonoanatomy, 110-111
    ultrasonographic picture, 111f
    ultrasound-guided injection technique, 111
Left glenohumeral joint, anteroposterior view, 228f
Left hip joint, ultrasound, 226f
Left L2 transforaminal epidural, 126f
Left shoulder
    superior view, 103f
    suprascapular fossa, muscle layers, 103f
    suprascapular nerve/branches, 102f
Legs
    external rotation, 69
    flexion, 70
        preservation, distal sciatic nerve block (usage), 70
    obturator nerve entry, 43
    positioning, 65
    saphenous nerve block sites, medial aspect, 72f
Lesion size/volume, increase (method), 187
Ligamentum flavum hypertrophy, 123f
Linear transducer, 201f
Local anesthetics, 17-18
    action
        duration, defining (difficulty), 17-18
        pKa/hydrophobocity, effects, 17t
    adverse reactions, 18
    blind infiltration, landmark-based techniques, 108
    blocks, false-positive rates, 137
    impact, 17
    metabolism, 18
    onset speed, 17
    properties, 17
    reactions, result, 18
    role, 39
    spread, short-axis transverse ultrasound image, 212f
    systemic toxicity, 18
    toxicity, 18
    usage, 217

Local anesthetic systemic toxicity (LAST)
  incidence
    epidemiological studies, 18
    reduction, 18
  practice advisory, 18t
  recognition, 18
Longus colli muscle
  anterior surface, contrast agent spread
    (anteroposterior view), 79f
  carotid sheath, contrast agent spread
    (anteroposterior view), 79f
  contrast agent spread, anteroposterior view,
    78f
Low back pain
  causes, 156t
  facet joint–mediated pain, impact, 205
  sacroiliac joint, impact, 8
  work time, loss, 185
Lower back (myofascial pain), muscles
  (involvement), 217
Lower limb blocks
  landmark-guided/ultrasound-guided
    approaches, 64
  landmark techniques, 66-67
  ultrasound technique, 67
Low-osmolality contrast media (LOCM),
  21
  protection, 24
  usage, 22-23
Lumbar discogenic pain, diagnosis/treatment,
  185
Lumbar discography, MRI (comparison),
  179
Lumbar epidural, iodinated contrast (usage),
  23f
Lumbar facet joint pain
  complication, avoidance, 161
  conservative management, 158
  description, 130
  diagnostic blocks, 159
    complications, 161
  false-negative blocks, 149
  guidelines, 158
  history, 156
  indications/contraindications, 159
  interventional management, 158
  intraarticular corticosteroid injections,
    158
  origination, 155-161
  outcomes evidence, 160
  patient management/evaluation, 160
  radiofrequency treatment, 158-159
    complications, 161
  Revel criteria, 156
  risk, avoidance, 161
  technique/equipment, 159-160
Lumbar facet joints
  anatomy, 156-158
  imaging, 158
  innervation, nerve fibers (impact), 138
  physical examination, 156
  radiofrequency treatment, 159-160
  target point, innervation, 205
Lumbar facet nerve block, 204-206
  history/literature, 204-205
  technique, 205-206
Lumbar facetogenic pain
  diagnosis, establishment, 130
  prevalence, 129-130
Lumbar facet pain
  interventional pain management, evidence,
    160t
  treatment, practice algorithm, 160f

Lumbar facets, 130, 133-134
  diagnosis, establishment, 155-156
  innervations, schematic, 131f
  intraarticular injection, 133f
  pain
    background, 155-156
    research, 149
Lumbar innervation, 138-139
Lumbar medial branch blocks (lumbar MBBs),
  143-144
  description, 7
  needle placement, 143-144
  outcomes evidence, 145-146
  positioning, 143
  possibility, 200
  risks/complications, 146
  ultrasound guidance, 204-205
Lumbar nerve root injection, 208
Lumbar paravertebral planes, 202-204
Lumbar paravertebral region, longitudinal
  sonogram, 65f
Lumbar percutaneous disc procedures, usage,
  185
Lumbar periradicular injections, 208
  possibility, 200
Lumbar plexus
  block, 64-65
    clinical utility, 65
  inguinal paravascular approach, 66
  location, 66f
  medial nerve, 67-68
Lumbar radicular pain, PRF application,
  175
Lumbar spinal column
  anatomy, 157f
  transverse histological section, 157f
Lumbar spine
  processus articularis superior, posterior
    enlargement, 156
  sonoanatomy, 202-204
  sonography, scanning sequence, 202-204
  structure, posterior view (illustration),
    137f
Lumbar sympathetic block, 82-86
  anatomy, 82-83
  bleeding, occurrence, 94
  bony contact, 84
  classic approach (paramedian), 84
  complications, 85-86
    list, 85
  description, 84
  illustration, 96f
  indications, 83-84
  injection, 84
  interventional pain medicine, 83-84
  lateral approach, 84
  needle placement, 85
  oblique radiographic view, 84f
  patient placement, prone position, 84
  skin temperature changes
    degree, 85
    evaluation, 85
  technique, 84-85
  temperature monitoring, 84-85
Lumbar sympathetic blockade, indication, 83
Lumbar sympathetic chain
  anatomy, 94
  blockage, 93-94
  location, 94
  preganglionic/postganglionic efferent fibers,
    82-83
  separation, 83
Lumbar sympathetic ganglia, 96f

Lumbar sympathetic neurolysis, 93-94
  aseptic meningitis, 94
  complications, 94
  efficacy, 94
  indications, 93-94
  neuraxial injection, accident, 94
  paraplegia, 94
  performing, fluoroscopy (usage), 95f
  postdural puncture headache, 94
  procedure, 94
  renal/ureter penetration, 94
Lumbar sympathetics, blockade, 84
Lumbar transforaminal epidural steroidal
  injections, 124-125
Lumbar zygapophyseal joints, referred pain,
  139
Lung pleural/parenchyma, puncture
  (avoidance), 90-91

M

Magnetic resonance imaging (MRI)
  lumbar discography, comparison, 179
  usage, 28
Magnus muscles, posterior branch, 68-69
Mandibular nerve block, 52-53
  anterior "foramen oval" approach, 53
  illustration, 54f
  lateral "pterygoid plate" approach, 53
  technique, 53
Maxillary artery injury, 31
Maxillary nerve block, 52-53
  contrast agent, spread, 53f
  needle direction, 53f
  technique, 52-53
Meckel's cavity, 50
Medial branch anatomy, 206f
Medial branch blocks (MBBs), 204-206
  anatomy, 137-138
  concordant response, 137
    prolongation, 137
  contraindications, 139-140
  diagnosis
    establishment, 136-137
    facilitation, injections (usage),
      136-137
  discordant prolongation response, 137
  discordant response, 137
  discrepant response, 137
  history, 136, 204-205
  imaging, 139
  indications, 139-140
  interventional pain management
    techniques, 153
  literature, 204-205
  pain referral patterns, 139
  patient management/evaluation, 144-145
  physical examination, 136
  purpose, 139-140
  response patterns, 137
  risks/complications, 146
  science, 139
  sonogram, transverse view, 207f
  spine phantom, immersion, 206f
  target point, needle placement
    anteroposterior view, 207f
    lateral view, 207f
  technique, 205-206
  usage, ease, 136
Medial branch displacement, C7 transverse
  process (impact), 141
Medial branches, referred pain, 139

Medial branch nerves, segmental level innervation, 138
Medial malleolus, identification, 73
Medial thigh, ultrasound images, 68f
Mediastinal infection, 82
Meniscoid entrapment, 136
Microvascular decompression (MVD), 50
Middle back pain (production), thoracic facets (impact), 139
Multidirectional C-arm fluoroscopy, requirement, 134
Multiple sclerosis (improvement), intrathecal steroids (usage), 5
Muscle layers, IL/IH nerves (presence), 108f
    color-flow Doppler, 108f
Myelinated fibers, classification, 39
Myofascial low back pain, indications/contraindications, 219-220
Myofascial pain, 217-218
    clinical diagnosis, 218
    contrast, 217
    diagnosis, establishment, 218
    discomfort, 217
    equipment, 219
    psoas muscle, involvement, 220

N

Neck
    blocks, importance, 46
    pain, classification, 152
    preganglionic fibers, impact, 77
Neck Disability Index, 154
Nephrogenic systemic fibrosis (NSF), 25
Nerve fibers, classification, 39
Nerve impulses (propagation), local anesthetic blockade, 39
Nerve root
    damage, risk (increase), 40
    proximity, annular tear, 180f
Nerve stimulator, 38
Nervus intermedius, SSN travel, 29
Neuraxial injections, 3-5
    accident, 94
Neuraxial steroids
    antiinflammatory potency, 19t
    side effects, 20
Neurological conduction loss (description), radiculopathy (usage), 122
Neurological symptoms, absence, 149
Neurolysis, complications, 52
Neurolytic injection, volume, 91
Neurolytic procedures, 50-52
Neuropeptide Y, presence, 137
Nociceptive structure, PRF application, 175
Non-ionic monomers, usage, 22
North American Spine Society (NASS), Position Statement on Discography, 178-179
Nuclear disc material (extraction), Dekompressor (usage), 189
Nuclear material, loss, 184
Nucleopasty
    clinical studies, 190t
    impact, 181
    plasma disc decompression, 9
    procedures, 188
Nucleotome (percutaneous disc decompression procedure), 190
Numeric rating scale (NRS), 171

O

Obturator nerve block, 68-69
    description, 69
    technique, 69
    usage, 68-69
Oral mucosa penetration, detection (prevention), 51-52
Organ radiation doses, 31t
Orthopedics, PMMA (usage), 193-194
Orthostatic hypotension, 91-93
Osteoarthritis, 136
Oswestry Disability Index (ODI), 171
    basis, 124
Out-of-plane (OOP) injections, needle insertion points, 201f

P

Pain
    control, spinal injections, 17
    etiology, determination (difficulty), 6
    interpretation (difficulty), complexity (impact), 7
    medicine
        ultrasonography, application, 101
        ultrasound, applications (comparison), 102t
    quality, description, 89
    referral patterns, 139
    relief
        PMMA, introduction, 10
        sympathetic nervous system, interruption, 6
    reproduction, annular disruption (correlation), 8
    spinal origin, evaluation, 178
    thoracic zygapophyseal joints, impact, 7
    types, classification, 38-39
Pain disability index (PDI), 171
Pain Medication Quantification, 154
Papaverine, usage, 24
Para-aminobenzoic acid (PABA) byproduct, 18
Paramidline lumbar approach, 5
Paraplegia
    lumbar sympathetic blocks, association, 94
Paraplegia, CPB complication, 93
Parasympathetic outflow, activation, 29
Paravertebral ganglia, existence, 83
Paravertebral sympathetic ganglia, postganglionic neurons (synapse), 82-83
Paresthesia, 59-60
    nerve-stimulating needle, usage, 53
Partial brachial plexus block, 82
Particulate steroids, complications, 19
Patella dance, 42
Pelvis, posterior view, 112f
Percutaneous balloon microcompression, 50
Percutaneous decompression (Dekompressor) technology, nuclear disc material extraction, 189
Percutaneous decompressive procedures, complication, 190-191
Percutaneous disc decompression (PDD), 9
    pain relief, 189-190
Percutaneous facet denervation, 153-154
Percutaneous Gasserian ganglion neuroablative procedures, complications, 52t
Percutaneous Gasserian ganglion neurolytic procedures, indications, 50

Percutaneous Gasserian ganglion neurolytic treatment, choice, 50
Percutaneous glycerol rhizolysis, 50
Percutaneous intradiscal RF thermocoagulation, 188
Percutaneous kyphoplasty (PK), 193-194
    acceptance/use rate, 195
    balloon placement, anteroposterior/lateral radiographs, 195f
    candidates, selection, 194
    coblation, 196-197
    complications, 196
        avoidance, 194-195
    cortoss cement, 197
    guidelines, summary, 194b
    outcomes/complications, 195-196
    procedural overview, 194-195
    technology, advancement, 196-197
Percutaneous lumbar discectomy, 9
Percutaneous minimally invasive intradiscal disc decompression, patient selection, 189
Percutaneous radiofrequency thermocoagulation, 50
Percutaneous vertebroplasty (PV), 193-194
    acceptance/use rate, 195
    balloon placement, anteroposterior/lateral radiographs, 195f
    candidates, selection, 194
    coblation, 196-197
    complications, 196
        avoidance, 194-195
    cortoss cement, 197
    efficacy, question, 195
    guidelines, summary, 194b
    outcomes/complications, 195-196
    procedural overview, 194-195
    technology, advancement, 196-197
Peripheral intraarticular injections, usage (success), 224
Peripheral joint injections, 230
    image guidance, usage, 224
Peripheral nerve block, 41
    association, 62
    landmark technique, 66-67
    ultrasound technique, 67
Peripheral neuropathy, 77
Periradicular hydrocortisone, usage, 4
Phantom limb pain, 6, 77
Pharyngoesophageal diverticulum (Zenker diverticulum), 80
Phenol
    benzene ring, substitution, 90
    injection, initial local anesthetic effect, 90
    usage, 90
Phrenic nerve block, 82
Picture archiving and communication system (PACS), 32
    components, 32
Piriformis injection, 114-115
    anatomy, 114
    equipment, 222
    guidelines, 222
    image-guided techniques, 114-115
    indications/contraindications, 222
    outcomes evidence, 223
    patient, prone position, 115
    patient management/evaluation, 222
    risk/complication avoidance, 223
    techniques, 114-115, 222
    ultrasonography, usage, 115
    ultrasound-guided injection technique, 115

Piriformis muscle, 112f
  anatomy, 222
  identification, 115
  imaging, 222
  MRI/CT, 222
  origination, 114
  outline
    contrast injection, 222f
    radiographic contrast, 115f
  pain
    diagnosis, establishment, 221
    evaluation/treatment, 221-223
  passage, 114
  proximal insertions, 222
  science, 222
Piriformis syndrome, 114
  complaint, 221
  diagnosis, 221
Piriformis tenderness, 221
Placebo-responsive pain, 38
Plasma disc decompression (nucleoplasty), 9
Plasma-mediated radiofrequency ablation
  (coblation), usage, 197
Platelet count, level, 194
Pneumothorax
  blind technique, 105
  CPB complication, 93
  risk, reduction, 142
Polymethyl methacrylate (PMMA) (Plexiglas),
  9-10
  anaphylaxis, 194
  injection, 194-195
  percutaneous use, 10
  usage, 10, 193-194
Popliteal artery (PA), sciatic nerve (proximity),
  71f
Popliteal block, technique, 40
Portable document format (PDF), 32
Postamputation stump pain, 77
Postdural puncture headache (PDPH), 5
  dural puncture, relationship, 94
  incidence, reduction, 6
  occurrence, reduction, 6
  risk, increase, 40
  symptoms, development, 5
  treatment, 5-6
Posterior left glenohumeral joint, ultrasound
  image, 228f
Posterior neural structure, posterior view
  (illustration), 137f
Posterior superior iliac spine (PSIS)
  ilium level, 112f
  SIJ dysfunction, 164-165
  ultrasound transducer placement, 113-114
Posterior tibial nerve
  blocking, 73
  color-flow Doppler, 74f
  ultrasound image, 73f
Postganglionic parasympathetic fibers,
  direction, 47
Postoperative trigeminal sensory loss, impact,
  52
Preganglionic sympathetic efferents,
  innervation impact, 77
Preganglionic sympathetic fibers, 82f
  cell body location, 76-77
Pressure caudal anesthesia, 4
Prevertebral fascia, anterior injection, 79
Primary dorsal rami, division, 138-139
Primary trigger points, 217
Probe, sterile covering, 202f
Procaine, trans-sacral (caudal) injections,
  17

Processus articularis superior, posterior
  enlargement, 156
Processus mamillaris, 156
Provocation discography (disc stimulation),
  8-9
Proximal anterior knee
  long-axis ultrasound view, 230f
  short-axis ultrasound view, 230f
Proximal patella, adductor canal (median
  distance), 72
Pseudogout, 136
Psoas compartment block
  Capdevila approach, 65
  landmark technique, 65-66
  ultrasound-guided technique, 65-66
Psoas major innervation, 220
Psoas muscle (PM), 64f
  arrangement, 220
  palpation, 220
  posterior part, lumbar plexus, 66f
Psoas stripe, MRI study, 64f
Psoas trigger point injections
  patient management/evaluation, 221
  ultrasound guidance, 221
Pterygopalatine fossa (PPF)
  maxillary artery, 48
  real-time fluoroscopy, usage, 48-49
  SPG location, 47
  target view, 47
  visualization, 48-49
Pudendal nerve, 112-114
  anterior/posterior urogenital area supply,
  112
  formation, 112
  path, 112
  technique, 113
  ultrasound-guided injection technique,
  113-114
  ultrasound image, optimization, 114
  ultrasound probe, positions, 112f
Pudendal neuralgia, 112
  anatomy, 112-113
  injection, transgluteal approach, 113
  sonoanatomy, 112-113
  transgluteal approach, 113
Pudendal neurovascular bundle, 112f
Pulsed fluoroscopy imaging, 32
Pulsed radiofrequency (PRF)
  applications, 175
    success, 175
  clinical efficacy, 175
  clinical uses, 175
  complications, 175
  controlled trials, 176t
  effect, mechanism, 174-175
  introduction/history, 174
  randomized controlled trials (RCTs), 175
  side effects, 175
  technique, 175
  treatment, proposal, 7
Purinergic receptors (P2X4), activation, 21f

Q

Quadratus lumborum
  anatomy, 218-219
    cadaver study, 218-219
  imaging, 219
  injections, 218-219
  muscle, injections (guidelines), 219
  myofascial pain, 220
  outcomes evidence, 219

Quadratus lumborum *(Continued)*
  patient management/evaluation, 219
  physical examination, 218
  risk/complication avoidance, 219
  shape, 218
  trigger point injections, 219
    fluoroscopic guidance, 219
Quadriceps twitch (patella dance), 42

R

Radiation neuritis, 77
Radiation safety, 31b
  fluoroscopy concern, 32
Radicular pain
  complaints, 9
  increase, 190
  occurrence, 122
Radiculopathy
  chymopapain chemonucleolysis injections,
  123-124
  intervertebral disc herniation, association,
  122
Radiofrequency ablation (RFA), 46-49
  complications, 49
  indications, 46-47
  needle, lateral view, 49f
  technique, 48-49
  usage, 49
Radiofrequency (RF) electrode, internal
  cooling, 187
Radiofrequency (RF) neurotomy, usage
  (success), 7
Radiofrequency (RF) posterior annuloplasty, 9
Radiofrequency thermocoagulation (RFT),
  52
Rami dorsales, cervical ramus medialis
  (radiofrequency treatment), 153f
Ramus dorsalis
  cervical ramus medialis, posterolateral
  approach, 153f
  L5, location, 156
  ramus medialis (medial branch)
    local infiltration, 155
    radiofrequency treatment, 155
Ramus medialis (medial branch)
  local infiltration, 155
  radiofrequency treatment, 155
Real-time fluoroscopy, usage, 48-49, 51
Referred pain, 139
  distribution, 139
  maps, 130f
Reflex bradycardia, occurrence, 49
Reflex sympathetic dystrophy, 77
Refractory cluster headache (treatment), RFA
  (usage), 49
Regional blocks, contraindications, 140
Renal penetration, 94
Residual limb pain, diagnosis, 6
Retropharyngeal hematoma, 79-80, 82
Revel criteria, 156
Right hip joint, anteroposterior view, 225f
Right SIJ arthrogram, 169f
RLN block, 82

S

S1, anteroposterior view, 145f
S1, lateral view, 144f
S1 needle placement, 144
S1 nerve root, granulation tissue, 123f

Sacral joint RF neurotomy, indications, 169
Sacroarthrogenic telagia, 164
Sacroiliac joint (SIJ)
  ablative procedures, 167
  anatomical features, uniqueness, 167-168
  anatomy, 165-167
  basic science, 167
  dysfunction, 164-165
  examination stress maneuvers, 166b
  guidelines, 168
  imaging, 167-168
  injections/procedures, 8
  innervation, 8, 167
  lesioning, 170
  ligamentous anatomy, 166f
  ligamentous structures, 166f
  low back pain source, 8
  needle placement, 169-170
  neurotomy, selection/exclusion criteria, 168b
  pathology, documentation, 164-165
  patient management/evaluation, 170
  physical examination, 165
  probe placement, 170
  target, identification, 169
Sacroiliac joint (SIJ) injections
  diagnosis, establishment, 164-165
  diagnostic/therapeutic injections, criteria, 168b
  equipment, 168b
  indications/contraindications, 168-169
  left L5/S1-S3 probe placement, 172f
  local anesthetic, usage, 168
  outcomes evidence, 171
  postprocedure instructions, 170, 171b
  risk/complication avoidance, 172
  steroids, usage, 168
  technique, 169-170
Sacroiliac joint (SIJ) pain
  cooled SIJ neurotomy, usage, 171
  management generator, 170
  referral, 165
    pattern, 165f
  treatment
    RF energy, usage (challenge), 167
    therapeutic interventions, 167
Sacroiliac pain, 164
Saphenous nerve
  bifurcation, 72f
  distal adductor canal, 71f
  medial aspect, blockade, 73
  terminal branch, 71
Saphenous nerve block, 71-72
  landmark techniques, 72
  sites, medial aspect, 72f
  success rate, infiltrated/fanned local anesthetic (usage), 72
  ultrasound technique, 72
Saw sign, 214f
Scapula
  lateral view, 104f
  superior margin, suprascapular notch (location), 102-103
Sciatica, treatment
  Clonidine
    effects, 22f
    usage, 20
  therapeutic epidural injections, usage, 121-122
Sciatic nerve (SN)
  approaches, description, 69
  block, 69-71
    popliteal approach, 70-71

Sciatic nerve (SN) *(Continued)*
    ultrasound probe, usage, 70-71
    ultrasound technique, 69-70
  formation, 69
  gluteal level, anatomy, 70f
  imaging, 70f
  injection, 70f
  landmark approach, 69
  local anesthetic, relationship, 70f
  pain, diagnosis, 6
  popliteal artery (PA), proximity, 71f
  posterior approach, 69
  variable innervation, 68-69
Sciatic pain, inflammation (impact), 4
Scotty dog eye, target point, 143-144
Scotty dog view, determination, 141-142
Short-axis transverse ultrasound images
  anterior tubercle, C5 transverse process, 212f
  anterior tubercle, C6 transverse process, 212f
  local anesthetic, spread, 212f
Single local anesthetic blocks, false-positive rates, 137
  double blocks, usage, 137
Skin depression, palpation, 69
Skin temperature changes
  degree, 85
  evaluation, 85
Society of Interventional Radiology (SIR), PV/PK techniques standards, 194
Sodium channel packing, 40
Soft tissue
  structures (direct real-time visualization), ultrasonography (usage), 210
Soft tissue, absence, 79
Somatic pain, 38
  diagnosis, 6
Sonoanatomy, knowledge, 201-202
Sonography
  diagnostic ultrasonography, 29
  scanning sequence, 202-204
Spermatic cord, cross section, 109f
Sphenopalatine ganglion (SPG)
  anatomy, 47
  approaches, 47
  infrazygomatic approach, 47
    anterior approach, 47
    coronoid approach, 47
  location, 47
  nasal wall, anteroposterior view, 48f
  neuroanatomy, 47
  origination, 47
  PPF location, 47
  radiofrequency ablation, efficacy, 49
  radiofrequency lesioning, 49
  radiofrequency thermocoagulation, stimulation, 49t
  RFA, efficacy, 49
  transnasal approach, 47
  transnasal blockade, 47
  transnasal endoscopic approach, 47
  transoral approach, 47
Sphenopalatine ganglion (SPG) block, 46-49
  anterior approach, 48f
  coronoid approach, 48f
  indications, 31, 46-47
  technique (infrazygomatic approach), 48
Spinal anesthesia
  cocaine injection, impact, 3
  procedure, application, 3-4

Spinal canal, dorsal aspect (caudal/translaminar approaches), 5
Spinal cord
  dorsal horn, visceral input (arrival), 89
  injury, avoidance, 3
Spinal injections, history, 17
Spinal pain
  commonness, 129
  controlled diagnostic blocks, local anesthetics (usage), 137
  diagnosis
    establishment, 136-137
    facilitation, injections (usage), 136-137
  history/physical examination, usage, 136
Spinal stenosis, 123f
  acquisition, 123
Spine anatomy, 137
Spine injections, history
  timeline, 4f
Spine phantom, immersion, 206f
Spinoglenoid notch (SGNo), suprascapular nerve entry, 103f
Spinous processes (SPs)
  median LAX (longitudinal view), 202
  median long-axis view (longitudinal view), 203f
Splanchnic nerves (visceral nerves), distribution, 83f
Steady state differential interruption, obtaining, 7
Stellate ganglion
  absolute contraindications, 77
  anatomical representations, 77f
  blockade
    indications, 77
  location, 77
  measurement, 77
Stellate ganglion block
  blind approach, 78f
  complications, 82
  performing, C7 location, 78
Stereotactic radiation therapy, 50
Sternal notch, needle direction, 60
Steroid injections, toxicity, 211
Steroid toxicity, etiology, 19-20
Stimulating needle, usage, 67, 69-70
Structures, visualization, 31
Stump pain, 6
Subarachnoid injection, 82
Subarachnoid space
  intrathecal spread, 31
  procaine hydrochloride, injection, 6t
Subcutaneous tissue, local anesthetic infiltration, 44
Substance P, presence, 137
Superficial peroneal nerve (block), subcutaneous fanning injection (usage), 73
Superior articular process (SAP), 125
  target location, 169
Superior cervical ganglion, somatic branches, 77
Superior hypogastric neurolysis
  single-needle transdiscal approach, 98f
  two-needle posterior-lateral approach, 97f
Superior hypogastric neurolysis, performing, 97f
Superior hypogastric plexus (SPH), 97f
  approaches, 95
  neurolytic block, consideration, 94

Superior hypogastric plexus (SPH) neurolysis, 94-96
  anatomy, 94
  complications, 96
  efficacy, 96
  indications, 94
  procedure, 95
Superior salivatory nucleus (SSN)
  efferent fibers, travel, 29
  SPG origination, 29
Supraclavicular block, 59
Supraclavicular brachial plexus, ultrasound
  image, 61f
Suprascapular artery, location, 103f
Suprascapular fossa
  imaging, ultrasonography (usage), 103
  muscle layers, 103f
Suprascapular nerve (SSN), 102-104
  anatomy, 102-103
  block, performing, 102
  branches, 102f
  injection, performing site, 103
  origination, 102
  PRF application, success, 175
  scapular spine floor
    ultrasonographic image, 104f
  sonoanatomy, 102-104
    nerve injection, relationship, 104
  targeting, disadvantages, 103-104
  techniques, 103-104
  ultrasonographic image, 103f-104f
  ultrasound-guided injection technique, 104
  ultrasound scanning, performing, 104
Suprascapular notch (SSNo)
  location, 102-103
  suprascapular nerve, ultrasonographic
    image, 103f
Sural nerve block, 73
  improvement, ultrasonography (usage), 73
Sweat glands, sympathetic pathway, 83f
Sympathectomy, consequences, 86
Sympathetic cell bodies, projection, 47
Sympathetic efferent fibers, interruption, 76
Sympathetic pain, 38
Synovial impingement, 136
Synovial inflammation, 136

T

T1, long-axis sonogram, 81f
T2 paracoronal T2-weighted MRI, 67f
T8, anteroposterior view, 143f
T8, lateral view, 143f
T9, anteroposterior view, 143f
T9, lateral view, 143f
T10, anteroposterior view, 143f
T11, anteroposterior view, 143f
T11/T12, medial branches, 138
T12, anteroposterior view, 143f
T12-L4, anterior rami, 64
Tamps (balloons), 193-194
Therapeutic epidural injections
  complication, avoidance, 126
  contraindications, 122-123
  diagnosis, establishment, 122
  equipment, 125-126
  false-positive scans, 123
  guidelines, 123-124
    American Society of Anesthesiologists
      update, 124
    American Society of Interventional Pain
      Physicians publication, 124

Therapeutic epidural injections *(Continued)*
  imaging, 123
  indications, 122-123
  infectious complications, 126
  ischemic complications, 126
  needle injuries, 126
  outcome measure, ODI basis, 124
  outcomes evidence, 124-125
  response, 122
  risk, 126
  technique, 125-126
  usage, 121-122
Therapeutic epidurals, usage, 122-123
Therapeutic SIJ injections, criteria, 168b
Therapeutic spinal injections, 17
  history, 17
Thermal annular procedures, development,
  187
Third occipital nerve
  cervical dorsal rami medial branches,
    comparison, 141
  cervical medial branch block, 213-214
  sonoanatomy, 213-214
Thoracic disc pathology, rarity, 9
Thoracic facet joints
  fluid accommodation, 131
  pain, 130
Thoracic facet pain, range, 130
Thoracic facets, 130, 133
  middle back pain, 139
Thoracic innervation, 138
Thoracic intraarticular zygapophyseal joint
  blocks, 7
Thoracic medial branch blocks (thoracic
  MBBs), 141-143
  needle placement, 141-143
  positioning, 141
Thoracic pain, anatomical approach (usage),
  42
Thoracic spine, facet joints (difference), 138
Thoracolumbar fascia, extension, 217
Three-in-one block, 66
  description, 67-68
Tibial nerve
  block (improvement), ultrasonography
    (usage), 73
  imaging, 73
Transcutaneous nerve stimulation (TENS),
  211
Transducer
  placement, 29
  relationship, 201f
Transforaminal lumbar epidural, 125-126
Transverse processes (TPs)
  needle tip position, 65f
  paramedian long-axis (longitudinal view),
    203
  paramedian long-axis view (longitudinal
    view), 204f
  paramedian short-axis (transverse view),
    203-204
  paramedian short-axis view (transverse
    view), 204f-205f
Transversus abdominis muscle, iliohypogastric
  nerve (interaction), 107
Trident sign, production, 65-66
Trigeminal ganglion thermal radiofrequency
  ablation, lateral view, 52f
Trigeminal nerve block, 50-52
  indications, 50
Trigeminal neuralgia
  management, algorithm, 51f
  treatment, 52

Trigger points
  fluoroscopic guidance, 220
  injections, 217-218
  palpation, 219-220
Tuffier's line, intersection, 65
Tumor necrosis factor (TNF), 20
Tumor necrosis factor-α (TNF-α), 122
Tuohy needle, usage, 42
Twitch response, 217

U

Ultra-fast computed tomography scanner, 30f
Ultrasonography
  imaging equipment, advantages/
    disadvantages, 102t
  real-time visualization, 210
  stimulator-guided block, combination, 73
  usage, 28
Ultrasonography in pain medicine (USPM),
  210
  application, 101-102
Ultrasound, 29
  disadvantages, 29
  frequency ranges, 202
  gel, characteristics, 29b
  image orientation, 201
  in-plane (IP) injections, needle insertion
    points, 201f
  kilohertz, level, 29f
  machines/transducers/knobology, 201
  medial longitudinal scan, 202f
  median long-axis view (longitudinal view),
    203f
  needles/techniques/sterility, 201
  out-of-plane (OOP) injections, needle
    insertion points, 201f
  paramedian long-axis view (longitudinal
    view), 203f
  paramedian short-axis (transverse view),
    203-204
  paramedian short-axis view (transverse
    view), 204f-205f
  production, 29
  safety concerns, 29
  system, diagnostic tool, 32f
  technique, 39
  training, knowledge, 201-202
Ultrasound-guided atlanto-axial joint
  injection, 215
Ultrasound-guided cervical facet intraarticular
  injections, literature review, 213
Ultrasound-guided cervical nerve root block,
  211-212
  literature review, 211
  technique, limitations, 211
Ultrasound-guided cervical sympathetic block,
  79-80
Ultrasound-guided cervical sympathetic chain
  (stellate ganglion) block, 210
Ultrasound-guided femoral nerve block, 66
Ultrasound-guided glenohumeral joint
  injections, 227-228
Ultrasound-guided hip joint injection, 226
Ultrasound-guided injections
  principles, 201
Ultrasound-guided knee joint injection,
  229-230
Ultrasound-guided left glenohumeral joint
  injection, needle placement, 228f
Ultrasound-guided left hip injection, needle
  tip placement, 226f

Ultrasound-guided lumbar spine injections, 200
  applications, 208
  development, 208-209
Ultrasound-guided medial branch block
  in-plane needle insertion, 207f
  out-of-plane needle control, 207f
Ultrasound-guided stellate ganglion block, safety improvement, 79
Ultrasound-guided third occipital nerve, literature review, 213
Ultrasound-guided tibial nerve block, performance time, 73
Ultrasound probe
  positions, 112f
  schematic diagram, 107f
  sterile covering, 202f
Ultrasound transducer
  caudal movement, 213
  lateral end, blunt-tip needle (introduction), 211-212
  orientation, 211f
Upper extremity
  complex regional pain syndrome (CRPS), 42
  peripheral nerve blockade, 62
    risk/complication avoidance, 62
  regional anesthetic techniques, 60t
Upper extremity blockade
  outcomes evidence, 62
  performing, 58
Upper extremity peripheral nerve blockade, 37
Upper lumbar facet joints (T12-L2), orientation, 138

Ureter penetration, 94
U.S. Preventive Services Task Force criteria, basis, 136

V

Vagus nerve block, 82
Vascular anatomy, color Doppler scan, 80-81
Vascular bundle, saphenous nerve, 71f
Vascular structures, absence, 79
Ventral rami
  preganglionic sympathetic fibers, relationship, 82f
  thoracic nerves, 105
Vertebrae, articular pillars, 131
Vertebral artery
  injection, complication, 56-57
  location, 79
  short-axis sonogram, C7 location, 80f
  sonogram, 56f
Vertebral augmentation, 9-10
Vertebral body (VB)
  bisecting, 125-126
  percutaneous injection, 193-194
  PMMA injections, 194-195
  void, creation (lateral fluoroscopic images), 197f
Vertebral column
  components, 131
  intercristal (Tuffier's) line, intersection, 65
  paravertebral ganglia, existence, 83

Vertebral compression fractures (VCFs), 10
  result, 193
Vertebral levels, identification, 133
Vertebral osteonecrosis, 189
Vertebroplasty
  clinician training, requirement, 194
  general anesthesia, usage, 194
  invasiveness, minimum, 193-194
  kyphoplasty, contrast, 196, 196b
  monitored anesthetic care (MAC), usage, 194
Villonodularsynovitis, 136
Visceral ganglia, 91f
Visceral input, arrival, 89
Visceral nerves (splanchnic nerves), distribution, 83f
Visceral pain, 38-39
  complaint, 89
  treatment, 89

Z

Zenker diverticulum, 80
Zygapophyseal joints
  diagnosis, history/physical examination (unreliability), 136
  facet joints, targeting (injections/procedures), 7
  pain (diagnosis), history/physical examination usage (avoidance), 136
  term, origination, 137